Dictionary for Nurses (English-Hindi)

AF557864

Disclaimer

Medical Science is an everchanging science. As new research and clinical experience broaden our knowledge, changes in treatment and drug therapy are required. The Authors and the Publisher of this work have checked with suitable sources believed to be reliable in their efforts to provide information that is complete and generally in accordance with the standards accepted at the time of publication. However, in view of the possibility of human error or changes in medical sciences, neither the authors nor the publisher and any other party who has been involved in the preparation or publication of this work warrants that the information contained herein is in every respect is accurate or complete, and they disclaim all responsibility for any errors or omissions or for the results obtained from use of the information contained in this work. Readers are encouraged to confirm the information contained herein with other sources.

Dictionary for Nurses (English-Hindi)

Vishal Tak MSc (N)
Principal
Ganadhipati Purushottam Shekhawati
College of Nursing
Jaipur, Rajasthan, India

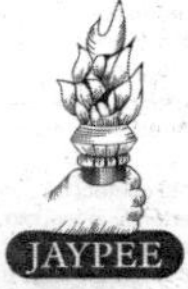

JAYPEE BROTHERS MEDICAL PUBLISHERS
The Health Sciences Publisher
New Delhi | London

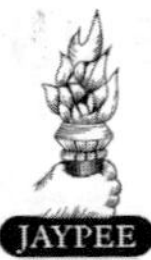

JAYPEE **Jaypee Brothers Medical Publishers (P) Ltd**

Headquarters
Jaypee Brothers Medical Publishers (P) Ltd
23/23-B, Ansari Road, Daryaganj
New Delhi 110 002, India
Phone: +91-11-23272143, +91-11-23272703
+91-11-23282021, +91-11-23245672
E-mail: jaypee@jaypeebrothers.com

Corporate Office
Jaypee Brothers Medical Publishers (P) Ltd.
4838/24, Ansari Road, Daryaganj
New Delhi 110 002, India
Phone: +91-11-43574357
Fax: +91-11-43574314
E-mail: jaypee@jaypeebrothers.com

Overseas Office
J P Medical Ltd
83 Victoria Street, London
SW1H 0HW (UK)
Phone: +44 20 3170 8910
E-mail: info@jpmedpub.com

EU GPSR Authorised Representative
Logos Europe, 9 rue Nicolas Poussin
17000, La Rochelle, France
Phone: +33 (0) 6 67 93 73 78
E-mail: Contact@logoseurope.eu

Website: www.jaypeebrothers.com
Website: www.jaypeedigital.com

© 2018, Jaypee Brothers Medical Publishers

The views and opinions expressed in this book are solely those of the original contributor(s)/author(s) and do not necessarily represent those of editor(s) of the book.

All rights reserved. No part of this publication may be reproduced, stored or transmitted in any form or by any means, electronic, mechanical, photocopying, recording or otherwise, without the prior permission in writing of the publishers.

All brand names and product names used in this book are trade names, service marks, trademarks or registered trademarks of their respective owners. The publisher is not associated with any product or vendor mentioned in this book.

Medical knowledge and practice change constantly. This book is designed to provide accurate, authoritative information about the subject matter in question. However, readers are advised to check the most current information available on procedures included and check information from the manufacturer of each product to be administered, to verify the recommended dose, formula, method and duration of administration, adverse effects and contraindications. It is the responsibility of the practitioner to take all appropriate safety precautions. Neither the publisher nor the author(s)/editor(s) assume any liability for any injury and/or damage to persons or property arising from or related to use of material in this book.

This book is sold on the understanding that the publisher is not engaged in providing professional medical services. If such advice or services are required, the services of a competent medical professional should be sought.

Every effort has been made where necessary to contact holders of copyright to obtain permission to reproduce copyright material. If any have been inadvertently overlooked, the publisher will be pleased to make the necessary arrangements at the first opportunity. The **CD/DVD-ROM** (if any) provided in the sealed envelope with this book is complimentary and free of cost. **Not meant for sale**.

Inquiries for bulk sales may be solicited at: jaypee@jaypeebrothers.com

Dictionary for Nurses (English-Hindi)

First Edition: 2018

Reprint 2024, 2025, **2026**

ISBN: 978-93-86150-39-4

Printed at: Sterling Graphics Pvt. Ltd.

Dedicated to

My beloved family members, my parents, loving wife, brother, sister-in-law, my loving son and daughter, all loving friends, colleagues, my students and all those who touched ours lives.

In memory of

My youngest brother late Ankit Tak
and
My grandparents

Preface

The objective of this dictionary is to visualize, with consistent terminology, quantitative, qualitative, and mixed methods of medical words in nursing education in a way that medical, paramedical and non-medical students can readily and easily understand and precisely relate it in their studies.

This dictionary is designed to improve one's ability to conceptualize, construct, test, problem-solving, acquiring knowledge with useful words and their meaning in the language which is understandable.

As nursing is the backbone of comprehensive medical care, nursing work is difficult but humanitarian. For the same purpose to keep their knowledge afresh this dictionary has been compiled for nurses.

Through my experience, I realized there are many inconsistencies and variations of terminologies in the medical and paramedical studies. I believe that the terminologies should be clearly illustrious and understandable with the appropriate language, which is so easy and to the point. With this effort, I would not hesitate in admitting the fact that this work does not cover the whole range of medical terminology, but most of those only which we find most frequently used in our day-to-day life.

Many figures have been added to make things more clear.

I hope that the members of this profession would welcome my efforts and give a place to it in their routine studies and work. Any suggestion made will be appreciated from the readers and efforts will be made for the betterment and improvement and addition of new terminologies too for this dictionary in upcoming editions.

Suggestions are most welcome, we can incorporate your valuable suggestions in next edition.

Vishal Tak

Acknowledgments

First I would like to express my warm gratitude to Dr Jogendra Sharma (President Awardee and Principal), SMS Government College of Nursing, Jaipur, Rajasthan, India; Dean, Rajasthan University of Health Sciences; Ex-Registrar, Rajasthan Nursing Council.

My heartiest thanks to Dr Mahipal Singh Fenin, Principal cum Director, Akhil Bharati Vidyapeeth College of Nursing, Sikar, Rajasthan for providing his valuable insight, thoughts and suggestions for the overall dictionary.

I would also like to thank Mr Sunil Sharma, Principal, Upchar College of Nursing, Jaipur and Mr Kailash Khandelwal, Principal, Soni College of Nursing, Jaipur, expert in their respective areas and ultimately helped me in delivering strength in the entire project.

A very special thanks goes to Mrs Anita Choudhary and Mrs Deepika Sharma, without you this dictionary would never find its way of selection of words; Mr Anil Choudhary and Mr Harimohan Choudhary for their support and dedication. At the same time I pay my sincere thanks to Mr Rohitash Kumar Dewanda and Mr Jitendra Kumar Sharma for successfully completing the project.

Thanks specially for motivation for this task to Dr SS Joshi, Director, Ganadhipati Purushottam Shekhawati Hospital and Research Center, Jaipur.

A number of reviewers provided useful and valuable feedback, which ultimately shaped the dictionary, particularly.

- Dr Sanjay Biyani, Director, Biyani Group of Colleges, Jaipur
- Dr Manish Jain, Director, Shri Navkar Hospital, Jaipur
- Dr Sanjay Mittal, Director, Mittal Skin Clinic, Jaipur
- Dr Ratna Chhaya Singh, Principal, Mansarovar Group of Institute, Bhopal, Madhya Pradesh
- Mr Hanock Rubel, Principal, SJB College of Nursing, Bengaluru, Karnataka
- Mr Sanjay Joshi, Principal, RR College of Nursing, Gurugram, Haryana.

Last but not least I would like to thanks to all my friends from nursing field, and those who have been with me over this project and whose names I have failed to mention.

Plate 1

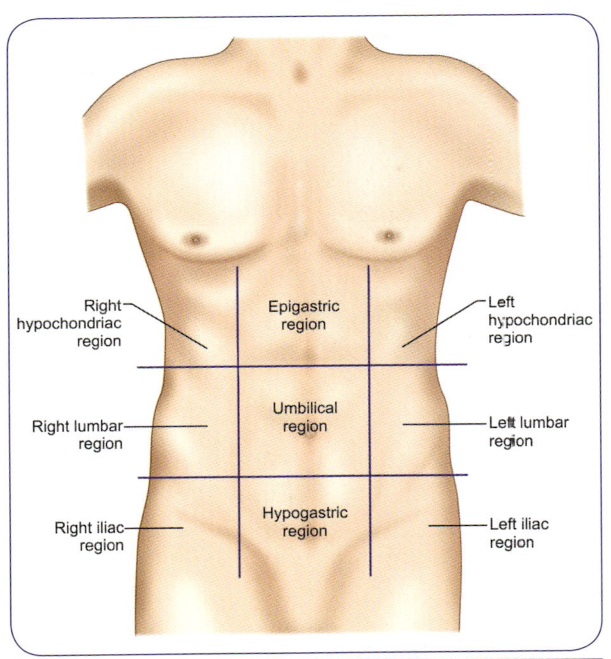

Abdominal nine regions

Plate 2

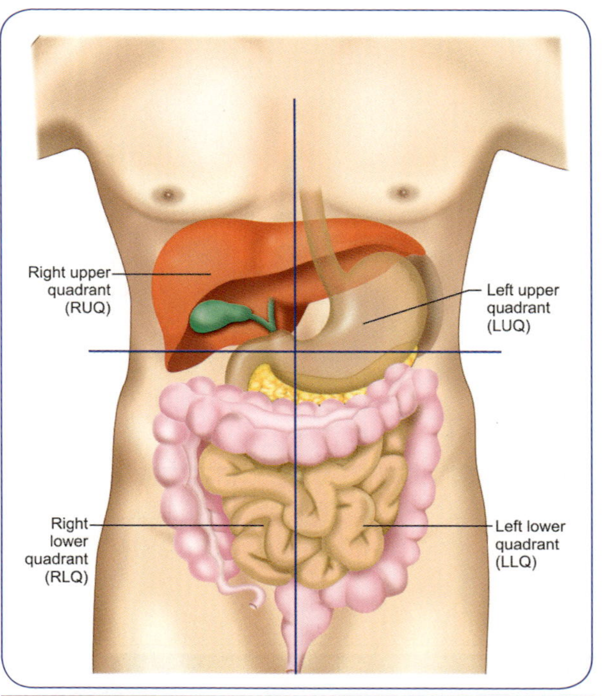

Abdominal regions

Plate 3

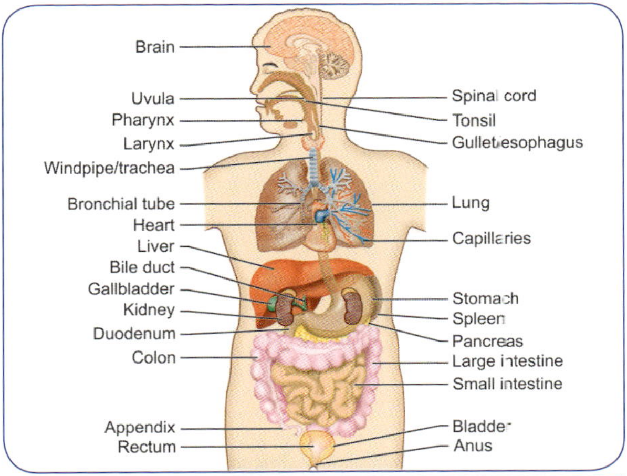

Brain
Uvula
Pharynx
Larynx
Windpipe/trachea
Bronchial tube
Heart
Liver
Bile duct
Gallbladder
Kidney
Duodenum
Colon
Appendix
Rectum
Spinal cord
Tonsil
Gullet/esophagus
Lung
Capillaries
Stomach
Spleen
Pancreas
Large intestine
Small intestine
Bladder
Anus

Body internal organs

Hypothalamus
Pineal gland
Pituitary gland
Thyroid gland
Thymus gland
Liver
Stomach
Duodenum
Pancreas
Kidney
Adrenal glands
Ovaries
Placenta
Uterus
Testes

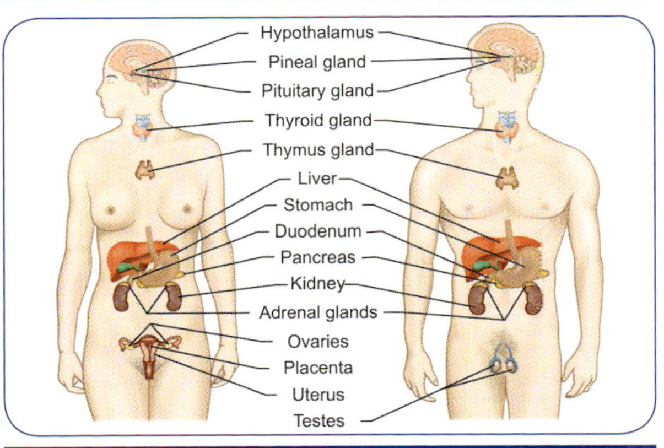

Endocrine system

Plate 4

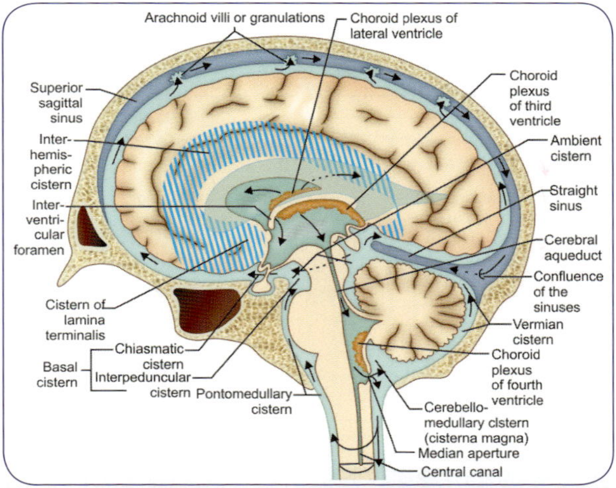

Arachnoid villi or granulations
Choroid plexus of lateral ventricle
Superior sagittal sinus
Choroid plexus of third ventricle
Inter-hemis-pheric cistern
Ambient cistern
Straight sinus
Inter-ventri-cular foramen
Cerebral aqueduct
Confluence of the sinuses
Cistern of lamina terminalis
Vermian cistern
Chiasmatic cistern
Basal cistern
Interpeduncular cistern
Pontomedullary cistern
Choroid plexus of fourth ventricle
Cerebello-medullary cistern (cisterna magna)
Median aperture
Central canal

CSF flow

Motor cortex (movement)
Central sulcus
Sensory cortex (pain, heat, and other sensations)
Frontal lobe (judgment, foresight, and voluntary movement)
Parietal lobe (comprehension of language)
Broca's area (speech)
Temporal lobe (hearing)
Frontal lobe (smell)
Occipital lobe (primary visual area)
Temporal lobe (intellectual and emotional functions)
Wernicke's area (speech compehension)
Brainstem (swallowing, breathing, heartbeat, wakefulness center and other involuntary function)
Cerebellum (coordination)

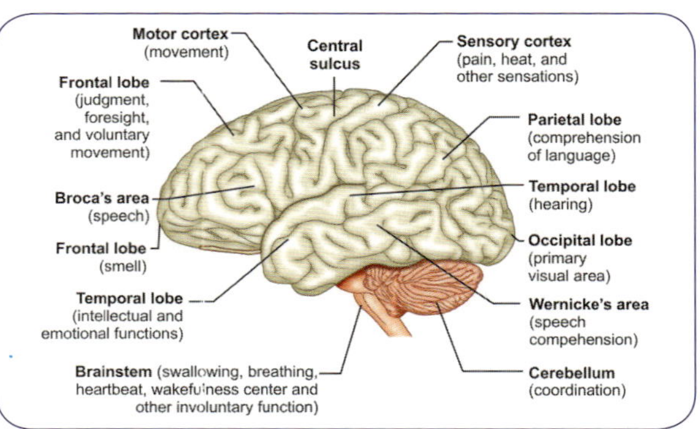

Brain

Plate 5

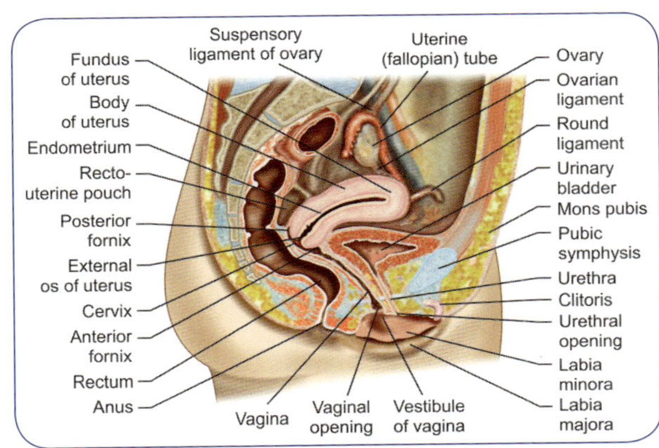

Female reproductive system

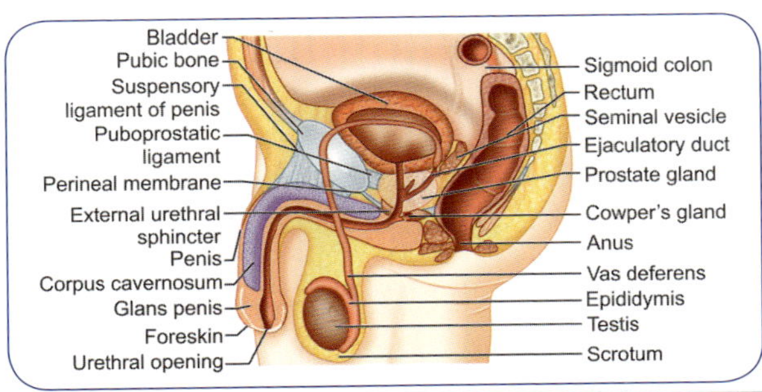

Male reproductive system

Plate 6

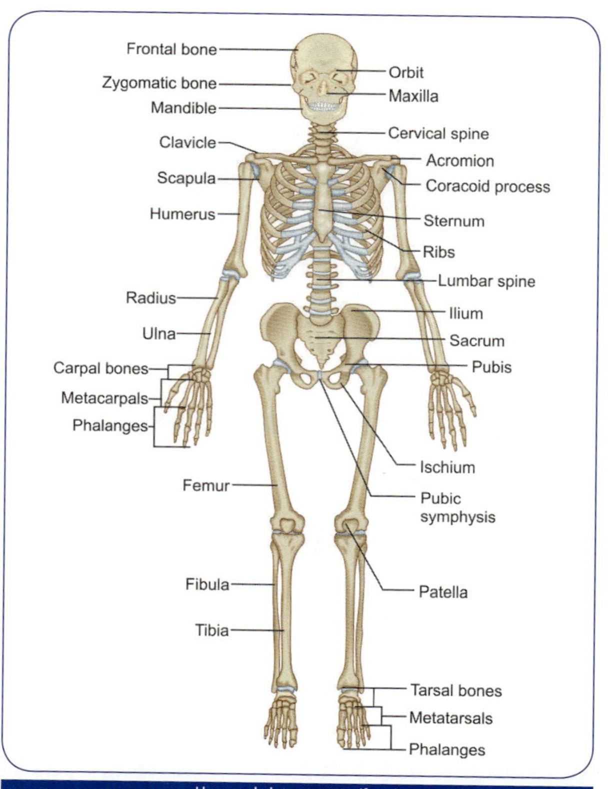

Human skeleton system (front)

Plate 7

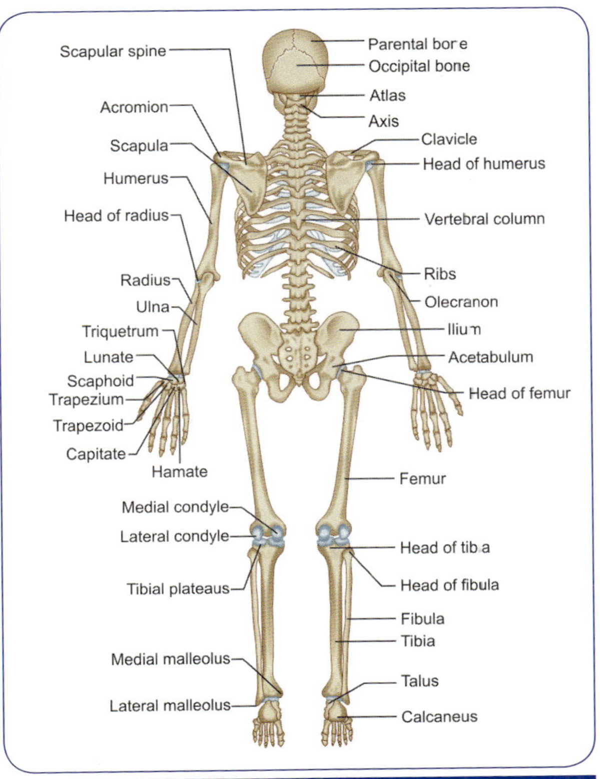

Human skeleton system (back)

Plate 8

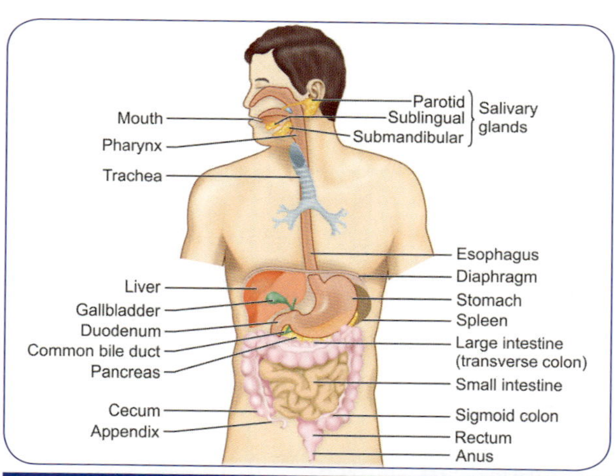

Digestive system

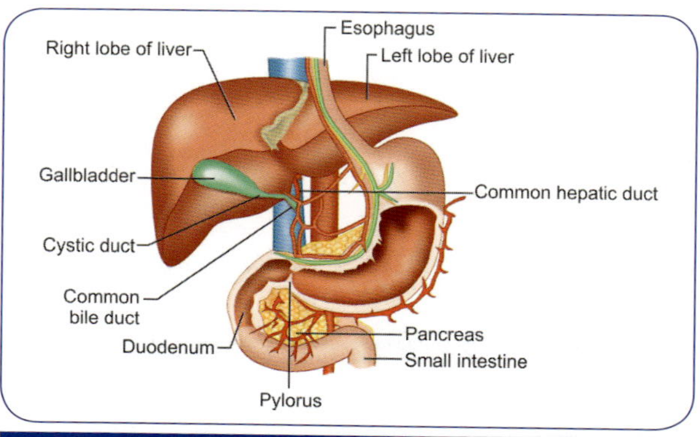

Liver

Plate 9

Anterior vena cava
Posterior vena cava
Liver
Portal vein
Kidney
Capillary bed
Lung
Heart
Stomach
Aorta
Spleen
Intestine

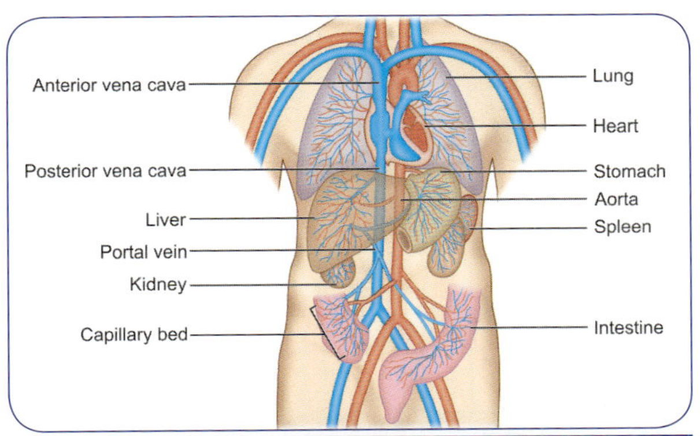

Circulatory system

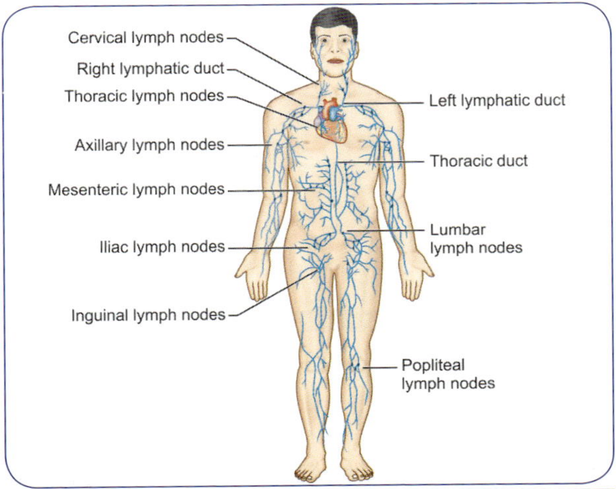

Cervical lymph nodes
Right lymphatic duct
Thoracic lymph nodes
Axillary lymph nodes
Mesenteric lymph nodes
Iliac lymph nodes
Inguinal lymph nodes
Left lymphatic duct
Thoracic duct
Lumbar lymph nodes
Popliteal lymph nodes

Lymphatic system

Plate 10

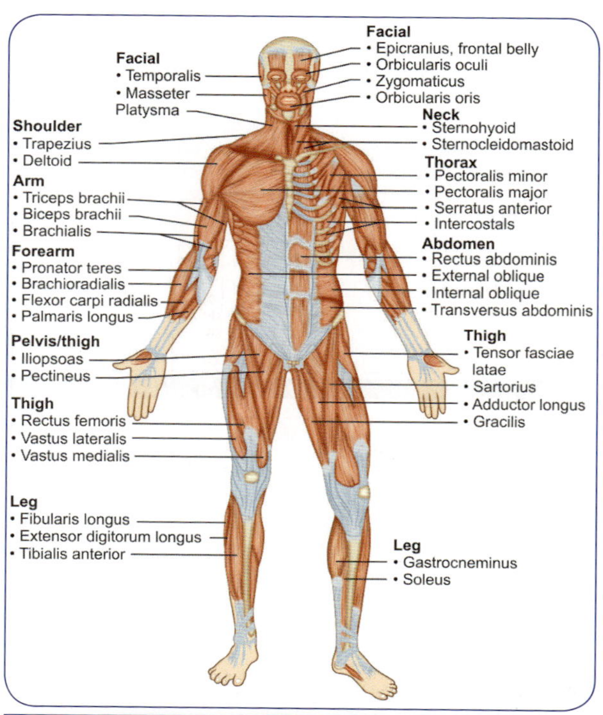

Muscular system anterior view

Plate 11

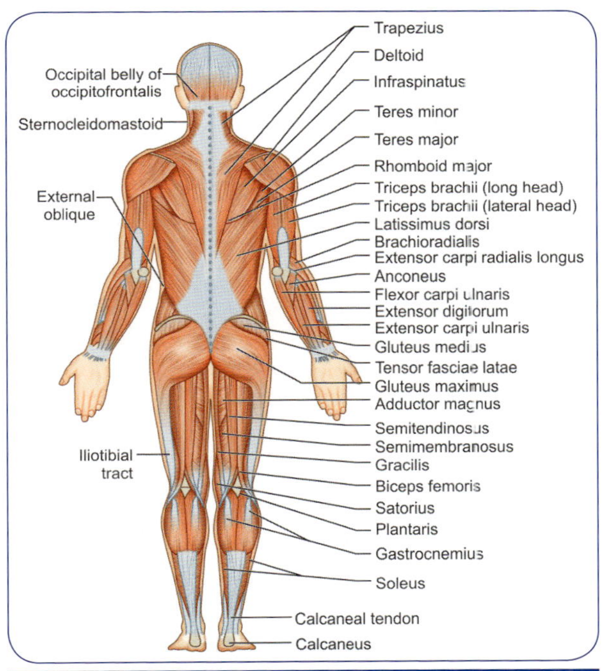

Muscular system posterior view

Plate 12

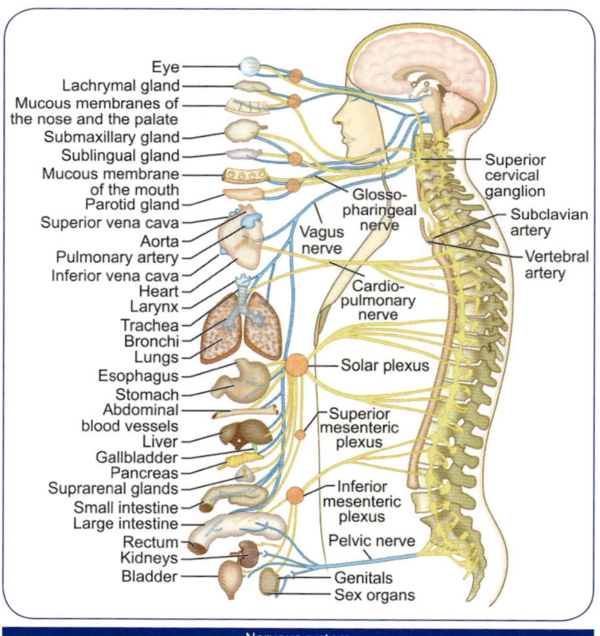

Nervous system

Plate 13

Vertebrae	Areas and parts of the body	Possible symptoms
Cervical		
C1	• Back of the head	Headaches including migraines, aches or pain at the back of the head, behind the eyes or in the temples tension across the forehead, throbbing or pulsating discomfort at the top or back of head
C2	• Various areas of the head	
C3	• Side and front of the neck	
C4	• Upper back of the neck	
C5	• Middle of neck and upper part of arms	Jaw muscle, or joint aches or pains
C6	• Lower part of neck, arms and elbows	Dizziness, nervousness, vertigo
C7	• Lower part of arms, shoulders	Soreness, tension and tightness left in back of the neck and throat area
Dorsal		
D1	• Hands, wrists, fingers, thyroid	Pain, soreness and restriction in the shoulder area
D2	• Heart, its valves and coronary arteries	Bursitis, tendonitis
D3	• Lungs, bronchial tubes, pleura, chest	Pain and soreness in arms, hands, elbows and/or fingers Chest pain, tightness or constriction, asthma, difficulty breathing
D4	• Gallbladder, common duct	
D5	• Liver, solar plexus	Middle or lower mid-back pain, discomfort and soreness
D6	• Stomach, mid-back area	Various and numerous symptoms from trouble or malfunctioning of:
D7	• Pancreas, duodenum	• Thyroid
D8	• Spleen, lower mid-back	• Heart
D9	• Adrenal glands	• Lungs • Gallbladder
D10	• Kidneys	• Liver • Stomach
D11	• Ureters	• Pancreas • Spleen
D12	• Small intestine, upper/lower back	• Adrenal glands • Kidneys
Lumbar		• Small and large intestines • Sex organs
L1	• Ileocecal valve, large intestine	• Uterus • Bladder
L2	• Appendix, abdomen, upper leg	• Prostate glands
L3	• Sex organs, uterus, bladder, knees	Low back pain, aches and soreness
L4	• Prostate gland, lower back	Trouble walking
L5	• Sciatic nerve, lower legs, ankles, feet	Leg, knee, ankle and foot soreness and pain
Sacro	• Hip bones, buttocks	Sciatica, pain or soreness in the hip and buttocks
Coxis	• Rectum, anus	Rectal trouble

Nervous system

Plate 14

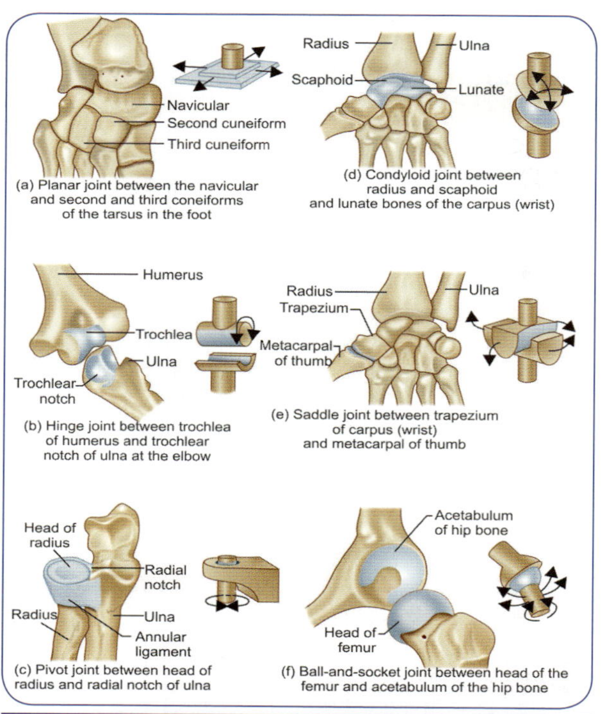

(a) Planar joint between the navicular and second and third coneiforms of the tarsus in the foot

(d) Condyloid joint between radius and scaphoid and lunate bones of the carpus (wrist)

(b) Hinge joint between trochlea of humerus and trochlear notch of ulna at the elbow

(e) Saddle joint between trapezium of carpus (wrist) and metacarpal of thumb

(c) Pivot joint between head of radius and radial notch of ulna

(f) Ball-and-socket joint between head of the femur and acetabulum of the hip bone

Human body joints

Plate 15

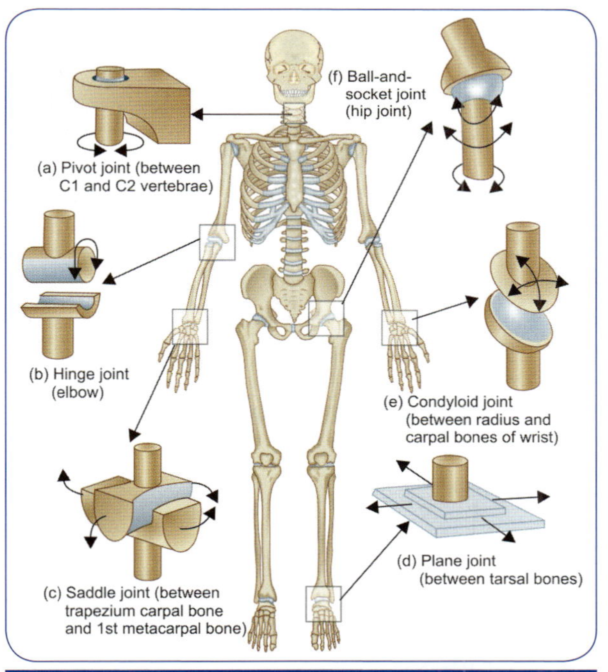

Types of synovial joints

Plate 16

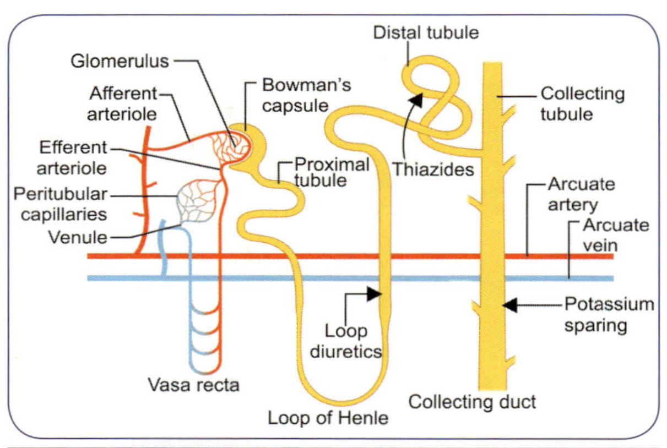

Nephron

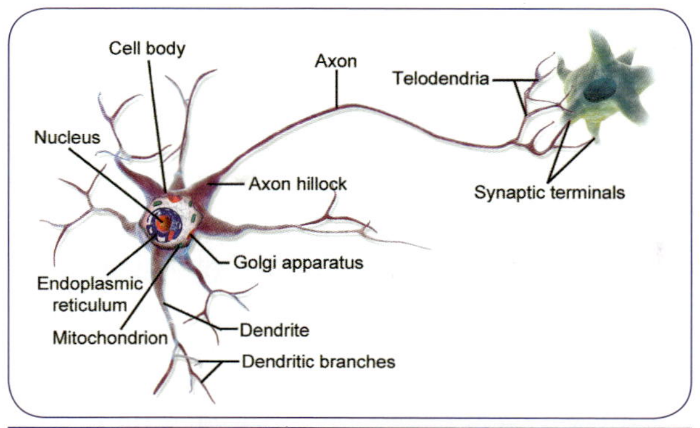

Neuron

Plate 17

Facial nerve
Parotid gland
Lymph nodes
Hypoglossal nerve
Sublingual gland
Lingual nerve
Submandibular gland

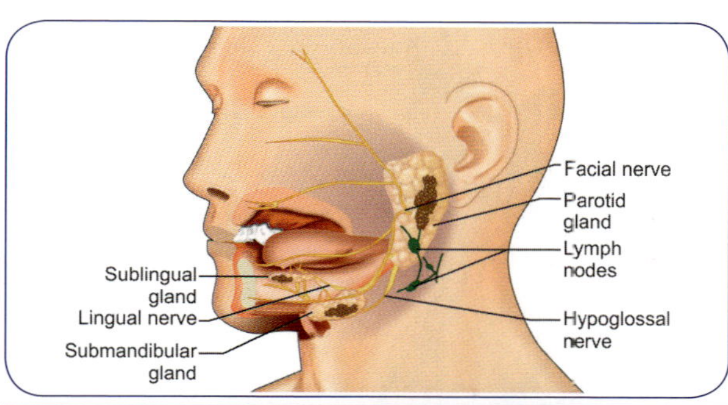

Salivary glands

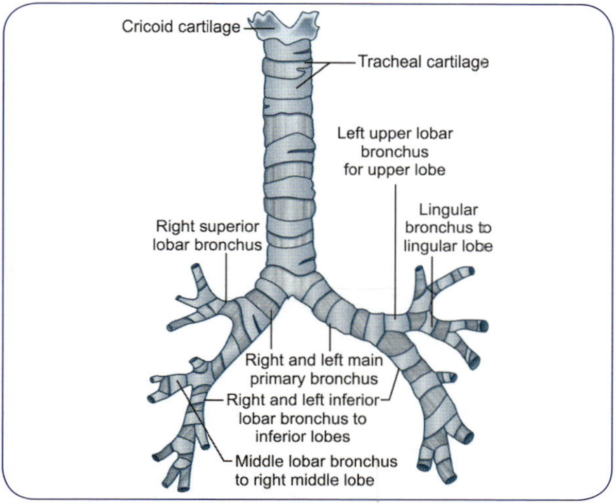

Cricoid cartilage
Tracheal cartilage
Left upper lobar bronchus for upper lobe
Lingular bronchus to lingular lobe
Right superior lobar bronchus
Right and left main primary bronchus
Right and left inferior lobar bronchus to inferior lobes
Middle lobar bronchus to right middle lobe

Tracheobronchial tree

Plate 18

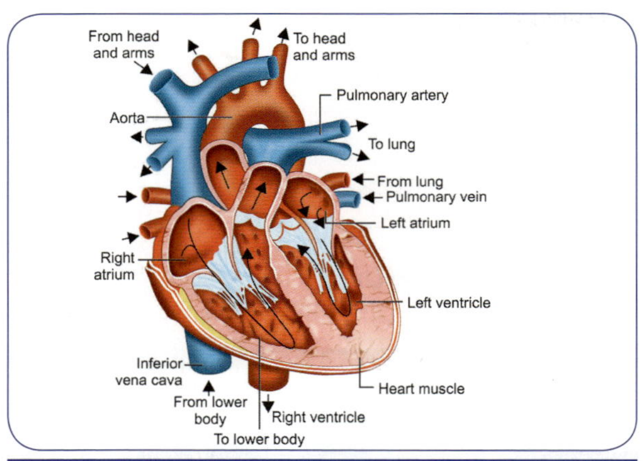

Heart

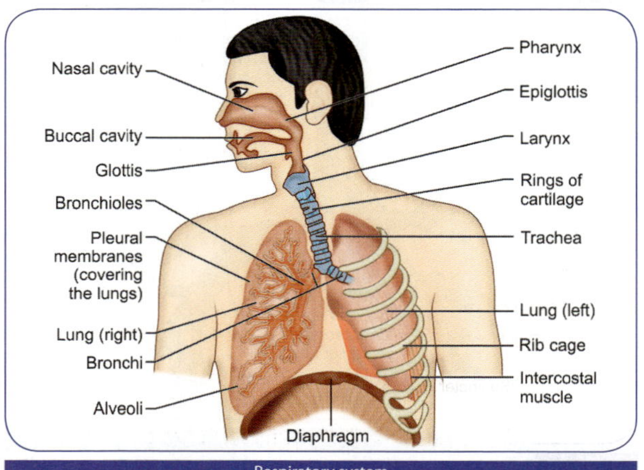

Respiratory system

Plate 19

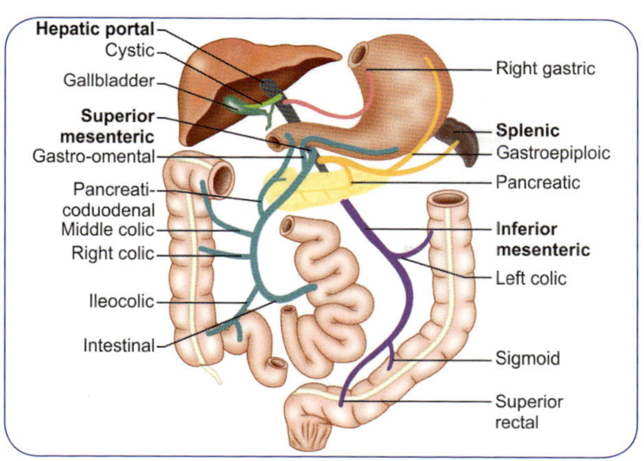

Hepatic portal circulation

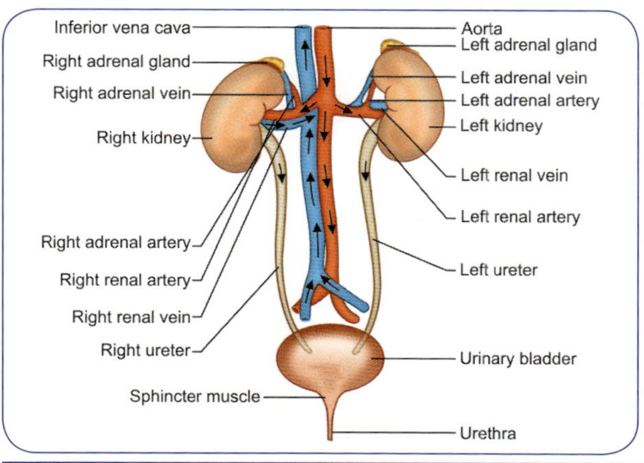

Urinary system

Plate 20

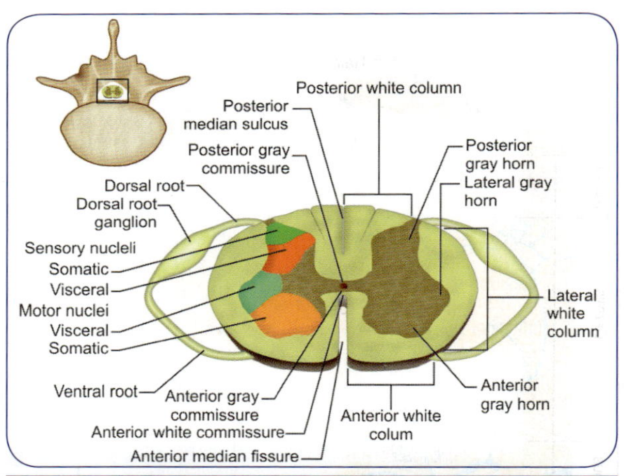

Spinal cord sectional

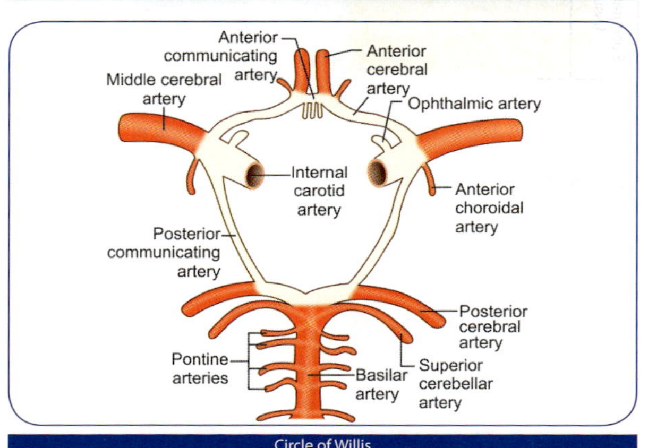

Circle of Willis

Plate 21

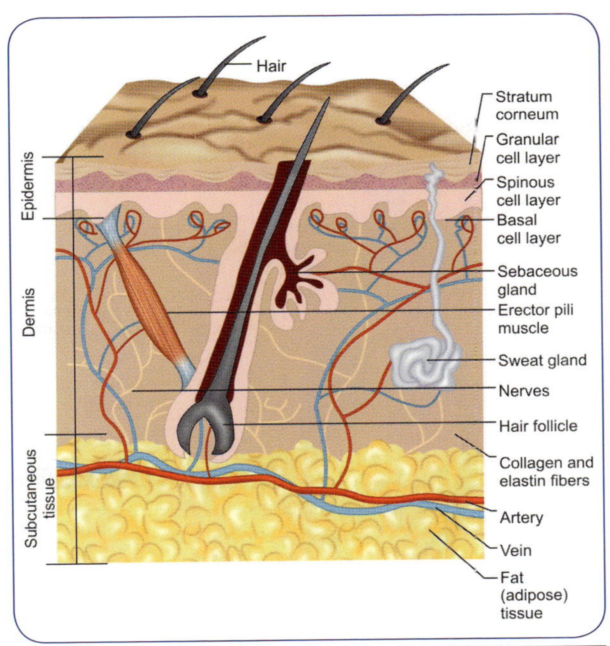

Human skin

Plate 22

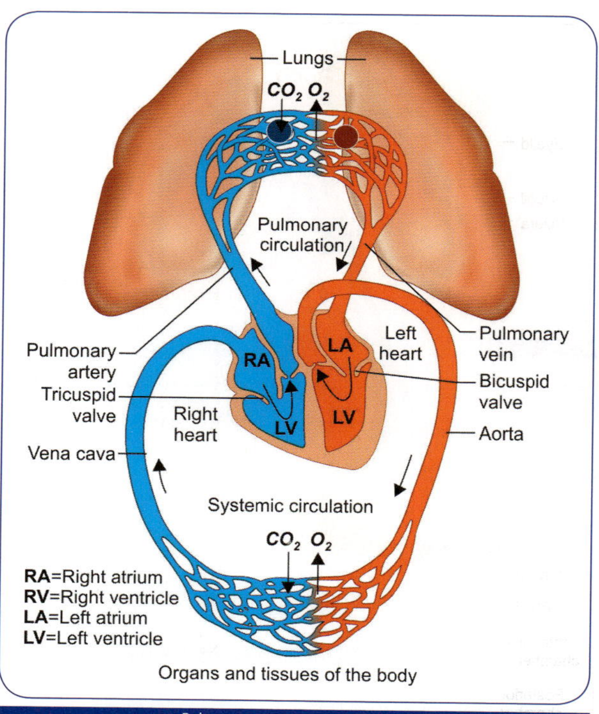

Pulmonary vs systemic circulation

Plate 23

Eyelid
Pupil
Sclera
Iris
Lacrimal duct

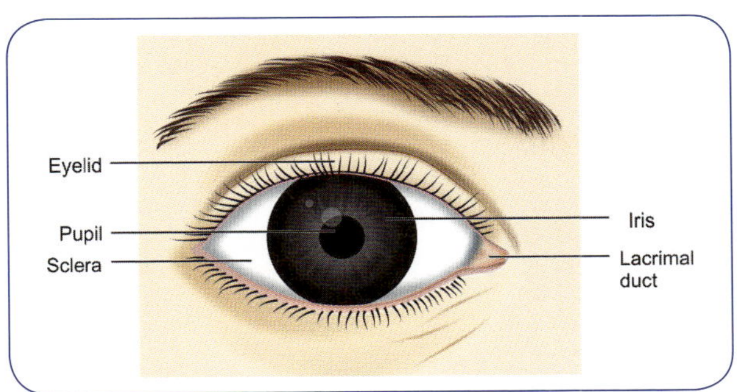

Eye diagram

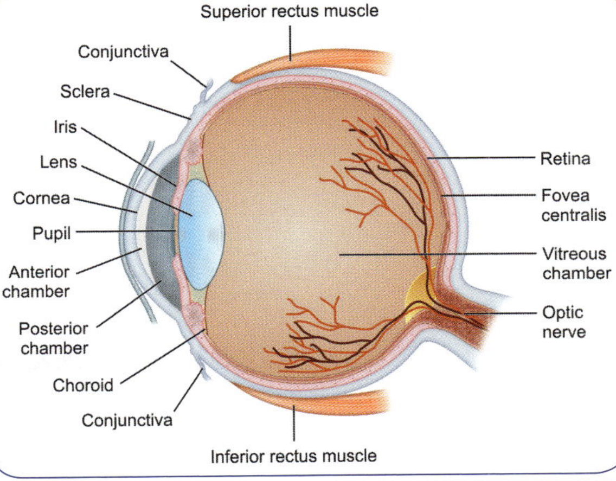

Superior rectus muscle
Conjunctiva
Sclera
Iris
Lens
Cornea
Pupil
Anterior chamber
Posterior chamber
Choroid
Conjunctiva
Inferior rectus muscle
Retina
Fovea centralis
Vitreous chamber
Optic nerve

Parts of eye

A

A (अ) अभाव सूचक उपसर्ग। Prefix meaning or absences of.

Ab (एब) से और से दूर। Away from and from.

Abacterial (एबैक्टिरियल) जीवाणुहीन, बिना बेक्टीरिया के। Without the bacteria, bacteria Furs.

Abactio (एबेक्टीयो) कृत्रिम गर्भपात। Artificial abortion.

Aband (एबेन्ड) एक्टिन एवं मायोसिन की मांसपेशियों पर परत। A dark color band in muscle representing covering of actin and myosin filaments.

Abacavir (एबाकेवीर) एक एच.आई.वी की श्रेणी की दवा। An anti-HIV drug.

Abaissement (अबैशमेन्ट) अवसाद, विषाद का भाव व उदासी। Depression and despondency.

Abalienation (अबेलीनेशन) शारीरिक एवं मानसिक शक्ति का क्षय, ह्रास। Decay of physical and mental power.

Abalienation Mentis (अबेलीनेशन मेन्टीस) मानसिक विपक्षन, मनोभ्रंश। The mental, abalienation, decay.

Abandon (एबेन्डन) किसी प्राणी या वस्तु को सदा के लिए छोड़ देना, परित्याग करना। To leave, to sales, to give up to another's control.

Abandonment (अबेन्डोनमैन्ट) अधिकार का परित्याग। Renunciation of a claim, self-surrender.

Abanet (एबानैट) कमरबंद पट्टी। Girdle-shaped bandage.

Abaptistion (एबाप्टिस्टन) कपालकर्तक यन्त्र। An instrument of perforation of the skull.

Abarognosis (एबारोग्नोसिस) भार अनुभूति का ह्रास, वजन का ज्ञात न होना। Loss of sense of weight.

Abarthrosis (एबारथ्रोसिस) उन्मुक्त रूप से घुमने वाला जोड़। Freely moveable joints.

Abarticular (एबार्टिकुलर) जोड़ से दूर, अलग। Distance from a joint.

Abarticulation (एबार्टिकुलेशन) जोड़ का अपने स्थान से हट जाना। Dislocation of a joint.

Abasia (ऐबसिया) चलने के योग्य न होना, चलने में असमर्थ होना। Inability to walk. (*i*) **Abasia Astasia** (ऐबसिया एस्टेसिया) खड़ा रहने या चलने मे असमर्थता। Loss of walking and standing power. (*ii*) **Abasia Atactica** (ऐबसिया एटेक्टिका) चलने में अनिश्चित गति। Uncertainty of movements in walking. (*iii*) **Abasia Choreic** (ऐबसिया कोरिक) पैरों का कोरिया रोग के कारण चलने में असमर्थता। Inability to walk due to choreg. (*iv*) **Abasia Paralytic** (ऐबसिया पैरालाइटिक) पैरों में लकवा होने के कारण चलने में असमर्थता। Inability to walk due to paralysis. (*v*) **Abasia Spastic** (ऐबसिया स्पास्टिक) पैरों में कठोरता के कारण चलने में असमर्थता। Inability to walk due to stiffing of legs.

Abasic (ऐबेसिक) चलने में असमर्थ व्यक्ति। The person unable to walk.

Abatement (एबेटमेन्ट) दर्द में कमी होना। Decrease in the pain or disease.

Abater (एबेटर) आराम पहुँचाने वाला कारक। The palliative agent.

Abats (एबेट) कम करना। To decrease or lessen.

Abattoir (एबेट्वार) वधशाला, बूचड़खाना। Slaughter house, place killing of animal.

Abaxils (एबेक्सियल) शरीर के किसी भाग की अक्ष रेखा में स्थित नहीं रहने वाला। Not situated in the axis of the body or any part.

Abbreviation (एबरीवेशन) छोटा रूप, संक्षिप्त। Shorting.

Abdicate (एबडिकेट) परित्याग करना, छोड़ देना। To renounce, to leave.

Abdomen (एबडोमन) पेट, उदर, छाती से नीचे का भाग। The cavity, the thorax and pelvis. (*i*) **Acute Abdomen** (एक्यूट एबडोमन) पेट में स्थित कोई रोग से दर्द होना। Severe pain which require sudden surgery. (*ii*) **Pendulous Abdomen** (पेन्ड्यूल्स एबडोमन) पेट का ढीलापन। Reloud condition of abdominal wall. (*iii*) **Tumid Abdomen** (ट्यूमिड एब्डोमन) पेट का फूलना। Swollen of abdomen.

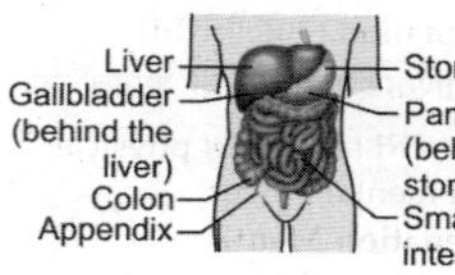

Abdominal (एबडोमिनल) उदर, उदर सम्बंधी। Pertaining to the abdomen.

Abdominal angina (एबडोमिनल एन्जाइना) तीव्र पेट दर्द, उदर के किसी भी भाग में दर्द होना। Severe abdominal pain. (*i*) **Abdominal aneurysm** (एबडोमिनल एन्यूरिजम) पेट की धमनी का बड़ा होना। Large abdominal aorta. (*ii*) **Abdominal Crises** (एबडोमिनल क्राइसिस) पेट में तेज दर्द होना। Severe pain in the abdomen. (*iii*) **Abdominal Reflexes** (एबडोमिनल रिफ्लैक्सेज) उदर-पेशियों की निरंकुश ऐंठन, उदरप्रतिवर्त। Involuntary sparm of the abdominal muscles.

(*iv*) **Abdominal respiration** (एबडोमिनल रेस्पाइरेशन) उदर-श्वास। That carried on by the diaphragm and the abdominal muscles.

Abdominocyesis (एबडोमिनोसाइसिस) उदरीय गर्भावस्था। Abdominal pregnancy.

Abdominogenital (एबडोमिनोजैनाइटल) उदर तथा जननांगों से सम्बन्धित। Pertaining to the abdomen and the genital organ.

Abdominoposterior (एबडोमिनोपोस्टीरियर) उदरपश्च, पश्चोदरी, पाश्चाद्वर्ती उदर, पश्चोदर। Having the abdomen backward.

Abdominous (एबडोमिनस) बड़े पेट वाला, तोन्दू। Having a large belly.

Abducent Nerves (एबडूसैन्ट नर्वस) अपकर्षिणी तंत्रिकायें, अपवर्तनी तंत्रिकायें। Nerves drawing from the median line.

Abduct (एबडक्ट) मध्य रेखा से दूर ले जाना, अपावर्तन। To draw from the mediar plane.

Abduction (एबडक्शन) हाथ-पैरों का शरीर के मध्य तल से दूर पार्श्व में जाना या सिर अथवा धड़ का पार्श्व में झुक जाना। अंगुलियों का किसी भुजा की अक्षीय (केन्द्रीय) रेखा से दूर जाना। The lateral movement of the limbs away from the median plane of the body or the lateral bending of the head or trunk, movement of the digits away from the axial line of a limb.

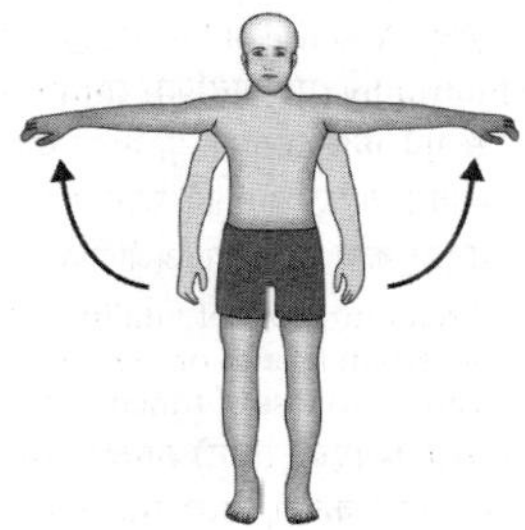

Abductor (एबडक्टर) मध्याक्ष या केन्द्र से दूर खींच ले जाने वाली पेशी, अपकर्षी (पेशी), अपवर्ती (पेशी), अपवर्तनी (पेशी)। An abducent muscle.

Aberrant (एबेरेन्ट) असामान्य, विपथन। Abnormal.

Aberration (एबेरेशन) सामान्य से विचलित होना, प्रकाश का किरणों का अपूर्ण अपवर्तन, विपथन। Deviation from the normal. Imperfect refraction of light rays.

Abevacuation (एबइवाकुएशन) अपूर्ण मलोत्सर्ग, अपूर्ण मल विसर्जन। Incomplete evacuation.

Abeyance (एबइयान्स) अभाव, निलम्बन, दुविधा या लटकाव। Absence suspension.

Abiogenesis (एबायोजेनेसिस) जीवों की निर्जीव पदार्थों से उत्पत्ति। The production of livings from nonliving matters.

Abiosis (एबायोसिस) अजीवता, मृत्यु। Absence of life, death.

Abiotrophy (एबायोट्रॉफी) समय से पूर्व कुछ ऊतकों या अंगों की जीवन शक्ति कम हो जाने से उनका कार्य न करना, अजीवीपोषण। Premature loss of vitality of certain tissues or organs leading to loss of function.

Abirritate (एबीर्रीटेट) शान्त करना, उपशमन करना, उत्तेजना कम करना। To sooth, to diminish or ameliorate irritation.

Ablatio Placenta (एबलेशियो प्लेसेन्टा) अपरा-वियोजन, अपरा-पृथक्करण, अपरा हटा कर अलग कर देना। Detachment of the placenta.

Ablation (एबलेशन) कटकर अलग हो जाना, अंशोच्छेदन। Removal by cutting.

Ablepharous (एब्लेफेरस) बिना आँखों की पलकों वाला। Without eyelids.

Ablepsia (एब्लेप्सिया) दृष्टिहीनता, अन्धापन। Blindness.

Abluent (एब्लुइन्ट) स्वच्छकारी, निर्मलकारी, परिमार्जक, शोधक, प्रक्षालक। An agent possessing cleansing quality; A detergent.

Ablution (एब्लुशन) शोधन, प्रक्षालन। A cleansing or washing.

Abnormal (एबनॉर्मल) असामान्य, अपसामान्य, असाधारण, अस्वाभाविक, अस्वस्थ। Not normal; not according to rule, irregular, unhealthy.

Aborad (एबारोड) मुख से दूर। Away from the mouth.

Abort (एबोर्ट) गर्भस्राव करना, किसी रोग का विकास करना। To expel fetus before it is viable, to arrest the development of a disease.

Aborticide (एबोर्टिसाइड) गर्भनाशक, गर्भपातक, गर्भपाती, गर्भस्रावक, गर्भस्रावी, गर्भनाशी। The killing of a fetus within the uterus.

Abortifacient (एबोर्टिफेसिएन्ट) कोई भी वस्तु जिससे गर्भस्राव हो जाता है। गर्भस्रावक। Anything that induces abortion.

Abortion (एबोर्शन) गर्भस्राव, छः माह से पूर्व गर्भ का गिर जाना। Termination of pregnancy before six months. (*i*) **Accidental abortion** (एक्सीडैन्टल एबोर्शन) दुर्घटनावश हो जाने वाला गर्भस्राव। Abortion caused by an accident. (*ii*) **Complete abortion** (कम्पलीट एबोर्शन) पूर्ण गर्भस्राव, गर्भाशय से सम्पूर्ण भ्रूण का बाहर निकल जाना। Abortion in which complete products of conception have been expelled. (*iii*) **Criminal abortion** (क्रीमिनल एबोर्शन) आपराधिक गर्भस्राव Illegal abortion. (*iv*) **Habitual abortion** (हैबिचुअल एबोर्शन) पुनर्पुनः गर्भपात, पुनरावर्ती गर्भपात। Recurrent abortion. (*v*) **Incomplete abortion** (इनकम्पलीट एबोर्शन) अपूर्ण गर्भस्राव, भ्रूण के कुछ भाग का अन्दर गर्भाशय् में ठहर जाना। Abortion in which part of the products of conception has been retained in the uterus. (*vi*) **Inevitable abortion** (इनइवाइटेबल एबोर्शन) अपरिहार्य गर्भस्राव, ऐसा गर्भस्राव जिसे रोका न जा सके। An abortion that cannot be prevented. (*vii*) **Missed Abortion** (मिस्ड एबोर्शन) अलक्षित या लीन गर्भस्राव, मृत भ्रूण का उसकी मृत्यु के पश्चात् कम से कम चार माह तक गर्भाशय में ठहरे रहना। Retention of a dead fetus in the uterus for at least four months after its death.

Abortionist (एबोर्शियोनिस्ट) गर्भस्रावक, वह व्यक्ति जो गर्भस्राव कराता है। One who performs an abortion.

Abortus (एबोर्टस) पतित-भ्रूण, गिरा हुआ गर्भ। An aborted fetus.

Abrachia (एब्रेकिया) जन्म से बाहों का न होना। Congenital absences of the arms.

Abrachius (एब्रेकियस) भुजाहीन भ्रूण। An armless fetus.

Abrasion (एब्रेजन) खरोंच, रगड़न, घर्षण, अपघर्षण। A scarping of the skin, excoriation; abrade; abrasia.

Abrosia (एब्रोसिया) निराहार रहना, व्रत रखना, क्षय, क्षरण, विनाश। Fasting; abstaining from food; a wasting away.

Abruptio (एबरप्शियो) पृथक्करण या अलग होना जैसे अपरा का काल-पूर्ण पृथक्करण या अलग होना, हड्डी का आड़ा टूटना। Separation as premature detachment of the placenta; transverse fracture of a bone.

Abscess (एबसेस) वियाधि, व्रण या फोड़ा। A localized collection of pus in any part of the body

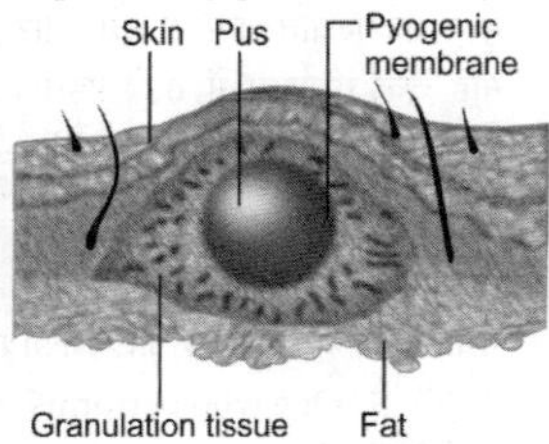

(*i*) **Amebic abscess** (अमीबिक एबसेस) आँत की पेचिश के पश्चात् उपद्रव स्वरूप उत्पन्न होने वाला जिगर का फोड़ा जिसमें अमीबा होते हैं। An abscess of the liver as a complication of amebic dysentery containing ameba. (*ii*) **Axillary Abscess** (एक्जीलरी एबसेस) बगल में होने वाला फोड़ा। Abscess in the axilla. (*iii*) **Brodie's Abscess** (ब्रोडिस एबसेस) जीर्ण अस्थिपेशी शोध, पर्यस्थि व्रण, रक्त संक्रमण से उत्पन्न अस्थिव्रण। Chronic asteomylitis; bone abscess.

(*iv*) **Cold Abscess** (कोल्ड एबसेस) यह पुराना फोड़ा होता है जो अधिकतर तपेदिक की बीमारी में होता है और स्पर्श करने पर ठण्डा प्रतीत होता है। Chronic abscess usually tuberculous which feels cold to touch.

(*v*) **Faucal Abscess** (फिकल एबसेस) मलाशय अथवा बड़ी आँत का फोड़ा, आँत-विद्रधि। One in the rectum or large intestine.

(*vi*) **Ovarian abscess** (ओवेरियन एबसेस) ग्रन्थि-विद्रधि। An abscess of the ovary.

(*vii*) **Primary abscess** (प्राइमरी एबसेस) प्रारम्भिक विद्रधि, मूल व्रण, प्रमुख व्रण। One arising at the seat of infection.

Absence (एबसेन्स) वातावरण से अनभिज्ञता, अभाव, कमी, मिर्गी। Inattention to surroundings, want, epilepsy.

Absorb (एब्जोर्ब) अवशोषण करना। To suck in.

Absorbefocient (एब्जौर्बिफेसिएन्ट) जो अवशोषण का कारक है। Which cause absorption.

Absorbent (एब्जौर्बेन्ट) वह पदार्थ जो अवशोषण करता है, अवशोषक। The substance which absorb.

Absorption (एब्जौरप्शन) किसी पदार्थ का शरीर की किसी सतह से घुस कर शरीर के भीतर ऊतकों एवं तरलों में पहुँच जाना,

अवशोषण। The passage of a substance through some surface of the body into the tissues and body fluids.

Absorptive (एब्जौरप्टिव) अवशोषक। Absorbent.

Abstain (एब्सटेन) परित्याग करना, परहेज करना। To keep oneself away; to retrain.

Abstergent (एब्सटरजेन्ट) शोधक, सफाई करने वाला। Cleansing agent.

Abstinence (एब्सटीनेन्स) भोजन, शराब, उत्तेजक पदार्थों के सेवन अथवा लैंगिक ससंर्ग से परहेज। Refraining from indulgence in food, alcohol, stimulants, or sexual intercourse.

Abstraction (एब्सट्रैक्शन) किसी मिश्रण अथवा यौगिक से उसके किसी घटक को पृथक करना। Separation of a constituent from a mixture or compound.

Abulia (एबूलिया) इच्छाशक्ति का अभाव। Loss or deficiency of willpower.

Abulomania (एबूलोमैनिया) इच्छा शक्ति की दुर्बलता के कारण होने वाला मनोविकार। Mental derangement by weaken willpower.

Abuse (एब्यूज) दुरूपयोग जैसे किसी औषधि या शराब आदि का। Misuse as that of a drug or alcohol.

Acalculia (एकेल्कुलिया) परिकलन-अक्षमता, गणित का हिसाब लगाने में असमर्थता। Inability to solve mathematical problems.

Acanthesthesia (एकेन्थेस्थीसिया) शरीर में सुई चुभने जैसी अनुभूति होना। A sensation as of a pin pricking the body.

Acanthion (एकेन्थियोन) अग्र नासा-शूल के आधार पर स्थित एक बिन्दु। A point at the base of the anterior nasal spine.

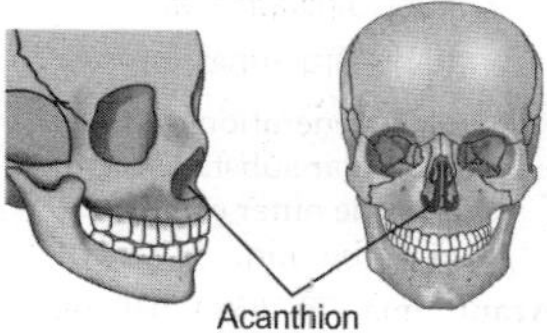

Acanthocyte (एकेन्थोसाइट) कांटेदार लाल रक्त कोशिका, ऐसी रक्त कोशिका जिससे जीवद्रव्य के प्रक्षेपण निकल आने के कारण उसकी कांटेदार आकृति हो जाती है। Thorny red blood cell. RBC with protoplasmic projections giving it thorny appearance.

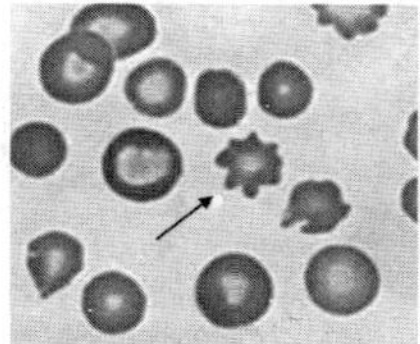

Acanthocytosis (एकेन्थोसाइटोसिस) रक्त में कांटेदार लाल रक्त कोशिकाओं के होने की दशा। A condition characterized by the presence of acanthocytes in the blood.

Acanthoid (एकेन्थोइड) कष्टकी, मेरूदण्डवत्, रीढ़ की हड्डी जैसा। Thorny, spiny; of a spinous nature.

Acantholysis (एकेन्थोलाइसिस) त्वचा की बाह्य अथवा कंटकीय परत की कोशिकाओं के अन्तर्कोशिकीय पदार्थ का ह्रास। Degeneration of the intercellular substance of the cells of the outer or horny layer of the skin.

Acanthoma (एकेन्थोमा) त्वचा का सुदम अबुर्द, कणिका-बुर्द। Benign tumor of the skin.

Acarbia (एकार्बिया) रक्त में बाइकार्बोनेट की मात्रा कम हो जाना। Diminution of bicarbonate in the blood.

Acardia (एकार्डिया) ह्रदय का जन्म-जात अभाव। Congenital absence of the heart.

Acardiacus (एकार्डियाकस) अह्रदयभ्रूण, अह्रदयगर्भ A fetus with no heart.

Acariasis (एकारियेसिस) कुटकी द्वारा उत्पन्न कोई भी रोग। Any disease caused by a mite.

Acarid (एकारिड) किलनी या कुटकी, जूं। Tick or mite.

Acaridiasis (एकारीडिएसिस) जूं पड़ने की बीमारी। Any disease due to the itch mites.

Acarodermatitis (एकारोडर्मेटाइटिस) जूं पड़ने के कारण चमड़ी का प्रदाह होना। Dermatitis due to mites.

Acaroid (एकारॉयड) कुटकी से मिलता-जुलता। Resembling a mite.

Acarophobia (एकारोफोबिया) कुटकियों, किलनियों या किड़ो का रोगोंत्पादक मय। Morbid fear of mites, ticks or worms.

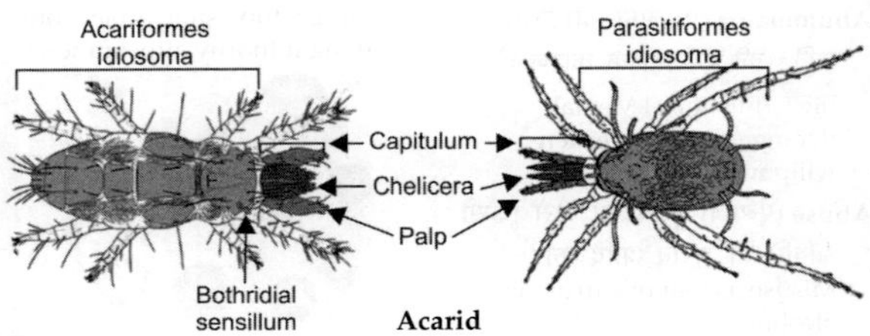

Acarid

Acataleptic (एकेटालेप्टीक) मूढ़चित्त, मन्दबुद्धि, संशयग्रस्त, शंकालु, शकी। Mentally deficient, one affected with catalepsy, suspicious.

Acataphasia (एकेटाफेसिया) मस्तिष्क में क्षति हो जाने के कारण अपने विचारों को सम्बद्ध प्रकार से व्यक्त करने में असमर्थता, तुतलाना। Inability to express the thoughts in connected manner due to cerebral lesion.

Acathexia (एकेथेक्सिया) शरीर में उत्पन्न स्रावों को धारण करने की अक्षमता।
Inability to retain the secretions of the body.

Acathexis (एकेथेक्सिस) एक मानसिक विकार जिसमें किसी वस्तु या विचार के प्रति भावावेगी अनुक्रिया नहीं होती जो सामान्यतया उस व्यक्ति के लिए बहुत महत्वपूर्ण होती है। A mental disorder in which there is lock of emotional response toward a thing or idea which is normally very important to the individual.

Acathisia (एकेथिसिया) बैठने में परेशानी महसूस होना। Feeling of discomfort on sitting.

Acaudal (एकौडल) बिना पूंछ वाला। Having no tail.

Accentuation (एकेन्थुएशन) बोलने में किन्ही शब्दों पर अधिक जोर देना, प्रबलन। Emphasis.

Accessory (एसेसरी) सहायक, आनुषंगिक, अनुषंगी। Auxiliary; accessories; assisting.

Accident (एक्सीडैन्ट) आकस्मिक घटना, दुर्घटना। An unexpected event, mishap.

Accommodation (एकोमोडेशन) समायोजन या अनुकूलन, नेत्र का विभिन्न दूरियों की वस्तुओं को देखने के लिए समायोजन। Adjustment or adaptation; adjustment of the eye for seeing objects at various distances.

Accouchee (एकाऊची) वह स्त्री जिसने बच्चे को जन्म दिया हो, प्रसूता। The woman who delivered a child.

Accouchement (एकाऊचमेंट) प्रसव, बच्चे का जन्म लेना। Delivery of a child.

Accoucheur (एकाऊचीयर) प्रसूति-तन्त्र-विशेषज्ञ या मिडवाइफ, दाई। An obstetrician or midwife.

Accretion (एक्रोशन) किसी पदार्थ के जोड़ने से हुई वृद्धि, संचय, प्राकृतिक रूप से अलग हुए भागों का आपस में जुड़ जाना। Growth by addition of material, Accumulation, coherence of the parts naturally separated.

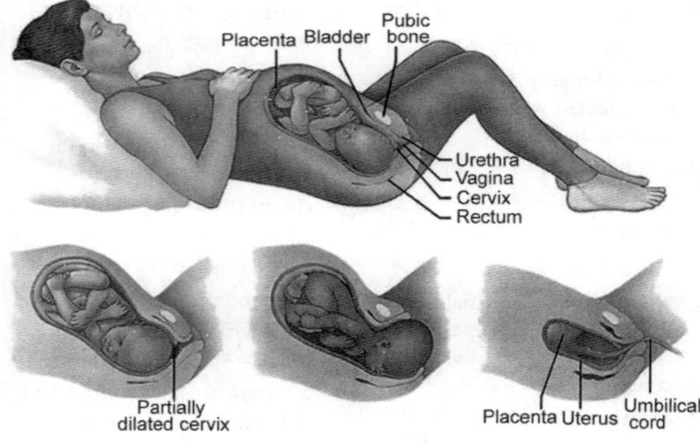

Accouchement

Acenesthesia (एसेनेस्थीसिया) अपने को स्वस्थ महसूस न करना। Loose of feeling of well-being.

Acephalia (एसिफेलिया) जन्म से सिर का न होना। Congenital absence of the head.

Acephalochiria (एसिफेलोकाइरिया) जन्मजात सिर एवं हाथों का न होना। Congenital absence of the head and the hands.

Acephalopodius (एसिफेलोपोडियस) बिना सिर तथा पांवों वाला भ्रूण। A fetus without a head and feet.

Acerate (एसिरेट) तेज, नुकीला। Sharp, pointed.

Acestoma (एसिस्टोमा) क्षतांकुर, कणिकी-ऊतक, कण पुंज। Granulation tissue.

Acetabuloplasty (एसीटाबुलोप्लास्टी) प्लास्टिक सर्जरी द्वारा उल्खल या एसीटाबुलम की मरम्मत करना। Repair of the acetabulum by plastic surgery.

Acetabulum (एसीटाबुलम) कुल्हे की हड्डी के पार्श्व तल पर स्थित प्यालेनुमा गड्ढ़ा जिसमें फीमर हड्डी का सिर फिट रहता है। उलुखल।

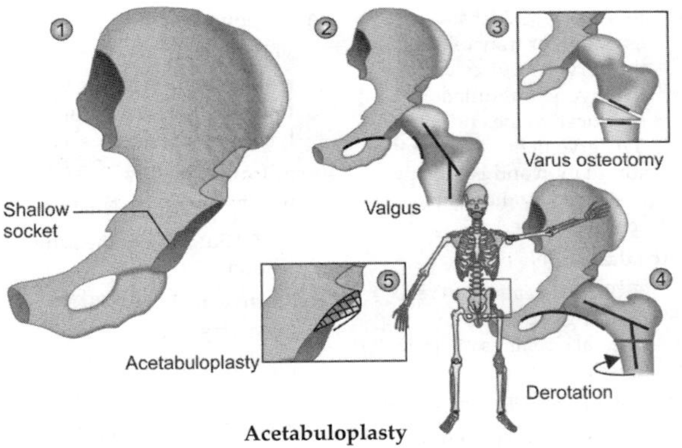

Acetabuloplasty

The cup-shaped cavity on the lateral surface of the hip bone, in which the head of the femur is fitted.

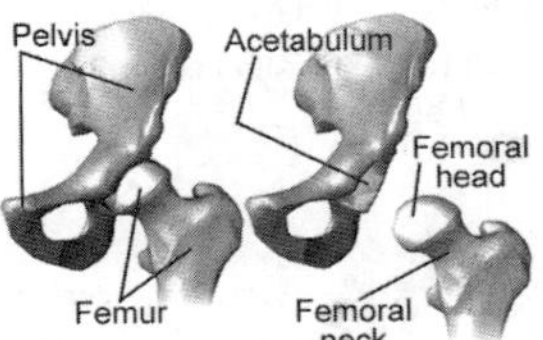

Acetate (एसीटेट) शौक्त, शुक्ल, सिरका।
A salt of acetic acid, vinegar.

Acetic (एसीटिक) सिरके से सम्बन्धित, खट्टा। Pertaining to vinegar, sour.

Acetify (एसीटिफाइ) शुक्ताम्लोत्पादन, सिरकोत्पादन।
To produce acetic fermentation or vinegar.

Acetone (एसिटोन) बहुमूत्ररोग में पेशाब तथा खून में पाया जाने वाला एक पदार्थ।
A substance found in the urine and blood in diabetes.

Acetonuria (एसिटोन्यूरिया) पेशाब में ऐसिटोन पदार्थ का पाया जाना, एसिटोनमेह। Excessive acetone bodies in the urine.

Acetylcholine (एसिटाइलकोलीन) पेशी-तंत्रिका संगम पर तंत्रिका तंतुओं के सिरों पर उद्दीपन के फलस्वरूप उत्पन्न होने वाला एक पदार्थ जो तंत्रिका आवेगों के संचारण के लिए आवश्यक होता है तथा शीघ्र ही कोलीनेस्टेरेज नामक एन्जाइम द्वारा नष्ट

हो जाता है। A substance essential for transmitting the nerve impulses at the myoneural function, produced at the endings of the nerve fibers as a result of stimulation and is quickly destroyed by the enzyme cholinesterase.

Achalasia (एकालैसिया) अशिथिलता। Failure to relax, referring especially to visceral openings or sphincter muscles.

Acheilia (ऐकीलिया) एक या दोनों होठों का जन्म-जात अभाव। Congenital absence of one or both lips.

Acheilous (ऐकीलस) जन्मजात एक या दोनों होठों के अभाव से युक्त अथवा इस विकार से सम्बन्धित। Characterized by or relating to acheilia.

Achillobursitis (एकिलोबसाईटिस) एकिलस टेन्डन के ऊपर स्थित बर्सा या श्लेषपुटी का शोथ। Inflammation of the bursa lying over the achilles tendon.

Achillorrhaphy (एकिलौरैहफी) एकिलस टेन्डन की सिलाई करना। Suturing of the achilles tendon.

Achlorhydria (एक्लोरहाइड्रिया) आमाशयिक स्राव में हाइड्रोक्लोरिक एसिड की अनुपस्थिति, जठर-अम्लता। Absence of hydrochloric acid in gastric reaction.

Acholia (एकोलिया) अपित्त, पित्त की कमी। Absence or want of bile.

Acholic (एकोलिक) अपैत्रिक, अपित्तता सम्बन्धी। Pertaining to acholia.

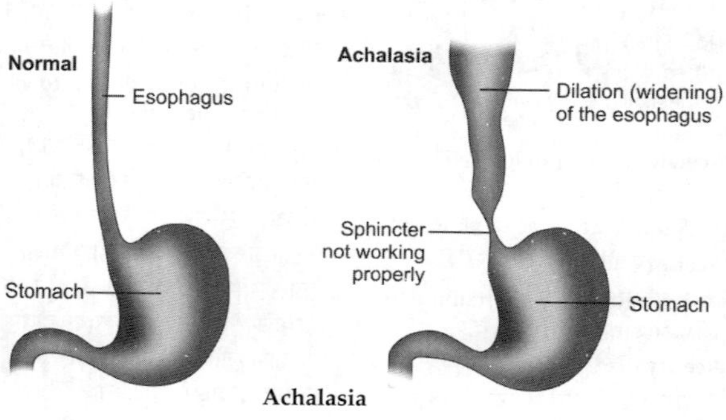

Achalasia

Acholuria (एकोलूरिया) मूत्र में बाइल से रहित। Without bile in urine.

Achondroplasia (एकॉन्ड्रोप्लेसिया) लम्बी हड्डियों के अधिवर्ष पर उपास्थि के बनने में दोष उत्पन्न होना जिससे एक प्रकार का बौनापन पैदा हो जाता है, उपास्थि-अविकासन। Chondrodystrophy, defect in the cartilage formation at the epiphyses of long bones producing a type of dwarfism.

Achromasia (एक्रोमेसिया) त्वचा की सामान्य वर्णकयुक्तता की कमी। Lack of normal skin pigmentation.

Achromate (एक्रोमेट) वर्णान्ध, रंगान्ध (व्यक्ति) Color-blind.

Achromatic (एक्रोमेटिक) कठिनाई के साथ अभिरंजित होने वाला विशेषकर ऊतक एवं कोशिकाएँ, रंगहीन। Staining with difficulty, especially the tissues and cells, colorless.

Achromatolysis (एक्रोमेटोलाइसिस) कोशिका के क्रोमेटिन के घुलने अथवा नष्ट होने की क्रिया। Dissolution of the achromatin of a cell.

Achromatopsia (एक्रोमेटोप्सिया) पूर्ण वर्णान्धता, रंग पहचानने में पूर्ण असमर्थता। Complete color blindness.

Achromatosis (एक्रोमेटोसिस) प्राकृतिक वर्णकयुक्तता रहित होने की दशा। Condition of being without natural pigmentation.

Achromaturia (एक्रोमेचूरिया) रंगहीन मूत्र। Colorless urine.

Achylia (एकाइलिया) वसातसीका अथवा अन्य पाचक रसों का अभाव जैसे जठर-रस अथवा अग्नाशयी रस का पूर्ण अभाव अथवा उनकी कमी, श्रवणहीनता। Absence of chyle or other digestive juices, e.g. the absence or deficiency of the gastric or the pancreatic juice.

Achylous (एकाइलस) किसी भी प्रकार के पाचक रस की कमी वाला। Deficient in any kind of digestive secretion.

Acid (एसिड) किसी धातु से प्रतिक्रिया करके कोई लवण बनाने वाला तथा नीले लिटमस पेपर को लाल करने वाला पदार्थ, अम्ल या तेजाब, खट्टा। The substance which form a salt reacting with a metal and twin blue litmus paper to red, sour.
(*i*) **Ascorbic Acid** (एस्कोर्बिक एसिड) विटामिन सी। Vitamin C. (*ii*) **Citric Acid** (साइट्रिक एसिड) यह नींबू नें पाया जाता है। It is found in lemon.
(*iii*) **Hydrochloric Acid** (हाइड्रोक्लोरिक एसिड) नमक का

तेजाब। (*iv*) **Nicotinic Acid** (निकोटिनिक एसिड) विटामिन बी कॉमप्लैक्स का एक घटक। A member of the vitamin B complex. (*v*) **Pantothenic Acid** (पैन्टोथैनिक एसिड) विटामिन बी कॉमप्लैक्स का एक घटक। A member of the vitamin B complex.

Acidemia (एसिडीमिया) रक्त में अम्ल की अधिकता, अम्लरक्तता। Excess of acid in the blood.

Acid Fast (एसिड फास्ट) अम्ल अप्रभावी, अम्ल स्थायी, अम्ल से अभिरंजित करने पर रंगहीन न होने वाला, इसका अधिकतर जीवाणुओं के परिक्षण में प्रयोग किया जाता है। Not decolorized by staining with acids, usually used for examination of bacteria.

Acidifiable (एसिडीफायबिल) अम्ल बन जाने योग्य। Capable of being made an acid.

Acidify (एसिडीफाइ) खट्टा बनाना, किसी अम्ल में परिवर्तित करना। To make sour, to convert into an acid.

Acidimetry (एसिडीमीट्री) किसी तरल की अम्लता का पता लगाना। Determination of the acidity.

Acidophil (एसिडोफिल) कोशिका अथवा ऊतक जो अम्ल रंजकों द्वारा अभिरंजित हो जाते हैं या अम्लरागी। The cell or the tissue capable of being stained with acid dyes.

Acidosis (एसिडोसिस) अम्लों के संचित हो जाने से अथवा क्षार जैसे कार्बोनेट के अत्यधिक मात्रा में शरीर से रक्त की अत्यधिक अम्लता हो जाना। Excessive acidity of the blood due to accumulation of acids or excessive loss of alkali as bicarbonate from the body. (*i*) **Carbondioxide Acidosis** (कार्बनडाइऑक्साइड एसिडोसिस) पानी में डूबने से अथवा श्वसन अपर्याप्तता में कार्बनडाईऑक्साइड के शरीर में रूक जाने के फलस्वरूप होने वाली अम्लरक्तता। Acidosis resulting from retention of CO_2 in the body as in drowning or due to respiratory insufficiency.

Aciduric (एसिड्रिक) अम्ल माध्यम में वृद्धि करने वाला जैसे कुछ जीवाणु। Capable of growing in acid medium as some bacteria.

Aciniform (एसिनीफॉर्म) अंगूर की शक्ल का। Shaped like grapes.

Acinous (एसिनस) अंगूरों के गुच्छे से मिलती-जुलती ग्रन्थियों से सम्बन्धित। Pertaining to glands resembling a bunch of grapes, aciniform.

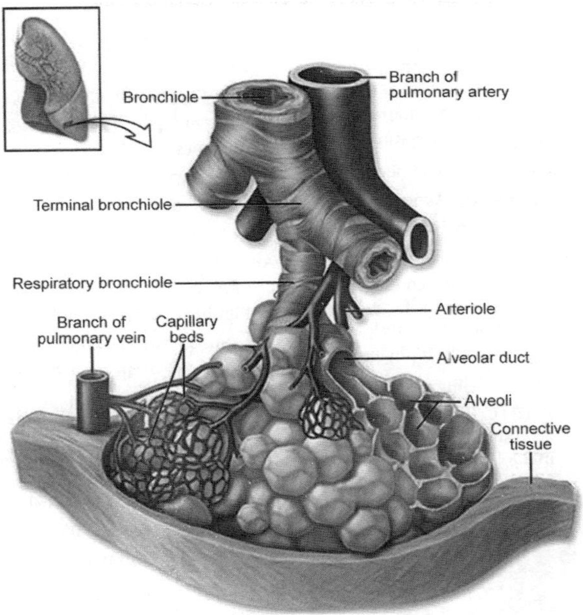

Acinus

Acinus (एसिनस) किसी ग्रन्थि का सबसे छोटा भाग, कोष्ठक। The smallest portion of a gland.

Acme (एक्मी) रोग चर्मोत्कर्ष, दारूणावस्था। Climax of a disease.

Acne (एक्नी) मुहांसा, मुहासे, पनसिका, चेहरे की फुन्सी। Pimple; comedones. (*i*) **Atrophica Acne** (एट्रोफिका एक्नी) इस प्रकार के मुहासे जिनके निकलने के पश्चात् त्वचा पर गड्ढे एवं खुरट के निशान बन जाते है। शोधक पनसिका।
Acne after which pits and signs of scars are formed on the skin.

(*ii*) **Ciliaris Acne** (सिलयरीस एक्नी) पलकों के किनारें होने वाली फुन्सी, वर्त्मान्त पनसिका। Acne of the edges of the eyelids. (*iii*) **Neonatrum Acne** (नियोनेट्रम एक्नी) नवजात पनसिका। Acne in newborn. (*iv*) **Rosacea Acne** (रोजैसिया एक्नी) रक्तिम पनसिका, चेहरे पर निकलने वाले गुलाबी मुहासे। Chronic congestion of the skin of the face; Acne erythematasa. (*v*) **Vulgaris Acne** (वल्गैरिस एक्नी) सामान्य पनसिका, सामान्य प्रकार के मुहासे। Common acne, acne simplex, common in adolescence appearing usually on face, neck and upper part of chest and back.

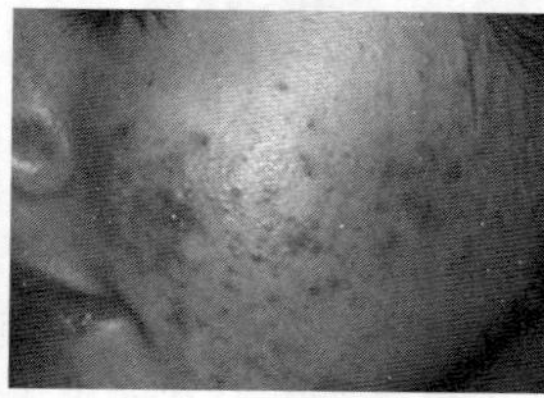

Acnegenic (एक्नेजेनिक) मुहांसे उत्पन्न करने वाला। Producing acne.

Acnemia (एक्नीमिया) जंघापिण्डिकाक्षय। Wasting of the calves.

Acognosia (एकोग्नोसिया) औषधिज्ञान, भेषजज्ञान। Knowledge of drugs.

Acology (एकोलॉजी) औषधिविज्ञान, चिकित्सा शास्त्र। The science of remedies.

Acomia (एकोमिया) खल्वाटता, गंजापन, बाल गिरना। Baldness; alopecia.

Acompsia (एकेम्पसिया) अकड़ाहट, किसी हाथ या पैर में सख्तीपन। Rigidity of a part or limb.

Aconite (एकोनाइट) एकोनाइटम नेपीलस की सुखी जड़ों से प्राप्त होने वाली विषैली औषधी। A poisonous drug derived from the dried roots of *Aconitum napellus*.

Acorea (एकोरिया) आँख की पुतली का अभाव। Absence of the pupil.

Acoria (एकोरिया) अतिक्षुधा, बहुत भूख लगना, राक्षसी भूख। Canine or insatiable hunger.

Acostate (एकोस्टेट) बिना पसलियों वाला। Having no ribs.

Acoumeter (एक्यूमीटर) सुनने की तीक्ष्णता को मापने वाला यन्त्र। An instrument for measuring the acuteness of hearing.

Acoustic (एकोस्टिक) ध्वनि अथवा सुनने से सम्बन्धित, ध्वनिक। Pertaining to sound or hearing.

Acoustic Agraphia (ऐकोस्टिक एग्रेफिया) सुने गये शब्दों को लिखने की अक्षमता। Inability to write the words which are heard.

(*i*) **Motor Agraphia** (मोटर एग्रेफिया) पेशीय असमंजन के कारण लिखने में असमर्थता। Inability to write due to muscular incoordination.

(*ii*) **Optic Argraphia** (ऑप्टिक एग्रेफिया) शब्दों की नकल करने में असमर्थता। Inability to copy the words.

Acoustics (एकोस्टिक्स) ध्वनि का अथवा श्रवण का विज्ञान। The science of sound or of hearing.

Acquired (एक्वायर्ड) अवंशानुगत, उपार्जित, अर्जित। Not inherited.

Acral (एक्रल) भुजाओं से सम्बन्धित अथवा उन्हें प्रभावित करने वाला। Pertaining to or affecting the extremities.

Acrania (एक्रेनिया) कपाल का आंशिक अथवा पूर्ण रूप से जन्मजात अभाव। Partial or complete absence of the cranium congenitally.

Acrasia (एक्रेसिया) आत्म-नियंत्रण की कमी। Lack of self-control.

Acridity (एक्रीडिटी) तीखापन, कड़वाहट। Sharpness, bitterness.

Acriflavine (एक्रीफ्लैविन) तारकोल से प्राप्त एक रंजक। A dye; a derivation obtained from coal-tar.

Acritical (एक्रीटिकल) संकट रहित। Without crisis.

Acrobrachycephaly (एक्रोब्रेकीसिफेली) सिर के आगे-पीछे से छोटे होने की अवस्था। The condition of the head being short in anteroposter or dimension.

Acrocephaly (एक्रोसिफेली) नुकीले सिर का होना, शंकुशीर्षता। The condition of having a pointed head.

Acrocynosis (एक्रोसायनोसिस) भुजाओं का नीला पड़ जाना, शाखाश्यावता। Cyanosis of the extremities.

Acrodynia (एक्रोडाइनिया) भुजाओं का ज्ञान होना। Sensory recognition of the limbs.

Acrohypothermy (एक्रोहाइपोथर्मी) भुजाओं का असामान्य रूप से ठण्डा होना। Abnormal coldness of the limbs.

Acrokinesia (एक्रोकाइनोसिया) भुजाओं का असामान्य रूप से गति करना। Abnormal movements of the extremities.

Acromastitis (एक्रोमैस्टाइटिस) चुचूकशोथ। Inflammation of the nipple.

Acromegaly (एक्रोमेगैली) पीयूष ग्रन्थि के वृद्धि हार्मोन के अधिक मात्रा में स्रावित होने से शरीर का

अनावश्यक रूप से बढ़ जाना, महाकायता या महांगता। Undue enlargement of the body due to hypersecretion of the pituitary growth hormone.

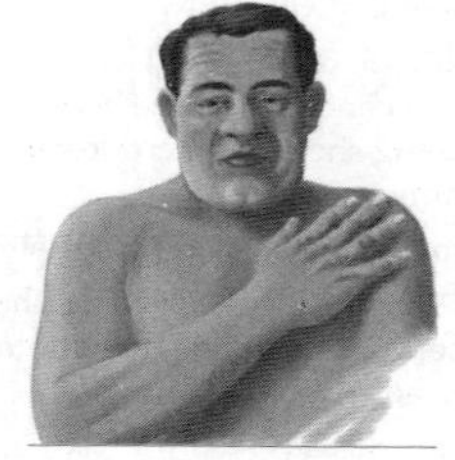

Acromelalgia (एक्रोमेलल्जिया) वह अवस्था जिसमें वाहिका-विस्फार होने के कारण हाथों-पैरों की त्वचा लाल, गर्म तथा वेदनायुक्त हो जाती है। The condition in which the skin of the hands and feet becomes reddened, worm and painful due to vasodilatation.

Acromicria (एक्रोमिक्रिया) भुजाओं का जन्म से ही छोटा होना। Congenital shortness of the limbs.

Acromion (एक्रोमियन) स्कैपुला हड्डी के कंटक का पार्श्विक त्रिकोणिय प्रक्षेप जिससे कन्धे का सबसे ऊपरी बिन्दु बनता है जहाँ पर यह क्लैविकल हड्डी से जुड़कर संधि बनाता है। The lateral triangular projection of the spine of the scapula bone forming the highest point of the shoulder where it articulates with the clavicle bone.

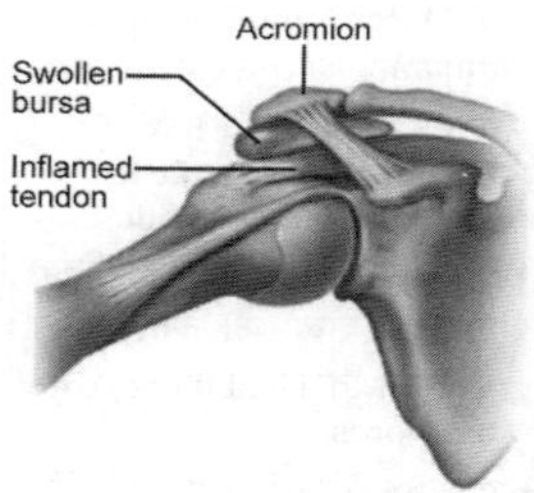

Acromionectomy (एक्रोमियोनेक्टॉमी) एक्रोमियन को काट कर अलग कर देना। Excision of the acromion.

Acromyotonia (एक्रोमायोटोनिया) भुजाओं की पेशीतानता। Myotonia of the extremities.

Acroneurosis (एक्रोन्यूरोसिस) भुजाओं का कोई भी तंत्रिका-रोग। Any nervous disease of the extremities.

Acropachy (एक्रोपैकी) उँगलियों का किनारा मोटा हो जाना। A thickened state of finger tips.

Acropathy (एक्रोपैथी) भुजाओं का कोई भी रोग। Any disease of the extremities.

Acrophobia (एक्रोफोबिया) ऊँचे स्थानों का अस्वस्थ कर देने

वाला भय। Morbid fear of high place.

Acrosome (एक्रोसोम) अग्रपिण्डक। The anterior end of the head of the spermatozoon.

Acrotism (एक्रोटिज्म) नाड़ी का अभाव अथवा उसका महसूस न होना। Absence or imperceptibility of the pulse.

Actin (एक्टिन) पेशी की दो प्रोटीनों में से एक, दूसरी मायोसिन होती है जिसके साथ मिलकर यह पेशी को संकुचित करने एवं शिथिल करने का कार्य करती है। One of the two proteins of the muscle, the other being the myosin, along with which it is responsible for contraction and relation of the muscles.

Actinic (एक्टिनिक) रसायनविकारी, रसायन-विकारण, क्रियाशील। Having the power of exciting chemical action.

Actinomycosis (एक्टिनोमाइकोसिस) एक्टिनो माइक्रोसिस इसराइली नामक जीवाणु जो मुख में रहते हैं, उनके द्वारा उत्पन्न मनुष्य में एक जीवाणु जनित रोग है। A bacterial disease in man caused by the bacteria actinomyces israeli, present in the mouth.

Actinoneuritis (एक्टिनोन्यूराइटिस) रेडियम अथवा एक्स-रे के सम्मुख अनावृत होने के कारण उत्पन्न एक अथवा कई तंत्रिकाओं का शोथ। Inflammation of a nerve or nerves due to exposure to radium or X-rays.

Action (एक्शन) किसी कार्य को करना अथवा प्रक्रिया जैसे किसी औषधि की, या किसी प्रभाव की प्राप्ति। Performance of a function or process as of a drug or the attainment of an effect.

Activation (एक्टिवेशन) सक्रिय बनना। To render active.

Activator (एक्टिवेटर) वह पदार्थ जो किसी निष्क्रिय पदार्थ को सक्रिय पदार्थ में परिवर्तित कर देता है। उत्प्रेरक। A substance which converts an inactive substance into an active substance.

Active (एक्टिव) सक्रिय, क्रियाशील, चेतन। Energetic, the reverse of passive.

Acu (एक्यू) सुई। Needle.

Acuity (एक्यूटी) तीव्रता, स्पष्टता अथवा तीक्ष्णता जैसे दृष्टि, तीक्ष्णता। Severity, cleanness or sharpness as of vision.
(*i*) **Visual Acuity** (विजुअल एक्यूटी) दृष्टि-तीक्षणता। Acuteness of vision.

Acuminous (एक्यूमिनस) तेज बुद्धि वाला। Possessing sharp wit.

Acupuncture (एक्यूपंक्चर) शरीर के किसी विशेष स्थान का पतली

एवं लम्बी सूईयों द्वारा दर्द दूर करने, शरीर के उस स्थान को संज्ञाहीन करने एवं कुछ रोग जैसे दमें की चिकित्सा करने के लिए परिसरीय तंत्रिकाओं के साथ-साथ त्वचा में से होकर छेदन करना। The Piercing of a specific area of the body through the skin along with the peripheral nerves with fine and long needles to relieve pain, to an-esthesize the body area and to treat some disease as asthma.

Acuteness (एक्यूटनैस) तेजी या नूकीलापन, उग्रता या तीव्रता। Sharpness, severity.

Acyanoblepsia (एस्यानोबलेप्सिया) नीले रंगों को न पहचान सकना। Achromatopsia inability to distinguish the blue color.

Acyesis (एसाइसिस) स्त्री बन्ध्यता, गर्भावस्था का अभाव। Sterility in woman, nonpregnancy.

Acystia (एसिस्टिया) मूत्राशय का जन्मजात अभाव। Congenital absence of the urinary blader.

Adacrya (एडाक्राइया) आंसूओं का अभाव होना। Absence of tears, tearlessness.

Adamantine (एडामैन्टाइन) दाँतों के इनैमल अथवा दन्त-वल्क से सम्बन्धित। Pertaining to the enamel of teeth.

Adamantinoma (एडामैन्टीनोमा) जबड़े विशेष रूप से निचले जबड़े का अबुर्द जो इनैमल बनाने वाली कोशिकाओं से उत्पन्न होता है। A tumor of the jaw, especially of the lower jaw, that arises from the enamel-farming cells.

Adamas-S tokes syndrome (एडैम्स-स्टोकस सिण्ड्रोम) मस्तिष्क में रक्त प्रवाह की कमी होने के कारण बेहोश हो जाना एवं दौरे पड़ना। Unconsciousness with convulsion due to decreased blood flow of the brain.

Adapter (एडेप्टर) किसी उपकरण के एक भाग को दूसरे भाग से जोड़ने वाला साधन। A device for connecting one part of an apparatus to another.

Adaxial (एडेक्सियल) मध्य तक की ओर। Towards the medial plane.

Addict (एडिक्ट) व्यसनी, आसक्त, नसेड़ी, आनिसेव, बुरी आदत वाला।
One who habitually uses narcotics.

Addiction (एडिक्शन) व्यसन, आसक्ति, लत, अभ्यस्तता। Bad habits.

Addison's disease (एडिसन्स डिजीस) एड्रीनल ग्रन्थि के कॉर्टेक्स से उत्पन्न होने वाले हार्मोन की कमी से होने वाला रोग जिसमें त्वचा की अतिवर्णकता

हो जाती है तथा कमजोरी हो जाती है और वजन घटने लगता है। A disease caused by the deficiency of adrenocortical hormones characterized by hyper-pigmentation of the skin with debility and loss of weight.

Additive (एडिटीव) योगशील। A substance not essentially part of a material, but is deliberately added to fulfill some specific purpose.

Adducent (एडयूसेन्ट) अभिवर्तनकारी, अभिवर्तक। Causing adduction.

Adduction (एडक्शन) किसी अंग का शरीर की मध्य रेखा की ओर गति करना अथवा अंगुलियों के मामले मे उनका भुजा की अक्षीय रेखा की ओर गति करना, अभिवर्तन। Movement of an organ towards the middle line of the body or in case of digits towards the axial line of a limb.

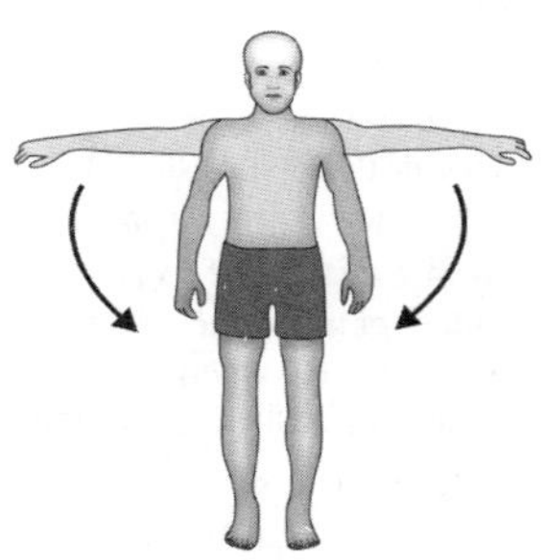

Adductor (एडक्टर) जो शरीर की मध्य रेखा या किसी केन्द्र की ओर खींचता है, इसे पेशी के लिए प्रयोग किया जाता है, अभिवर्तनी। Which draws toward the middle line of the body or towards a center, said of a muscle.

Adenalgia (एडीनेल्जिया) किसी ग्रन्थि में दर्द होना। Pain in a gland.

Adenectopia (एडीनेक्टोपिया) किसी ग्रन्थि का असामान्य स्थिती में पाया जाना। The presence of a gland in an abnormal position.

Adenia (एडीनिया) शोथ के कारण उत्पन्न किसी ग्रन्थि की जीर्ण वृद्धि। Chronic enlargement of a lymin gland due to inflammation.

Adenitis (एडीनाइटिस) किसी ग्रन्थि का सूजन। Inflammation of a gland.

Adenoblast (एडीनोब्लास्ट) ग्रन्थि प्रसू, सक्रिय ग्रन्थि-कोशिका। Any active gland cell.

Adenocarcinoma (एडीनोकार्सिनोमा) ग्रन्थि केन्सर, ग्रन्थिककेटता। A cancer arising from glandular tissue, as in the breast, stomach, etc. adenocanthoma.

Adenocyst (एडीनोसिस्ट) किसी ग्रन्थि से उत्पन्न होने वाला पुटीय अबुर्द । A cystic tumor arising from gland.

Adenocystoma (एडीनोसिस्टोमा) ग्रन्थिपुटी-अबुर्द । A cystous adenoma.

Adenodynia (एडीनोडाइनिया) किसी ग्रन्थि में दर्द होना । Pain in a gland.

Adenography (एडीनोग्राफी) ग्रन्थियों का एक्स-रे लेना । X-ray of the glands.

Adenohypophysis (एडीनोहाइपोफाइसिस) पीयूष ग्रन्थि का अग्र खण्ड । Anterior lobe of the pituitary gland.

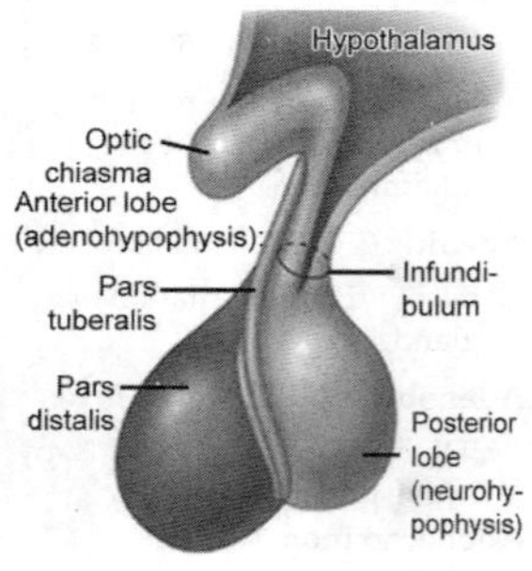

Adenoid (एडीनॉयड) ग्रन्थि से मिलता–जुलता, ग्रन्थ्याभ, कण्ठशालूक । Resembling a gland.

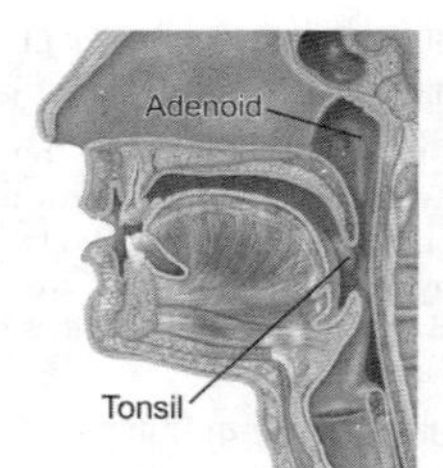

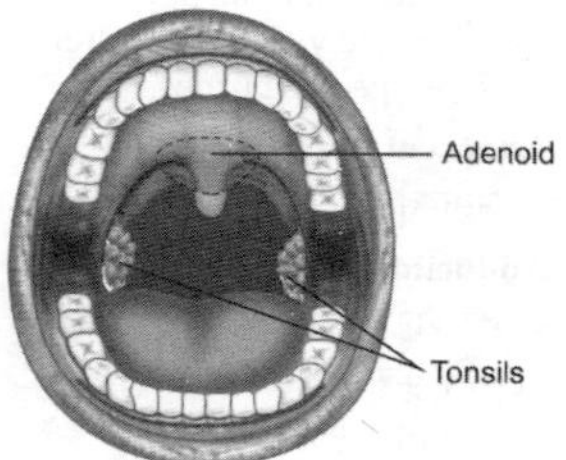

Adenoiditis (एडीनॉयडाइटिस) एडीनॉयड की सूजन । Inflammation of the adenoid.

Adenology (एडीनोलॉजी) ग्रन्थिविज्ञान । The doctrine of the glands.

Adenoma (एडीनोमा) किसी ग्रन्थि की उपकला-कोशिकाओं का सुदम अबुर्द ग्रन्थ्यबुर्द । A benign tumor of the epithelial cells of a gland (*i*) **Acidophilic Adenoma** (एसिडोफिलिक एडीनोमा) पीयूष ग्रन्थि के अग्र खण्ड की अल्फा कोशिकाओं का अबुर्द

जिससे अधिक मात्रा में वृद्धि हार्मोन स्रावित होता है जिससे अतिकायता या महाकायता रोग उत्पन्न होता है। A tumor of the alpha cells of the anterior lobe of the pituitary gland which secrets the growth hormone in excess causing acromegaly or gigantism. (*ii*) **Sebaceum Adenoma** (सीबैसियम एडीनोमा) त्वग्वसीय ग्रन्थ्यबुद। A fatty tumor of face composed of sebaceous glands.

Adenomalacia (एडीनोमैलेशिया) किसी ग्रन्थि का मुलायम हो जाना। Softening of a gland.

Adenomatous (एडीनोमेटस) ग्रन्थ्यबुर्द या एडीनॉयड अथवा कण्ठषालूक से सम्बन्धित। Pertaining to adenoma or adenoid.

Adenomegaly (एडीनोमेगैली) किसी ग्रन्थि का बढ़ जाना। Enlargement of a gland.

Adenomyosis (एडीनोमायोसिस) अन्तर्गभाशयकला में सुदम वृद्धि का उत्पन्न होना जो बढ़कर गर्भाशय के पेशी अस्तर को प्रभावित करती है। Benign growth of the endometrium invading into the myometrium of the uterus.

Adenopathy (एडीनोपैथी) किसी ग्रन्थि का कोई भी रोग। Any disease of a gland.

Adenosarcoma (एडीनोसार्कोमा) ग्रन्थिल एवं सार्कोमा तत्वों दोनों से बना दुर्दम अबुर्द। A malignant tumor composed of both glandular and sarcomatous elements.

Adenosis (एडीनोसिस) किसी ग्रन्थि विशेषकर लसीका ग्रन्थि का कोई रोग, ग्रन्थिलता। Any disease of a gland, especially the lymph gland.

Adenotome (एडीनोटोम) कण्ठशालूओं को काटकर अलग कर देने वाला यंत्र। An instrument for excisioning the adenoids.

Adenovirus (एडीनोवाइरस) विशाणुओं का बड़ा समूह जिसके द्वारा ऊपरी श्वसन पथ में संक्रमण होता है। Any of a large group of viruses causing infection of the upper respiratory tract.

Adermia (एडर्मिया) त्वचा का जन्मजात दोषयुक्त होना अथवा इसका अभाव होना। Congenital defect or absence of the skin.

Adherence (एडहोयरैन्स) किसी वस्तु पर चिपकने की क्रिया अथवा चिपकने का गुण होना। The act or quality of sticking to something.

Adhesiotomy (एडहीजियोस्टॉमी) चिपकावों को शल्यक्रिया द्वारा अलग कर देना। Surgical division of adhesions.

Adiaphoresis (एडियाफोरेसिस) पसीने की कमी अथवा पसीना बिल्कुल न आना। Deficiency or absence of sweat.

Adiaphoretic (एडियाफोरेटिक) पसीना रोकने या कम करने वाला। Preventing or reducing perspiration.

Adipic (एडिपिक) वसा सम्बन्धी। Pertaining to fat.

Adipocele (एडिपोसील) ऐसा बहिःसरण अथवा हर्निया जिसमें वसीय ऊतक होता है। A hernia containing fatty tissue.

Adipocere (एडिपोसीयर) मृत जन्तुओं के शरीर के विघटन के दौरान उत्पन्न होने वाला मोम जैसा पदार्थ। A waxy substance produced during decomposition of dead animal bodies.

Adipofibroma (एडिपोफाइब्रोमा) वसाबुर्द जिसमें तन्तुमय ऊतक होते हैं। A lipoma with fibrous tissues.

Adipogenic (एडिपोजैनिक) वसा या मोटापा उत्पन्न करने वाला। Producing fat or fatness.

Adipolysis (एडिपोलाइसिस) वसा का पाचन। Digestion of fat.

Adiposis (एडिपोसिस) मोटापा या शरीर में अत्यधिक वसा का संचित हो जाना, वसामयता। Obesity or excessive accumulation of fat in the body.

Adipositis (एडिपोजाइटिस) वसा-ऊतकों का शोथ। Inflammation of the fatty tissue.

Adipsia (एडिप्सिया) प्यास न लगना। Absence of thirst.

Adjuvant (एडजुवैन्ट) वह पदार्थ जो किसी औषधि के साथ मिलाने पर उसके गुण को बढ़ा देता है। सहायक। A substance which on adding to a medicine enhances its property, assisting.

Adnerval (एडनर्वल) किसी तंत्रिका की ओर। Towards a nerve.

Adnexal (एडनेक्सल) उपांगीय, उपांगों सम्बंधी। Pertaining to the appendages.

Adolescence (एडोलेसैन्स) किशोरावस्था, यौवनावस्था, प्रौढ़ता की शुरूआत। Youth, the period between puberty and maturity.

Adoral (एडोरल) मुख की ओर या मुख के पास। Toward or near the mouth.

Adrenal (एड्रीनल) एड्रीनल ग्रन्थि अथवा इसके स्रावों के सन्दर्भ में प्रयुक्त शब्द। वृक्क के पास अथवा उसके ऊपर। The word used in reference to the adrenal gland or its secretion, near or upon the kidney.

Adrenalectomy (एड्रीनलेक्टॉमी) एक या दोनों एड्रीनल ग्रन्थियों को काटकर निकाल देना। Excision of one or both adrenal glands.

Adrenaline (एड्रीनलीन) इपिनेफ्रीन। Expinephrine.

Adrenalism (एड्रीनालिज्म) एड्रीनल ग्रन्थि के कार्य में गड़बड़ी होने से उत्पन्न रोग। Illness due to adrenal dysfunction.

Adrenalitis (एड्रीनालाइटिस) एड्रीनल ग्रन्थियों की सूजन। Adrenitis, Inflammation of the adrenal glands.

Adrenergic (एड्रीनार्जिक) वे तंत्रिका तन्तु जो उत्तेजित होने पर अपने सिरों पर इपिनेफ्रीन मुक्त करते हैं। Nerve fibers which on stimulation release epinephrine at their ending.

Adrenocortical (एड्रीनोकॉर्टिकल) एड्रीनल ग्रन्थि के कॉर्टेक्स से सम्बन्धित अथवा उससे उत्पन्न होने वाला। Pertaining to or arising from adrenal cortex.

Adrenocorticotropin (एड्रीनोकॉर्टिकोट्रॉपिन) पीयूष ग्रन्थि के अग्र खण्ड से स्रावित होने वाला एक हार्मोन जो एड्रीनल कॉर्टेक्स के विकास एवं उसके निरन्तर कार्य करने के लिए आवश्यक होता है। A hormone secreted by the anterior lobe of the pituitary gland which is necessary for the development and continued function of the adrenal cortex.

Adrenogenous (एड्रीनोजीनस) एड्रीनल ग्रन्थि से उत्पन्न होने वाला। Arising from the adrenal gland.

Adsorb (एडजार्ब) अपनी सतह पर अन्य पदार्थ को चिपका लेना अधिशोषण करना। To adhere other material on its surface.

Adsorbent (एडजॉरबेंट) वह पदार्थ जो अन्य पदार्थों के कणों को अपनी सतह पर चिपकाता है, अधिशोषक। A substance which adheres the particles of other materials on its surface.

Adult (एडल्ट) पूर्णतया विकसित एवं परिपक्व व्यक्ति अथवा जीव। Fully developed and mature person or organism.

Adulterant (एडल्टेरेन्ट) मिलावट करने के लिए किसी बनाई गई वस्तु में मिलाया जाने वाला अशुद्ध एवं सस्ता पदार्थ। An impure and cheap substance used to add to a product for adulteration.

Adulteration (एडल्टेरेशन) ठगने के लिए किसी बनाई गई वस्तु में अशुद्ध (एवं सस्ते पदार्थ को मिलाना) मिलावट। Addition of an impure and cheap substance to a product to cheat, admixture.

Adventitia (एडवेन्टीशिया) बाह्यास्तर, रक्तवाहिनियों का बाहरी आवरण, बाह्यकंचुक। The external coat of the blood vessels.

Adventitious (एडवेन्टीशियस) असामान्य स्थान पर स्थित, अपस्थानिक। Situated at an abnormal place.

Adynamia (एडायनैमिया) अगतिकता, क्षीणता, दुर्बलता, निर्बलता, कमजोरी, जैवी शक्तियों का अभाव। Weakness caused by disease.

Adynatus (एडायनैट्स) रूग्ण, बीमार। Sickly, weakly.

Aerated (ऐरेटेड) वायु अथवा किसी गैस से युक्त। Containing air or a gas.

Aerial (ऐरियल) वायवी, वायु सम्बन्धी। Belonging to air.

Aerobe (ऐरोब) वातापेक्षी, वायुजीवी, हवा पर जीवित रहने वाला। One of the aerobia, aerobion.

Aerobiosis (ऐरोबायोसिस) ऑक्सीजन से युक्त वातावरण में रहना। Living in an environment containing oxygen.

Aerocele (ऐरोसील) वायु के भरने से बना कोई अबुर्द अथवा किसी गुहा का गैस से फूल जाना। A tumor formed by air filling a pouch, or distention of a cavity with gas.

Aerocalpas (ऐरोकोल्पस) वायु अथवा गैस द्वारा योनि का फूल जाना। Distention of the vagina with air or a gas.

Aerocoly (ऐरोकोली) गैस से कॉलन या बड़ी आँत का फूल जाना। Distention of the colon with gas.

Aerodynamics (ऐरोडाइनामिक्स) वायु गति-विज्ञान। The science of air or gases in motion.

Aerometer (ऐरोमीटर) गैसों का घनत्व मापने वाला एक उपकरण। An apparatus for measuring the density of gases.

Aerophagia (ऐरोफेजिया) वायु का निगलना। Swallowing of the air.

Aerophobia (ऐरोफोबिया) वायु का रोगोत्पादक भय। Morbid fear of air.

Aerophore (ऐरोफोर) नवजात शिशु के फेफड़ो में हवा भरने वाला उपकरण। An apparatus for inflating the lungs of the newborn child.

Aeroscope (ऐरोस्कोप) वायुशुद्ध तादर्शी यंत्र, हवा की शुद्धता मापने वाला यंत्र। An instrument for examination of air dust.

Aerosis (ऐरोसिस) ऊतकों में गैस इकट्ठी हो जाना। Accumulation of gas in the tissues.

Aerotoxis (ऐरोटोक्सिस) जीवों का वायु से दूर अथवा वायु की ओर गति करना। Movement of the organisms away from or towards the air.

Aestivalis (ऐस्टिवेलिस) ग्रीष्मकालीन, गर्मियों में प्रकट होने वाला। Occurring in the season of summer.

Afebrile (एफेब्राइल) ज्वर रहित। Without fever.

Affect (अफैक्ट) दुषप्रभाव पड़ना, भाववृत्ति, अनुभाव। A feeling directed towards anything.

Afferent (अफेरेन्ट) किसी केन्द्र की ओर ले जाने वाला, अन्तर्गामी, अभिवाही। Carrying towards a center.

Affinity (अफिनीटी) सम्बन्ध, नाता, आकर्षण, खिंचाव। Relationship, a synonym for attraction.

Affusion (अफ्यूजन) परिषेक जैसे जलपरिषेक, गीला करना। A pouring upon, as water on the body.

Afibrinogenemia (एफाइब्रिनोजेनीमिया) रक्त में फाइब्रिनोजन की कमी अथवा इसका अभाव। Deficiency or absence of fibrinogen in the blood.

After birth (आफ्टर बर्थ) अपरा एवं झिल्लियां जो बच्चे के जन्म के पश्चात् गर्भाशय से बाहर निकलते है। The placenta and the membranes which are expelled from the uterus after child birth.

After care (आफ्टर केयर) अनुरक्षण, उपचारोत्तर देखभाल। The care given during convalescence and rehabilitation.

Afterimage (आफ्टरइमेज) किसी प्रतिबिम्ब को उत्पन्न करने वाले उछीपन के समाप्त हो जाने पर भी प्रतिबिम्ब का बने रहना। Image that persists after cessation of the stimulus causing it.

Afterpains (आफ्टरपेन्स) बच्चा पैदा होने के बाद पहले कुछ दिनों के भीतर गर्भाशय के संकोचों के द्वारा उत्पन्न होने वाले ऐंठन के समान दर्द। Cramp like pains due to contractions of the uterus occurring during first few days after child birth.

Afterpotential (आफ्टरपोटैन्शियल) अनुविभव। Small changes in electrical potential in a stimulated nerve which follow the main potential.

Agalactia (एगैलेक्टिया) बच्चा पैदा होने के बाद दुग्धस्राव न होना, अस्तन्यता। Absence of milk secretion after child birth.

Agalactous (एगैलेक्टस) दुग्धरोधी, दुग्धरोधक, दूध का बहाव रोकने वाला। Checking the secretion of milk.

Agammaglobulinemia (एगामाग्लोबुलिनीमिया) रक्त में गामा ग्लोबुलिन की कमी। Deficiency of gamma globulins in the blood.

Agamous (एगैमस) जननांगो से रहित। Without sex organs.

Aganglionosis (एगैंगलियोनोसिस) परानुकम्पी गैंगलियोन कोशिकाओं का जन्मजात अभाव। Congenital absence of parasympathetic ganglion cells.

Agastria (एगैस्ट्रिया) आमाशय का अभाव। Absence of the stomach.

Age (ऐज) वय, आयु, उम्र, वयस, जीवनकाल। Length of life.

Agent (एजेन्ट) जो किसी प्रभाव को उत्पन्न करता है। Something producing an effect.

Ageusia (एग्यूसिया) स्वाद की अनुभूति का पूर्ण अथवा आंशिक प्रभाव। Absence or partial loss of the sense of taste.

Agglutinate (एग्लूटिनेट) चिपकना, चिपकाना। To unite with glue.

Agglutination (एग्लूटिनेशन) जख्म भरने में चिपकाव द्वारा सतहों के जुड़ने की क्रिया। The process of union of the surfaces by adhesion in wound healing.

Agglutinin (एग्लूटिनिन) रक्त के सीरम में विद्यमान कोई एण्टीबॉडी या पदार्थ जो अपने एंटिजन से मिलकर एंटिजन तत्वों को एक दूसरे से चिपका कर गुच्छों के रूप में बना देता है, समूहिक। An antibody or a substance present in the serum of the blood which combining with its antigen causes the antigen elements to adhere to one another in clumps. (*i*) **Cold Agglutinin** (कोल्ड एग्लुटिनिन) ऐसा समुहिका या एग्लुटिनिन जो केवल नीचे तापमान (0–20 °से.) पर ही कार्य करता है। An agglutinin which acts only in low temperature (0–20 °C).

Agglutinogen (एग्लुटिनोजन) कोई भी पदार्थ जो एग्लुटिनिन के उत्पादन को प्रोत्साहित करता है,

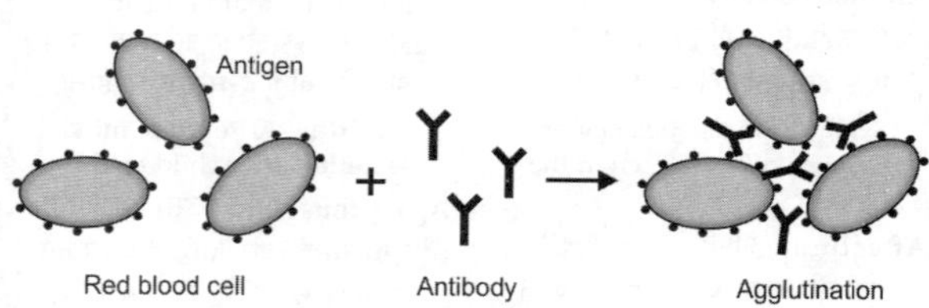

Agglutinate

एक प्रकार का एंटिजन की भांति कार्य करता है जैसे एग्लुटिनोजन आर एच, समूहजन। Any substance which stimulates the production of agglutinin, thereby acting as an antigen, e.g. agglutinogen RH.

Agglutinophilic (एग्लुटिनोफिलिक) शीघ्र ही गुच्छों के रूप में एकत्रित हो जाने वाला। Readily agglutinating.

Aggregate (एग्रीगेट) समुच्चय करना। To group or arrange in clusters.

Agitographia (एजिटोग्राफिया) असामान्य रूप से तेज बोलना जिसमें शब्द ठीक प्रकार से नहीं बोले जाते। Abnormally rapid speech in which words are spoken imperfectly.

Aglossia (एग्लोसिया) जिह्वा का जन्मजात अभाव। Congenital absence of the tongue.

Aglutition (एग्लुटिशन) निगलने में अक्षमता। Inability to swallow.

Agnathia (एग्नेथिया) निचले जबड़े का जन्मजात अभाव। Congenital absence of the lower jaw.

Agnosia (एग्नोसिया) पहचानने में असमर्थता। Inability to recognize.

Agonal (एगोनल) अन्तकाल, आसन्न मृत्युकाल, मृत्यु से पूर्व का समय। The period just preceding death.

Agonist (एगोनिस्ट) एगोनिस्ट पेशी की एक किस्म होती है जो किसी भाग को संकुचित करती है तथा दूसरी पेशी द्वारा इसके विपरीत कार्य किया जाता है। प्रचालक। Agonist is a type of muscle which contracts a part and is opposed by another muscle as in being the elbow, the biceps brachii muscle is the agonist.

Agoraphobia (एगोराफोबिया) भीड़ से बहुत डर लगना। Morbid fear of being of crowds.

Agrammatism (एग्रामैटीज्म) अशुद्ध वाक्, अशुद्ध शब्दों का प्रयोग करना। An inability to form grammatic sentences.

Agranulocyte (एग्रेनुलोसाइट) कणिकाओं से रहित श्वेत कोशिका। A WBC without granules.

Aganulocytosis (एग्रेनुलोसाइटोसिस) रक्त में कणिका कोशिकाओं की संख्या में कमी से उत्पन्न होने वाली दशा जिसमें तेज बुखार हो जाता है तथा मुख एवं अन्य श्लेष्मिक झिल्लियों में जख्म बन जाते हैं, कणीश्वेत कोशिकाहीनता। A condition occurring due to decrease in the number of granulocytes in the blood characterized by high fever, ulceration of the mouth and other mucous membranes.

Agraphia (एग्रेफिया) लिखने की अक्षमता। Inability to write.

Agromania (एग्रोमेनिया) एकान्त स्थान पर रहने की तीव्र इच्छा। Keen desire to live in a lonely place.

Ague (एग्यू) मलेरिया बुखार या ठण्ड लगना। Malarial fever or chill.

Aichmophobia (ऐक्मोफोबिया) नुकीली वस्तुओं अथवा अंगुलियों के स्पर्श का रोगोत्पादक भय। Morbid fear of being touched by pointed objects or fingers.

AID (ए.आई.डी.) दाता द्वारा कृत्रिम शुक्रसेचन। Artificial insemination by donor.

AIDS (ऐड्स) एक्वायर्ड इम्यून डेफिसियन्सी सिण्ड्रोम। Acquired immune deficiency syndrome.

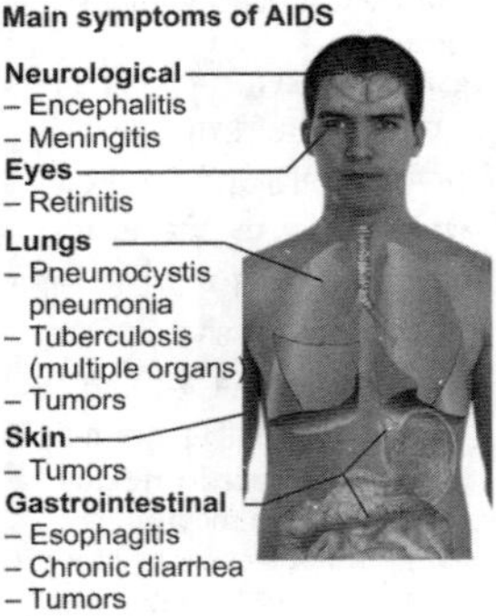

Main symptoms of AIDS

Neurological
– Encephalitis
– Meningitis
Eyes
– Retinitis
Lungs
– Pneumocystis pneumonia
– Tuberculosis (multiple organs)
– Tumors
Skin
– Tumors
Gastrointestinal
– Esophagitis
– Chronic diarrhea
– Tumors

Ailment (ऐलमेन्ट) एक छोटी बीमारी। A minor disease.

Air (एयर) पृथ्वी को चारों ओर से घेरे रहने वाली दिखाई न देने वाली, स्वादहीन एवं गन्धहीन गैसों का मिश्रण, वायु, पवन, वात, हवा। The mixture of invisible tasteless and odorless gases surrounding the earth.

(*i*) **Complement Air** (कॉमप्लीमैन्ट एयर) अन्तःश्वसनीय आरक्षित आयतन, वायु का वह आयतन जिसे वायु के उस आयतन से अधिक सांस के साथ अन्दर खींचा जा सकता है जो प्रत्येक सामान्य श्वसन में फेफड़ों के भीतर जाता है वहां से बाहर आता है। Inspiratory reserve volume, the volume of the air that can be respired over the volume of air which flows in and out of the lungs with each normal respiration.

(*ii*) **Residual Air** (रेजीडुअल एयर) पूर्ण निश्वसन के पश्चात् फेफड़ों में बची रहने वाली वायु जो युवा व्यक्ति में लगभग 1500 घ.से. होती है। Air remaining in the lungs after the full expiration which is about 1500 cc in the adult.

(*iii*) **Supplemental Air** (सप्लीमैन्टल एयर) वायु का आयतन जिसे पूर्ण सामान्य

निःश्वसन के पश्चात् सांस के साथ बाहर निकाला जा सकता है जो किसी युवा में लगभग 1500 घ.से. होता है। The volume of air that can be expired after a full normal expiration which is about 1500 cc in an adult. (*iv*) **Tidal Air** (टाइडल एयर) प्रत्येक सामान्य श्वसन के साथ फेफड़ों के भीतर जाने तथा वहां से बाहर आने वाली वायु का आयतन जो पुरूष के लिए लगभग 500 घ.से. होता है। Tidal volume. The volume of air that flows in and out of the lungs with each normal respiration which is about 500 cc for a man.

Air Embolism (ऐयर एम्बोलिज्म) एक वायु का बुलबुला जो किसी रक्त वाहिनी को अवरूद्ध कर देता है। An air bubble obstructing a blood vessel.

Air Hunger (ऐयर हन्गर) सांस फूलना। Dyspnea.

Air Way (ऐयर वे) नासा-रन्ध्रो या मुख से फेफड़ो में विद्यमान अन्तिम सूक्ष्म श्वासनलिकाओं तक का मार्ग जिसके द्वारा वायु फेफड़ों के भीतर प्रवेश करती है तथा वहाँ से बाहर निकलती है। श्वास मार्ग में अवरोध उत्पन्न होने को रोकने के लिए प्रयोग में लाया जाने वाला उपकरण जिसका विशेषकर नशा सुंघाते समय प्रयोग किया जाता है। The passage from the nares or mouth to the terminal bronchioles in the lungs by which the air enters and leaves the lungs. An apparatus used to prevent that obstruction of respiratory passage, especially during anesthesia.

AK (ए.के.) घुटने से ऊपर। Above knee.

Akathisia (एकेथीसिया) मनोव्यथा, अशान्ति और चिन्ता की दशा। A state in which the patient feels a distressing inner restlessness.

Akinesia (एकाइनेसिया) पूर्ण या आंशिक गत्याभाव या अगति। Acinesia, complete or parital loss of movements.

Alacrima (एलेक्राइमा) आँसुओं की कमी अथवा उनका पूर्ण अभाव। Deficiency or absence of tears.

Alalia (एलैलिया) वाक्-अंगों में दोष उत्पन्न हो जाने अथवा उनका पक्षाघात हो जाने के कारण उत्पन्न वाक्-अक्षमता। Aphasia, inability to speak due to defect or paralysis of the vocal organs.

Alar (एलर) किसी पक्षक पंख से सम्बन्धित अथवा पंख के समान। Pertaining to an ala, or wing, or like a wing.

Alba (एल्बा) सफेद अथवा मस्तिष्क का श्वेत द्रव्य। White or white substance of the brain.

Albinism (एल्बीनिज्म) मेलेनिन के बनने में दोष उत्पन्न होने के कारण त्वचा, बालों तथा आँखों में वर्णकयुक्तता का जन्मजात पूर्ण अथवा आंशिक अभाव, अवर्णकता। Congenital total or partial absence of pigmentation in the skin, hair and eyes due to defect in melanin formation.

Albino (एल्बिनो) अवर्णता से पीड़ित व्यक्ति। A person suffering from albinism.

Albugineous (एल्बूजीनियस) व्यूनिका एल्बूजीनिया से सम्बन्धित अथवा मिलता-जुलता। Pertaining to or resembling tunica albuginea.

Albumen (एल्ब्युमिन) एक प्रकार की प्रोटीन जो पौधों एवं जन्तुओं में पाई जाती है। यह रक्त सीरम में पाई जाती है जिसे सिरम एल्ब्युमिन कहते है। A kind of protein found in plant and animal tissues. It is found in blood serum as serum albumin.

Albuminemia (एल्ब्युमिनेमिया) रक्त में एल्ब्युमिन की अधिकता। Excess of albumin in the blood.

Albuminoid (एल्ब्युमिनॉयड) एल्ब्युमिन के समान। एक प्रोटीन। Resembling albumin, a protein.

Albuminuria (एल्ब्युमिनुरिया) मूत्र में सीरम एल्ब्युमिन का पाया जाना। Presence of serum albumin in the urine. (*i*) **Cyclic Albuminuria** (साइक्लिक एल्ब्युमिनुरिया) चक्रिय अन्नसारमेह, क्रियात्मक अन्नसारमेह, प्रवेगी अन्नसारमेह। Albuminuria accuring at stated times in the day; functional albuminuria; paroxysmal albuminuria. (*ii*) **Dietetic Albuminuria** (डाइटेटिक एल्ब्युमिनुरिया) कुछ भोज्य पदार्थों का सेवन करने के पश्चात् उत्पन्न होने वाला एल्ब्युमिनमेह। Albuminuria accuring following ingestion of certain foods. (*iii*) **Febrile Albuminuria** (फेब्राइल एल्ब्युमिनूरिया) ज्वर के साथ होने वाला एल्ब्युमिनूरिया। Albuminuria associated with fever. (*iv*) **Pathological Albuminuria** (पैथोलॉजिकल एल्ब्युमिनुरिया) किसी रोग के द्वारा उत्पन्न एल्ब्युमिनमेह। Albuminuria caused by a disease.

Alcohol (एल्कोहॉल) एल्कोहॉल एक रंगहीन, गंधहीन, उड़नशील तथा ज्वलनशील द्रव्य है जो शुगर या शर्करा युक्त खाद्य पदार्थों जैसे अंगूर, सिरका, अनाज आदि के किण्वन एवं आसवन

द्वारा प्राप्त होता है। मद्यसार, सुरासार। Alcohol is a colorless, volatile and flammable liquid obtained by the fermentation and distillation of sugar containing food materials such as grapes, vineger and grains. (*i*) **Absolute Alcohol** (एब्सोल्यूट एल्कोहॉल) शुद्ध सुरासार। Spirit containing no water.
(*ii*) **Denatured Alcohol** (डिनेचर्ड एल्कोहॉल) ऐसा एल्कोहॉल जिसमें विषैले पदार्थ मिलाकर उसे पीने के अयोग्य बना दिया जाता है। Alcohol which is made unfit for drinking by adding toxic substance.

Alcoholemia (एल्कोहॉलेमिया) रक्त में एल्कोहॉल का पाया जाना। Presence of alcohol in the blood.

Alcoholism (एल्कोहॉलिज्म) मदात्य, शराब का नशा। Alcohol intoxication.

Alcoholomania (एल्कोहॉलोमैनिया) शराब पीने की अत्यधिक इच्छा करना। मद्योन्माद। Excessive craving for alcohol.

Alcoholophilia (एल्कोहॉलोफिलिया) शराब की अत्यधिक लालसा। Morbid craving for alcohol.

Alcoholuria (एल्कोहॉलूरिया) मूत्र में एल्कोहॉल का पाया जाना। Presence of alcohol in the urine.

Aldosterone (एल्डोस्टेरोन) एड्रीनल ग्रन्थि के कॉर्टेक्स से उत्पन्न होने वाला एक मिनरलोकोर्तिकॉयड हार्मोन जो सोडियम क्लोराइड तथा पोटेशियम के चयापचय को नियमित करता है। A mineralocorticoid hormone secreted by the adrenal cortex which regulates the metabolism of sodium, chloride and potassium.

Aldosteronism (एल्डोस्टेरोनिज्म) रक्त में अधिक मात्रा में एल्डोस्टोरोन हार्मोन होने की दशा। A condition in which the blood contains a large amount of aldosterone hormone.

Aleukocytic (एल्यूकोसाइटिक) जिसमें श्वेत रक्त कोशिकायें न हो। Showing no leukocytes.

Alexia (एलेक्सिया) पढ़ने में असमर्थता या लेखान्धता अथवा शब्दान्धता। Inability to read, or word blindness.

Algefacient (एल्गीफेसिएन्ट) ठण्डा करने वाला। Refrigerant or cooling.

Algesia (एल्जेसिया) दर्द के लिए अत्यधिक संवेदनशीलता होना। Hypersensitiveness to pain.

Algesic (एल्जेसिक) वेदनायुक्त। Painful.

Algesimeter (एल्जेसिमीटर) आर्तिमापी, पीड़ामापी। An instrument for measuring cutaneous sensitiveness.

Algid (एल्जिड) ठण्डा। Cold or Chilly.

Algogenic (एलगोजेनिक) पीड़ाजनक, दर्दकारी, दर्द पैदा करने वाला, तापोशामक, ताप कम करने वाला। Causing pain, lowering temperature.

Algolagnia (एल्गोलैग्निया) दर्द का अनुभव करके लैंगिक संतुष्टि होना। Sexual satisfaction occurring by feeling pain.

Algophobia (एल्गोफोबिया) दर्द का रोगोत्पादक भय। Morbid fear of pain.

Algor (एल्गर) शीतानुभूति, कंपकंपी, शिशिर, ज्वरजनित शीत। An unusual feeling of coldness, rigor or chill.

Alienate (एलाइनेट) स्वयं को अलग करना। To isolate oneself.

Alienate (एलाइनेट) प्लीहा का अभाव। Absence of the spleen.

Aliform (एलीफार्म) पंख के आकार का। Wing-shapes.

Alimentary (एलीमेन्टरी) भोजन या पोशक पदार्थ अथवा पाचक अंगों से सम्बन्धित। Pertaining to food or nutritive material or to the digestive organs.

Aliphatic (एलीफेटीक) वसा सम्बन्धी, चर्बी सम्बन्धी। Relating to a fat; fatty.

Alkalemia (एल्केलीमिया) रक्त में बढ़ी हुई क्षारता, क्षरक्तता। Increased alkalinity of the blood.

Alkaline (एल्कालाइन) किसी क्षार की प्रतिक्रिया से युक्त, क्षारीय। Having the reaction of an alkali.

Alkalinuria (एल्कालीनूरिया) क्षारीय मूत्र। Alkaluria, alkaline urine.

Alkalitherapy (एल्कलीथिरैपी) क्षारों द्वारा रोगों की चिकित्सा। Treatment of disease with alkaline.

Alkaloid (एल्केलॉयड) कार्बनिक क्षारीय पदार्थों के समूह में से एक जो पौधों से प्राप्त होता है, एल्केलॉयड अम्लों के साथ प्रतिक्रिया करके लवण बनाते हैं। जिनका औषधि में प्रयोग किया जाता है। One of a group of organic alkaline substance obtained from the plants. Alkaloids react with the acids to form salt which are used in medicine.

Alkalosis (एल्केलोसिस) रक्त में एल्कली रिजर्व के बढ़ जाने से उत्पन्न दशा, क्षारमयता। A condition caused by a rise of alkali reserve in the blood.

Allantoic (एलेन्टॉइक) अपरापोशिका से सम्बन्धित। Pertaining to allontois.

Allele (अलील) दो या अधिक भिन्न जीनों में से एक जो जोड़ीदार समजात गुण सूत्रों के अनुरूप स्थानों पर स्थित होते है जिसके कारण आनुवांशिक लक्षण परिवर्तित हो जाते हैं। One of two or more different genes occupying the corresponding sites on homologous paired chromosomes, due to which the hereditary characters are altered.

Allenthesis (एलेन्थेसिस) किसी बाह्य पदार्थ का शरीर में प्रवेश होना। Introduction of a foreign substance into the body.

Allergen (एलर्जेन) एलर्जी उत्पन्न करने वाला कोई भी पदार्थ, प्रत्यूर्जतोत्पादक। Any substance causing allergy.

Allergic (एलर्जिक) किसी एलर्जेन से सम्बन्धित, उससे संवेदनशील अथवा किसी एलर्जेन द्वारा उत्पन्न। Pertaining to, sensitive to or caused by allergen.

Allergy (एलर्जी) किसी पदार्थ के प्रति उत्पन्न होने वाली अतिसुग्राही प्रतिक्रिया नहीं होती। यह कोशिकाओं से हिस्टामिन अथवा हिस्टामीन की भांति पदार्थो के मुक्त होने से होती है। एलर्जी में पित्ती उछलना, स्तब्धता, दमा, एलर्जी जनक नासाशोध या प्रतिश्याय (जुकाम) और एक्जिमा या छांजन आदि अवस्थायें उत्पन्न हो जाती है। प्रत्यूर्जता। A ccurence of a hypersensitive reaction to a substance which does not normally causes any reaction. It is due to the release of histamine or histamine like substances from the damage cells. Allergic condition includes urticaria, shake, bronchial asthma, allergic, rhinitis or coryza and eczema, etc.

Allochezia (एलोकीजिया) किसी असामान्य छिद्र से होकर मल का विसर्जित होना। Excretion of feces through an abnormal opening.

Allochroism (एलोक्रोइज्म) रंग में परिवर्तन। Change in color.

Allograft (एलोग्राफ्ट) उसी जाति के प्राणी से उपलब्ध प्रतिरोपित किया जाने वाला ऊतक। Transplant tissue obtained from the same species.

Allolalia (एलोलेलिया) मस्तिष्क में हुई क्षति से उत्पन्न वाक्-दोष। Speech defect due to brain lesion.

Allopath (एलोपैथ) एलोपैथी में प्रैक्टिस करने वाला व्यक्ति। The person who practices in allopathy.

Allopathy (एलोपैथी) कोई विकृतिजनक प्रतिक्रिया उत्पन्न करके जो रोग के विपरीत होती है, किसी रोग की चिकित्सा करने की एक पद्धति। A system of treatment of disease by producing a pathological reaction which is antagonistic to the disease.

Alloploidy (एलोप्लॉयडी) ऐलोप्लॉयड होने की दशा। The condition of being alloploid.

Allorhythmia (एलोरिह्दमिया) नियमित हद्स्पन्द या नाड़ी का अनियमित हो जाना। Irregularity of the regular heart beat or pulse.

Allosome (एलोसोम) लिंग गुणसूत्र। One of the chromosome differing in appearance or behavior from the ordinary chromosome.

Allotriogeustia (एलोट्रॉयोग्यूस्टिया) स्वाद का बदल जाना। Perverted sense of taste.

Alloy (एलोय) मिश्रधातु, दो या दो से अधिक धातुओं का मिश्रण। A combination of two or more metals.

Alopecia (एलोपीसिया) गंजापन, त्वचा से विशेषकर सिर की त्वचा से बालों का लुप्त हो जाना, खालित्य या खल्वाटता। Baldness, loss of hair from the skin especially of the head. (*i*) **Alopecia Areata**

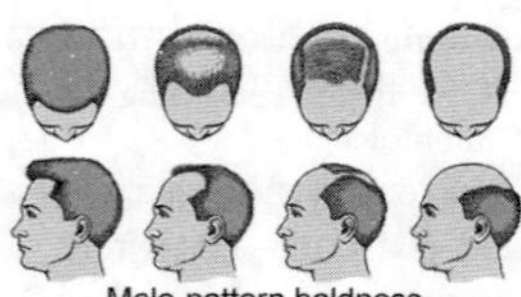

Male-pattern baldness

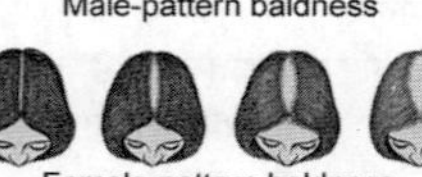

Female-pattern baldness

(एलोपीसिया एरियेटा) स्पष्ट दिखने वाले चकत्तों के रूप में बालों का उखड़ जाना। ऐसा अधिकतर खोपड़ी अथवा दाढ़ी पर होता है, सीमित खालित्य। Loss of hair appearing in well-defined patches usually involving the scalp or beard. (*ii*) **Alopecia Senilis** (एलोपीसिया सैनाइलिस) वृद्धावस्था में होने वाला गंजापन। Baldness occurring in old age.

Alter (अल्टर) अण्डकोश निकाल देना या बधिया करना, बदलना। To castrate, to change.

Altitude Sickness (आल्टीट्यूड सिक्नैस) वायुमण्डलीय ऑक्सीजन की कमी से उत्पन्न होने वाला रोग जैसे हवाई यात्रा करने या पहाड़ो पर चढ़ने पर ऑक्सीजन की कमी से होता है जिसमें सिर में दर्द होता है, सांस फूलता है, घबराहट होती है, बहोशी हो जाती है और यहाँ तक कि गम्भीर स्थिति में मृत्यु तक हो जाती है।

A disease caused by decreased atmospheric oxygen as on flying or climbing on mountain and characterized by headache, dyspnea, malaise, fainting and even death if severe.

Alum (एलम) फिटकरी। Alumen.

Aluminum (एल्यूमिनियम) एक धातु, जिसके बर्तन बनते है। Whitish metal with a low specific gravity.

Alveolalingual (एल्वियोलोलिंगुअल) दन्त उलूखल-प्रवर्ध तथा जिह्वा सम्बन्धी। Pertaining to the alveolar process and the tongue.

Alveolar (एल्वियोलर) किसी वायुकोष्ठ अथवा दन्त उलूखल से सम्बन्धित। Pertaining to an alvelus.

Alveolate (एल्वियोलेट) शहद की मक्खी के छत्ते के समान, गड्ढो वाला। Honeycombed, pitted.

Alveolitis (एल्वियोलाइटिस) दन्तउलूखल अथवा वायुकोष्ठ की सूजन। Inflammation of an alveolus.

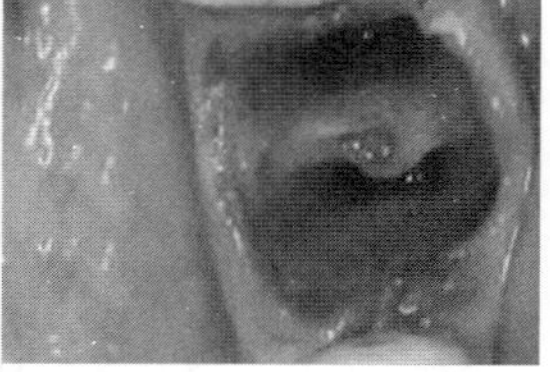

Alveus (एल्वियस) एक नलिका या खातिका। A canal or groove.

Alymphoplasia (एलिम्फोप्लेसिया) लसीका ऊतक के विकसित होने में अक्षमता। Failure of lymph tissue to develop.

Amalgam (एमल्गाम) एक मिश्रण जिसमें पारा होता है जो दन्त-चिकित्सा में दाँतों को पुनःस्थापित करने के लिए प्रयोग में लाया जाता है, पारदमिश्र, पारद धातुयौगिक। An alloy containing mercury which is used in dentistry to restore teeth.

Amaurosis (एमौरोसिस) अंधता, अन्धापन विशेषकर जो आँख में किसी खराबी के कारण नहीं होता। Blindness, especially that which is not due to any lession of the eye.

(*i*) **Congenital Amaurosis** (कॉन्जेनाइटल एमौरोसिस) जन्म से अंधापन। Blindness since birth

(*ii*) **Fugax Amaurosis** (फ्यूगेक्स एमौरोसिस) रेटिना में अपर्याप्त रक्त प्रवाह होने के कारण उत्पन्न होने वाली अस्थायी अंधता जो 10 मिनट तक रह सकती है। Temporary blindness occurring due to insufficient blood flow to the retina which may last for up to 10 minutes.

(*iii*) **Toxic Amaurosis** (टॉक्सिक एमौरोसिस) जीवविषों द्वारा उत्पन्न

दृष्टि-तंत्रिका के शोथ के कारण होने वाली अंधता। ये जीव–विष अन्तर्जात हो सकते है। जैसे मधुमेह में अथवा बहिर्जात हो सकते है जैसे एल्कोहॉल या तम्बाकू में। Blindness due to optic neuritis caused by toxins which may be endogenous (such as in diabetes) or exogenous (as in alcohol or tobacco).

Amaurotic (एमौरोटिक) अंधेपन से सम्बन्धित अथवा इससे पीड़ित। Pertaining to amaurosis or suffering from it.

Ambidextrous (एम्बीडैक्सट्रस) किसी भी हाथ से ठीक से कार्य करने में सक्षम। Capable of working effectively with either hand.

Ambisexual (एम्बीसैक्सुअल) दोनों लिंगों से सम्बन्धित। Pertaining to both sexes.

Amblyacousia (एम्बलीएकाउसिया) श्रवण-मन्दता, सुनाई कम देना। Dullness of hearing.

Amblygeustia (एम्बलीज्यूसटीया) विरसता, बदला हुआ स्वाद। Diminished sense of taste.

Amblyoscope (एम्बलीयोस्कोप) मन्ददृष्टिता वाली आँख में दृष्टि बढ़ाने वाला यंत्र। An instrument for increasing the vision in an amblyopic eye.

Ambulant (एम्बुलैन्ट) चलने योग्य, जो बिस्तर पर न लेटा हो। Able to walk, not confined to bed.

Amebiasis (एमीबियेसिस) अमीबिकता, अमीबा-रूग्णता। State of being infected by ameba, amebism.

Amebocyte (एमीबोसाइट) अमीबा के समान गति करने वाली कोई भी कोशिका। Any cell showing ameboid movements.

Ameboid (अमीबॉयड) अमीबा की आकृति वाला, अमीबा से मिलता-जुलता। Amebiform, resembling an ameba.

Ameboma (अमीबोमा) अमीबारूग्णता द्वारा उत्पन्न आँत में स्थित अबुर्द के समान एक पिण्ड। A tumor-like mass in the intestine caused by amebiasis.

Amelia (एमेलिया) एक या अधिक भुजाओं का जन्मजात अभाव। Congenital absence of one or more limbs.

Amelioration (एमेलियोरेशन) सुधार, ह्रास, उपशम। Becoming better, improvement in the stages of a disease.

Ameloblastoma (एमीलोब्लास्टोमा) जबड़े, विशेषकर निचले जबड़े का अबुर्द जिसमें इनैमल की विशिष्टता होती है। A tumor of the jaw, especially of the lower jaw, which is characteristic of the enamel.

Amelus (अमीलस) अंगहीन जीव, बिना अंगों का जीव। A monster without limbs.

Amenomania (अमीनोमैनीय) हास्येन्माद, हँसते रहने का पागलपन। Mental disorder of a pleasing character.

Amenorrhea (एमेनोरिह्या) अनार्तव, मासिक धर्म अथवा आर्तव स्राव का अभाव अथवा उसका रूक जाना। Absence or stoppage of menstruation.

Amensalism (एमीनसालिज्म) सहजीविता जिसमें एक को हानि पहुँचती है और दूसरा लाभान्वित होता है। Symbiosis in which one is harmed and the other is benefited.

Amentia (एमेन्शिया) जन्मजात मन्दबुद्धिता। Congenital mental deficiency.

Ametria (एमीट्रिया) गर्भाशय का जन्मजात अभाव। Congenital absence of the uterus.

Ametropic (एमीट्रोपिक) अपसामान्य दृष्टि से पीड़ित व्यक्ति, असामान्य-दृष्टिक। The person suffering from ametropia.

Amino Acids (अमीनो एसिड्स) ये प्रोटीन पाचन के अन्तिम उत्पाद होते हैं एवं शरीर का निर्माण करने वाले होते है। These are the end products of protein digestion and are body-builders.

Ammonia (अमोनिया) प्रोटीनों एवं अमीनो एसिडों के विघटन से बनने वाली एक क्षारीय गैस। An alkaline gas formed by the decomposition of proteins and amino acids, (NH_3).

Amnesia (एम्नेसिया) स्मृतिलोप, याददाश्त खत्म हो जाना। Loss of memory. (*i*) **Anterograde Amnesia** (एन्ट्रोग्रेड एम्नेसिया) किसी चोट लगने के पश्चात् होने वाली घटनाओं का भूल जाना, घटनोत्त स्मृतिलोप। Loss of memory for the event occurring after receiving an injury. (*ii*) **Retrograde Amnesia** (रीट्रोग्रेड एम्नेसिया) किसी चोट लगने से पहले होने वाली घटनाओं को भूल जाना, घटनापूर्व स्मृतिलोप। Loss of memory for the events occurring before receiving an injury. (*iii*) **Visual Amnesia** (विजुअल एम्नेसिया) वस्तुओं की आकृति की याद न रहना अथवा छपे हुए शब्दों का ज्ञान न रहना। Inability to remember the appearance of the objects to have a knowledge or the printed words.

Amniocentesis (एम्नियोसेन्टेसिस) उल्वोदक को खींचकर बाहर निकालने के लिए सूई एवं सिरिंज का प्रयोग करके उल्वकोष का पार-उदरीय छेदन करना।

Transabdominal puncture of the amniotic sac using a needle and syringe in order to aspirate the amniotic fluid.

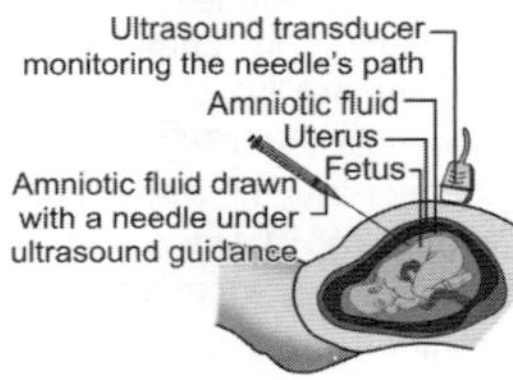

Amnion (एम्नियोन) उल्व, भ्रूणावरण। The thin but strong membrane enclosing the fetus in the womb.

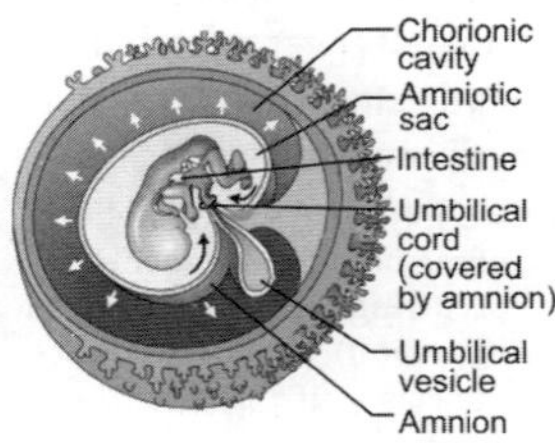

Amnionitis (एम्नियोनाइटिस) उल्व-शोथ। Inflammation of the amnion.

Amniorrhexis (एम्नियोरैहक्सिस) उल्व का फटना। Rupture of the amnion.

Amniotic Cavity (एम्नियोटिक केविटी) द्रव से भरी उल्व की गुहा। The cavity of the amnion filled with fluid.

Ampere (एम्पिरी) विद्युत धारा की इकाई। The unit of electric-current strength.

Amphi (एम्फी) दोनों ओर, सभी ओर तथा दुगुने का संकेत देने वाला उपसर्ग। Prefix indicating on both sides, on all sides, double.

Amphigonadism (एम्फीगोनाडिज्म) डिम्बग्रन्थि-ऊतक एवं शुक्र ग्रन्थि-ऊतक दोनों का पाया जाना। Possession of the ovarian and testicular tissue.

Amphocyte (एम्फोसाइट) ऐसी कोशिका जो अम्लीय अथवा क्षारीय अभिरंजकों से अभिरंजित हो जाती है। A cell staining with either acid or basic stains.

Amphoric (एम्फोरिक) खाली घड़े में बोलने की ध्वनि के समान। Similar to the sound produced by blowing into a hollow jar.

Amphoteric (एम्फोटेरिक) अम्ल एवं क्षार दोनों प्रकार की प्रतिक्रियायें करने की क्षमता रखने वाला, अभयधर्मी। Capable of reacting both as an acid and a base.

Amplification (एमप्लीफिकेशन) वृद्धि। Increasement.

Ampule (एमप्यूल) कांच का एक छोटा-सा पात्र जो ठीक प्रकार से सील बन्द किया होता है तथा जिसमें इन्जैक्शन द्वारा प्रयोग में लाई जाने वाली विसंक्रमित औषधि रहती है।

A small perfectly sealed glass container containing sterilized medicine for use by injection.

Ampulla (एम्प्यूला) किसी नली के आकार की संरचना का चौड़ा भाग, तम्बिका। The dilated portion of a tubular structure.

Amputation (एम्पुटेशन) किसी भुजा, भाग अथवा अंग को सामान्यता शल्य-क्रिया द्वारा शरीर से अलग कर देना, अंगोच्छेदन। Removal usually by surgery of a limb, part or organ, from the body.

Amusia (एम्यूजिया) संगीत उत्पन्न करने अथवा उसे पहचानने में अक्षमता। Inability to produce or recongnize music.

Amyelia (एमाइलिया) सुशुम्ना रज्जु का जन्मजात अभाव। Congenital absence of the spinal cord.

Amygdala (एमाइग्डेला) गलतुण्डिका, टांसिल। A tonsil, a lobe of the cerebellum.

Amygdalolith (एमाइग्डेलोलिथ) टॉन्सिल में स्थित पथरी। Stone in a tonsil.

Amygdalotome (एमाइग्डेलोटोम) टान्सिल को काटकर निकाल देने वाला यंत्र। An instrument for excising a tonsil.

Amylase (एमिलेज) श्वेतसार को शर्करा में बदलने वाला पदार्थ। An enzyme which converts starches into sugars.

Amyloid (एमाइलॉयड) श्वेतसाराभ, श्वेतसारिक, मण्डभ। A starch is wax like in appearance.

Amyloidosis (एमाइलॉयडोसिस) यह एक ऐसा रोग है जिसमें एमाइलॉयड ऊतकों एवं अंगों में कोशिकाओं से बाहर जमा हो जाता है। यह रोग बिना किसी कारण के प्राथमिक भी हो सकता है, जीर्ण रोगों जैसे सिफिलिस सन्धिशोथ के द्वितीयक भी हो सकता है। It is disease in which amyloid is deposited

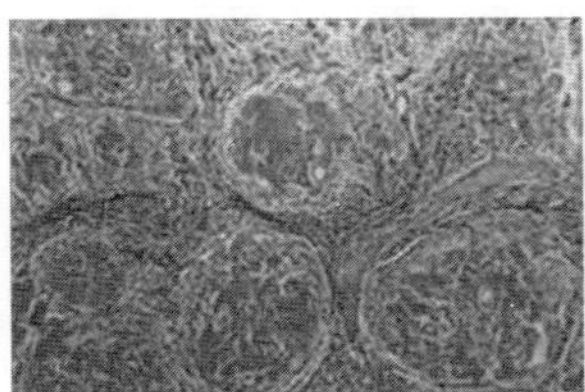

H and Z Source: TUSDM

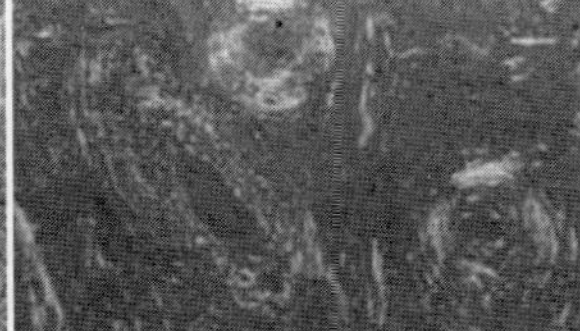

Polarized light Source: TUSDM

Amyloidosis

extracellulary in tissues and organs. The disease may be primary without any cause, secondary to chronic disease such as syphilis.

Amylophagia (एमाइलोफेजिया) स्टार्च की अत्यधिक लालसा। Excessive desire for starch.

Amyluria (एमाइलूरिया) स्टार्च का अधिक मात्रा में मूत्र में पाया जाना। An excess of starch in the urine.

Amyoplasia (एमायोप्लेसिया) पेशी का न बनना। Absence of muscle formation.

Amyotonia (एमायोटोनिया) पेशीय अतानता। Lack of muscular tone.

Amyotrophy (एमायोट्रॉफी) पेशीय शोथ। A trophy of the muscles.

Amyxorrhea (एमिक्सोरिह्या) श्लेश्मा स्राव का न होना। Absence of mucous secretion.

Anabasis (एनोबेसिस) किसी रोग में हालत बिगड़ जाने का समय। period of increased severity of a disease.

Anabolism (एनाबोलिज्म) उपचय, निर्माणक चयापचय। Constructive metabolism.

Anaclitic (एनेक्लाइटिक) झुकने अथवा निर्भर रहने वाला। Leaning or depending upon.

Anacousia (एनाकाऊजिया) पूर्ण बधिरता। Anakusis, total deafness.

Anadipsia (एनाडिप्सिया) प्यास अधिक लगना। Intense thirst.

Anaerobe (एनेरोब) ऑक्सीजन के अभाव में जीवित रहने एवं वृद्धि करने वाला जीव, वातनिरपेक्षी। An organism that can live and grow in the absence of oxygen.

Anaerogenic (एनेरोजेनिक) कम अथवा बिल्कुल ही गैस न बनने वाला। Producing little or no gas.

Anagenesis (एनाजेनेसिस) ऊतक की मरम्मत। Repair of the tissue.

Anal (एनल) गुदा सम्बन्धी। Pertaining to the anus.

Analgesia (एनलजेसिया) वेदना की अनुभूति न होना, वेदना असंवेदिता, वेदनाहरण। Absence of sensation of pain.

Analgia (एनाल्जिया) वेदनाभाव, वेदनाहीनता, पीड़ा का अभाव। painlessness, analgis.

Analogous (एनालोगस) कार्य अथवा आकृति में एक समान परन्तु उद्‌गम (उत्पत्ति स्थान) या संरचना में भिन्न। Similar in function or appearance but different in origin or structure.

Analogue (एनालोग) दो अंग जो एक सा कार्य करते हैं परन्तु रचना में भिन्न होते हैं। समधर्मी। Two organs similar in function but different in structure.

Analysis (एनालाइसिस) विश्लेषण, पृथक्करण, किसी पदार्थ के घटक, लक्षण या स्वरूप का निर्धारण। The resolution of a body into its elements.

Analyte (एनालाइट) रासायनिक विश्लेषण द्वारा ज्ञात कोई पदार्थ। A substance determined by a chemical analysis.

Analyze (एनालाइज) भागों में विभाजित होना। To separate into parts.

Anamnesis (एनेम्नेसिस) किसी रोग का पिछला चिकित्सीय इतिहास, पूर्ण इतिवृत्त। The past medical history of a patient.

Anaphase (एनाफेज) अर्धसूत्री विभाजन अथवा सूत्री विभाजन में केन्द्रक के विभाजन की तृतीय अवस्था। The third stage of division of the nucleus in either meiosis or mitosis.

Anaphoria (एनाफोरिया) नेत्र गोलकों के ऊपर घूम जाने की प्रवृत्ति। Anatropia, tendency of eyeballs to turn upward.

Anaphrodisiac (एनाफ्रोडिसियाक) लैंगिक इच्छा के दबाने वाली कोई भी वस्तु, अबाजीकर। An agent repressing sexual desire.

Anaphylactoid (एनाफाइलैक्टॉयड) तीव्रता सम्बन्धी अथवा इसके समान। Pertaining to or resembling anaphylaxis.

Anaphylaxis (एनाफाइलैक्सिस) तीव्र ग्राहिता, अतिरंजित प्रतिक्रिया। Oversusceptibility.

Anaplasia (एनाप्लेसिया) कोशिकाओं की भिन्नता का समाप्त हो जाना जो कि बहुत से केंसर अबुर्दों की विशिष्टता होती है। अविकसन। Dedifferentiation, loss of differentiation of cells, characteristic of most malignancies.

Anapneic (एनाप्नीक) श्वास कष्ट में आराम पहुँचाने वाला। Relieving dyspnea.

Anarthria (एनार्थरिया) साफ-साफ न बोल सकना, अस्पष्ट उच्चारण। Inability to speak distinctly.

Anastomasis (एनास्टोमोसिस) दो भागों विशेषकर तंत्रिकाओं अथवा रक्त वाहिनियों का संयोजन, सम्मिलन। The union of two parts, especially of the nerves or the blood vessels.

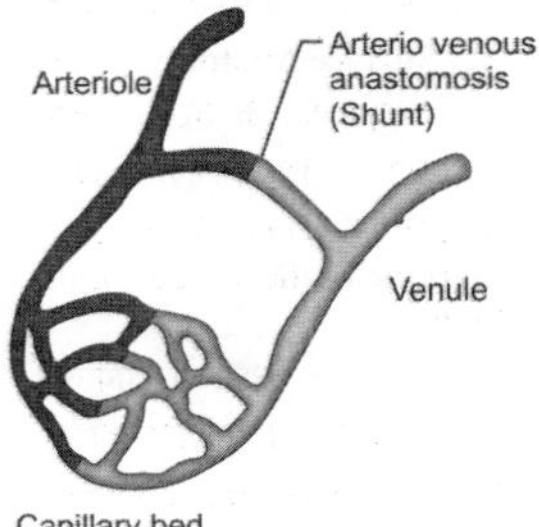

Anatomy (एनाटॉमी) प्राणियों की शरीर-रचना का विज्ञान, शरीर-रचना विज्ञान। The science of the structure of the organisms. (*i*) **Applied Anatomy** (एप्लाइड एनाटॉमी) रोग निदान एवं चिकित्सा विशेषकर शल्य-चिकित्सा में प्रयुक्त शरीर-रचना विज्ञान। Anatomy applied to the diagnosis and treatment, especially surgical treatment. (*ii*) **Comparative Anatomy** (कम्परेटिव एनॉटोमी) शरीर-रचना विज्ञान जिसमें विभिन्न जन्तुओं की समजात संरचनाओं की तुलना की जाती है। Anatomy in which homologous structures of different animals are compared. (*iii*) **Morbid Anatomy** (मोर्बिड एनाटॉमी) आसामान्य, रोगग्रस्त अथवा क्षतिग्रस्त संरचनाओं का अध्ययन। Study of the abnormal, diseased or injured structures. (*iv*) **Surface Anatomy** (सर्फेस एनाटॉमी) शरीर के तल के रूप एवं उस पर स्थित अंकनों का अध्ययन। Study of form and marking of the surface of the body.

Anatripsis (एनाट्रिप्सिस) चिकित्सा में रगड़ने अथवा मालिश का प्रयोग। The use of rubbing or massage in the treatment.

Anchorage (एन्कोरेज) किसी विस्थापित अंग को शल्यक्रिया द्वारा स्थिर करना। Surgical fixation of a displace organ.

Ancylostoma (एन्किलोस्टोम) मानवकृमि, अंकुशकृमि। Human hookworm, ankylostoma. **Ancylostoma Duodenale** (एन्किलोस्टोम ड्योडिनेल) अंकुशकृमि। Hookworm.

Androgen (एण्ड्रोजन) कोई भी पदार्थ जो पुरूष विशिष्टताओं को उत्पन्न करता है या उनके विकास को प्रोत्साहित करता है जैसे टैस्टोस्टेरोन एवं एण्ड्रोस्टेरोन हार्मोन। Any substance which produce or stimulates the development of male characteristics, such as the hormones testosterone and androsterone.

Androgenous (एण्ड्रोजीनस) पुरूष बच्चों को जन्म देने वाली। Giving birth to males.

Androgynoid (एण्ड्रोगाइनॉयड) ऐसा पुरूष जो स्त्री से मिलता-जुलता हो अथवा जिसमें नारी की विशिष्टताएँ पायी जाती है। A male resembling a female or possessing female characteristics.

Andrology (एण्ड्रोलॉजी) नरविज्ञान, पुरूष विज्ञान। The science of man.

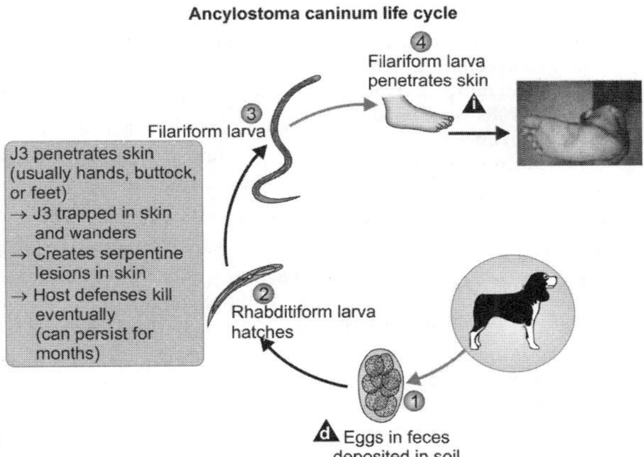

Andromania (एण्ड्रोमैनिया) स्त्रीकामोन्माद, स्त्रियों में पाया जाने वाला कामोन्माद। Nymphomania.

Andropathy (एण्ड्रोपैथी) कोई भी रोग जो विशेषकर पुरूष को ही होता है। Any disease peculiar to the male.

Androphobia (एण्ड्रोफोबीया) नरांतक, नरभीति, पुरूषों का भय, पुरूष भीति। A morbid for men.

Anemia (अनीमिया) रक्त ऑक्सीजन वाहन की क्षमता में कमी हो जाना जो रक्त में लाल रक्त कोशिकाओं की संख्या अथवा हीमोग्लोबिन की मात्रा में सामान्य से नीचे कमी हो जाने पर होती है। Reduced oxygen carrying capacity of the blood which may be due to reduction in the number or RBC or quantity of hemoglobin in the blood, below normal. (*i*) **Folic Acid Deficiency Anemia** (फोलिक एसिड डिफिशियन्सी) अनीमिया फोलिक एसिड की कमी के परिणामस्वरूप उत्पन्न रक्ताल्पता। Anemia resulting from deficiency of folic acid. (*ii*) **Hyperchromic Anemia** (हाइपरक्रोमिक अनीमिया) ऐसी रक्ताल्पता जिसमें औसत कणिका-हीमोग्लोबिन सान्द्रता सामान्य से अधिक होती है जिससे लाल रक्त कोशिकाएं सामान्य से अधिक

अभिरंजित होती है। Anemia in which mean corpuscular hemoglobin concentration is greater than normal, so the red blood cells are stained darker than normal. (*iii*) **Hypochromic Anemia** (हाइपोक्रोमिक अनीमिया) ऐसी रक्ताल्पता जिसमें हीमोग्लोबिन की कमी होती है। जो लाल रक्त कोशिकाओं की संख्या में कमी होने की अपेक्षा कहीं अधिक होती है। Anemia in which there is hemoglobin deficiency which is much greater than the decrease in number of RBCs. (*iv*) **Iron-Deficiency Anemia** (आयरन-डेफिसियन्सी अनीमिया) रक्त सीरम में लोहे की कमी, लौह अल्पताजन्य रक्ताल्पता। Anemia due to iron deficiency in the blood serum. (*v*) **Macrocytic Anemia** (मैक्रोसाइटिक अनीमिया) ऐसी रक्ताल्पता जिसमें लाल रक्त कोशिकाएं असामान्य रूप से बढ़ जाती है। Anemia in which the RBC are abnormally enlarged. (*vi*) **Megaloblastic Anemia** (मैगालोब्लास्टिक अनीमिया) ऐसी रक्ताल्पता जिसमें रक्त में मैगालोब्लास्ट पाये जाते हैं। Anemia in which megaloblasts are found in the blood. (*vii*) **Septic Anemia** (सैप्टिक अनीमिया) तीव्र संक्रमणों द्वारा उत्पन्न रक्ताल्पता। Anemia caused by severe infections.

Anemophobia (एनीमोफोबिया) वायु अथवा हवा के झोंके का रोगोत्पादक भय। Morbid fear of wind or draught.

Anencephalic (एननसिफेलिक) मस्तिष्कहीन। Having no brain.

Anephric (एनैफ्रिक) गुर्दों से रहित। Without kidneys.

Anergy (एनर्जी) विशिष्ट एन्टीजनों के प्रति प्रतिक्रिया करने की क्षमता में कमी होना, प्रतिक्रिया-हीनता। Diminished ability to react to specific antigens.

Aneroid (एनेरॉयड) तरल से रहित कार्य करने वाला जैसे एनेरॉयड स्फीइग्मोमैनोमीटर जिसमें पारद (तरल) नहीं होता और रक्त दाब या रक्त-चाप को मापने के लिए प्रयोग में लाया जाता है। Operating without fluid as aneroid sphygmomanometer which does not contain mercury (fluid) and used to measure the BP.

Anerythropsia (एनइरिथ्रोप्सिया) लाल रंग पहचानने में असमर्थता। Inability to recognize the red color.

Anesthesia (एनीस्थिसिया) बेहोशी के साथ अथवा इसके बिना संवेदना का आंशिक अथवा पूर्ण रूप से लुप्त हो जाना जो किसी

रोग, आघात अथवा शल्य-क्रिया करने के लिए किसी संवेदनाहारी पदार्थ या औषधि का इन्जैक्शन द्वारा अथवा सुंघाकर प्रयोग करने से होता है। संज्ञाहरण। Partial or complete loss of sensation with or without loss of consciousness as a result of some disease injury or administration of an anesthetic agent usually by injection or inhalation for the performance of surgery.

Anesthesiologist (एनीस्थीसियोलॉजिस्ट) संवेदनाहरण-विज्ञान विशेषज्ञ। Specialist in anesthesiology.

Aneurysm (एन्यूरिज्म) किसी रक्त वाहिनी के जन्मजात दोष अथवा उसकी दीवारों के कमजोर हो जाने के कारण स्थानीय रूप से विस्फारित हो जाने से बनने वाली थैलीनुमा रचना जैसे महाधमनी का एन्जूरिज्म। Formation of a sac by localized dilatation of blood vessels due to congenital defect or weakness of the wall of the blood vessel, e.g. aneurysm of the aorta.

Aneurysmectomy (एन्यूरिज्मेक्टॉमी) शल्यक्रिया द्वारा किसी एन्यूरिज्म को काटकर निकाल देना। Removal of an aneurysm by surgery.

Anfractuous (एनफ्रक्चुअस) कुण्डलित, संवालित, मरोड़ या लपेट वाला। Convoluted.

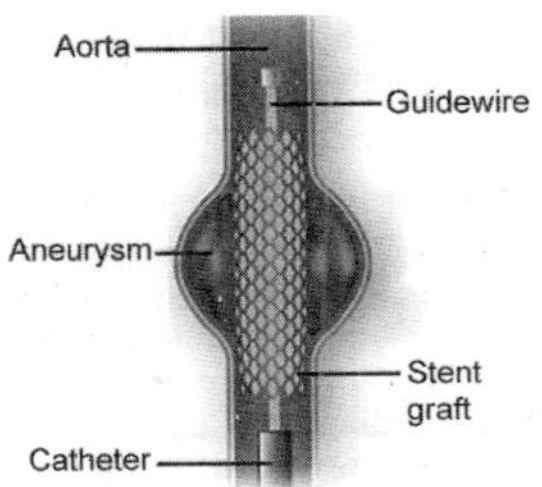

Aneurysm

Angiectasia (एन्जिएक्टेसिया) किसी रक्त अथवा लसीका वाहिनी का विस्फारण (चौड़ा हो जाना)। Dilatation of a blood or lymph vessels.

Angiectomy (एन्जिएक्टॉमी) किसी रक्त वाहिनी को काट कर निकाल देना। Excision of a blood vessel.

Angina (एन्जाइना) पेशियों में अचानक होने वाला तेज दर्द। Sudden severe pain in the muscles.

Angina Acuta (एन्जाइना एक्यूटा) सामान्य कण्ठदाह। Simple sore-throat; acute angina; angina simplex.

Angina Maligna (एन्जाइना मैलिग्ना) सांघातिक गलप्रदाह। Malignant inflammation of the throat.

Angina Pectoris (एन्जाइना पैक्टोरिस) हृद्शूल, हृदयार्ति। Severe heart-pains, cardiac neuralgia.

Anginophobia (एन्जाइनोफोबिया) हृद्शूलभीति । A morbid fear of angina pectoris.

Angioblastoma (एन्जियोब्लास्टोमा) वाहिकाप्रसू अबुर्द । A tumor of a particular blood vessel of the brain, or of the meninges of the brain or the spinal cord.

Angiocardiogram (एन्जियोकार्डियोग्राम) किसी रेडियो अपारदर्शक रंजक के अन्तःशिराभ इन्जैक्शन के पश्चात् हृदय एवं बड़ी रक्त वाहिनियों का लिया गया एक्स-रे चित्र। वाहिकाहृदयचित्र । X-ray film of the heart and the great blood vessels taken after intravenous injection of a radiopaque dye.

Angiocholitis (एन्जियोकोलाइटिस) पित्तनलीशोथ, पित्तनली का प्रदाह । Inflammation of the bile duct.

Angioedema (एन्जियोइडीमा) एन्जियोन्यूरोटिक इडीमा, वाहिकाशोफ । Angioneurotic edema.

Angiogenesis (एन्जियोजेनेसिस) भ्रूण में रक्त वाहिनियों का विकास होना, वाहिकजनन । Development of the blood vessels in the embryo.

Angiography (एन्जियोग्राफी) वाहिकाचित्रण, वाहिकालेख । A description of the vessels.

Angioid (एन्जियोऑयड) रक्त वाहिनियों जैसा । Resembling blood vessels.

Angiokeratoma (एन्जियोकेराटोमा) त्वचा का एक रोग जो मुख्यतया पैरों एवं पंजों पर होता है, जिसमें वाहिकास्फीतियां अथवा अधिमांस-वृद्धियाँ उत्पन्न हो जाती है तथा साथ ही बाह्यत्वचा मोटी हो जाती है । A skin disease occurring chiefly on the legs and feets, characterized by the formation of telangiectases or warty growth, together with epidermal thickening.

Angiolipoma (एन्जियोलिपोमा) वाहिकाबुर्द एवं वसाबुर्द से बना अबुर्द । A tumor composed of angioma and lipoma.

Angiolith (एन्जियोलिथ) शिरा का पथरी, शिराश्मरी । A venous calculus.

Angiology (एन्जियोलॉजी) वाहिका विज्ञान, रक्तनलिका विज्ञान । The doctrine of the vascular system.

Angioma (एन्जियोमा) वाहिकाबुर्द, रक्त वाहिनियों में बनने वाली रसौली । A tumor formed of the blood vessels.

Angiomalacia (एन्जियोमैलेसिया) रक्त वाहिनियों की दीवारों का मुलायम हो जाना । Softening of the walls of the blood vessels.

Angiomatosis (एन्जियोमेटोसिस) ऐसा रोग जिसमें बहुत से वाहिकाबुर्द बन जाते हैं। A disease in which multiple angiomas are formed.

Angiomyolipoma (एन्जियोमायोलाइपोमा) एक सुदम अबुर्द जिसमें वाहिकामय, वसीय तथा पेशीय ऊतक होते हैं। A benign tumor containing vascular, fatty and muscular tissues.

Angionoma (एन्जियोनोमा) किसी वाहिनी में जख्म बनना। Evisceration of a vessels.

Angiopathy (एन्जियोपैथी) किसी रक्त अथवा लसीका वाहिनी का कोई भी रोग। Any disease of a blood or lymph vessels.

Angioplasty (एन्जियोप्लास्टी) प्लास्टिक सर्जरी द्वारा रक्त वाहिनियों की मरम्मत करना। Repair of the blood vessels by plastic surgery.

Angiopoiesis (एन्जियोपॉयसिस) रक्त वाहिनियों का बनना। The formation of blood vessels.

Angiorrhexis (एन्जियोरैह्क्सिस) किसी वाहिनी का फट जाना। Rupture of a vessels.

Angiosclerosis (एन्जियोस्केलेरोसिस) रक्त वाहिनीयों की दीवारों का कठोर हो जाना।

Angiospastic (एन्जियोस्पास्टिक) वाहिका-आकर्ष से सम्बन्धित। Pertaining to giospasm.

Angiotensin (एन्जियोटैन्सिन) यह वृक्क से मुक्त एक एन्जाइम रेनिन की एन्जियोटैन्सिनोजन पर क्रिया होने से उत्पन्न होता है जो वाहिकासंकीर्णन करके रक्त-चाप को बढ़ाता है। It is produced by

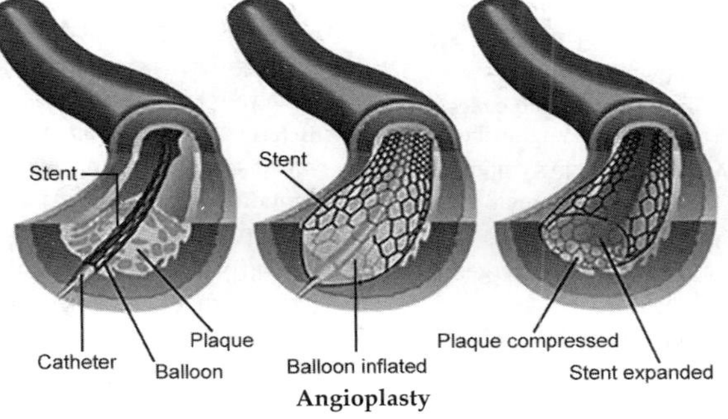

Angioplasty

the action of an enzyme renin released from the kidney, on angiotensinogen. It raises the blood pressure by causing vasoconstriction.

Angiotensinogen (एन्जियोटैन्सिनोजन) यह एन्जियोटैन्सिन का पूर्वगामी होता है। यह यकृत में बनता है, रक्त सीरम में मुक्त होता है तथा वृक्क से मुक्त हुए रेनिन की क्रिया से एन्जियोटैन्सिन में परिवर्तित हो जाता है।
It is the precursor of angiotensin. It is formed in the liver, released into the blood serum and converted to angiotensin by the action of renin released from the kidney.

Angiotonic (एन्जियोटॉनिक) धमनी-तनाव को बढ़ाने वाला। Increasing arterial tension.

Angiotripsy (एन्जियोट्राइप्सी) एन्जियोट्राइब का प्रयोग करके रक्तस्राव को रोकना।
To (arrest) stop the bleeding by using an angiotribe.

Angitis (एन्जाइटिस) वाहिकाशोथ Vascular inflammation.

Angle (एन्गल) कोण।
The degree of divergence of two lines.

Angor-Animi (एन्गर-एनीमि) मरणांतक, मृत्यु का भय। Fear of death.

Angstrom unit (एंग्सट्राम यूनिट) तरंग-दैर्ध्य की एक अन्तर्राष्ट्रीय ईकाई जो 10^{-10} मीटर या 1 नैनोमीटर के बराबर होती है। An international unit of wavelength equal to 10^{-10} meter or 1 nonometer.

Anhedonia (एन्हीडोनिया) ऐसे कार्यों में खुशी न होना जिनसे सामान्यतया खुशी होती है। Feeling no pleasure in the acts which are normally pleasurable.

Anhidrosis (एनहाइड्रोसिस) पसीने की कमी, स्वेदाल्पता। A deficiency sweating.

Anhidrotic (एनहाइड्रोटिक) पसीना रोकने वाला पदार्थ, अस्वेदकारी। An agent that checks sweating.

Anhydremia (एनहाइड्रीमिया) रक्त में प्लाज्मा की कमी। Deficiency of plasma in the blood.

Anhydrous (एनहाइड्रस) जल रहित, जलमुक्त, शुष्क। Containing no water.

Anicteric (एनइक्टैरिक) कामला या पीलिया रहित। Without jaundice.

Animal (एनीमल) जीव, प्राणी, जीवधारी, जन्तु। An organism being with life and power of motion.

Animation (एनिमेशन) चेतन, सजीवता, प्राण-संचरण।

Enlivenment, state of being alive or active.

Animation suspended (एनिमेशन सस्पैन्डेड) प्राणभूत अथवा जैव क्रियाओं का अल्पकालिक रूक जाना जिससे बेहोशी हो जाती है। Temporary cessation of the vital functions with loss of consciousness.

Anion (एनॉयन) एक ऋणात्मक आयन जो किसी विद्युत सैल से धनात्मक इलेक्ट्रोड (एनोड) की ओर आकर्षित होता है। A negatively charged ion, which is attracted to the positive electrode in an electrolytic cell.

Aniridia (एनाइराइडिया) परितारिका का जन्मजात अभाव। Irideremia congenital absence of the iris.

Anisocoria (एनीसोकोरिया) आँखों की पुतलियों का परिमाण में बराबर न होना। Inequality of the size of the pupils of the eyes.

Anisocytosis (एनीसोसाइटोसिस) लाल रक्त कोशिकाओं के आकार की असमानता, विशमकोशिकता। Abnormal equality in the size of the red blood cells.

Anisodactyly (एनीइसोडैक्टाइली) दोनों हाथों की अनुरूप अंगुलियों की असमान लम्बाई। Unequal length of the corresponding fingers of both the hands.

Anisognathous (एनीसोग्नेथस) वह व्यक्ति जिसका ऊपरी जबड़ा निचले जबड़े से चौड़ा होता है। Having the upper jaw wider than the lower jaw.

Anisometropia (एनीसोमीट्रोपीया) ऐसा रोग जिसमें दोनों आँखों की अपवर्तन-शक्ति असमान होती है, असमदृष्टिता। The condition in which the refractive power of the eyes is unequal.

Anisopiesis (एनीसोपाइसिस) शरीर के दो पार्श्वो में रक्त-चाप में असमानता। Unequality of blood pressure on the two sides of the body.

Anisosthenic (एनीसोस्थेनिक) असमान शक्ति वाला, विषम-शक्ति। Of unequal strength.

Ankle-jerk (एन्किल जर्क) एकिलस टैण्डन पर ठोकने से पिण्डली की पेशियों के सिकुड़ जाने के फलस्वरूप पंजे का फैल जाना। Contraction of the calf muscles resulting in extension of the foot, following a slow upon the achilles tondon.

Anklyosis (एन्किलोसिस) किसी जोड़ की निश्चलता तथा स्थिरता, जकड़ाहट, अस्थिसमेकन। Immobility and fixation of a joint, stiffness.

Ankyloblepharon (एन्किलोब्लेफेरोन) ऊपरी एवं

निचली पलको के किनारों का आपस में चिपक जाना, बद्धवर्तम। Adhesion of the edges of the upper and lower eyelids to each other.

Ankylocheillia (एन्किलोकीलिया) जीभ का मुख के तल से जुड़ा रहना, जिह्वा-बद्धता। Tongue-tie, congenital shortening of the frenulum of the tongue.

Ankyloproctia (एन्किलोप्रोक्सिया) मलांत्रसंकीर्णता, मलाशय का सिकुड़ जाना। Stricture of the rectum.

Annexa (एनेक्सा) किसी संरचना के सहायक भाग। Accessory part of a structure.

Annexitis (एनेक्साइटिस) गर्भाशय के सहायक अंगों का शोथ। Inflammation of the adnexa of the uterus.

Annoy (एनोय) खिझाना, चिढ़ना, उद्विग्न करना या होना। To irritate.

Annular (एन्यूलर) अंगूठी के आकार का। Ring-shaped.

Annulorrhaphy (एन्यूलोरैहफी) हर्निया के छल्ले को सीकर बन्द करना। Closure of a hernial ring by suture.

Annulus (एन्यूलस) वलय, मुद्राकार, घेरे वाला। A ring shaped object, structure, or region.

Annulus (एन्यूलस) शरीर के रीढ की हड्डी का छल्ले के आकार या अंगूठी के आकार का हो जाना। Ring-shaped or encircling structure of the vertebral body.

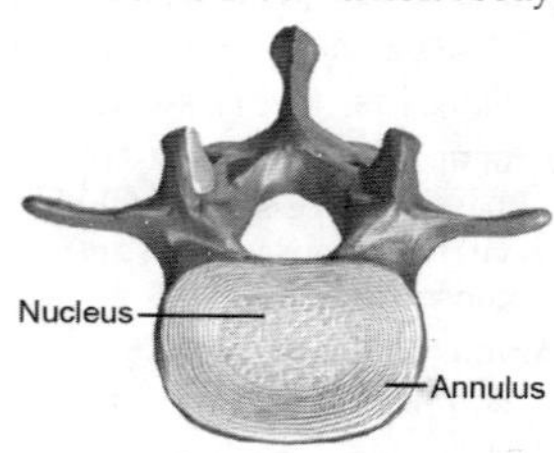

Anode (एनोड) किसी विद्युत स्रोत का धनात्मक ध्रुव जिसकी ओर ऋणात्मक आयन आकर्षित होते है। The positive pole of an electrical source to which the negative ions are attracted.

Anodontia (एनोडोन्शिया) कुछ अथवा सभी दाँतों का जन्मजात अभाव। Congenital absence of some or all of the teeth.

Anodynia (एनोडाइनिया) दर्द दूर होना। Cessation of pain.

Anomaloscope (एनोमैलोस्कोप) वर्णान्धता का पता लगाने के लिए प्रयोग में लाया जाने वाला उपकरण। An apparatus used to detect the color blindness.

Anomaly (एनोमैली) असंगति, अनियमितता। That which is anomalous.

Anomia (एनोमिया) वस्तुओं के नाम याद करने में असमर्थता।

Inability to remember the names of the objects.

Anoperineal (एनोपेरिनियल) गुदा एवं मूलाधार दोनों से सम्बन्धित। Pertaining to both the anus and the perineum.

Anorchid (एनॉर्किड़) वृषणहीन। Without testicles.

Anorchism (एनोर्चिज्म) एक या दोनों शुक्रग्रन्थियों का जन्मजात अभाव। Congenital absence of one or both testes.

Anorexia (एनोरेक्सिया) भूख न लगना। Loss of appetite.

Anorexigenic (एनोरेक्सीजेनिक) भूख खत्म करने वाला। Causing loss of appetite.

Anoscope (एनोस्कोप) गुदा एवं मलाशय के निचले भाग का परीक्षण करने वाला वीक्षक (स्पेकुलम)। A speculum for examining the anus and the lower rectum.

Anosmia (एनोस्मिया) सूंघने का ज्ञान न होना, अघ्राणता। Loss of sense of smell.

Anospinal (एनोस्पाइनल) गुदा एवं रीढ़ की हड्डी संबंधी। Relating to the anus and the spine.

Anostosis (एनोस्टोसिस) हड्डी का दोषयुक्त निर्माण। Defective formation of bone.

Anotus (एनोटस) कर्ण रहित भ्रूण। A fetus without ears.

Anovulatory (एनोव्यूलेटरी) जो किसी डिम्ब के उत्पन्न होने और उसके विसर्जित होने से सम्बद्ध नहीं होता, डिम्बाक्षरणी। Not associated with the production and discharge of an ovum.

Anoxemia (एनोक्सीमिया) रक्त में ऑक्सीजन का सामान्य स्तर से नीचे हो जाना। Reduction of oxygen in the blood below normal level.

Anoxia (एनोक्सिया) अनॉक्सिकता, ऊतकों को ऑक्सीजन की आपूर्ति न होना, इस शब्द का प्रयोग अक्सर अल्पऑक्सीजन के लिए भी किया जाता है जिसका अर्थ न्यून ऑक्सीजन आपूर्ति से होता है। Absence of oxygen supply to the tissues, the term is often used to indicate hypoxia which means reduced oxygen supply. (*i*) **Altitude Anoxia** (एल्टीयूड एनोक्सिया) ऊँचाइयों पर पहुँचने पर वायुमण्डल में ऑक्सीजन की कमी से होने वाली अनॉक्सिकता। Anoxia due to reduced oxygen in the atmosphere at the high altitudes.

(*ii*) **Anemic Anoxia** (एनीमिक एनोक्सिया) रक्त में हीमोग्लोबिन की मात्रा अथवा लाल रक्त कोशिकाओं की संख्या कम होने से उत्पन्न अनॉक्सिकता।

Anoxia due to decrease in the amount of hemoglobin or the number of red blood cells in the blood. (*iii*) **Anoxic Anoxia** (एनोक्सिक एनोक्सिया) ऑक्सीजन आपूर्ति में बांधा पड़ जाने से उत्पन्न अनॉक्सिकता जो फेफड़ों के रोगों में हो सकती है। Anoxia due to interference in the oxygen supply which may be in pulmonary disease.

Ansa (एन्सा) फंदे के आकार का। Loop-shaped.

Ansiform (एन्सीफॉर्म) पाशकार, पाशरूप। Of the form of a loop, ansate.

Antacid (एन्टेसिड) अम्लता विशेषकर आमाशय की अम्लता को उदासीन करने वाला पदार्थ अथवा औषधि। An agent neutralizing the acidity, especially in the stomach.

Antagonism (एन्टागोनिज्म) एक सी वस्तुओं का आपस में विरोध होना अथवा इनका एक दूसरे के विपरीत कार्य करना जैसा कि पेशियों, औषधियों अथवा जीवों के बीच होता है। Opposition or contrary action between similar things as between muscles, medicines or organisms.

Antagonist (एन्टोगोनिस्ट) वह पेषी जो दूसरी पेषी के कार्य की काट करती है। A muscle counteracting the action of another muscle.

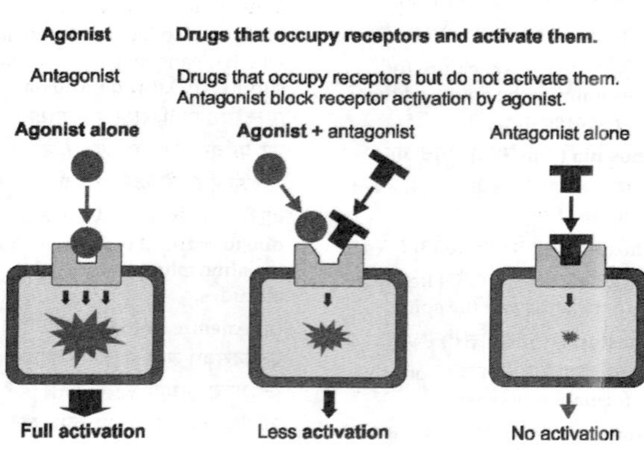

Antagonist

Antaphrodisiac (एन्टेफ्रोडिसियाक) सम्भोग की उत्तेजना को शान्त करने वाला पदार्थ, कामनाशक। An agent that diminishes sexual desire.

Antasthenic (एन्टेस्थेनिक) कमजोरी दूर करने वाला। Relieving weakness.

Ante (एन्टी) उपसर्ग जिसका अर्थ के पहले या के सामने होता है। Prefix meaning before.

Antebrachium (एन्टिब्रेयम) कोहनी से लेकर कलाई तक का हिस्सा, भुजा, बाजू। The Forearm.

Antecedent (एनटेसेडेन्ट) पूर्वगामी। Precursor.

Antecubital (एन्टिक्यूबिटल) कोहनी के सामने। In front of the elbow.

Anteflexion (एन्टिफ्लैक्सीयन) अग्रकुंचन। A bending forward.

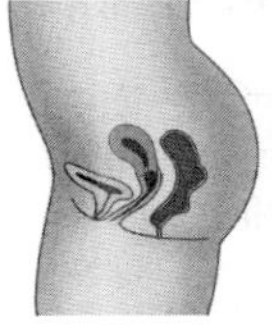

Antiflexed retroverted

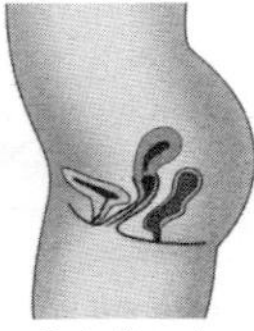

Retroflexed retroverted

Antegrade (एन्टिग्रेंड) सामान्य गति की दिशा में जैसा कि रक्त प्रवाह या क्रमाकुंचन में। In the direction of normal movement, as in blood flow or peristalsis.

Antemortem (एन्टिमॉर्टम) मृत्यु से पहले। Before death.

Antenatal (एन्टिनेटल) बच्चे के जन्म से पूर्व होने वाला। Occurring before child birth.

Antepartum (एन्टिपार्टम) प्रसव के प्रारम्भ होने से पूर्व उत्पन्न होने वाला जिसे मां के सन्दर्भ में प्रयोग किया जाता है। Occurring before the onset of labor, used with reference to the mother.

Anteprandial (एन्टिप्रडियल) प्रधान भोजन से पूर्व का। Before dinner.

Anterior (एन्टिरियर) पहले अथवा सामने स्थित, पश्च को विपरीत, अग्र। Situated before or infront of, opposite of posterior.

Anterograde (एन्टिरॉग्रेड) आगे की ओर गति करने वाला। Moving forward.

Anterolateral (एन्टिरालेट्रल) अग्रपार्ष्विक। In front and to the side.

Anteromedian (एन्टिरॉमीडियन) सामने एवं मध्यतल की ओर स्थित।
Situated in front and towards the medium plane.

Anteroposterior (एन्टीरोपोस्टीरियर) सामने से पीछे की ओर जाता हुआ।
Passing from the front to the back.

Anterosuperior (एन्टिरोसुपीरियर) सामने एवं ऊपर की ओर स्थित। Situated in front and above.

Anteversion (एन्टिवर्जन) किसी अंग का बिना मुड़े पूर्ण रूपेण आगे की ओर घूम जाना। Turning forward of a organ as a whole without bending.

Anthelmintic (एन्थैलमिन्टिक) कृमिनाशक। Destroying worms.

Anthoma (एन्थौमा) वसीय त्वम्बुद्धि, चर्बी चढ़ाना। Fatty enlargement of skin.

Anthophobia (एन्थोफोबिया) पुष्पभीति, फूलों से भय। A morbid fear of flowers.

Anthracosis (एन्थ्रेकोसिस) फुस्फुसकालिमा, फेफड़ों का काला पड़ना। Black pigmentation of lungs due to inhalation of carbon particles.

Anthrax (एन्थ्रेक्स) संक्रमित जन्तुओं जैसे भेड़, घोड़े आदि के सम्पर्क से बेसीलस एन्थ्रेक्स नामक जीवाणु द्वारा उत्पन्न एक विशिष्ट तीव्र संक्रामक रोग। A specific acute infections disease caused by bacillus anthracis due to contact with the infected animals such as sheep, horses, etc.

Anthropoid (एन्थ्रोपॉयड) मनुष्य से मिलता हुआ। Resembling man.

Anthropology (एन्थ्रोपोलॉजी) नृविज्ञान, मानवविज्ञान। The Science of man.

Anthropometry (एन्थ्रोपोमीट्री) मानव शरीर एवं इसके भागों को मापने का विज्ञान। Science of measuring the human body and its parts.

Anti (एण्टी) एक उपसर्ग जिसका अर्थ विरूद्ध या प्रतिकूल होता है। Prefix meaning against.

Ante cibum (एन्टी सीबम) नुस्खे लिखने मे इसका प्रयोग किया जाता है जो भोजन से पहले को दर्शाता है, भोजन पूर्व। It is used in prescription writing to indicate before meals.

Antiadrenergic (एन्टिएड्रीनार्जिक) एड्रीनालिन-धर्मोत्तेजक क्रिया को रोकने अथवा इसके विपरीत कार्य करने वाला। Preventing or counteracting the adrenergic action.

Antiagglutinin (एन्टिएग्लूटिनिन) किसी एग्लूटिनिन की क्रिया का विरोध करने वाली एण्टीबॉडी। An antibody opposing the action of an agglutinin.

Antiamebic (एण्टीएमीबिक) अमीबा, विशेषकर एण्टेमीबा हिस्टोलीटिका के संक्रमण को रोकने अथवा उसकी चिकित्सा करने के लिए प्रयोग में लायी जाने वाली औषधि। The medicine used to prevent or treat the infection of ameba, especially *Entamoeba histolytica.*

Antiandrogen (एन्टिएण्ड्रोजन) एण्ड्रोजन की क्रिया को कम करने अथवा रोकने वाला कोई भी पदार्थ। Any substance inhibiting or preventing the action of androgen.

Antiarthritic (एन्टिआर्थराइटिक) सन्धिशोथ में आराम पहुंचाने वाला। Relieving arthritis.

Antibechic (एन्टिबेचिक) कफशामक, कफ अथवा खांसी से मुक्ति दिलाने वाला। Relieving cough.

Antibiosis (एन्टिबायोसिस) दो जीवों की समबद्धता जिसमें से एक दूसरे के लिए हानिकारक होता है। The association of two organisms in which one is harmful to the other.

Antibiotic (एन्टिबायोटिक) किसी सूक्ष्मजीव द्वारा उत्पन्न एक रासायनिक पदार्थ जो अन्य सूक्ष्मजीवों की वृद्धि को कम करता अथवा उन्हें नष्ट करता है। प्रतिजीवी। A chemical substance produced by a microorganism which is capable of inhibiting the growth or to destroy the other microorganism.

Antibody (एन्टिबॉडी) प्रतिरक्षी, रोगप्रतिकारक, प्रतिपिण्ड, प्रतिविष। Specific substance produced in the blood as a reaction to an antigen.

Anticalculous (एण्टिकेल्कुलस) पथरियों के बनने को रोकने वाला। Suppression the formation of calculi.

Anticholinergic (एन्टिकोलीनार्जिक) आवेगों के परनुकम्पी तंत्रिकाओं से होकर गुजरने के मार्ग को अवरूद्ध करने वाला। Parasympathalytic; blocking the passage of impulses through the parasympathetic.

Anticoagulant (एन्टिकौगुलैन्ट) खून में बनने वाले थक्कों को रोकने वाला, प्रतिस्कन्दी स्कन्दनरोधी। An agent which prevents or retards clotting of blood.

Anticonvulsant (एन्टिकन्वलजैन्ट) आक्षेपों को रोकने अथवा उनमें आराम पहुँचाने वाला। Preventing or relieving convulsion.

Antidepressant (एन्टिडिप्रेसेन्ट) अवसाद को रोकने अथवा उसमें आराम पहुँचाने वाला। Preventing or relieving depression.

Antidinic (एन्टिडाइनिक) चक्कर रोकने वाली औषधि, भ्रमरोधी। A remedy used in vertigo.

Antidote (एन्टिडोट) किसी विश के प्रभाव को उदासीन करने वाला पदार्थ, प्रतिकारक। A substance which neutralizes the effect

of a poison. (*i*) **Chemical antidote** (केमिकल एन्टिडोट) ऐसा प्रतिकारक जो विष से प्रतिक्रिया करके एक हानिरहित रासायनिक यौगिक बनाता है। Antidote which reacts with the poison forming a harmless chemical compound.
(*ii*) **Mechanical antidote** (मैकेनिकल एन्टिडोट) विष के अवशोषण को रोकने वाला प्रतिकारक। Antidote which prevents absorption of the poison.

Antiemetic (एन्टिएमेटिक) जी मिचलाने एवं उल्टी को रोकने वाला। Preventing nauseas and vomiting.

Antiestrogen (एन्टिइस्ट्रोजन) ईस्ट्रोजन के कार्य में अवरोध उत्पन्न करने वाला पदार्थ। The substance which blocks the action of estrogen.

Antifebrile (एन्टिफेब्राइल) ज्वररोधी, बुखार को रोकने वाली (औषधि)। An agent that allays fever.

Antifungal (एन्टिफन्गल) कवकरोधी, फफूंदी की वृद्धि को रोकने वाला पदार्थ। Preventing fungus.

Antigen (एन्टिजन) प्रतिजन, प्रतिपिण्डों की उत्पत्ति करने वाला पदार्थ। Substance introduced in the blood to stimulate production of antibodies.

Antihelix (एन्टिहेलिक्स) प्रतिकुण्डलिका, प्रतिकर्ण शुष्कुली। Semicircular ridge of the external ear, opposite the helix.

Antihemolytic (एन्टिहीमोलाइटिक) रक्तस्राव को रोकने अथवा उसे बन्द करने वाला। Preventing or arresting hemorrhage.

Antihypnotic (एन्टिहिप्नोटिक) निद्राहर, निद्रारोधक। Preventing sleep.

Anti-icteric (एन्टि-इक्टेरिक) कामला या पीलिया को रोकने अथवा उसे कम करने वाला। Preventing or relieving jaundice.

Anti-inflammatory (एन्टि-इन्फ्लेमेटरी) शोथ को कम करने वाला कारक। An agent diminishing the inflammation.

Antiluetic (एन्टिल्यूइटिक) उपदंशरोधक, उपदंश-निवारक। Any agent which prevents or cures syphilis.

Antilytic (एन्टिलाइटिक) अपघटन को रोकने अथवा उसे कम करने वाला।
Preventing or inhibiting the lysis.

Antimetabolite (एन्टिमेटाबोलाइट) चयापचय-रोधी। Against a metabolite.

Antimony (एन्टिमनी) सीसा, अंजन। A metal commonly found associated with sulfur.

Antinarcotic (एन्टिनार्कोटिक) प्रतिस्वादक, निद्राहारी। Preventing sleep.

Antineoplastic (एन्टिन्योप्लास्टिक) अबुर्दों के विकास को कम करने अथवा उसे रोकने वाला। Inhibiting or preventing the development of tumors.

Antineuralgic (एन्टिन्यूराल्जिक) नाड़ीशूल का शमन करने वाला। Relieving neuralgia.

Antioxidant (एन्टिऑक्सीडैन्ट) ऑक्सीकरण को रोकने अथवा उसे कम करने वाला कारक। An agent preventing or inhibiting oxidation.

Antipathy (एन्टिपैथी) अरूचि, घृणा। Aversion; Dislike.

Antiperistalsis (एन्टिपैरिस्टेल्सिस) पुरवसरणरोधी, कृमिकुंचनरोधी। Abnormal movement of bowels towards stomach.

Antiplastic (एन्टिप्लास्टिक) व्रण विरोहण (जख्म भरना) को रोकने अथवा कम करने वाला। Preventing or inhibiting wound healing.

Antiprostate (एन्टिप्रोस्टेट) कॅपर ग्रन्थि। Cowper's gland.

Antipruritic (एन्टिप्रुराइटिक) खुजली को रोकने वाला। Prevent itching.

Antipyretic (एन्टिपाइरेटिक) बुखार को कम करने वाला। Reducing fever.

Antirachitic (एन्टिरैकिटिक) बालास्थिविकार रोग को ठीक करने वाला। Curing rickets.

Antiscabietic (एन्टिस्केबीटिक) पामा की रोकथाम अथवा उसका शमन करने के लिए लाभकारी। Effective in the prevention or relief of scabies.

Antiseptic (एन्टिसेप्टिक) पूतिरोधक, रोगाणुरोधक। Agent counteracting putrefaction.

Antisialic (एन्टिसियालिक) थूक या लार के स्राव को रोकने वाला। Checking the secretion of saliva.

Antisyphilitic (एन्टिसिफिलिटिक) सिफिलिस रोग से मुक्ति दिलाने अथवा उसमें आराम पहुँचाने वाला कारक। An agent curing or relieving syphilis.

Antithyroid (एन्टिथाइरॉयड) अवटु ग्रन्थि की क्रिया मंद करने वाला (तत्व), प्रत्यवतु। Any agent used to decrease the activity of thyroid gland.

Antitoxin (एन्टिटॉक्सिन) किसी जीवविष की अनुक्रिया में शरीर में उत्पन्न एक एण्टीबॉडी जो उस जीवविष के प्रभाव को उदासीन कर देती है। An antibody produced in the body in response to a toxin, which neutralize the effect of the toxin.

Antitussive (एन्टिटुसिव) खांसी को रोकने अथवा उसमें आराम पहुँचाने वाला। Preventing or relieving cough.

Antivenin (एन्टिवेनिन) एक सीरम जिसमें विशेष रूप से किसी जन्तु अथवा कृमि के विष के लिए प्रतिजीवविष होता है जो रोगक्षमीकृत किए गए जन्तुओं के सीरम से तैयार किया जाता है। A serum that contains anti-toxin specific for an animal or insect venom, which is prepared from the serum of the immunized animals.

Antivitamin (एन्टिविटामिन) किसी विटामिन के कार्य के विरूद्ध कार्य करने वाला। Opposing the action of a vitamin.

Antixerotic (एन्टिजीरोटिक) त्वचा की शुष्कता को रोकने वाला। Preventing dryness of the skin.

Antrectomy (एन्ट्रेक्टॉमी) किसी कोटर को काट कर निकाल देना। Excision of an antrum.

Antritis (एन्ट्राइटिस) किसी कोटर का शोथ। Inflammation of an antrum.

Antropyloric (एन्ट्रोपाइलोरिक) जठर निर्गमीय कोटर से सम्बन्धित अथवा उसे प्रभावित करने वाला। Pertaining to or affecting the pyloric antrum.

Antrostomy (एन्ट्रोस्टॉमी) निकास के लिए किसी कोटर में छिद्र बनाना। To make an opening in an antrum for drainage.

Antrotomy (एन्ट्रोटॉमी) किसी कोटर में चीरा लगाना, कोटर छेदन। To take an incision in an antrum.

Antrum (एन्ट्रम) गुहा, कोष्ठ, खास तौर पर अस्थिकोष्ठर। A cavity, especially in the bone.

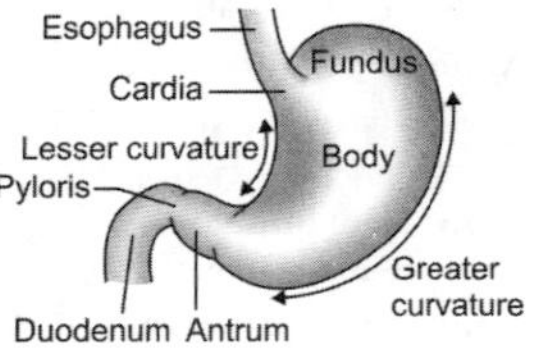

Anuresis (एन्यूरेसिस) मूत्र त्याग न होना। Absence of urination.

Anus (एनस) मलद्वार, गुदा, गुद। External opening of the rectum.

Anxiety (एन्जाइटी) आशंका या भय प्रतीत होना, मानसिक बेचैनी, घबराहट। A feeling of apprehension, uneasiness of mind.

Anxiety neurosis (एन्जाइटी न्यूरोसिस) एक मानसिक विकार जिसमें अत्यधिक चिन्ता होती है। जिसके साथ शारीरिक लक्षण जैसे दिल की धड़कन का महसूस होना, हृदय शूल, अपच, सिर में दर्द, ठण्डा पीसना

आना तथा साथ ही हाथों पैरों में कम्पन होना, आदि हो जाते हैं। चिन्ताधि। A mental disorder characterized by excessive anxiety associated with physical symptoms such as palpitation, cardiac pain, dyspepsia, headache, cold sweating with tremulousness of the extremities.

Anxiolytic (एन्जियोलाइटिक) चिन्ता को दूर करने अथवा कम करने वाला जिसे औषधिय अथवा मनोवैज्ञानिक चिकित्सा द्वारा किया जा सकता है। Counteracting or diminishing anxiety which may be done by the medicinal or psychological treatment.

Aorta (एओरटा) शरीर की धमनीय प्रणाली का मुख्य धड़ जो बांये निलय से निकलता है, महाधमनी। The main trunk of the arterial system of the body arising from the left ventricle.

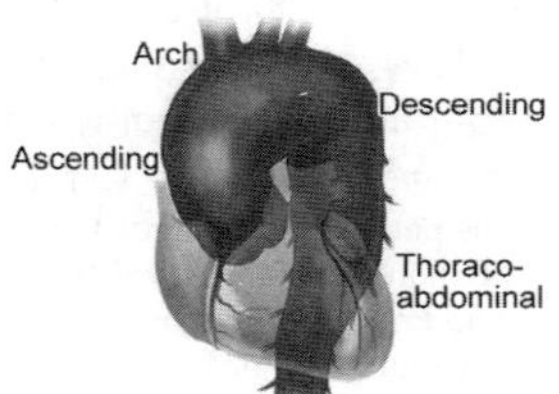

Aortalgia (एओर्टेल्जिया) महाधमनी क्षेत्र में दर्द होना। Pain in the region of the aorta.

Aortasclerosis (एओरटोस्क्लेरोसिस) महाधमनी का कठोर हो जाना। Sclerosis of the aorta.

Aortitis (एओरटाइटिस) महाधमनीशोथ। Inflammation of the aorta.

Aortoclasia (एओरटे क्लासिया) महाधमनी का फट जाना। Rupture of the aorta.

Aortography (एओरटोग्राफी) महाधमनी चित्रण। A description of the aorta.

Aortolith (एओर्टोलिथ) महाधमनी की दीवार में पथरियों का जमा हो जाना। Depositicn of the calculi in the wall of the aorta.

Aortopathy (एओर्टपैथी) महाधमनी का कोई भी रोग। Any disease of the aorta.

Aortotomy (एओटोटॉमी) महाधमनी में चीरा लगाना। To make an incision in the aorta.

Apathetic (एपैथेटिक) उदासीन, किसी बात में कोई रूचि न लेने वाला। Indifferent, having no interest.

Apepsia (एपेप्सिया) पाचन न होना, बदहजमी Cessation of digestion.

Aperient (एपीरियन्ट) एक मृदु विरेचक। A mild laxative.

Aperitive (एपेरिटिव) भूख बढ़ाने वाला। Increasing the appetite.

Apert's Syndrome (एपर्टस सिन्ड्रोम) एक जन्मजात रोग जिसमें सिर चोंच के समान होता है तथा हाथ-पैरों की अंगुलियों के बीच जाल होता है। A congenital condition in which the head is peaked and the fingers and toes are webbed.

Aperture (एपरचर) मुख या छिद्र। An opening or orifice.

Apex (एपैक्स) किसी शंक्वाकार संरचना का नुकीला सिरा। The pointed end of a conical structure.

Apex beat (एपैक्स बीट) हृदशिखरस्पन्द। The point of maximum impulse of the heart against the chest wall.

Aphakia (एफेकिया) आँख में लैंस का अभाव। Absence of the lens of the eyes.

Aphalangia (एफेलेन्जिया) हाथ या पैरों की अंगुलियों का अभाव। Absence of fingers or toes.

Aphasia (एफेजिया) मस्तिष्क-केन्द्र के आघात अथवा उनके किसी रोग के कारण बोलकर, लिखकर या संकेतों द्वारा विचारों को अभिव्यक्त करने में अक्षमता, वाचाघात। Inability to express thoughts by speech writing and signs, due to injury or disease of the brain centers.

(*i*) **Amnesic Aphasia** (एम्नेसिक एफेजिया) शब्दों के लिए स्मृति लोप हो जाना। Loss of memory for words.

(*ii*) **Anomic Aphasia** (ऐनोमिक एफेजिया) वस्तुओं के नाम लेने (एवं उनके गुणों के विषय में बताने में असमर्थता। Inability to name the objects and their qualities. (*iii*) **Global Aphasia** (ग्लोबल एफेजिया) पूर्ण वाचाघात जिसमें सम्पर्क स्थापित करने के सभी साधन बेकार हो जाते है, रोगी बोल नहीं सकता, समझ नहीं सकता, पढ़ और लिख नहीं सकता। Total aphasia involving the failure of all means of communication, the patient cannot speak, understand, read and write.

(*iv*) **Motor Aphasia** (मोटर एफेजिया) ऐसा वाचाघात जिसमें रोगी लिखे हुए एवं बोले गये शब्दों को समझता है और जानता है कि वह क्या कहना चाहता है परन्तु वह शब्दों का उच्चारण नहीं कर सकता। Aphasia in which the patient understands the written and spoken words and knows what he wants to say, but he cannot utter the words. (*v*) **Nominal Aphasia** (नौमिनल एफेजिया) वस्तुओं का नाम लेने में असमर्थता। Inability to name the objects.

Aphemia (एफीमिया) केन्द्रीय तन्त्रिका-तंत्र में क्षति हो जाने से वाक्शक्ति का नष्ट हो जाना, वाक्प्रेरणाघात। Loss of power to speak due to a lesion in the central nervous system.

Aphephobia (एफीफोबिया) छू जाने का विकृत भय। Morbid fear of being touched.

Apheresis (एफेरेसिस) एक कार्य-विधि जिसमें रक्त के घटकों जैसे श्वेत रक्त कोशिकाओं लाल रक्त कोशिकाओं तथा प्लेटलेट्स आदि को रक्त से अलग किया जाता है। A procedure in which the components of blood, as white blood cells, RBC and platelets, etc. are separated from the blood.

Aphonia (एफोनिया) वाणीलोप, स्वरहानि, गला बैठना, आवाज बिल्कुल बन्द हो जाना। Inability to use the voice except in a whisper.

Aphrasia (एफ्रेजिया) बोलने अथवा बोले हुए शब्दों को समझने में असमर्थता। Inability to speak or understand the spoken words.

Aphthe (एफ्थी) मुखव्रण-मुखक्षत, छाले। Roundish, whitish vesicles found in the sore mouth; thrush.

Aphthous (एफ्थस) एफ्थी से सम्बन्धित अथवा उनसे युक्त। Pertaining to or characterized by aphthae.

Apicectomy (एपिसेक्टॉमी) टैम्पोरल हड्डी के अश्म अथवा पिड्स भाग के शिखाग्र को काट कर निकाल देना। Excision of the apex or the petrous portion of the temporal bone.

Apicitis (एपिसाइटिस) किसी शिखाग्र जैसे किसी फेफड़े के अथवा दन्तमूल के शिखाग्र का शोध। Inflammation of an apex as of a lung or roof of a tooth.

Aplasia (एप्लेसिया) किसी अंग अथवा ऊतक के सामान्य विकास में कमी, विकासरोध, अविकसन। Lack of normal development of an organ or tissue.

Aplastic (एप्लास्टिक) अविकसन सम्बन्धित, अविकासी। Pertaining to aplasia.

Apnea (एप्निया) कुछ समय के लिए सांस रूक जाना, अश्वसन। Cessation of respiration for sometime.

Apneumatic (एन्यूमेटिक) वायु से मुक्त जैसे किसी पिचके हुए फेफड़े में होता है। Free of air, as in a collapsed lung.

Apochromatic (एपोक्रोमेटिक) एक ऐसा लैन्स जो गोलाकार एवं वर्णक दोनों विपथनों को सही करता है। A lens that corrects both spherical and chromatic aberrations.

Apocrine (एपोक्राइन) यह एक प्रकार की श्वेदग्रन्थि होती है जो बगल, जघन-क्षेत्र, स्तन ग्रन्थि एवं बृहत भगोष्ठ में पाई जाती है तथा सीधे त्वचा के तल पर खुलने के बजाय जैसा कि एक्रीन स्वेद ग्रन्थियां करती है, रोमकूप में खुलती है। It is a type of sweat gland located in the axilla, pubic region, mammary gland and labia majora, which opens into the hair follicle instead of opening directly onto the surface of the skin like eccrine sweat gland.

Apodal (एपोडल) पंजो से रहित। Having no feet.

Apogee (एपोजी) किसी रोग की सबसे अधिक गम्भीर अवस्था। The state of greatest severity of a disease.

Aponeurosis (एपोन्यूरोसिस) तन्तु-कला की एक चादर जो किसी पेशी को उसके द्वारा गति करने वाले अंगों से जोड़ती है, कंडराकला। A sheet of fibrous membrane connecting a muscle with the parts it moves.

Aponeurotome (एपोन्यूरोटोम) कंडराकला को काटने वाला यंत्र। An instrument for cutting an aponeurosis.

Apophysis (एपोफाइसिस) एक अतिवृद्धि विशेषक किसी हड्डी की, अस्थिविवर्धन। An outgrowth especially of bone.

Apophysitis (एपोफाइसाइटिस) किसी विवर्ध का शोथ। Inflammation of an apophysis.

Apoplexy (एपोप्लेक्सी) किसी अंग में प्रचुर मात्रा में रक्त परिस्रवण होना जैसे उदरीय, फुस्फुसीय अथवा गर्भाशयी रक्ताघात हो जाना, रक्ताघात। Copious extravasation of blood into an organ, as abdominal, pulmonary or uterine apoplexy.

Apostaxis (एपोस्टैक्सिस) मामूली रक्तस्राव होना। Slight hemorrhage.

Apparatus (एपारेटस) यंत्र उपकरण। An instrument for performing a common purpose in medical profession.

Appendectomy (एपेन्डेक्टॉमी) उण्डुकपुच्छ को काटकर निकाल देना। Excision of the vermiform.

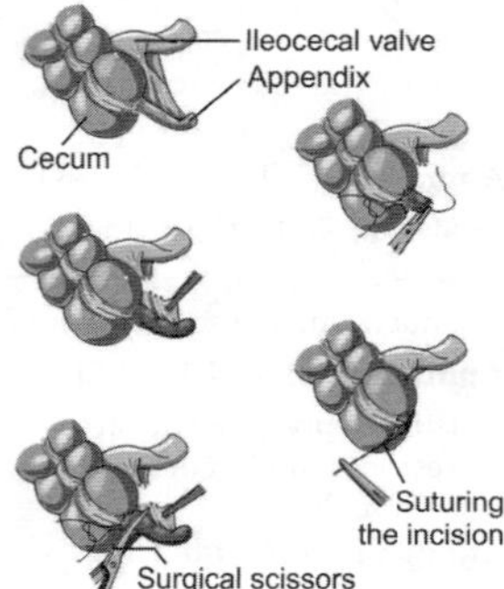

Appendicitis (एपेण्डिसाइटिस) उण्डुकपुच्छ का शोथ। Inflammation of the vermiform appendix.

Appendicolysis (एपेण्डिकोलाइसिस) वर्मीफार्म एपेण्डिक्स को शल्यक्रिया द्वारा आसंजनो (चिपकावों) से पृथक करना। To separate the vermiform appendix from the adhesion by surgery.

Appendicostomy (एपेण्डिकोस्टॉमी) बडी आँत को सींचने अथवा उसमें से पानी बहाने के लिए शल्यक्रिया द्वारा वर्मीफार्म एपेण्डिक्स में एक छेद बनाना। To make an opening into the vermiform appendix by surgery to irrigate or drain the large intestine.

Appendix (एपेण्डिक्स) मुख्य संरचना से जुड़ा एक अतिरिक्त अथवा सहायक अंग जैसे वर्मीफार्म एपेण्डिक्स जो सीकम के अन्ध सिरे से जुड़ा कीड़े के समान लगभग 9 से.मी. लम्बा एक प्रक्षेपण (उभार) होता है तथा असिरूप प्रवर्ध आदि। पुच्छ। A supplementary or accessory part attached to a main structure, e.g. vermiform appendix, which is a worm like projection about 9 cms long from the blind end of the cecum; and xiphoid process, etc.

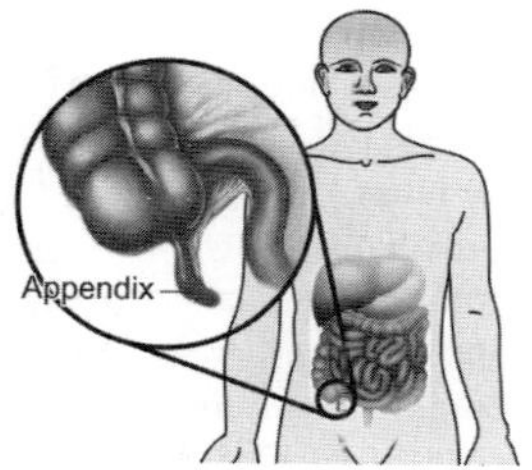

Appestat (एपीस्टेट) मस्तिष्क का वह क्षेत्र जो भूख को अनियन्त्रित करने से सम्बन्धित होता है। The area of the brain concerned in controlling the appetite.

Appetite (एपीटाइट) क्षुधा, भूख। Desire for food.

Appetizer (एपीटाइज़र) भूख बढ़ाने वाला। Promoting the appetite.

Appliance (एप्लायन्स) किसी कार्य विशेष को आसान बनाने के लिए प्रयोग में लाया जाने वाला उपकरण जैसे दन्त-चिकित्सा में कृत्रिम दन्तावली। A device used to facilitate a particular function, such as artificial denture in dentistry.

Applicator (एप्लीकेटर) किसी भाग में दवाई लगाने के लिये प्रयुक्त किया जाने वाला यंत्र, साधित्र। An instrument for supplying medicines to a part.

Apposition (एपोजिशन) सन्निधान, पार्श्वस्थापन। The act of fitting together.

Apprehensive (एप्रीहैन्सिव) अधीर, आतंकित, भविष्य के प्रति चिन्तातुर। Anxious or fearful for future.

Approach (एप्रोच) शल्य-क्रिया सम्बन्धी कार्यविधियां जिनसे कोई अंग अथवा भाग अनावृत होता है। Surgical procedures by which an organ a part is exposed.

Apraxia (एप्रैक्सिया) संवेदी अथवा प्रेरक किसी प्रकार की कोई बाधा न होने पर उद्देश्यपूर्ण गतियाँ करने में अक्षमता, चेष्टा अक्षमता। Inability to perform purposeful movements in the absence of sensory or motor impairment.

Apron (एप्रन) एक प्रकार का कोट जो शरीर रचना विज्ञान में व्यवच्छेदन करते समय, शल्य-क्रिया के समय, कुछ परिचर्या के कार्यों में तथा प्लास्टर आदि करते समय कपड़ों के बचाव के लिए पहना जाता है। A type of coat which is put on during anatomy dissection, surgery, certain nursing procedure, while plastering, etc. for protecting the clothes.

Aptitude (एप्टीट्यूड) सीखने या शारीरिक अथवा मानसिक कार्य करने में स्वाभाविक योग्यता अथवा निपुणता। Inherent ability or skill in learning or performing physical or mental works.

Aptyalism (एटायलिज्म) मुख शुष्कता, थूक की कमी अथवा इसका पूर्ण अभाव। Xerostomia, deficiency or absence of saliva.

Apus (एपस) पाँवों से रहित। The person having no feet.

Apyogenous (एपायोजीनस) जो पस या मवाद के कारण न हो। Not due to pus.

Aqua (एक्वा) जल जैसे आस्तुत जल, विसंक्रमित जल, औषधियुक्त जल। Water e.g. distal water, sterilized water, medicated water.

Aquapuncture (एक्वापंक्चर) जल का अवत्वक् इन्जैक्शन। Subcutaneous injection of water.

Aqueduct (एक्वीडक्ट) नलिका। Conal or channel.

Aqueous (एक्युअस) जलीय, जल द्वारा तैयार किया गया। Watery, prepared by water.

Aqueous humor (एक्युअस ह्यूमर) नेत्र के अग्र एवं पष्च कोष्ठों में भरा रहने वाला पारदर्षक तरल, नेत्रोद, चक्षु जल। Transparent liquid contained in the anterior and posterior chambers of the eye.

Arachnoid (एरेक्नॉयड) मस्तिष्कावरक झिल्ली, जो

मकड़ी के जाल जैसी होती है। Resembling a web.

Arc (आर्क) एक वक्र रेखा तथा किसी वृत्त का कोई भाग। A curved line or the portion of a circle.

Arch (आर्च) वृत्तखण्ड अथवा धनुष के आकार की संरचना, मेहराब, चाप, तोरणिका। A curved or bow-like structure.

(*i*) **Alveolar arch** (एल्वियोलर आर्च) प्रत्येक जबड़े में दन्तउल्खल प्रवर्ध एवं दॉंतों द्वारा बना चाप। The arch formed by the alveolar process and the teeth in each jaw. (*ii*) **Palmar arch** (पामर आर्च) हथेली में बना चाप। Arch formed in the palm.

(*iii*) **Plantar arch** (प्लान्ट आर्च) पैर के तलुपे में बना चाप। Arch formed in the flam of the foot. (*iv*) **Mandibular arch** (मैन्डिबुलर आर्च) अधोहनुचाप। The first branchial arch, developing into the lower jaw. (*v*) **Zygomatic arch** (जाइगोमैटिक आर्च) गण्ड चाप। That formed by the malar and temporal bones.

Archaff's nodes (अशोफ'स नोड्स) अशोफ पर्व, गठिया रोग में हृदय-पेशी में पाई जाने वाली पर्विकाऐं। Nodes in the myocardium in rheumatism.

Archipallium (आर्काईपैलियम) आद्य-प्रमस्तिष्क प्रावारक। The rhinencephalon.

Architis (आर्काइटिस) मलाशयशोथ, मलांत्रशोथ। Inflammation of the rectum.

Arctation (आर्कुटेशन) किसी छिद्र तथा नली का सिकुड़ना। Narrowing of any opening or canal.

Arcuate (आर्क्रुएट) चापाकार, धनुषाकार, टेढ़ा। Bent like anarch; arciform.

Arcus (आर्कुस) चाप, मेहराब। Arch.

Ardor (आर्डर) प्रचण्ड, ताप, जलन। Voilent heat, burning.

Area (एरिया) क्षेत्र, क्षेत्रफल, सीमित स्थल। Any space with boundaries.

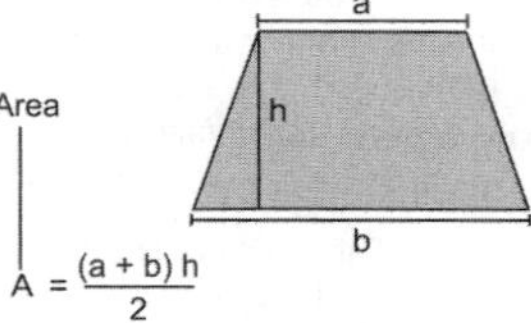

Areflexia (एरिफ्लैक्सिया) प्रतिवर्त क्रियाओं का अभाव। Absence of the reflex actions.

Areola (एरियोला) वृन्त, परिवेष, मण्डल, चक्कर। The pigmented area around the nipple of the breast.

Areometer (एरियोमिटर) द्रवघन्त्वमापी। An instrument

for measuring the specific gravity of fluids.

Argentation (आरजेन्टेशन) किसी रजत लवण के साथ संसेचन। Impregnation with a silver salt.

Argyll Rebertson Rupil (आर्जिल रोबर्टसन प्यूपिल) चक्षुपटलास्थिरता, आँखों की पुतलियों की अस्थिरता, जो मस्तिष्क रोगों में पाई जाती है। Loss of the rupil reflex to light, found in the brain disease.

Argyria (आर्जइरिया) लम्बे समय तक रजत लवणों का प्रयोग करते रहने से उत्पन्न रोग जिसमें त्वचा एवं श्लेष्मिक कलाओं का रंग नीला हो जाता है। A condition caused by prolonged administration of silver salts in which the skin and the mucous membranes become blue.

Argyrophil (आर्जीरोफिल) रजत लवणों से संयुक्त होने की क्षमता रखने वाली कोशिका। The cell capable to bind with the silver salts.

Armamentarium (आर्मामेन्टेरियम) चिकित्सा साधन उपचारक साधन। A doctors outfit of medicines or instruments. Armarium, therapeutic armamentarium.

Aroma (एरोमा) सुगन्ध, वास। Agreeable odor.

Aromatic (एरोमेटिक) सुगन्ध वाला। Having agreeable odor.

Arousal (एराउजल) कार्य करने के लिए तैयार रहने की अवस्था, लैंगिक उत्तेजना। The state of being prepared to act, sexual excitement.

Arrest (एरेस्ट) रूक जाना जैसे किसी क्रिया अथवा रोग प्रक्रिया का रूक जाना। Stoppage, as of a function or a disease process. (*i*) **Cardiac Arrest** (कार्डियक एरेस्ट) अचानक हृदय की धड़कन का रूक जाना। Sudden cessation of the heart beat. (*ii*) **Epiphyseal arrest** (एपीफिजियल एरेस्ट) अधिवर्ध रोध। Early and premature fusion between epiphysis and diaphysis.

Arrhemoblastoma (एरीह्मोब्लास्टोमा) डिम्ब ग्रन्थि का अबुर्द। A tumor of the ovary.

Arseniasis (आर्सेनिएसिस) जीर्ण आर्सेनिक विषाक्तता। Chronic arsenic poisoning.

Arsenicophagy (आर्सेनिकोफेजी) आर्सेनिक आदतन खाना। Habitual eating of arsenic.

Arteralgia (आर्टिरेल्जिया) धमनीशूलता। Pain in the artery.

Arterial (आर्टीरियल) धमनी सम्बन्धी। Pertaining to an artery.

Arterial varix (आर्टीरियल वैरिक्स) एक बड़ी एवं ऐंठी हुई धमनी।

An enlargement and twisted artery.

Arteriectasis (आर्टीरिएक्टेसिस) धमनी-विस्फारण। Dialation of an artery.

Arterioatony (आर्टीरियोएटोनी) किसी धमनी की दीवारों की तान कम हो जाना। Lack of tone in the walls of an artery.

Arteriogram (आर्टीरियोग्राम) किसी रेडियो अपारदर्शक पदार्थ का इन्जैक्शन लगाकर किसी धमनी का लिया गया एक्स-रे चित्रण। X-ray film of an artery after injection of a radiopaque substance.

Arteriography (आर्टिरियोग्राफी) धमनी चित्रण। A description of the arteries.

Arteriole (आर्टीरियोल) एक सूक्ष्म धमनी जो एक कोशिका के रूप में अग्रसर हो जाती है। A minute artery which leads to a capillary.

Arteriolith (आर्टिरियोलिथ) किसी धमनी में स्थित अश्मरी। A calculus in an artery.

Arteriolitis (आर्टिरियोलाइटिस) धमनिकाओं की सूजन। Inflammation of the arterioles.

Arteriolosclerotic (आर्टीरियोलोस्क्लेरोटिक) धमनीकाकठिन्य से सम्बन्धित या धमनिका-काठिन्य के लक्षणों से युक्त। Pertaining to or characterized by arteriolosclerosis.

Arteriomalacia (आर्टीरियोमैलेशिया) धमनियों का असामान्य रूप से ढीला या मुलायम हो जाना। Abnormal softening of the arteries.

Arterionecrosis (आर्टीरियोनेक्रोसिस) धमनियों का परिगलन। Necrosis of arteries.

Arterioplasty (आर्टीरियोप्लास्टी) प्लास्टिक सर्जरी द्वारा किसी धमनी की मरम्मत करना। Repair of an artery by plastic surgery.

Arteriosclerosis (आर्टिरियोस्क्लेरोसिस) धमनीकाठिन्य, धमनी-प्राचीर की कठोरता। Thickening of the coats of the arteries promoting blood pressure.

Arteriospasm (आर्टीरियोस्पाज्म) किसी धमनी में ऐंठन आ जाना। Spasm of an artery.

Arteritis (आर्टीराइटिस) किसी धमनी की सूजन। Inflammation of an artery.

Artery (आर्टरी) रक्त वाहिनियों में से एक जो हृदय से आक्सीजनित रक्त को लेकर शरीर के सभी भागों में पहुँचाती है, धमनी। One of the blood vessels carrying oxygenated blood from the heart to all the parts of the body.

Arthralgia (आरथ्रेल्जिया) किसी जोड़ में दर्द होना। Pain in a joint.

Arthrempyesis (आर्थ्रेमपाइसिस) किसी सन्धि में पूयवा। Suppuration in a joint.

Arthresthesia (आर्थ्रेस्थीसिया) सन्धि गतियों का बोध होना। The perception of joint movements.

Arthritis (आर्थराइटिस) सन्धिशोथ। Inflammation of a joint.

Arthrocace (आर्थ्रोकेस) जोड़ो की हड्डी गलना, सन्धि-अस्थिक्षय। Caries of joints.

Arthrocentesis (आर्थ्रोसेन्टेसिस) किसी सन्धि अवकाश में संचित तरल का चूषण करने के लिए सुई के द्वारा उसमें वेधन करना। Puncture of a joint space by a needle to aspirate the fluid accumulated therein.

Arthrochondritis (आर्थोकॉण्डराइटिस) किसी जोड़ की उपास्थि का शोथ। Inflammation of the cartilage of a joint.

Arthrodesis (आर्थ्रोडेसिस) शल्यक्रिया सम्बन्धी कार्य से किसी जोड़ को अचल बनाना। कृत्रिम सन्धिग्रह। To immobilize a joint by surgical procedure, artificial ankylosis.

Arthrodysplasia (आर्थ्रोडिसप्लेसिया) बहुत से जोड़ों की आनुवंशिक विकृति। Hereditary deformity of various joints.

Arthrogram (आथ्रोग्राम) सन्धिलेख, सन्धिचित्र। An X-ray film demonstrating a joint.

Arthrogryposis (आथ्रोग्राइपोसिस) संकुचित अवस्था में किसी जोड़ का स्थिर हो जाना जो आसंजनो द्वारा हो सकता है। Fixation of a joint in contracted position which may be due to adhesions.

Arthrolysis (आथ्रोलाइसिस) किसी सन्धिग्रहित जोड़ मे शल्य-क्रिया द्वारा आंसजनों को ढीला करने की क्रिया। The process of loosening the adhesions in an ankylosed joint by surgery.

Arthropathy (आर्थ्रोपैथी) कोई भी सन्धि रोग। Any disease of a joint.

Arthroplasty (आर्थ्रोप्लास्टी) किसी जोड़ की प्लास्टिक सर्जरी द्वारा मरम्मत करना। Repair of a joint by plastic surgery.

Arthroscope (आर्थ्रोस्कोप) किसी जोड़ के भीतर का परीक्षण करने वाला एण्डोस्कोप। An endoscope for examination of the interior of a joint.

Arthroscopy (आर्थ्रोस्कोपी) एण्डोस्कोप के द्वारा किसी जोड़ के भीतर का परीक्षण करना।

Examination of the interior of a joint with an endoscope.

Arthrosis (आर्थ्रोसिस) कोई जोड़, किसी जोड़ का कोई रोग। A joint, a disease of a joint.

Arthrotome (आर्थ्रोटोम) किसी जोड़ में चीरे लगाने वाला चाकू। To knife for making incisions into a joint.

Articulate (आर्टिकुलेट) आपस में जोड़ देना जैसे किसी जोड़ को। To joints together as a joint.

Articulation (आर्टिकुलेशन) कंकाल की दो या अधिक हड्डियों के मिलने का स्थान। The place of junction of two or more bones of the skeleton.

Articulo Mortis (आर्टिकुलो मोर्टिस) मृत्यु के क्षण। At the moment of death.

Artificial (आर्टिफिसियल) कृत्रिम, नकली। Not natural, made or imitated by art.

Articulus (आर्टिकुलस) उंगली की गांठ या कोई जोड़। A knuckle or a joint.

Arytenoiditis (आरीटीनॉयडाइटिस) आरीटीनॉयड उपास्थि अथवा पेशी का शोध। Inflammation of arytenoid cartilage or muscle.

Asafoetida (एसएफेटिडा) हींग। A fetid gum resin with garlic and like odor, asafoetida.

Ascariasis (एस्केरिएसिस) एस्केरिस लम्बी कॉयडस नामक गोलकृमियों के संक्रमण के द्वारा उत्पन्न रोग। The condition occurring from the infection of the roundworms, Ascaris lumbricoides.

Ascaris (एस्केरिस) गोलकृमि। Roundworm.

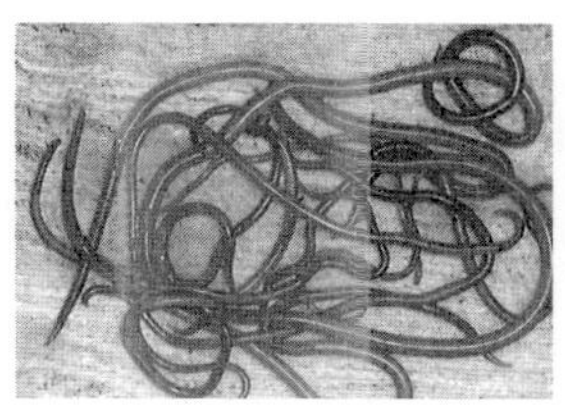

Aschner's Phenomenon, Reflex Sign (एस्कनर्स फिनोमैनन, रिफ्लैक्स साइन) नेत्रगोलक या केरोटिड साइनस पर दबाव डालने से नाड़ी का धीमा हो जाना। Oculocardiac reflex. Slowing of the pulse following pressure applied to the eyeball or the carotid sinus.

Ascites (एसाइटिस) उदरीय गुहा में सीरमी तरल का संचित होना, जलोदर। The accumulation of serous fluid in the abdominal cavity.

Ascitic (एसाइटिक) जलोदर सम्बन्धी। Pertaining to ascites.

Asemia (एसीमिया) शब्दज्ञान-अक्षमता, चिन्ह ज्ञान-अक्षमता।

Inability to comprehend words or signs; asymbolia.

Aseptic (एसेप्टिक) अपूतित। Pertaining to masked by asepsis.

Ash (एश) भस्म, राख। Residue of combustion.

Asialia (एसियालिया) थूक का कम बनना, लार हीनता। Deficient secretion of saliva.

Asitia (एसिटिया) भोजन से घृणा होना। Aversion to food.

Asoma (एसोमा) अधूरे बने धड़ एवं सिर से युक्त विकृत भ्रूण। Deformed fetus with imperfectly formed trunk and head.

Asonia (एसोनिया) संगीत ध्वनियों को सुनने के लिए बधिरता बहरापन। Deafness to the musical sounds.

Aspergillosis (एस्पर्जिलोसिस) एस्पर्जिलस नामक कवक के संक्रमण द्वारा उत्पन्न रोग जिसमें त्वचा, कान, नेत्रगुहा तथा मस्तिष्कावरणों में शोधज कणिका गुल्मीय विक्षतियां उत्पन्न हो जाती हैं।

A disease caused by the infection of the fungus aspergillus characterized by inflammatory granulomatous lesion in the skin, ear, orbit and meninges.

Aspergillus (एस्पर्जिलस) एक प्रकार का कवक। A kind of fungus.

Aspermatism (एस्पर्मेटिज्म) वीर्य का न बनना अथवा उसका स्खलित न होना। Lack of formation or non-ejaculation of semen.

Aspermia (एस्पर्मिया) अशुक्राणुता, बीजाभाव, वीर्यहीनता, अशुक्रता। Lack of seminal discharge; aspermatism.

Aspersion (एस्पर्जन) छिड़काव। The act of besprinkling.

Asphyxia (एस्फाइक्सिया) अपर्याप्त ऑक्सीजन के ग्रहण करने से उत्पन्न दशा, श्वासरोध, अनॉक्सी श्वसन। The condition caused by insufficient intake of oxygen. Suffocation.

Asphyxiant (एस्फाइक्सिएन्ट) श्वसावरोध उत्पन्न करने वाला। Causing asphyxia.

Asphyxiate (एस्फाइक्सिएट) श्वसावरोध उत्पन्न करना। To cause asphyxia.

Aspirate (एस्पिरेट) चूषण के द्वारा अन्दर या बाहर की ओर खींचना। To draw in or out by suction.

Aspirator (एस्पिरेटर) चूषण द्वारा किसी गुहा से किसी तरल अथवा गैसों के निकालने वाला उपकरण। An apparatus for removing the fluids or gases from a cavity by suction.

Asplenia (एस्प्लेनिया) प्लीहा का अभाव। Absence of the spleen.

Assay (एसे) विश्लेषण, निर्धारण। Analysis, to subject to analysis.

Assimilate (एसिमिलेट) स्वांगीकरण करना, आत्मसात करना। To convert nutritious substance furnished by the food into flesh or other tissues of the body.

Assimilation (एसिमिलेशन) अवशोषित भोजन का शरीर की कोशिकाओं में ऑक्सीकरण होना तथा इसका जीवद्रव्य में परिवर्तित होना। Oxidation of the absorbed food in the cells of the body and its conversion into protoplasm.

Astasia (एस्टेसिया) प्रेरक असमंजन होने के कारण सीधे खड़े होने अथवा सीधा बैठने में असमर्थता। Inability to stand or sit erect due to motor incoordination.

Astatic (एस्टेटिक) सामान्य ढंग से खड़े होने में असमर्थ। Unable to stand in normal manner.

Astereognosis (एस्टेरीयोग्नोसिस) वस्तुओं को छूकर उन्हें पहचानने में असमर्थता। Inability to recognize the objects by touch.

Asterion (एस्टेरियोन) बिन्दुतारक (सन्धि), तारक सन्धि। The junction of occipital, parietal and temporal bones.

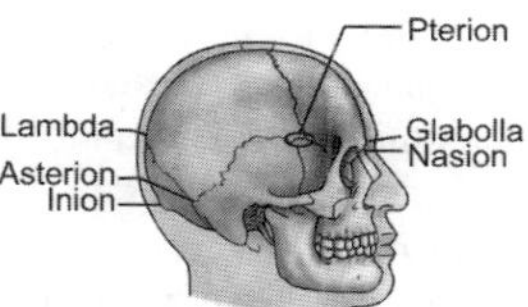

Asterixis (एस्टेरिक्सिस) असामान्य रूप से पेशी कम्पन्न होना जिसमें विशेषकर हाथों में स्वतः झटके आने लगते हैं। Abnormal muscle temor consisting of involuntary jerky movements, especially in the hands.

Asteroid (एस्टीरॉयड) तारकरूप। Star-shaped.

Asthenia (एस्थीनिया) दुर्बलता, कमजोरी। Weakness.

Asthenometer (एस्थीनोमीटर) पेशीय शक्ति मापक यन्त्र। An instrument for determining the muscular strength.

Asthenope (एस्थीनोप) नेत्रावसाद से प्रभावित व्यक्ति। The person affected with asthonopia.

Asthenospermia (एस्थीनोस्पर्मिया) वीर्य में शुक्राणुओं की स्वतः गतिशीलता घट जाना। Reduction of motility of spermatozoa in semen.

Asthma (एस्थमा) दमा, खासरोग। Violent oppression of breathing; paroxysmal dyspnea with appression. (*i*) **Allergic asthma** (एलर्जिक एस्थमा)

प्रत्यूर्जतात्मक दमा। One due to allergens. (*ii*) **Cardiac Asthma** (कार्डियक एस्थमा) हृदय रोग जैसे रक्ताधिक्यज हृदय-पात में सांस फूलना। Dyspnea associated with heart disease such as congestive heart failure. (*iii*) **Renal Asthma** (रीनल एस्थमा) वृक्कज दमा। That sometimes accompanying Bright's disease.

Asthmogenic (एस्थमोजेनिक) दमा उत्पन्न करने वाला। Causing asthma.

Astigmatism (एस्टिग्मेटिज्म) प्रत्यावर्तन-तलों अर्थात नेत्र के कॉर्निया एवं लैन्स के तलों की वक्रता में विभिन्न रेखाओं में अन्तर होने से उत्पन्न एक दोषयुक्त दृष्टि जिसमें प्रत्यावर्तित प्रकाश किरणों विस्तृत क्षेत्र में फैल जाती हैं और ठीक रेटिना पर केन्द्रित नहीं होती, दृष्टिवैषम्य। Defective vision in which the refracted light rays are spread over a diffused area and not focused sharply on the retina due to the differences in the curvature in different meridians of the refractive surfaces, i.e. the surface of the cornea and the lens of the eye. (*i*) **Compound Astigmatism** (कम्पाउण्ड एस्टिग्मेटिज्म) ऐसी दोषयुक्त दृष्टि अथवा दृष्टिवैषम्य जिसमें सभी रेखाओं में दूरदृष्टिता अथवा निकटदृष्टिता हो जाती है। Defective vision in which these is hypermetropia or myopia in all meridians (*ii*) **Lenticular Astigmatism** (लैन्टीकुलर एस्टिग्मेटिज्म) लैन्स की खराबी से होने वाला दृष्टिवैषम्य। Astigmatism due to defect of the lens. (*iii*) **Simple Astigmatism** (सिम्पिल एस्टिग्मेटिज्म) एक ही दिशा रेखा में होने वाला दृष्टिवैषम्य। Astigmatism along one meridian only.

Astomatous (एस्टोमेटस) बिना मुंह वाला अथवा मुख छिद्र रहित। Without mouth or oral aperture.

Astragalar (एस्ट्रागैलर) घुटने की हड्डी से सम्बन्धित। Relating to the astragalus.

Astraphobia (एस्ट्राफोबिया) बादलों की गर्जना एवं बिजली के चमकने से डर लगना। Fear of thunder and lightening.

Astringent (एस्ट्रिन्जैन्ट) रक्त वाहिनियों को संकुचित करके रक्तस्राव को रोकने वाला अथवा स्राव की प्रोटीन को जमाकर उसे रोकने वाला। An agent checking the hemorrhage by constricting the bloodvessels, or the secretion by coagulating its portein.

Astrocyte (एस्ट्रोसाइट) तार के आकार की तन्त्रिका बन्ध सम्बन्धी एक कोशिका, तारिका कोशिका। A star-shaped neuroglial cell.

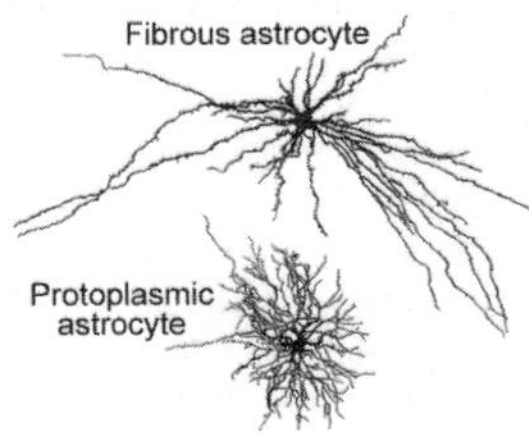

Astrocytoma (एस्ट्रोसाइटोमा) तारिका कोशिकाबुर्द। A slowly growing tumor of the glial tissue of the brain.

Astrophobia (एस्ट्रोफोबिया) तारों एवं स्वर्गलोक का विकृत भय। Morbid fear of stars and the heaven.

Asylum (एसाइलम) आश्रयस्थल, शरणास्थल, शरण स्थल। An institution for the care of the incapables and destitutes.

Asymmetry (एसिमेट्री) असमरूपता। Lack of symmetry.

Asymptomatic (एसिमप्टोमेटिक) लक्षणों से रहित, अलक्षणी। Having no symptoms.

Asynclitism (एसिनक्लीटिज्म) प्रसव में भ्रूण के सिर की तिर्यक प्रस्तुति। Oblique presentation of the fetal head in labor.

Asynergia (एसिनर्जिया) शरीर के भागों अथवा अंगों में असमन्वय जो सामान्यता एक दूसरे से मिलकर कार्य करते हैं। In coordination of parts or organs of the boсy normally acting in harmony.

Asynovia (एसाइनोविया) किसी जोड़ केश्लेषक-तरल के स्राव की कमी। Deficiency of secretion of synovial fluid of a joint.

Asyntaxia (एसिनटैक्सिया) भ्रूण के उचित विकास में कमी हो जाना। Lack of proper development of the embryo.

Asystolic (एसिस्टोलिक) हृदय-अप्रकुंचन से सम्बन्धित। Pertaining to asystole.

Atactiform (एटेक्टीफार्म) गतिविभ्रम के समान। Similar to ataxia.

Ataraxia (एटारैक्सिया) बिना अवसाद अथवा संज्ञाहीनता (बेहोशी) के मानसिक शान्ति होने की अवस्था। A state of mental calmness without depression or unconsciousness.

Atavism (एटाविज्म) निकट पितर लोगों की अपेक्षा किसी दूरस्थ पितर के किसी लक्षण का प्रकट होना, पूर्वजता। The appearance of a character from remote ancestor rather than the immediate ones.

Ataxia (एटेक्सिया) पेशीय समन्वय का दोषयुक्त होना अथवा

पेशीय क्रिया की अनियमितता, गतिविभ्रम। Defective muscular coordination or irregularity of muscular action.

(*i*) **Alcoholic Ataxia** (एल्कोहॉलिक एटेक्सिया) पुराने शराब पीने वाले लागों में अपनी स्थिति या आसन एवं गतियों का ज्ञान न रहने से उत्पन्न गति विभ्रम। Ataxia due to loss of sense of the position and movements in chronic alcoholism.

(*ii*) **Hysterical ataxia** (हिस्टीरिकल एटेक्सिया) हिस्टीरिया के कारण पैर की पेशियों में होने वाला गतिविभ्रम। Ataxia of the muscles of the leg due to hysteria.

(*iii*) **Motor Ataxia** (मोटर एटेक्सिया) प्रेरक गतिभंग, चलते समय पेशियों में सामंजस्य रखने की असमर्थता। Inability to coordinate the muscles in walking.

Ataxiameter (एटेक्सियामीटर) गति-विभ्रम को मापने वाला उपकरण। An apparatus of measuring ataxia.

Ataximnesia (एटेक्सिम्नेसिया) गतिविभ्रम के साथ स्मृतिलोप। Ataxia with amnesia.

Atelectasis (एटेलेक्टेसिस) जन्म के समय भ्रूण के फेफड़ो का पूर्ण अथवा आंशिक रूप से विस्तारित न होना। किसी युवा व्यक्ति का चिपका हुआ अथवा वायु रहित फेफड़ा होना। Total or partial absence of expansion of the lungs of a fetus of collapsed or airless lung of an adult.

Atelia (एटीलिया) अपूर्ण विकास। Imperfect or incomplete development.

Atelocardia (एटीलोकार्डिया) हृदय का जन्मजात अपूर्ण विकास। Congenital incomplete development of the heart.

Atelocephaly (एटीलोसिफेली) सिर का अपूर्ण विकास। Incomplete development of the head.

Atelocheiria (एटीलोचीरिया) हाथ का अपूर्ण विकास। Incomplete development of the head.

Atelomyelia (एटीलोमाइलिया) सुषुम्ना रज्जु का अपूर्ण विकास। Incomplete development of the spinal cord.

Ateloprasopia (एटीलोप्रोसोपिया) चेहरे का अपूर्ण विकास। Incomplete development of the face.

Atelostomia (एटीलोस्टोमिया) मुख का अपूर्ण विकास। Incomplete development of the mouth.

Athelia (एथीलिया) चुचुकों का जन्मजात अभाव। Congenital absence of the nipples.

Atherogenesis (एथीरोजेनेसिस) धमनियों की दीवारों में मेदाबुर्द

एथीरोमा का बनना। Formation of atheroma in the walls of the arteries.

Atheroma (एथीरोमा) मेदाबुर्द। A disease which involves degeneration of blood vessels, chiefly to arteries.

Atherosclerosis (एथीरोस्क्लेरोसिस) धमनी कला काठिन्य।

A disease affecting the lining membranes of the arteries.

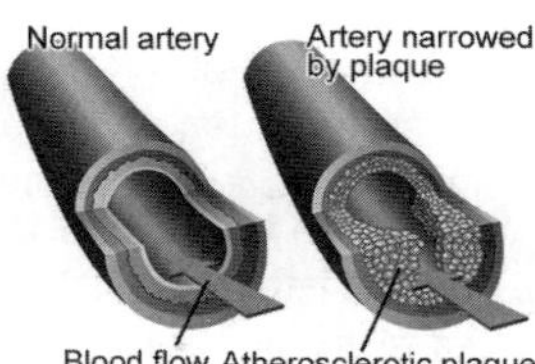

Athetoid (एथिटॉयड) वलन के समान अथवा उससे पीड़ित। Resembling or affected with athetosis.

Athetosis (एथिटोसिस) वलन, हाथ-पैरों की अँगलियों की धीमी, मन्द गति।

Slow, steady movement of the fingers and toes.

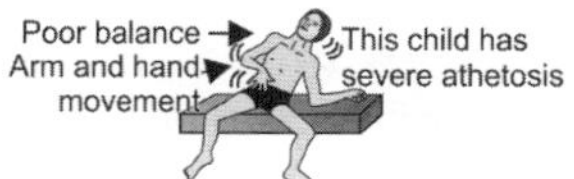

Athlete (एथलेट) पहलवान, कुश्ती लड़ने वाले, खिलाड़ी। A robust person.

Athlete's Foot (एथलेट्स फूट) पैर का कवक संक्रमण। Tinea pedis. Fungus infection of the foot.

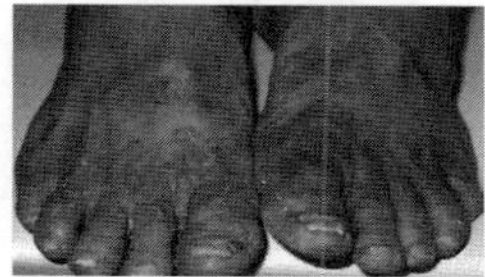

Athlete's Heart (एथलेट्स हार्ट) महाधमनी-शैथिल्य। Aortic incompetence from strain.

Athrepsia (एथेरेप्सिया) सूखा रोग। Marasmus.

Athymia (एथाइमिया) थाइमस ग्रन्थि अथवा इसके स्राव का अभाव। Absence of thymus gland or its secretion.

Athyroidemia (एथाइरॉयडीमिया) रक्त से थाइरॉयड हार्मोन का अभाव। Absence of thyroid hormone from the blood.

Atlantad (एटलेन्टाड) एटलस हड्डी की ओर। Towards the atlas bone.

Atlantoaxial (एटलेन्टोएक्सियल) एटलस एवं अक्ष से सम्बन्धित। Pertaining to the atlas and the axis.

Atlas (एटलस) प्रथम ग्रीवा-कशेरूका। The first cervical vertebra.

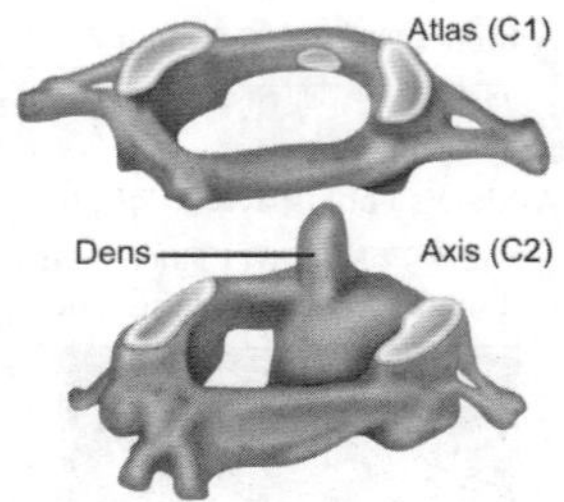

Atmospheric (एटमोस्फेरिक) वातावरण सम्बन्धी। Pertaining to the atmosphere.

Atocia (एटोसिया) स्त्री में बन्ध्यता। Sterility in the female.

Atom (एटम) परमाणु, अणु, कण। The ultimate unit of an element.

Atomization (एटोमाइजेशन) किसी तरल को फुहार अथवा वाष्प में बदलने की क्रिया। The process of converting a liquid into a spray or vapor.

Atomizer (एटोमाइजर) कणित्रण तरल पदार्थों को सूक्ष्म कणों में बदल देने वाला यंत्र। A spraying instrument.

Atonic (एटोनिक सामान्य तनाव अथवा तनाव से रहित। Without normal tension or tone.

Atopic (एटोपिक) जिसका स्थान बदल गया हो। Displaced.

Atopy (एटोपी) एलर्जी उत्पन्न होने की आनुवंशिक प्रवृत्ति। Hereditary tendency to develop allergy.

Atresia (एट्रेसिया) अविवरता, अछिद्रता, नलिकारोध, मार्गरोध। A blocking of a cannal or passage, as the ear. (*i*) **Anal atresia** (एनल एट्रेसिया) अछिद्री गुदा। Imperforate anus. (*ii*) **Mitral atresia** (माइट्ल एट्रेसिया) माइट्स कपाट छिद्र का जन्म से बंद रहना। Congenital closure of the mitral valve opening. (*iii*) **Urethral atresia** (यूरेथ्रल एट्रेसिया) मूत्रमार्ग-छिद्र का बन्द रहना। Closure of the urethral opening. (*iv*) **Vaginal atresia** (वैजाइनल एट्रेसिया) योनि का जन्म से बन्द रहना अथवा उसका अभाव। Congenital absence or closure of the vagina.

Atresic (एट्रेसिक) अछिद्रता से सम्बन्धित। Pertaining to atresia.

Atreto (एट्रीटो) किसी छिद्र के अभाव को प्रदर्शित करने वाला उपसर्ग। Prefix denoting the absence of an opening.

Atrial fibrillation (एट्रियल फिब्रीलेशन) अलिन्दी विकम्पन या एट्रियल फिब्रीलेशन में शिरानाल-अलिन्दी पर्व अथवा साइनो एट्रियल नोड से आवेग न उठकर जो सामान्यतया अलिन्दनिलयी पूलिका या बण्डल

ऑफ हिज से होकर निलयों में पहुँचते हैं। 350-600 प्रति मिनट की गति से अलिन्द से उठते हैं, अतः केवल अलिन्द ही तेजी से तथा अनियमित रूप से संकुचित होते हैं, निलय नहीं, अलिन्दी विकम्पन। Inatrial fibrilation the impulses arise in the atrium at the rate of 350–600 per minute instead of the sinoatrial node from which they are normally conducted along the bundles of His to the ventricles, so the atria only contract rapidly and irregularly and not the ventricles.

Atrial Flutter (एट्रियल फ्लटर) यह एक ऐसा रोग है जिसमें आलिन्दों के शीघ्रगामी एक नियमित उत्तेजन के परिणाम स्परूप अलिन्दों में शीघ्रगामी और नियमित उत्तेजन के परिणाम स्परूप आलिन्दों में शीघ्रगामी और नियमित संकुचन होते है तथा हृदय गति 200 से 350. सामान्यतः 300 प्रति मिनट हो जाती है। सामान्यतः हृदरोध पाया जाता है। जिससे अलिन्दों एवं निलयों के आवेगों की संख्या का अनुपात 2:1 हो जाता है अर्थात नाड़ी गति 100 से 175 सामान्यतः 150 हो जाती है। It is a condition characterized by rapid and regular atrial contractions and the heart rate becomes 200 to 350, usually 300 per minute, resulting from rapid and regular stimulation of the atria. Heart block is generally present causing the atria and the ventricles to be ratio of the number of the impulses of the atria and the ventricles to be 2:1, i.e. pulse rate becomes 100 to 175, usually 150.

Atrichia (एट्रिकिया) गंजापन या बालों का अभाव। Alopecia or absence of hair.

Atrioseptopexy (एट्रियोसेप्टोपैक्सी) अंतरा अलिन्दी मध्यपत में स्थित दोष की प्लास्टिक सर्जरी द्वारा मरम्मत करना। Repair of a defect in the interatrial septum by plastic surgery.

Atriotomy (एट्रियोटॉमी) शल्य-क्रिया द्वारा किसी अलिन्द को खोलना। Surgical opening of an atrium.

Atrioventricular bundle (एट्रियोवेन्ट्रिकुलर बण्डल) बण्डल ऑफ हिज। हृदय पेशी तन्तुओं की एक पूलिका जो अलिन्द-निलयपर्व से आरम्भ होकर अंतरा-निलयी मध्यपत में कुछ दूर तक जाकर दो शाखाओं में विभाजित हो जाती है जो दोनों निलयों को तन्तुओं की आपूर्ति करती है। यह अपनी शाखाओं पकिन्जी तन्तुओं के द्वारा अलिन्द-निलय-पर्व से आवेगों को हृदय के निलयों को संचालित

करती है। Bundle of His. A bundle of cardiac muscle fibers extending from the atrioventricular (A-V) node up to a short distance in the interventricular septum and then dividing into two branches which supply fibers to both the ventricles it conducts the impulses from the atrioventricular node to the ventricles, of the heart through its branches the purkinje fibers.

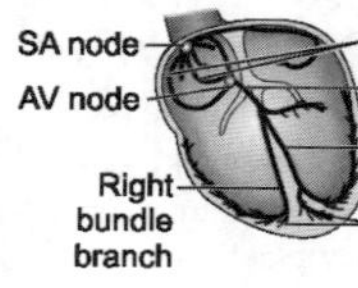

Atrium (एट्रियम) एक कोष्ठ अथवा गुहा जो दूसरी संरचना, अंग अथवा कोष्ठ से जुड़ा होता है जैसे हृदय के ऊपरी भाग में प्रत्येक ओर स्थित एक छोटा कोष्ठ-अलिन्द। A chamber or cavity communicating with another structure, organ or chamber, e.g. upper smaller chamber on each side of the heart.

Atrophic (एट्रॉफिक) अपक्षय से सम्बन्धित अथवा अपक्षय से ग्रस्त। Pertaining to or characterized by atrophy.

Atrophoderma (एट्रॉफोडर्मा) त्वचा का अपक्षय। Atrophy of the skin.

Atrophy (एट्रॉफी) शरीर के किसी ऊतक, अंग अथवा भाग का परिमाण में घटना। A decrease in sized of a tissue, organ or part of the body. (*i*) **Acute yellow atrophy** (एक्यूट यलो एट्रॉफी) यकृतशोथ का एक उपद्रव जिसमें यकृत सिकुड़ा हुआ एवं पीले रंग का हो जाता है तथा साथ ही कामला या पीलिया भी हो जाता है। Shrunken yellow liver with jaundice, as a complication of hepatitis. (*ii*) **Muscular atrophy** (मस्कुलर एट्रॉफी) पेशियों का अपक्षय। Atrophy of the muscles. (*iii*) **Optic atrophy** (ऑप्टिक एट्रॉफी) दृष्टि-नाड़ी के ह्रास से होने वाला दृष्टि-चक्रिका का अपक्षय। Atrophy of the optic disk due to degeneration of the optic nerve. (*iv*) **Sudeck's atrophy** (सुडेक्स एट्रॉफी) चोट लगने के स्थान पर किसी हड्डी में होने वाला शोध। Atrophy of a bone at the site of injury.

Attack (ऐटेक) आक्रमण। Occu-rrence of some disease or episode often with a dramatic onset.

Attic (ऐटिक) अधिमध्यकर्ण, मध्यकर्ण-कुहर का एक भाग। The portion of the tympanum above the atrium.

Atticitis (एटिसाइटिस) अधिमध्यकर्ण का शोथ। Inflammation of the attic of the ear.

Attitude (एटिट्यूड) शरीर का आसन अथवा उसकी स्थिति, प्रसूति-तंत्र में भ्रूण के शरीर के विविध भागों का एक दूसरे से सम्बन्ध व्यवहार, स्वभाव। A posture or position of the body in obstetrics; the relation of the various parts of the body of the fetus to one another.

Attolens (एटोलैन्स) ऊपर उठाने वाला। Raising or lifting up.

Attrition (एट्रीशन) रगड़ से त्वचा का घिस जाना। The wearning away of the skin by friction or rubbing.

Atypical (एटिपिकल) सामान्य से विचलित हो जाने वाला। Deviating from the normal.

Audible (ऑडिबिल) सुनाई दिया जाने वाला। Capable of being heard.

Audile (ऑडाइल) सुनने से सम्बन्धित। Pertaining to hearing.

Audiogenic (ऑडियोजेनिक) ध्वनि से उत्पन्न। Produced by sound.

Audiologist (ऑडियोलॉजिस्ट) श्रवणविज्ञान का विशेषज्ञ। The person specialist in audiology.

Audiometry (ऑडियोमीटरी) सुनने के ज्ञान का परीक्षण करना, श्रवणमिति। Testing of the hearing sense.

Audiosurgery ऑडियोसर्जरी कान की शल्य-चिकित्सा करना। Surgery of the ear.

Audito oculo gyric reflex (ऑडिटो ऑकलो गाइरिक रिफ्लैक्स) किसी भयप्रद ध्वनि की ओर अचानक सिर एवं आँखों का घूम जाना। The sudden turning of the head and the eyes in the direction of an alarming sound.

Auditory Agnosia (ऑडिटरी एग्नोसिया) ध्वनि, शब्दों या संगीत को पहचानने में असमर्थता। Inability to recognize.

(*i*) **Color Agnosia** (कलर एग्नोसिया) रंग को पहचानने में असमर्थता। Inability to recognize color. (*ii*) **Tactile Agnosia** (टैक्टाइल एग्नोसिया) छूकर वस्तुओं को पहचानने में असमर्थता। Inability to recognize the objects by touch. (*iii*) **Visual Agnosia** (विजुअल एग्नोसिया) वस्तुओं को देखकर उन्हें पहचानने में असमर्थता। Inability to recognize the things by sight.

Auditory epilepsy (ऑडिटरी ऐपिलेप्सी) ऐसा मिर्गी रोम जिसका कुछ ध्वनियाँ सुन कर दौरा पड़

जाता है। The epilepsy that is triggered off by certain sounds.

Auditory nerve (ऑडिटरी नर्व) आठवीं कपालीय तंत्रिका। The 8th cranial nerve.

Auditory reflex (ऑडिटरी रिफ्लैक्स) अचानक किसी आवाज के पैदा होने से आँखों का फड़ फड़ाना। Blinking of the eyes upon sudden production of a sound.

Augmentation (ऑग्मैन्टेशन) जोड़ने अथवा बढ़ाने की क्रिया। The process of adding or increasing.

Aura (औरा) किसी रोगाक्रमण से पूर्व होने वाला उसका आभास जैसा कि मिर्गी रोग में होता है, पूर्वाभास। A subjective sensation before an attack of a disease, as occurs in epilepsy.

Aural (औरल) कान अथवा किसी पूर्वाभास से सम्बन्धित। Pertaining to the ear or to an aura.

Auriasis (औरिएसिस) स्वर्ण देने के पश्चात् त्वचा पर भूरे रंग के चकते पड़ जाना। Occurring of gray patches on the skin after administration of gold.

Auricle (ऑरिकिल) बाह्य कर्ण का सिर से बाहर रहने वाला भाग, पल्ला या कर्ण पाली। The portion of the external ear remaining outside the head, the flap or the pinna.

Auricular (ऑरिकुलर) कान की कर्णपाली से सम्बन्धित। Pertaining to the auricle of the ear.

Auriform (ऑरिफार्म) कान की आकृति वाला। Ear-shaped.

Aurigo (ऑरिगो) कामला, पीलिया, पाण्डुरोग। Jaundice.

Auris (ऑरिस) कान का बाहरी हिस्सा, बहिकर्ण। The external ear.

Auriscope (ऑरिस्कोप) कान के नेत्र परीक्षण के लिए प्रयोग में लाया जाने वाला यंत्र, कर्णदर्षी। Otoscope. An instrument used for visual examination of the ear.

Aurotherapy (औरोथिरैपी) स्वर्ण लवणों का प्रयोग करके रोगों जैसे रिह्यूमेटॉयड (गठिया रूप) सन्धिशोध की चिकित्सा करना। Treatment of disease like rheumatoid arthritis by administration of gold salts.

Auscultation (ऑस्कल्टेशन) विकृत अवस्थाओं अथवा गर्भावस्था का पता लगाने के लिए शरीर के भीतर की, अधिकतर वक्षीय अथवा उदरीय अंतरांगों की ध्वनि सुनने की क्रिया। इसे बिना किसी यंत्र की सहायता के कान लगाकर

या किसी यंत्र जैसे स्टेथोस्कोप की सहायता से किया जा सकता है, परिश्रवण। The process of listening for the sounds within the body, usually the sounds of thoracic or abdominal viscera, to detect some abnormal conditions or the pregnancy. It may be perform with the unaided ear or with an instrument such as stetoscope.

Auscultatory (ऑस्कल्टेरी) परिश्रवण से सम्बन्धित। Pertaining to auscultation.

Autacoids (ऑटेकोइड) अन्तःस्राव, आन्तरिक स्राव। Internal secretions.

Autism (ऑटिज्म) ऐसी मानसिक अवस्था जिसमें अपने में ही ध्यान केन्द्रित रहता है, स्वपरायणता। The self-centered mental state.

Autistic (ऑटिस्टिक) स्वपरायण, वह व्यक्ति जिसका अपने में ही ध्यान केन्द्रित रहता है, जो दिवास्वप्न देखता है तथा बाह्य जगत से कोई मतलब नहीं रखता। The person who is self-centered, day-dreaming and unaware of the outer world.

Auto (ऑटो) उपसर्ग जिसका अर्थ स्वयं होता है। Prefix meaning self.

Autoagglutinin (ऑटोएग्लुटिनिन) किसी व्यक्ति के रक्त में स्थित पदार्थ जो उसी व्यक्ति की लाल रक्त कोशिकाओं का समूहन करता है। The substance present in a person's blood which agglutinates that person's own red blood cells.

Autoamputation (ऑटोएमपुटेशन) शरीर के किसी भाग का स्वयं ही कट कर अलग हो जाना। Spontaneous amputation of a part of the body.

Autoanalyzer (ऑटोएनालाइजर) स्वतः विष्लेशण करने वाला एक यंत्र जो सामान्यतः रासायनिक विश्लेषण में प्रयोग में लाया जाता है। An instrument conducting analysis automatically, commonly used in chemical analysis.

Autoantibody (ऑटोएण्टीबॉडी) एक एण्टीबॉडी जो व्यक्ति के अपने ऊतकों के एन्टिजन की अनुक्रिया के फलस्वरूप बन्ती है तथा उसी के विरूद्ध प्रतिक्रिया करती है। स्वप्रतिपिण्ड। An antibody formed in response to an antigen of the person's own tissues and reacting against it.

Autoantitoxin (ऑटोएन्टीटॉक्सिन) स्वयं शरीर के द्वारा उत्पन्न प्रतिजीवविष। Antitoxin produced by the body itself.

Autocatheterism (ऑटोकेथेट्रिज्म) स्वयं ही नालशलाका प्रवेश विशेष

रूप से मूत्रमार्गीय नालशलाका प्रवेश करना। Catheterization by oneself, especially urethral catheterization.

Autoclasis (ऑटोक्लेसिस) शरीर के किसी भाग का किसी आन्तरिक कारण से नष्ट हो जाना। Destruction of a part of the body from some internal cause.

Autoclave (ऑटोक्लेव) वस्तुओं का वाष्पीय दाब में निर्जीवाणुकरण करने वाला उपकरण। An apparatus for the sterilization of materials by steam under pressure.

Autocytolysis (ऑटोसाइटोलाइसिस) कोशिकाओं का स्वतः ही पाचन अथवा स्वतः नष्ट हो जाना। Self-digestion or self-destruction of cells.

Autodigestion (ऑटोडाइजेशन) स्वपाचन, अपने ही स्रावों द्वारा ऊतकों का विघटन। Digestion of the gastric walls from disease of the stomach.

Autoecholalia (ऑटोइकोलालिया) किसी व्यक्ति का अपने शब्दों को बार-बार दुहराना। Repetition of one's own words.

Autoerotism (ऑटोएरोटिज्म) अपने शरीर को देखकर लैंगिक उत्तेजना होना जैसा कि हस्तमैथुन में होता है। स्वकामुकता। Sexual excitement by seeing one's own body, as in masturbation.

Autogenous (ओटोजीनस) शरीर में स्वतः उत्पन्न होने वाला। Self-generating within the body.

Autograft (ऑटोग्राफ्ट) रोगी के शरीर के किसी भाग से लिया गया ऊतक निरोप जिसे दूसरे किसी भाग पर स्थानान्तरित किया जाता है। A tissue graft taken from a part of the patient's body and transferred to the other part.

Autohemolysis (ऑटोहीमोलाइसिस) किसी व्यक्ति की लाल रक्त कोशिकाओं का उसी के अपने सीरम से अपघटन हो जाना। Hemolysis of a person's red blood cells by that person's own serum.

Autohemotherapy (ऑटोहीमोथिरैपी) रोगी के शरीर से रक्त खींचकर इसे इन्जैक्शन द्वारा उसकी पेशी में पहुँचाकर चिकित्सा करना, स्वरक्तोपचार। Treatment by with drawing the blood from patient's body and injecting into the muscles of the patient.

Autoimmunity (ऑटोइम्यूनिटी) स्वक्षमता, स्वरोगक्षमता। An abnormal immune reaction of unknown cause.

Autoinfection (ऑटोइनफेक्शन) स्वोपसर्ग। Self-infection by direct contagion, autoinfection.

Autoinfusion (ऑटोइनफ्यूजन) रक्तचाप बढ़ाने के लिए पट्टी या किसी दाब उपकरण का प्रयोग करके रक्त को भुजाओं से प्राणाधार अंगों को धकेलना जैसा कि सामान्यतः शरीर से रक्त या अन्य तरल की अत्यधिक हानि हो जाने पर किया जाता है। Forcing of blood from the extremities to the vital organs by applying bandage or pressure device to raise the blood pressure, which is usually done after excessive loss of blood or other fluid from the body.

Autoinoculation (ऑटोइनोकुलेशन) किसी व्यक्ति के शरीर से प्राप्त जीवों का उसी के शरीर में टीका लगाना, स्वसंरोपण। Inoculation with organisms obtained from one's own body.

Autointoxication (ऑटोइन्टॉक्सिकेशन) शरीर में उत्पन्न किसी विषैले पदार्थ द्वारा उत्पन्न विशाक्तता। Toxicosis poisoning caused by a poisonous substance produce within the body.

Autokeratoplasty (ऑटोकेरेटोप्लास्टी) किसी व्यक्ति के कॉर्निया का निरोपण उसी की दूसरी आँख से प्राप्त ऊतक द्वारा करना। Grafting of the cornea by the tissue obtained from the other eye of the same person.

Autokinetic (ऑटोकाइनेटिक) स्वेच्छा से चलने-फिरने योग्य। Capable of moving voluntarily.

Autologous (ऑटोलोगस) उसी जीव से सम्बन्धित। Related to the same organism.

Autolysin (ऑटोलाइसिन) किसी जीव से उत्पन्न एण्टीबॉडी जो उसी जीव की कोशिकाओं एवं ऊतकों को नष्ट कर सकती है। An antibody produced in an organism and capable of destroying the cells and tissues of the same organism.

Autolytic (ऑटोलाइटिक) स्वलयन सम्बन्धी। Pertaining to autolysis.

Automatism (ऑटोमेटिज्म) शरीर में स्वतः क्रियाओं का होना जिनका व्यक्ति को पता नहीं चलता जैसे रोमकों का हिलना-डुलना, स्वचलता। Occurrence of spontaneous activities in the body without the knowledge to the person, as the movements of the cilia.

Autonomic nervous system (ऑटोनोमिक नर्वस सिस्टम) तंत्रिका-तंत्र का वह भाग जो शरीर के अनैच्छिक कार्यों जैसे हृदय के कार्य के नियंत्रण से सम्बन्धित रहता है तथा दो

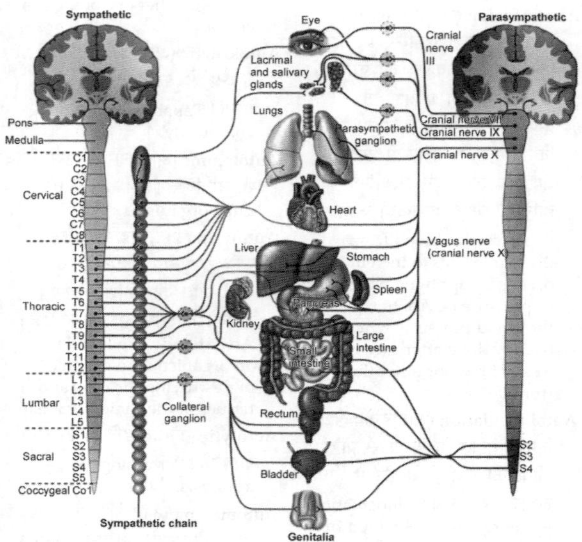

भागों-अनुकम्पी एवं परानुकम्पी तंन्त्रिका-तंत्र में विभाजित रहता है, स्वायत्त तंत्रिका-तन्त्र। The part of the nervous system which is concerned with the control of the involuntary functions of the body, such as the function of the heart and is divided into two parts sympathetic and parasympathetic nervous system.

Autopathy (ऑटोपैथी) बिना किसी स्पष्ट बाहय कारण के उत्पन्न होने वाला रोग। The disease originating without apparent external cause.

Autophagic (ऑटोफेजिक) स्वभक्षण से सम्बन्धित अथवा स्वभक्षण करने वाला। Pertaining to or characterized by autophagia.

Autophobia (ऑटोफोबिया) अकेले रहने का विकृत भय, स्वभिति, एकान्तभिति।
A morbid fear of being alone.

Autoplasmotherapy (ऑटोप्लाज्मोथिरैपी) रोगी में

उसके रक्तप्लाज्मा का इन्जैक्शन लगाकर चिकित्सा करना। Treatment by injecting patient's own blood plasma.

Autoplastic (ऑटोप्लास्टिक) स्वांग-संधान से सम्बन्धित। Pertaining to autoplasty.

Autopolyploidy (ऑटोपोलीप्लॉयडी) गुणसूत्रों के दो पूर्ण सैटों से अधिक होने की दशा। The condition of having more than two complete sets of chromosomes.

Autopsy (ऑटोप्सी) मरणोत्तर जांच, शवपरीक्षा। A postmortem examination.

Autopsychic (ऑटोसाइकिक) अपने व्यक्तित्व से अवगत रहने वाला व्यक्ति, स्वमानसिक। Aware of one's own personality.

Autopsychosis (ऑटोसाइकोसिस) एक मानसिक रोग जिसमें रोगियों के अपने बारे में विचार विकृत हो जाते है। A mental disease in which the patient's ideas about themselves are disordered.

Autoreinfusion (ऑटोरिइन्फ्यूजन) रोगी के रक्तस्राव वाले स्थानों जैसे उदरीय अथवा फुस्फुसीया गुहा से एकत्रित रक्त को अन्तःशिराभ मार्ग द्वारा उसी रोगी में पहुँचाना। The reinfusion of the blood to the patient intravenously collected from the bleeding sites such as abdominal or pleural cavity of the same patient.

Autosensitize (ऑटोसैन्सीटाइज) किसी व्यक्ति को उसके अपने शरीर की कोशिकाओं के प्रति सुग्राही बनाना। Isosensitize. To sensitize against one's own body cells.

Autoserodiagnosis (ऑटोसीरोडायग्नोसिस) रोगी के रक्त सीरम के द्वारा रोग निदान करना। Diagnosis through the serum from patient's blood.

Autoserotherapy (ऑटोसीरोथिरैपी) रोगी के अपने रक्त सीरम का इन्जैक्शन लगाकर चिकित्सा करना। Treatment by injection of the patient's own blood serum.

Autosmia (ऑटोस्मिया) किसी व्यक्ति का अपने शरीर से निकलने वाली दुर्गन्ध से अवगत कराना। Awareness of the odor of one's own body.

Autosome (ऑटोसोम) लिंग गुणसूत्रों के अतिरिक्त कोई भी गुणसूत्र, अलिंग गुणसूत्र, मनुष्य में ऑटोसोम के 22 जोड़े होते हैं। Any of the chromosome other than the sex chromosome, in man there are 22 pairs of autosomes.

Autosplenectomy (ओटोस्प्लीनेक्टॉमी) तन्तुमयता एवं सिकुड़न के कारण प्लीही का लगभग पूर्ण रूप से अन्तर्धान हो जाना। Almost complete disappearance of the spleen due to fibrosis and shrinkage.

Autosuggestion (ऑटोसजेशन) किसी व्यक्ति के मस्तिष्क में उठने वाले किसी विचार को उस व्यक्ति द्वारा स्वीकार कर लेना जिससे कोई शारीरिक अथवा मानसिक कार्य सम्पन्न होता है अथवा कोई परिवर्तन होता है। The acceptance of an idea arising from within one's own mind, bringing about some physical or mental action or change.

Autotherapy (ऑटोथिरैपी) स्वचिकित्सा, सोपचार। The spontaneous cure of disease.

Autotoxin (ऑटोटॉक्सिन) स्वविष, शरीर में स्वयमेव पैदा होने वाला विष-पदार्थ। Any poisonous substance produced in the body.

Autotransfusion (ऑटोट्रान्सफ्यूजन) रोगी के शरीर से रक्त लेकर उसी के शरीर पर चढ़ा देना। Reinfusion of a patient's own blood.

Autotrophic (ऑटोट्राफिक) अपना पोषण स्वयं करने वाला। स्वपोषी। Self-nourishing.

Autovaccination (ऑटोवैक्सीनेशन) ऑटोवैक्सीन द्वारा चिकित्सा करना। Treatment with autovaccine.

Autovaccine (ऑटोवैक्सीन) रोगी के शरीर से अलग किए गए विषाणुओं से तैयार की गई वैक्सीन। Vaccine prepared from the viruses isolated from the patient's own body.

Auxiliary (ऑक्जिलरी) सहायक, आनुशंगिक। Helping or asissting.

A-V block (ए-वी ब्लाक) ऐसा हृदयरोध जिसमें आवेग अलिन्द-निलयी पर्व पर रूक जाते है। A heart block in which the impulses are impeded at the atrioventricular node.

Avascular (एवैस्कुलर) रक्त वाहिनियों से रहित अथवा रक्तहीन जैसे उपास्थि। Locking of blood vessels or bloodless as cartilage.

Aviation (एवियेशन) विमानन, हवाई यात्रा करना। Travelling in airplane.

Avirulent (एवाइरूलैन्ट) अतिविष्णता से रहित। Without virulence.

Avulsion (एवल्सन) शरीर के किसी भाग अथवा रचना को चीर देना। The tearing away of a part or structure of the body.

Axanthopsia (एक्जेन्थोप्सिया) पीत वर्णान्धता। Yellow blindness.

Axenic (एक्जेनिक) रोगाणु रहित अथवा विसंक्रमित। Germ-free or sterile.

Axifugal (एक्सिफ्यूगल) केन्द्रापसारी, केन्द्र अथवा अक्ष से दूर। Centrifugal; Away from the axis.

Axilla (एक्जिला) बगल। Armpit.

Axis (एक्सिस) शरीर के केन्द्र से गुजरने वाली रेखा अथवा जिसके चारों और कोई संरचना घूमती है। द्वितीय ग्रैव कशेरूका। A line which runs through the center of a body or about which a structure revolves, second cervical vertebra.

Axocardia (ऐक्सोकार्डिया) अतिवृद्धि अथवा विस्फारण हो जाने के कारण हृदय का बढ़ जाना। Enlargement of the heart by hypertrophy or dilatation.

Axodendrite (एक्सोडेण्ड्राइट) अक्षतंतु से निकलने वाला प्रवर्ध। Process arising from an axon.

Axolemma (एक्सोलेमा) अक्षतंतु का बाह्य आवरण। The outer sheath of an axon.

Axon (एक्सोन) तन्त्रिका-कोशिका से निकलने वाला एक प्रवर्ध जो कोशिकाय से आवेगों को दूर ले जाता है। अक्षतंतु। Axis cylinder. A process of a neuron (nerve cell) which conducts the impules away from the cell body.

Axoneme (एक्सोनेम) गुणसूत्र का अक्षीय धागा। Axial thread of a chromosome.

Axonometer (एक्सोनोमीटर) दृष्टिवैषम्य के अक्ष का पता लगाने वाला उपकरण। A device for determining the axis of astigmatism.

Axonotmesis (एक्सोनोटमेसिस) संयोजी ऊतक को क्षति पहुँचे बिना अक्षतन्तु एवं माइलिन आवरण पर आघात पहुँचना। Injury of the axon and myelin sheath without damage of the connective tissue.

Axoplasm (एक्सोप्लाज्म) अक्षतंतु का कोशिका द्रव्य। The cytoplasm of an axon.

Axospongium (एक्सोस्पॉन्जियम) तन्त्रिका कोशिका के अक्षतंतु पदार्थ की बारीक तन्तु की जाली। The fine fibrillar network of the axon substance of a nerve cell.

Azoic (एजोइक) जीवित प्राणियों से रहित। Containing no living organisms.

Azotemia (एजोटीमिया) रक्त में नाइट्रोजन यौगिकों विशेषकर यूरिया की अधिक मात्रा में विद्यमानता। An excess of nitrogenous compounds, especially the urea in the blood.

Azotification (एजोटिफिकेशन) वायुमण्डल की नाइट्रोजन का स्थरीकरण। Fixation of the nitrogen at the atmosphere.

Azotobacter (एजोटोबैक्टर) वायुमण्डल की नाइट्रोजन का स्थिरीकरण करने वाला जीवाणु। Nitrogen fixing bacteria.

AZR (ए.जेड.आर) ऐश्चाहइम जौंडेक प्रतिक्रिया, गर्भ-ज्ञान के लिये की जाने वाली मूत्र-जांच की एक पद्धति। A pregnancy test where patient's urine is injected into female mice to induce ovulation.

Azygous (एज़ाइगस) अकेला, जोड़ीदार नहीं। Single, not paired.

Azymia (एजाइमिया) किण्व (फर्मेन्ट) अथवा एन्जाइम रहित होने की अवस्था। The condition of being without a ferment or enzyme.

B

B (ब) बीटा। Beta

Ba (बे) बेरियम का प्रतीक। Symbol of barium.

Babcock sentence test (बैबकॉक सेनटेन्स टेस्ट) मानसिक उन्माद को जांचने की प्रक्रिया।

This is a test for dementia pt.

Bacciform (बेसीफार्म) बेर का रूप। Shaped like a Berry.

Bacilliform (बेसीलीफार्म) जीवाणु का रूप। Shaped like a bacillus.

Bacilliparous (बेसीलीपेरस) जीवाणुओं को जन्म देने वाला। Producing bacilli.

Bacillophobia (बेसीलोफोबिया) जीवाणुओं से डर। A morbid fear of microbes.

Bacillum (बेसीलम) छड़।

A Stick.

Bacilluria (बेसील्यूरिया) मूत्र में जीवाणु अथवा बेसीलाई को विद्यमान होना। Presence of bacili in the urine.

Bacillus (बेसीलस) छड़ की आकृति का जीवाणु। Any rod-shaped bacterium.

Bacillus streptococcus pneumonia (बेसीलस स्ट्रेप्टोकॉकस न्यूमोनिया) इससे न्यूमोनिया रोग होता है। It causes pneumonia.

Backache (बैकैएक) कमर का दर्द। Pain in the back.

Backbone (बैकबोन) रीढ़ की हड्डी। The spinal column.

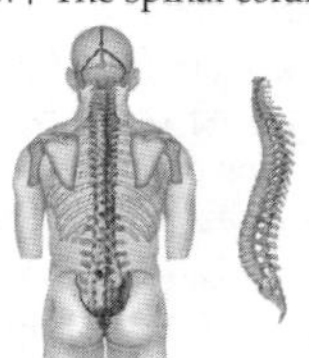

Backrest (बैकरेस्ट) पीठ को सहारा देना। Support the back in bed.

Bacteremia (बैक्टेरेमिया) जीवाणुओं का रक्त में पाया जाना। Presence of bacteria in the blood.

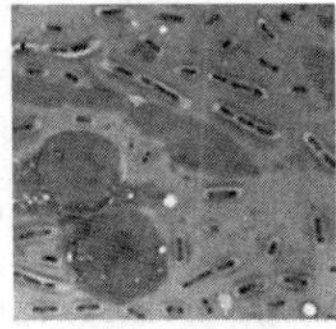

Bactericidal (बैक्टेरीसाइडल) जीवाणुओं को नष्ट करने वाला। Destroying bacteria.

Bactericide (बैक्टेरीसाइड) जीवाणुओं को नष्ट करने का साधन। An agent which destroys the bacteria.

Bactericidin (बैक्टेरीसाइडिन) जीवाणु को खत्म करने वाली एण्टीबॉडी। Antibody which kills bacteria.

Bacteriogenic (बैक्टेरियोजेनिक) जीवाणुओं द्वारा उत्पन्न। Caused by bacteria.

Bacteriogenous (बैक्टेरियोजीनस) जीवाणुओं को उत्पन्न करना। Producing bacteria.

Bacterioid (बैक्टेरिऑयड) जीवाणुओं के जैसा। Resembling bacteria.

Bacteriologic (बैक्टेरियोलॉजिक) जीवाणु विज्ञान द्वारा सम्बन्धित। Relating to bacteria or to bacteriology.

Bacteriologist (बैक्टेरियोलॉजिस्ट) जीवाणु-विज्ञान विशेषज्ञ। Specialist in bacteriology.

Bacteriology (बैक्टेरियोलॉजी) जीवाणुओं का वैज्ञानिक अध्ययन करना। Scientific study of bacteria.

Bacteriolysis (बैक्टेरियोलाइसिस) जीवाणुओं को खत्म करना। Destroy of bacteria.

Bacteriolytic (बैक्टीरियोलाइटिक) जीवाणुओं को नष्ट करने से सम्बन्धी। Pertaining to bacteriolysis.

Bacteriophage (बैक्टीरियोफेज) जीवाणुओं को नष्ट करने वाला वाइरस। A virus that destroys bacteria.

Bacteriosis (बैक्टीरियोसिस) जीवाणुओं के द्वारा होने वाला कोई भी रोग। Any disease which is caused by bacteria.

Bacteriostasis (बैक्टीरियोस्टेसिस) जीवाणुओं की वृद्धि होना। Multiplication of the bacteria.

Bacteriostatic (बैक्टीरियोस्टेटिक) जीवाणुओं की वृद्धि को रोकने वाला साधन। Inhibits the growth of bacteria.

Bacteriuria (बैक्टीरियूरिया) पेशाब में जीवाणुओं का पाया जाना। Presence of bacteria in the urine.

Bag (बैग) थैला। A cell.

Bag of waters (बैग ऑफ वाटर्स) पानी की थैली, गर्भाशय में स्थित झिल्ली की थैली जिसके भीतर भ्रूण विद्यमान करता है। Membrane enclosing the liquor amni and the fetus in uterus amnion.

Bagnio (बैगनिओ) स्नानागार। A bath house.

Balance (बैलेन्स) भार मापक। An apparatus for measuring weight.

Balanic (बैलेनिक) भ्रूण का मुण्ड सम्बन्धी। Pertaining to the glans penis or glans clitoris.

Balanitis (बैलेनाइटिस) भ्रूण के सिर का शोध। Inflammation of the glans penis.

Balanoposthitis (बैलेनोपोस्थाइटिस) भ्रूण के सिर के ऊपर स्थित आवरण। Inflammation of the prepuce.

Balanopreputial (बैलेनोप्रिप्यूशियल) लिंगमुण्ड और लिंगच्छप सम्बन्धी Relating to the glans penis and the prepuce.

Balanorrhea (बैलेनोरेह्रिया) शिष्नमुण्ड शोध जिसमें से पस निकलना। Pus discharge.

Balbuties (बालब्यूटिज) हकलाना, अटक-अटक कर बोलना। Stammering.

Bald (बैल्ड) गंजा। Without hair.

Baldness (बैल्डनैस) गंजापन। Absence of hair Alopexia.

Ballismus (बालिजमस) शरीर का हिलना, कंपन। A tremor.

Ballistics (बैलिस्टिक्स) प्रक्षेपणास्त्रों को नियंत्रित तथा मिसाइलों की गति की क्षमता का अध्ययन करना। The science of the motion and trajectory bullets bombs, rockets and guided missiles.

Ballistophobia (बैलिस्टोफोबिया) बंदूक से निकलने वाली गोली से डरना। Fear of a projectile or missile.

Ballooning (बैलूनिंग) फुलाव। Distention of a cavity.

Ballottement (बैलोटमेन्ट) गर्भावस्था का पता लगाने के लिए प्रयोग किया जाता है। Especially used to diagnose pregnancy.

Balm (बॉम) मालिश करने पर आराम पहुँचाने वाली दवा, मरहम। A soothing application or ointment.

Balneology (बालनियेलॉजी) नहाने से सम्बन्धित विज्ञान। The science of baths.

Balneum (बालनियम) स्नान। A bath.

Balsamic (बालसैमिक) सुगंधित। Pertaining to balsam.

Bandage (बैण्डेज) पट्टी। Bandage.

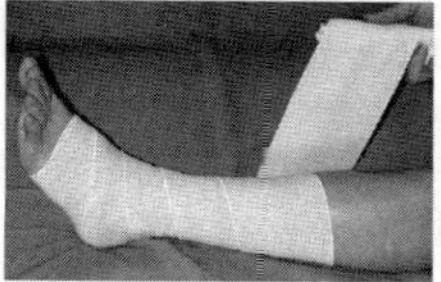

Banelet (बेनलेट) छोटी सी हड्डी। A little bone.

Bar (बार) डण्डा। A rod.

Baragnosis (बैरागनोसिस) भार को महसूस करने में अक्षमता। Loss of sense of weight or pressure.

Barber's itch (बारबर्स इच) दाढ़ी का दाद। Ringworm of the beard.

Baresthesia (बैरीस्थीसिया) भार का ज्ञान होना। Pressure sence.

Baresthesiometer (बेरीस्थीसियोमीटर) भार नापने वाला यंत्र। Instrument for testing the sence of pressure.

Baric (बैरीक) भार से सम्बन्धित। Pertaining to barometric, pressure or weight.

Barium (बेरियम) क्षारीय वर्ग की एक धातु। A metal of the alkaline group.

Bark (बार्क) छाल। Tree or shrub.

Barley (बारली) जौ। A cereal used for food.

Baro (बैरो) भारीपन का संकेत। Indicating heaviness.

Barograph (बैरोग्राफ) वायुमण्डल में होने वाले दाब परिवर्तन को मापना। Measure and record atmospheric pressure.

Baromacrometer (बैरोमैक्रोमीटर) शिशु को मापने वाला यंत्र। An instrument for weighing and measuring newborn infants.

Barophillic (बैरोफिलीक) वायुदाबप्रेमी। Thriving under high environmental.

Baroscope (बैरोस्कोप) वायु में होने वाले परिवर्तनों का पता लगाने वाला यंत्र। An instrument registers the changes in the density of air.

Barotrauma (बैरोट्रोमा) दाब के कारण पहुंचने वाला आघात। Injury due to pressure.

Barren (बरन) बांझ, निसंतान, संतान को जन्म देने में असक्षम। Sterile.

Barrenness (बैरेननैस) बांझपन। Sterility.

Barrier (बैरियर) बाधा। An obstruction.

Bartholinitis (बार्थोलीनाइटिस) बार्थोलिन ग्रन्थि का शोध। Inflammation of the bartholin gland.

Bary (बैरी) भारी। Prefix indicating heavy or hard.

Baryecoia (बैरीकोईया) कम सुनाई देना, बहरापन। Deafness.

Baryglossia (बैरीग्लोसिया) भारी आवाज में बोलना धीरे-धीरे। To speak slow and thick voice.

Barylalia (बैरीलेलिया) अस्पष्ट बोलना। Thickness of speech.

Baryphonia (बैरीफोनिया) बोलने में दिक्कत होना। Difficulty of speech.

Baryta (बैरीटा) एक जहरीला क्षार। Protoxide of barium.

Basad (बैसाड) आधार की ओर। Towards a base.

Bashful (बैसफूल) शर्मीला। Shy, Shamefull.

Basicranial (बेसीक्रेनियल) खोपड़ी के आधार से सम्बन्धित। The base of the skull.

Basifacial (बेसीफेशियल) चेहरे के निचले भाग से सम्बन्धित। To lower portion of the face.

Basil (बैसिल) तुलसी। A saered fragrant aromatic plant called tulsi.

Basiphobia (बेसीफोबिया) चलने-फिरने से डरना। Fearing of walking.

Basisphenoid (बेसीस्फेनॉयड) स्फेनाइड हड्डी से आधार से सम्बन्धित। To the base of sphenoid bone.

Bath (बाथ) नहाना। Balsem.

Bathophobia (बाथोफोबिया) गहरे स्थानों से भय। A morbid fear of depths.

Bathyanesthesi (बैथीएनीस्थीसिया) चेतनता का अभाव। Loss of deep sensibility.

BD (बी.डी.) दिन में दो बार। Two times a day.

BE (बी.ई.) कोहनी से नीचे। Below elbow.

Beard (बीयर्ड) दाढ़ी। Hair of the low or face.

Bearing down (बीयरिंग डाऊन) प्रसव पीड़ा जैसा अहसास। Labor like sensation.

Beat (बीट) धड़कन। As of pulse heart.

Bechic (बेकिक) खांसी से सम्बन्धित। Pertaining to cough.

Bedbug (बैडबग) खटमल। Insect that rainus in bed.

Beef (बीफ) पशु का मांस। The flesh of cattle.

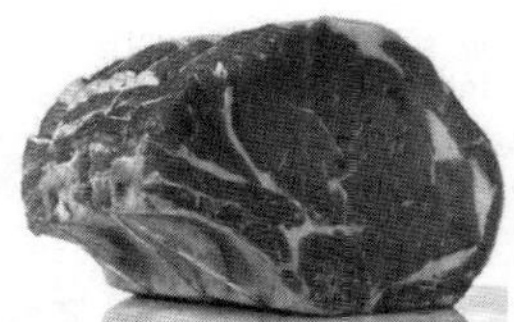

Belch (बेल्च) डकार लेना। To eructate.

Belly button (बैली बटन) नाभि। Umbilicus.

Bellyache (बैलीएक) पेट दर्द। Pain in the abdomen.

Belonephobia (बैलीनोफोबिया) तेज नुकीली वस्तुओ से डरना। Morbid fear of sharp. Pointed things.

Belonoid (बैलोनॉयड) सूई के आकार की। Needle shape.

Belt (बैल्ट) कमर का पट्टा। Weapones.

Beng (बैंग) भांग। Bhang.

Benign (बैनाइन) हल्का, कोमल। Mild, not malignant.

Bereavement (बिरियावेमैन्ट) शोक एवं दुःख की प्रतिक्रिया। Sadness and some financial loss.

BeriBeri (बैरीबैरी) विटामिन-बी, की कमी से होने वाला रोग। Due to deficiency of Vit-B.

Bestial form (बैसटियल फॉर्म) जानवर से मिलता जुलता रूप। Resembling an animal.

Bestiality (बेस्टियालिटी) जानवरों के साथ संभोग। Sexual intercourse with animals.

Beverage (बिवीरेज) शराब, पेय पदार्थ। A drink.

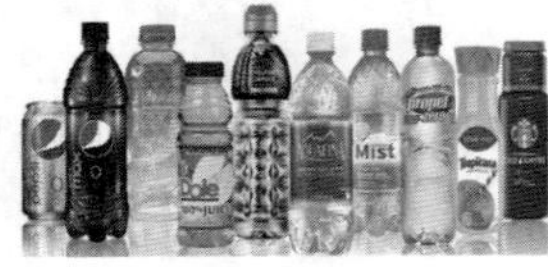

Biarticular (बाइआर्टिकुलर) दो जोड़ों सम्बन्धित। Pertaining to two joints.

Bias (बायस) भेदभाव करना। Partiality.

Biaxial (बाइएक्सियल) दो अक्षों वाला। Having two axes.

Bibliotherapy (बिबलियोथिरैपी) मानसिक रोगों में केवल पुस्तकें पढाकर ही इलाज करना। Treatment of some mental disease by teaching books only.

Bicapitate (बाईकाडेट) दो सिर वाला। Having two heads.

Bicapsular (बाइकैप्सूलर) दो सम्पुट वाला। Having two capsuler.

Bicaudate (बाइकॉडेट) दो पूंछ वाला। Having two tails.

Bicellular (बाइसैल्यूलर) दो कोशिकाओं वाला। Having two cells.

Bicentric (बाइसैन्ट्रीक) दो केन्द्रों वाला। Having two centers.

Bicollis (बाइकोलिस) दो गर्दन वाला। Having two necks.

Biconcave (बाइकोनकेभ) द्विअवतल वाला। Concave on hollow on both surface.

Bicornuate (बाइकोरन्यूएट) दो सींगों वाला। Having two horns.

Bicoronal (बाइकोरोनल) दो शिखरों से सम्बन्धित। Two coronas.

Bicorporate (बाइकोर्पोरेट) दो शरीरों वाला। Having two bodies.

Bicuspid (बाइकस्पिड) दो उभारों वाला। Having two cusps.

BID (बी.आई.डी.) दिन में दो बार। Two times a day.

Biennial (बाइनियल) दो वर्ष में होने वाला। Occurring every two years.

Bifid (बाइफिड) दो भागों में विभाजित, द्विखण्डी। Divided into two.

Bifid spine (बाइफिड स्पाइन) रीढ़ की हड्डी का जन्मजात फटना। Congenital fissure of the vertebral column.

Bifid tongue (बाइफिड टंग) फटी हुई जीभ। Cleft tongue.

Bifocal (बाइफोकल) चश्में का लैंस। As a lens.

Bifurcate (बाइफर्केट) दो शाखाओं में विभाजित। Divided into two branches.

Bigaster (बाइगैस्टर) दो तोंद वाला। Having two bellies.

Bigeminal (बाइजैमिनल) जोड़ी। Paired.

Bilateral (बाईलेट्रल) दोनों ओर से सम्बन्धित। Pertaining to both sides.

Bile (बाइल) पित्त, यकृत द्वारा वह स्राव जिसका काम पाचन करना होता है। Yellowish brown and green color gluid secreated by lengue.

Biliation (बाइलीएशन) पित्त का स्राव। Bile secreation.

Bilification (बाइलीफिकेसन) पित्त की रचना। The formation of bile.

Biligenesis (बाइलीजेनेसिस) पित्त का उत्पादन। Production of bile.

Bilious (बिलीअस) पित्त ज्वर। Partaking of the nature of bile.

Biliousness (बाइलीयसनेस) पित्त का ज्यादा होना। Due to excess of bile.

Bilirubinemia (बिलीरूबिनीमिया) रक्त में बिलीरूबिन की विद्यमानता। Presence of bilirubin in the blood.

Bilitherapy (बाइलीथिरैपी) पित्त लवणों द्वारा चिकित्सा। Treatment by bile or bile salt in the urine.

Biliuria (बाइलीयूरिया) मूत्र में पित्त लवणों का पाया जाना।
The Presence of bile or bile salt in the urine.

Bilobate (बाइलोबेट) दो खण्ड़ों वाला। Having two lobes.

Bilocular (बाइलोक्यूलर) दो भागों वाला। Having two cells or compartment.

Bimana (बाइमैना) दो हाथों वाला जन्तु। Having two hands animal.

Bimanual (बाइमैनुअल) दोनों हाथों से। With both hands.

Binary (बाइनरी) दो वर्णों में संकुचित विभाजित होने वाला। Compounded division of two element.

Binaural (बाइनौरल) दोनों कानों से सम्बन्धित।
Pertaining to both ears.

Binder (बाइनडर) पेट को बाँधने वाली पट्टी। One encircling the abdomen.

Binocular (बाइनोक्यूलर) दोनों आँखों से सम्बन्धित।
Pertaining to both eyes.

Binoculus (बाइनोक्यूलस) आँखों पर लगायी जाने वाली 'एक्स' आकार की पट्टी। An 'X' shaped bandage for both eyes.

Binovular (बाइनोव्यूलर) दो डिम्बों से सम्बन्धित। Derived from two separate ova.

Binucleolate (बाइन्यूक्लियोलेट) दो उपकेन्द्र वाला। Having two nucleoli.

Bio (बायो) जीवन से संबंध बताने वाला उपसर्ग। Prefix meaning life.

Biochemical (बायोकैमिकल) जीवन रसायन शास्त्र से सम्बन्धी। Pertaining to biochemistry.

Biocidal (बायोसाइडल) जीवित जीवों को मारने वाला। Destructive to life.

Bioclimatology (बायोक्लाइमेटोलॉजी) जलवायु के जीवन से सम्बन्ध का अध्ययन। Study of the relationship of climate of life.

Biodynamic (बायोडायनेमिक) जीव गति का विज्ञान। The science of vital force.

Biogenic (बायोजैनिक) जीव द्वारा उत्पन्न।

Produced by some living being.

Biohazard (बायोहर्जाड) पर्यावरण के लिए जो नुकसानदायक हो। Harmful to human-being or the environment.

Biolysis (बायोलाइसिस) मृत्यु। Death.

Biolytic (बायोलाइटिक) जीवन को खत्म करने वाला। Capable of destroying life.

Biomass (बायोमास) किसी जगह पर जीवों का इकट्ठा हो जाना। The collection of many living organism in a specified area.

Biometry (बायोमेटरी) जीवों का मापन। The measurement of life.

Bioparous (बायोपेरस) एक बार में दो बच्चे को जन्म देने वाली। Producing two offsprings at one birth.

Biophage (बायोफेज) जीवित वस्तुओं से जीने के लिए पोषण प्राप्त करना। Obtaining nourishment from living things for its existence.

Biopsy (बायोप्सी) जीवित ऊतकों की जांच। Observation of the living tissues.

Biostatics (बायोस्टेटिक्स) जीवों की संख्या का पता करना। Physics and mechanics of the living bodies.

Biotic (बायोटिक) जीवन से सम्बन्धित। Pertaining to the life.

Biped (बाइपेड) दो पैरों वाला। Having two feet.

Black (ब्लैक) काला। An absence of light.

Blain (ब्लैन) छाला। A blister or pustule.

Bland (ब्लैन्ड) कोमल। non-irritating.

Blastema (ब्लास्टेमा) कोशिका का गुच्छा। A cluster of cells.

Blepharostenosis (ब्लैफेरोस्टेनोसिस) पलकों का सिकुडना। Narrowing of the interpalpebral opening.

Blinking (ब्लींकिंग) पलकों का अपने आप खुलना-बंद होना। Momentary gleam or glimpses.

Bloated (ब्लोटेड) फूला हुआ। Swelled.

Blond (ब्लौंड) गोरी। Fair complexion.

Blood (ब्लड) रक्त। A liquid made of RBCs.

Blow (ब्लो) मुक्का मारना। A hard stroke.

Boat-belly (बोट-बैली) अन्दर को धंसा हुआ पेट। The seenleen appearance of the belly.

Bole (बोले) चिकनी मिट्टी। Fine clay.

Bone (बोन) हड्डी। A rigid hard connective tissue.

Botany (बोटनी) पौधों से सम्बन्धी विज्ञान। The science of plants.

Bow (बॉ) धनुष। Arc

Brain (ब्रेन) कपाल के भीतर केन्द्रीय तन्त्रिका तन्त्र का भाग। A larges soft mass in skull.

Bulimia (बूलीमिया) ज्यादा भूख लगना। Excessive hunger.

C

C (सी) कार्बन, सेल्सियस। Symbol for Carbon, Celsius.

Ca (कै) कैल्सियम का प्रतीक। Symbol for Calcium.

Cacatian (कैकेसन) मल त्यागना। Defecation.

Cacemia (केसीमिया) रक्त में दोष होना। A deprived condition of the blood.

Cachectic (केचेक्टिक) कमजोर। Weakness.

Cacoethes (केकोइथस) बुरी आदत। Any bad habit.

Cacogeusia (कैकोग्यूसिया) मुँह का स्वाद खराब होना। Bad taste in the mouth.

Cacosmia (कैकोस्मिया) बुरी बदबू। Bad odor.

Cacosomium (केकोसोमियम) लाइलाज रोगी का अस्पताल। A hospital for incurables.

Cacothanasia (केकोथेनासिया) दर्दनाक मौत। Miserable death.

Cadaver (केडेवर) मरा हुआ शरीर। Dead body.

Cainotophobia (केनोटोफोबिया) किसी नयी वस्तु से डर लगना। Fear of novelty newness.

Calcaneus (केलकेनियस) एड़ी की हड्डी। Bone of heel.

Calcarea (कैल्केरिया) चूना। Lime.

Calcariuria (कैल्केरीयूरिया) मूत्र में कैल्सियम के लवणों का पाया जाना। Presence of lime salts in the urine.

Calciferol (कैल्सिफैरोल) विटामिन डी$_2$ । Vitamin-D_2

Calcigerous (कैल्सिजेरस) कैल्सियम को उत्पन्न करने वाला। Producing or containing calcium.

Calcipenia (कैल्सिपीनिया) कैल्सियम की कमी आना। Deficiency of calcium.

Calciprivia (कैल्सिप्राइविया) कैल्सियम की हानि। Loss of calcium.

Calcis (कैलकिस) एड़ी की हड्डी। The heal bone.

Caldarium (कैलडेरियम) गरम पानी से नहाना। Taking hot bath.

Caligo (कैलिगो) आँखों से धुंधला दिखना। Dimness of vision.

Callous (केलस) कठोर। Hardened.

Calmative (कालमेटिव) बेचैनी को कम करने वाला। Sedative soothing.

Caloricity (केलोरीसिटी) ताप की एक इकाई। A unit of heat.

Calorific (केलोरीफिक) गर्मी पैदा करने वाला। Producing heat.

Calorigenic (केलोरीजैनिक) शक्ति के उत्पादन से सम्बन्धित। Producing of heat or energy.

Calorimeter (केलोरीमीटर) उष्मामापक यंत्र। An instrument used to measure the heat transfer between system and surroundings.

Calvities (केलवीटिज) गंजापन। Diffused or general baldness.

Camphol (कामपोल) कपूर का तेल। Oil of camphor.

Campylotropous (कामपायलोट्रोपस) टेढ़ा। Curved.

Canalization (कैनालाइजेशन) ऊतक में किसी नली का निर्माण होना। Formation of a canal in tissue.

Cancellous (केनसेलस) जालीनुमा Resembling lattice work.

Cancer (कैंसर) कर्क रोग। A malignant tumor spread rapidly.

Canceroid (केनक्रोइड) कैंसर। जैसा। Having the appearance of a cancer.

Cancrum (केनक्रम) कंकर। Inflammatory lesion.

Canities (केनाइटिस) बाल सफेद हो जाना। Greyness or whiteness of the hair.

Cannabis (केनेबिस) भांग। A genus of narcotic plant.

Capsicum (केपसीकम) लाल मिर्च का पौधा। African pepper.

Capsid fructus (केपसीड फ्रक्टस) लाल मिर्च। The red peppers.

Caput (केपुट) सिर। The head.

Caraway (केरावे) कालाजीरा। A genus of plants.

Carbohydraturia (कारबोहाइड्रेटयूरिया) पेशाब में सफेद सार जाना। An excess of carbohydrates in the urine.

Carboluria (कारबोलयूरिया) पेशाब में कार्बोलिक एसिड जाना। Carbolic acid in the urine.

Carcase (कारकेस) पशु का शव। Dead body of an animal.

Carcinogenesis (कार्सिनोजेनेसिस) कैंसर की उत्पत्ति। Production of cancer.

Carcinogenic (कारसिनोजेनिक) कैंसर पैदा करने वाला पदार्थ। A agent producing cancer.

Carcinolysis (कार्सिनोलाइसिस) कैंसर कोशिकाओं का नष्ट होना। Destruction of the cancer cells.

Carcinomatosis (कार्सिनोमेटोसिस) कैंसर की पूरे शरीर में फैल जाने की अवस्था। Spread of cancer in whole body.

Carbuncle (कारबन्कल) मांस का बढ़ा हुआ भाग। Fleshy projection.

Cardamom (कारडेमोम) इलायची। The fruit of elettaria cardamom.

Cardiaectasia (कार्डिएक्टेसिया) हृदय का चौड़ा होना। Dialatation of the heart.

Cardiagra (कारडिएग्रा) हृदय का गठिया। Gout of the heart.

Cardialgia (कार्डियाल्जिया) हृदय क्षेत्र में दर्द। Pain in the heart region.

Cardiant (कार्रडयेन्ट) हृदय को प्रभावित करने वाली दवाई। A heart remedy.

Cardiectasis (कारडियेस्टेसिस) हृदय का फैलना। Dilation of the heart.

Cardiomalacia (कार्डियोमेलेसिया) हृदय पेशी का मुलायम होना। Softening of the heart muscle.

Cardiomegaly (कार्डियोमेगैली) हृदय की वृद्धि होना। Enlargement of the heart.

Cardiomotility (कारडियोमोटिलीटी) हृदय की गति। Movement of the heart.

Cardiophone (कारडियोफोन) हृदय की आवाज सुनने योग्य बनाने वाला यंत्र। Stethoscope for listening to sound of the heart.

Cardiorrhexis (कार्डियोरैह्क्सिस) हृदय का फट जाना। Rupture of the heart.

Cardiosclerosis (कार्डियोस्क्लेरोसिस) हृदय-पेशी का कठोर होना। Hardening of the cardiac muscle.

Cardiostenosis (कार्डियोस्टेनोसिस) हृदय का संकुचित हो जाना। Constriction of the heart.

Cardiotomy (कार्डियोटॉमी) हृदय में चीरा लगाना। Incision of the heart.

Cardiotonics (कार्डियोटोनिक) हृदय को मजबूती देने वाली दवाईयाँ और पौष्टिक तत्व। Nutrient's and Drugs used to increase the efficiency and improve the contraction power of heart muscle.

Carcinogenic (कार्सिनोजेनिक) कैंसर रोग पैदा करने वाला। Any substance involve in producing cancer.

Carnia (कारनिया) रीढ़। The spine.

Carotid (केरोटिड) गर्दन की परक। The principal artery of the neck.

Carpagra (कारपेग्रा) कलाई का दर्द। Pain in the wrist.

Carpi (कारपी) कलाई। The wrist.

Carus (केरस) गहन मूर्च्छा बेहोशी। Complete insensibility.

Casein (केसिन) दूध में पाया जाने वाला थक्केदार प्रोटीन।

The clotted protein of milk.

Caseous (केसियस) पनीर जैसा। Having the nature of cheeze.

Castor oil (केस्टर आयल) अरण्ड का तेल। A purgative.

Casualty (केजुएल्टि) घायल। Accidental injury.

Catamenia (केटेमेनिया) मासिक धर्म। The menses.

Cataracta brunescence (केटेरेक्टा ब्रुनेससेंस) भूरा मोतियाबिंद। The brown cataract.

Cataracta coerulea (केटेरेक्टा कोरयूला) नीला मोतियाबिंद। The blue cataract.

Catarrh (केटेर्ह) सर्दी जुकाम। Inflammation of the mucous membrane.

Catgut (कैटगट) भेड़ की आंतों से तैयार किया जाने वाला धागा। A ligature substance made from sheep's intestine.

Catharsis (कैथारसिस) दस्त हो जाना। Purgation.

Catheter (कैथेटर) पेशाब कराने की नली। A tube to drain from body.

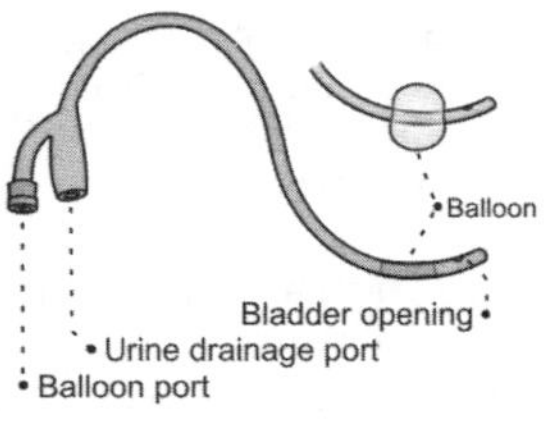

Catheterization (कैथेटेराइजेशन) कैथेटर को शरीर के किसी भी गुहा में प्रवीष्ट करना। Passage of catheter in body.

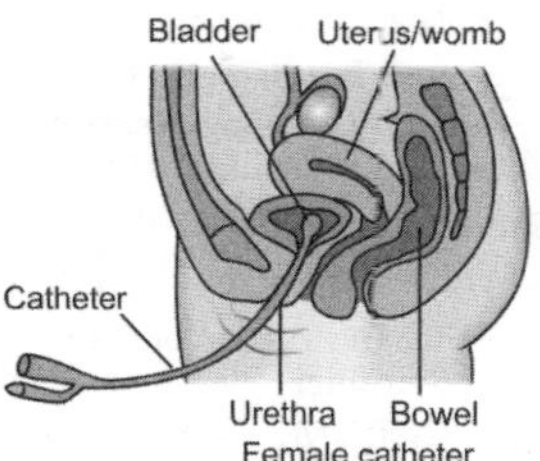

Female catheter

Bladder
Catheter
Male catheter

Cauda (कौडा) पूंछ अथवा पूंछ के समान रचना। A tail or tail-like structure.

Caudate (कौडेट) पूंछ वाला। Having a tail.

Caudocephalad (कॅडोसिफैलाड) पूंछ के सिरे से सिर की ओर गति करने वाला।

Moving from the tail end toward the head

Caudotomy (कौडोटॉमी) मेरूरज्जु की पूंछ में चीरा लगाना। Incision of the cauda equina.

Caustic (कॉस्टिक) ऐसा पदार्थ जो जलाकर जिन्दा ऊतकों को खत्म कर देता है। The substance destroys the living tissues by burning as an alkali.

Cauterization (कॉटेराइजेशन) कॉटरी द्वारा ऊतक को नष्ट करना। Destruction of tissue with a cautery.

Cava (केवा) शरीर में स्थित खोखला स्थान। Hollow area or a body cavity.

Cavernous (कैवरनस) खाली स्थानों से युक्त। Containing hollow spaces.

Cavitory (कैविटरी) गुहा से सम्बन्धित। Pertaining to a cavity.

CBC (सी.बी.सी.) सम्पूर्ण रक्त जाँच। Complete blood count.

CC (सी.सी.) मुख्य शिकायत। Chief complaint.

Cecal (सीकल) अंधान्त्र से सम्बन्धित। Pertaining to the cecum.

Cecectomy (सीकेक्टॉमी) अंद्यान्त्र को काटकर निकाल देना। Excision of the cecum.

Cecitis (सीकाइटिस) अंद्यान्त्र का शोध। Inflammation of the cecum.

Cecocolostomy (सीकोकोलोस्टॉमी) ऑपरेशन द्वारा सीकम और कोलान को जोड़ देना। An operation of joining the cecum to the colon.

Cecoileostomy (सीकोइलियोस्टॉमी) ऑपरेशन द्वारा सीकम और इलियम को जोड़ना। An operation for joining the cecum.

Cecoptosis (सीकोप्टोसिस) सीकम का नीचे को गिर जाना। Falling down of the cecum.

Cecosigmoidostomy (सीकोसिग्मॉयडोस्टॉमी) ऑपरेशन द्वारा सीकम और सिग्मोइड कोलोन को जोड़ना। To make a connection between the cecum and the sigmoid colon by an operation.

Cel (सील) सूजन, हर्निया का संकेत देने वाला उपसर्ग। Swelling or hernia.

Celiocentesis (सिलियोसेन्टेसिस) पेट में छेद होना। Puncture in the abdomen.

Celioenterotomy (सीलियोएन्ट्रोटामी) उदर में चीरा लगाकर आंत में चीरा लगाना। Incision through the abdominal wall into the intestine.

Cell (सेल) कोशिकाएं। Basic structure of plants, animals.

Cellalgia (सेलागिया) पेट का दर्द। Abdominal pain.

Cellula (सेल्यूला) बहुत छोटी कोशिका। A very small cell.

Cellularity (सैल्युलैरिटी) कोशिका की दशा, गुणवत्ता। Condition and quality of cells present.

Cellulicidal (सेल्यूलीसाइडल) कोशिकाओं को खत्म करने वाला। Destroyer of the cells.

Cellulifugal (सेल्यूलीफ्यूगल) कोशिका से दूर गति करने वाला। Moving away from a cell.

Cellulipetal (सेल्यूलीपिटल) कोशिका की ओर गति करना। Moving towards a cell.

Cellulotoxic (सैल्यूलोटॉक्सिक) कोशिकाओं के विष से उत्पन्न होने वाला। Poisonous to cells.

Celoscopy (सीलोस्कोपी) शरीर गुहा का प्रकाश यंत्र द्वारा अध्ययन, परीक्षण करना। Examination of body cavity with an optical instrument.

Cementitis (सीमेन्टाइटिस) दांत-सीमेंट का शोध। Inflammation of the dental cement.

Cenesthesia (सिनेस्थीसिया) चेतना का आभास। Normal feeling of being alive.

Cenesthopathia (सिनेस्थेपैथिया) स्वस्थ महसूस नहीं करना। Not feeling well.

Cenosis (सिनोसिस) गंदा स्राव। Morbid discharge.

Cenotophobia (सिनोटोफोबिया) नये विचारों से डर लगना। Morbid fear of new things and new ideas.

Census (सेनसस) जनगणना। Official counting of the population.

Centenarian (सेन्टीनेरियन) 100 वर्ष से ज्यादा उम्र का व्यक्ति। Person over the age of 100 years.

Centesis (सेन्टेसिस) गुहा में छेद में से तरल बाहर निकालना। Puncture of a cavity and aspiration of fluid from it.

Centigram (सेन्टीग्राम) ग्राम का सौंवा भाग। Hundredth part of a gram.

Centiliter (सेन्टीलीटर) लीटर का सौंवा भाग। Hundredth part of a liter.

Centimeter (सेन्टीमीटर) मीटर का सौंवा भाग। Hundredth part of a meter.

Centrifugal (सैन्ट्रीफ्यूगल) केन्द्र से दूर जाने वाला। Moving away from the center.

Cephalagra (सिफैलेग्रा) सिर का गठिया। Gout in the head.

Cephalalgia (सिफैलैल्जिया) सिर में दर्द। Headache.

Cephalocentesis (सिफैलोसेन्टेसिस) सर्जरी द्वारा सिर में छेद करना। Surgical pumetive of the head.

Cephalogenesis (स्फैलोजेनेसिस) भ्रूणीय अवस्था में सिर का बनना। Formation of the head in the embryonic stage.

Cephalogram (सिफैलोग्राम) सिर का एक्स-रे। X-ray picture of the head.

Cephaloid (सिफैलॉयड) सिर से मिलता-जुलता। Resembling the head.

Cephalomegaly (सिफैलोमिगैली) सिर का बढ़ना। Enlargement of a head.

Cephalomeningitis (सिफैलोमैनिनजाइटिस) सिर और उसकी झिल्ली में मवाद भरना, प्रदाह होना। Inflammation of the brain membrane.

Cephalometer (सिफैलोमीटर) सिर को मापने वाला यंत्र। An apparatus for measuring the head.

Cephalopagus (सिफैलोपेगस) दो बच्चों का सिर जुड़ा होना आपस में और शरीर अलग-अलग होना। Two twins conjoined with fused head but body part separately.

Cephalopathy (सिफैलोपेथी) सिर की कोई बीमारी। Any disease of the head.

Cephalotractor (सेफेलोट्रेक्टर) प्रसव के समय भ्रूण के सिर को बाहर निकालने की चिमटी। Forceps for extracting the head of fetus.

Cephalotribe (सिफैलोट्राइव) भ्रूण के सिर को कुचलने का यंत्र। An instrument to crush the fetal head.

Cephalotripsy (सिफैलोट्रिपसी) भ्रूण का सिर कुचलना। The crushing of the fetal head.

Cera (सीरा) मोम। Wax.

Cereals (सीरीयल्स) अनाज। Grains.

Cerebral anoxia (सेरीब्रल अनॉक्सिया) सिर में O_2 की कमी आना। Lack of O_2 in the brain.

Cerebrasthenia (सेरेब्रसथेनिया) दिमागी कमजोरी। Weakness of mind.

Cerebration (सेरेब्रेसन) मानसिक सक्रियता। Mental activity.

Cerebrifugal (सेरीब्रीफ्यूगल) सेरीब्रम से दूर जाने वाला। Proceeding away from the cerebrum.

Cerebripetal (सेरीब्रीपीटल) सेरीब्रम की ओर जाने वाला। Proceeding towards the cerebrum.

Cerebritis (सेरीब्रइटिस) सिर का प्रदाह, सूजन। Inflammation of the brain.

Cerebroid (सेरीब्रॉयड) सेरीब्रम से मिलता-जुलता। Resembling the cerebrum.

Cerebromalacia (सेरेब्रोमलेसिया) दिमाग, सिर की कोमलता। Softening of the brain.

Cerebropathy (सेरीब्रोपेथी) सिर का रोग। Any disease of the brain.

Cerebrosclerosis (सेरेब्रोसक्ले. रोसिस) सिर की कठोरता। Hardening of the brain.

Cerebrotomy (सेरीब्रोटोमी) सिर में चीरा लगाना। To make an incision in the brain.

Cerebrum (सेरीब्रम) अनुमस्तिष्क। The posterior brain.

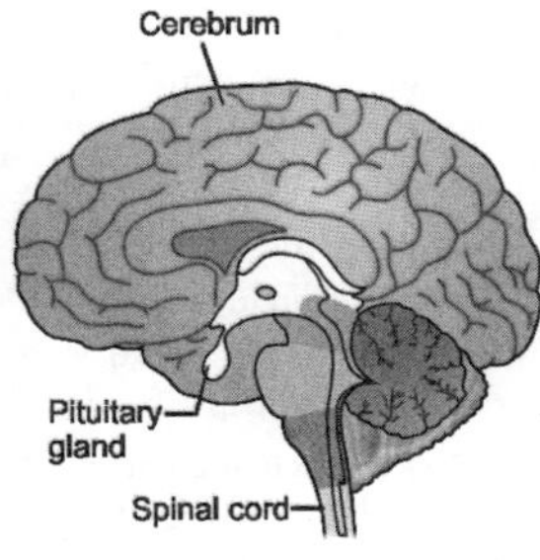

Cerumen (सेरूमेन) कान का मैल। Earwax.

Ceruminolytic (सेरूमिनोलाइटिक) कान के मैल को मुलायम करने के लिए डाला जाने वाला पदार्थ। A substance instilled into the ear to soften the wax.

Ceruminosis (सेरूमिनोसिस) कान में ज्यादा मैल बनना। Excessive secreation of cerumen.

Cervical (सरवाइकल) गर्दन। Pertaining to the neck or to the cervix.

Cervicectomy (सर्विसेक्टॉमी) गर्भाशय ग्रीवा को काटकर निकाल देना। Excision of the cervix of the uterus.

Cervicocolpitis (सर्वाइकोकोलपाइटिस) गर्भाशय ग्रीवा एंव योनि का सूजन। Inflammation of the cervix and the vagina.

Cervicodynia (सर्वाइकोडाइनिया) गर्दन में दर्द होना। Pain in the neck.

Cervicoplasty (सर्वाइक्लोप्लास्टी) गर्भाशय की प्लास्टिक सर्जरी करना। Plastic surgery of the uterine cavity.

Cervicovesical (सर्वाइकोवैसाइकल) गर्भावस्था ग्रीवा एंव मूत्राशय से सम्बन्धित। Pertaining to the cervix of the uterus and urinary bladder.

Cestode (कैस्टोड) एक प्रकार की फीताकृमि। A type of tapeworm.

Cestodiasis (कैस्टोडियासिस) फीताकृमि से उत्पन्न होने वाली बीमारी। Infestation with tapeworm.

Chagrin (केग्रीन) घोर निराशा। Acute disappointment.

Chalinoplasty (कैलिनोप्लास्टी) मुँह और होंठों की प्लास्टिक सर्जरी। Plastic surgery of the mouth and lips.

Chamber (चैम्बर) कोई भी बंद स्थान। Any closed space.

Chamecephalic (कैमेसिफैलिक) चपटे सिर वाला। Having a flat head.

Chameprosopic (कैमेप्रोसोपिक) चौड़े चेहरे वाला। Having a broad face.

Chapped (चैप्ड) सूजी हुई, खुरदरी, फटी हुई त्वचा।

The inflamed, rangened and fissured slam.

Charlatan (चारलेटान) वह व्यक्ति जो झूठी योग्यता का प्रदर्शन करता है। The person who pretends to have a special knowledge in medical line.

Chasma (कैज्मा) एक छिद्र अथवा दरार। An opening or a cleft.

Chastisment (कास्टीसमेन्ट) सजा। Punishment.

Cheese (चीज़) पनीर। The coagulum of milk compressed into a solid mass.

Cheesy (चीज़ी) पनीर से मिलता-जुलता। Resembling the cheese.

Cheilectropion (कीलेक्ट्रोपियोन) होंठ का बाहर की ओर उलट जाना। Eversion of the lip.

Cheilitis (कीइलाइटिस) होंठ की सूजन। Inflammation of the lip.

Cheilophagia (कीलोफेजिया) किसी का अपना होठ काटने की आदत। Habit of bitting one's own lip.

Cheiloplasty (कीलीप्लास्टी) होंठों की प्लास्टिक सर्जरी। Plastic surgery upon the lips.

Cheilorrhaphy (कीलीरैह्फी) फटे हुए होंठ की सर्जरी करके मरम्मत करना। Repair of the cleft lip by surgery.

Cheilotomy (कीलीटोमी) होंठ में चीरा लगना। Incision into the lip.

Cheiralgia (कीरैल्जिया) हाथ में दर्द होना। Pain in the hand.

Cheirathritis (कीरारथ्राइटिस) हाथों व अंगुलियों के जोड़ों में सूजन। Inflammation in the joints of hands and fingers.

Cheiroagra (कीरोएग्रा) हाथों का गठिया। Gout in the hands.

Cheiromegaly (कीरोमगैली) हाथों एवं अंगुलियों का असामान्य रूप से बढ़ जाना। Abnormal enlargement of the hands and fingers.

Cheiroplasty (कीरोप्लास्टी) हाथ पर प्लास्टिक सर्जरी करना। Plastic surgery on the hand.

Cheiropodalgia (कीरोपोडैल्जिया) हाथ व पैरों में दर्द। Pain in the hands and feet.

Chemical (केमीकल) रसायन विज्ञान सम्बन्धी। Relating to chemistry.

Chemocoagulation (कीमोकौगुलेशन) रासायनिक कारक द्वारा जमाना। To coagulate by some chemical agent.

Chemolysis (कीमोलाइसिस) रासायनिक क्रिया द्वारा नष्ट होना। Destruction by chemical action.

Chemoprophylaxis (कीमाप्रोफाइलेक्सिस) रासायनिक पदार्थो द्वारा बीमारी को रोकना। Prevention of disease by administration of chemicals.

Chemosensitive (कीमोसेनसिटिव) रासायनिक परिवर्तन के प्रति-प्रतिक्रिया करना। Reacting to a chemical charge.

Chemosis (कीमोसिस) आँखों की श्लेष्मा झिल्ली में सूजन। Inflammatory swelling of the conjunctiva.

Chemotherapeutics (कीमोथिराप्यूटिक) रसायन-चिकित्सा से सम्बन्धी। Pertaining to chemotherapy.

Chenopodium oil (कीनोपोडियम ऑयल) बथुये का तेल। An anthelmintic.

Chemosurgery (कीमोसर्जरी) किसी रासायनिक यौगिक द्वारा ऊतकों का नष्ट होना। Destruction of tissues by the use of a chemical compound.

Chest (चेस्ट) छाती या सीना। The thorax.

Chest thump (चेस्ट थम्प) दिल का काम करना बंद करने पर सीने पर मुक्का मारना। A sharp blow to the chest in the precordial area in an attempt to restore the normal heart beat in pts cardiac arrest.

Chiasma (कियाज्मा) एक-दूसरे को काटना। X-shaped crossing or decussation.

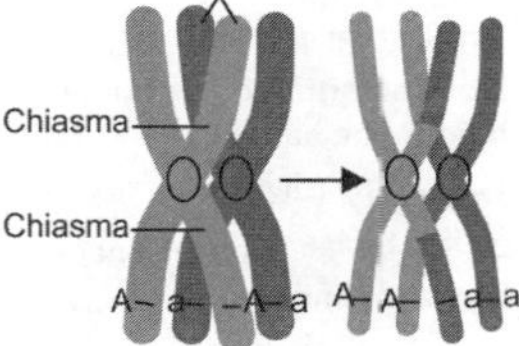

Chickenfat Clot (चिकनफेट क्लोट) खून का पीला थक्का। A yellowish blood clot.

Chickenpox (चिकन पौक्स) छोटी माता। A vesicular eruption of the body.

Chilalgia (कीलैल्जिया) होंठो में दर्द होना। Pain in lips.

Child bearing (चाइल्ड बियरिंग) गर्भ एवं प्रसव। Pregnancy and parturition.

Childbed fever (चाइल्डबैड फीवर) प्रसूति ज्वर। Puerperal sepsis.

Chill (चिल) ठंड लगने के साथ कांपना। A feeling of cold with shivering.

Chin (चिन) ठोढ़ी, निचले जबड़े को होंठ के नीचे का भाग। The portion of the lower jaw below the lip.

Chip (चिप) किसी वस्तु का छोटा टुकड़ा। Small piece of things.

Chiragra (चीराग्रा) हाथों का गठिया। Gout in the hands.

Chiralgia (चिराल्जिया) नाड़ी से सम्बन्धित हाथ में होने वाला दर्द। Nontraulantics or neuralgic pain in the hand.

Chiromegaly (चीरोमेगैली) हाथ-पैरों का बढ जाना। Enlargement of the hands and feet.

Chiroplasty (चीरोप्लास्टी) हाथ की प्लास्टिक सर्जरी। Plastic surgery of the hand.

Chiropodist (कीरोपोडिस्ट) पैरों की चिकित्सा करने वाला व्यक्ति। The person who practices in chiropody.

Chirospasm (चीरोस्पाज्म) लिखते समय हाथ का कांपना। Spasm of the muscles of the hand.

Chloral (क्लोरल) तेज गंध वाला वर्णहीन द्रव्य। Hypnotic.

Chloridorrhea (क्लोराइडोरिया) दस्त लगना, मल में क्लोराइड की मात्रा ज्यादा होना। Diarrhea, with an excess of chlorids in the stools.

Chloriduria (क्लोराइडयूरिया) मूत्र में क्लोराइड की अधिकता। Excess of chlorids in the urine.

Chloroform (क्लोरोफार्म) बेहोश करने वाला पदार्थ। Anesthetic and internally as a narcotic.

Chloroma (क्लोरोमा) हरे रंग की गाढ, गूमड़ी। The tumor having greenish color.

Chloropenia, Hypochloremia (क्लोरोपीनिया, हाइपोक्लोरीमिया) खून में क्लोराइड की कमी होना। Deficiency of chloride in the blood.

Chloropenic (क्लोरोपेनिक) क्लोरीन में कमी आना। Deficiency in chlorine.

Chlorophenothane (क्लोरोफीनोथेन) कीटनाशक डी. डी.टी. पाउडर। The insecticide DDT powder.

Chloropia, chloropsia (क्लोरोपिया, क्लोरोप्सिया) आँखों में दोष से सभी चीजें हरी दिखाई देना। Defect of vision in all things appear green.

Cholangiotomy (कोलन्जियोटॉमी) पथरी को निकालने के लिए पित्त नली में चीरा लगाना। Incision into a bile duct.

Cholecyst (कोलीसिस्ट) पित्ताशय। The gallbladder.

Cholecystalgia (कोलीसिस्टैल्जिया) पित्ताशय में दर्द उठना। Biliary colic.

Cholecystectomy (कोलीस्टिेक्टॉमी) ऑपरेशन से पित्ताशय को काटकर निकाल देना।

Removal of the gallbladder by operation

Cholecystocolotomy (कोलीसिस्टोकोलोटॉमी) पित्ताशय एवं बड़ी आंत में चीरा लगाना। An incision into the gallbladder and the colon.

Cholecystolithiasis (कोलीसिस्टोलिथिएसिस) पित्ताशय में पथरी। Stone in the gallbladder.

Cholecystoptosis (कोलीसिस्टोप्टो. सिस) पित्ताशय का अपने स्थान से नीचे की ओर हट जाना। Downward displacement of the gallbladder.

Cholecystorrhaphy (कोलीसिस्टोरैह्फी) पित्ताशय की सिलाई करना। Suture of the gallbladder.

Choledochectomy (कोलीडोकेक्टॉमी) पित्त वाहिनी के किसी भाग को काटकर निकाल देना। Excision of a part of the common bile duct.

Cholemesis (कोलीमेसिस) पित्त की उल्टी होना। Vomiting of bile.

Cholemia (कोलीमिया) खून में पित्त होना। Presence of bile or bile pigment in the blood.

Cholepoiesis (कोलेपोइसिस) पित्त का बढ़ना। The production of bile.

Cholepoietic (कोलोपोइटिक) पित्त पैदा करने वाला। Producing bile.

Choleric (कोलेरिक) बिना किसी कारण के चिड़चिड़ा होना। To become irritable with antomy apparent cause.

Choleriform (कॉलेरीफॉर्म) हैजे से मिलता-जुलता। Resembling cholera.

Choleromania (कोलेरोमेनिया) हैजे के दौरान होने वाला पागलपन। Madness occasionally seen in cholera.

Cholerophobia (कोलेरोफोबिया) हैजे से होने वाला डर। A morbid fear of cholera.

Cholestatic (कोलेस्टेटिक) पूरी तरह से रोक देना। Diminishing or stopping the flow of bile.

Cholestrol (कोलेस्ट्रोल) खून में वसा। The most abundant steroid in animal tissue.

Cholongiectasis (कोलन्जिएकटेसिस) पित्त वाहिनी का चौड़ा हो जाना। Dilatation of a bile duct.

Cholorrhea (कोलोरिह्या) पित्त का ज्यादा होना। Formation of bile in excess.

Chondric (कॉण्ड्रिक) किसी उपास्थि से सम्बन्धी। Pertaining to a cartilage

Chondralgia (कॉण्ड्रेल्जिया) किसी उपास्थि में दर्द। Pain in a cartilage.

Choroid (कोरोइड) आँख का मध्य भाग जो स्कलेस व रेटिना में स्थित होता है।
The pigmented vascular layer of the eyeball between the retina and the sclera.

Choroidal (कोरॉयडल) रंजितपटल से सम्बन्धित। Pertaining to the choroid.

Choroidoiritis (कोरॉयडोआइराइटिस) कोरॉयड एवं आइरिस का शोथ। Inflammation of the choroid and the iris.

Choroidoretinitis (कोरॉयडोरेटीनाइटिस) कोरॉयड एवं रेटिना का शोथ। Inflammation of the choroid and the retina.

Chromatic (क्रोमेटिक) रंग से सम्बन्धित। Pertaining to color.

Chromatin (क्रोमेटिन) रंग। Color.

Chromatinolysis (क्रौमेटिनोलाइसिस) क्रौमेटिन का नष्ट होना। Destruction of chromatin.

Chromatinorrhexis (क्रौमेटिनोरैह्क्सिस) क्रौमेटिन के टुकड़े-टुकड़े हो जाना। Fragmentation of the chromatin.

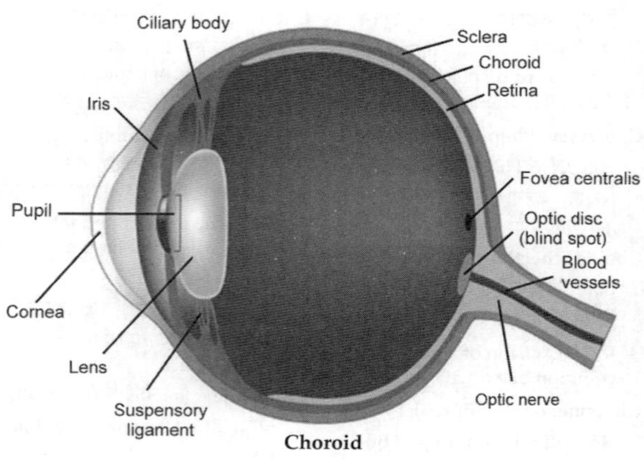

Choroid

Chromatism (क्रौमेटिज्म) रंग का बोध होने का वहम् होना। Hallucination for perception of color.

Chromatogenous (क्रौमेटोजीनस) रंग उत्पन्न करने वाला।
Producing color.

Chromatometer (क्रोमेटोमीटर) रंग मापक यंत्र। An instrument for measuring color perception or the intensity of the color.

Chromatopsia (क्रोमेटोपसिया) रंग-विशेष की अस्वभाविक अनुभूति। Abnormal sensation of color.

Chromatosis (क्रोमेटोसिस) त्वचा की अस्वभाविक रंजकता। An abnormal pigmentation of the skin.

Chromaturia (क्रोमेटूरिया) मूत्र का अप्राकृत वर्ण। Abnormal color of the urine.

Chromesthesia (क्रौमेस्थेसिया) रंग संवेदनाओं का शब्दों, स्वाद, गंध, आवाज सें सम्बन्धित। Association of color sensation of words, taste, smell or sounds.

Chromidrosis (क्रोमाइड्ररोसिस) रंगीन पसीना आना। The secretion of colored sweat.

Chromodacryorrhea (क्रोमोडेक्रीओरिहिया) खून से युक्त आंसूओं का बहना। The flow of bloody tears.

Chromogenesis (क्रोमोजेनेसिस) वर्णक का बनना। Formation of pigment.

Chromonychia (क्रोमोनिकीया) नाखूनों के रंग में असामान्यता। Abnormality in the color of the nails.

Chromophore (क्रोमोफोर) स्वयं को आँख में रंग के एक धब्बे की अनुभूति होना। Subjective sensation of a color spot on the eye.

Chromosomal (क्रोमोजोमल) गुणसूत्री। Pertaining to the chromosome.

Chromotherapy (क्रोनोथिरैपी) रंगीन प्रकाश द्वारा बीमारी की चिकित्सा। Treatment of disease by colored light.

Chuilitis (कीलाइटिस) होंठों की सूजन।
Inflammation of the lips.

Cilia (सीलिया) पलकें। The hair of the eyelids.

Ciliogenesis (सिलियोजेनेसिस) रोमों का बनना। Formation of cillia.

Cilosis (सीलियोसिस) ऊपर की पलकों में ऐठन से युक्त कम्पन होना। A spasmodic trembling of the upper eyelids.

Cinder (सीनडर) भस्म, राख। Ash.

Cinematics (साइनेमेटिक्स) गति-विज्ञान। Science of motion.

Cinematoradiography (साइनेमेटोरेडियोग्राफि) किसी अंग का गति करते हुए उसका एक्स-रे लेना। X-ray of an organ in motion.

Circadian (सर्कैडियन) लगभग 24 घंटे के अंतराल पर उत्पन्न होने वाला। Occuring at about 24 hrs intervals.

Circohoral (सकौरल) एक घण्टे में एक बार पैदा होने वाला। Occurring once in an hour.

Circoid (सर्कायड) सर्प की आकृति। Snake live.

Circulatory (सर्कुलेटरी) संचार सम्बन्धी। Pertaining to the circulation.

Circum (सर्कम) उपसर्ग जिसका अर्थ चारों ओर। Prefix meaning around.

Circumarticular (सर्कमआर्टिकुलर) किसी जोड़ के चारों ओर। Around a joint.

Circumcision (सर्कमसिजन) शिश्न के आगे की चमड़ी काटना। Excision of the prepuce or foreskin.

Circumflex (सर्कमफ्लेक्स) गोलमोल। Surrounding.

Circumoral (सर्कमओरल) मुँह के चारों ओर। Perioral around the mouth.

Cirrhotic (सिरोहटिक) सिरोहसिस से सम्बन्धित। Pertaining to cirrhoris.

Cirsoid (सिरसॉयड) चौड़ी व टेढ़ी-मेढ़ी शिरा के जैसा। Pertaining to or suffering from resembling varix, varicose.

Cirsomphalos (र्ससमफेलोस) नाभि की शिरा का फूल जाना।

The presence of varicose vein around and umbilicus.

Cirsotome (सिरसोटोम) अपस्फीत शिराओं को काटने वाला यंत्र। An instrument for cutting the varicose urine.

Cistern (सिस्टर्न) फैसला, तरल को इकट्ठा रखने वाला भाग। A dilation, a receptacle for storage of fluid.

Cisterna (सिस्टर्ना) एक थैली। A sac or cavity.

Citrus Aurantium (सिटरस ओरेनटियम) संतरे का पेड़। An orange tree.

Citrus limonia (सिटरस लिमोनीया) नींबू का पेड़। A lemon tree.

Clairvoyance (क्लायरवोयेन्स) दूर की सोचने वाला। The extrasensory perception of objective events.

Clammy (कलेमी) चिपचिपा। Sticky, Adhesive.

Clarificant (क्लेरीफिकेन्ट) शोषक। A substance for clearing a solution.

Clarification (क्लेरीफिकेशन) शोषण। The process of purifying or refining.

Clasp (क्लैस्प) ऐसा उपकरण जिसके द्वारा किसी वस्तु को पकड़ा जाता है। An apparatus by with something is hold.

Clastic (क्लेस्टीक) टुकड़े करने वाला। Divided into parts.

Clastothrix (क्लेस्टोथ्रिक्स) बालों का खंडन होना। Splitting of the hair.

Claudication (क्लाउडिकेशन) लंगड़ापन। Lameness.

Claustrophobia (क्लास्ट्ररोफोबिया) किसी घिरे हुए स्थान का आतंक। A morbid dread of an enclo-sed space.

Clavicle (क्लेवीकल) हॅसुली। Collar-bone.

Clavicles (क्लेवीकल्स) हॅसुली, कॉलरबोन। Collar bones, which makes shoulder joint.

Clavicotomy (क्लैविकोटॉमी) शल्य-क्रिया द्वारा कलेविमल हड्डी का विभाजन होना। Surgical division of the clavicle bone.

Clavipedis (क्लेवीपेडिस) कील। Corn.

Clavus (क्लेवस) नाखून। A nail.

Cleaver (क्लीयावर) काटने के लिए एक भारी चाकू। A heavy knife for cutting.

Cleft (क्लेफ्ट) दरार। A fissure.

Clenching (क्लैंचिग) दांत पीसने वाला। Grinding the teeth.

Click (क्लिक) बहुत ही कम समय के लिए उत्पन्न होने वाली आवाज। A sharp short sound heard during a joint movement.

Climacophobia (क्लाइमैंकोफोबिया) ऊपर चढने का डर। Morbid fear of climbing up.

Climacteric (क्लाइमेक्ट्रिक) स्त्री में जननकाल की समाप्ति, पुरूष में लैंगिक सक्रियता। The end of the reproductive in female, a diminution of sexual activity in the male.

Clinodactyly (क्लाइनोडेक्टेली) उंगलियों का अस्वभाविक टेढ़ापन। An abnormal flexure of fingers or toes.

Cliteridectomy (क्लाइटेरिडेक्टोमी) क्लाइटोरिस को काटकर निकाल देना। Excision of the clitoris.

Clitoritis (क्लाइटोराइटिस) क्लाइटोरिस की सूजन। Inflammation of the clitoris.

Clitoromegaly (क्लाइटोरोमेगैली) क्लाइटोरिस का बढ़ना। Enlargement of the clitoris.

Clitorplasty (क्लाइटोर्प्लास्टी) क्लाइटोरिस की प्लास्टिक सर्जरी। Plastic surgery of the clitoris.

Clonic (क्लोनिक) पेशियों का सिकुड़ना। Pertaining to clonus.

Clonicity (क्लोनीसिटी) अवमोटनीय होने की दशा। Condition of being clonic.

Clot (क्लोट) थक्का जमना। A mass of thickened blood.

Clounism (क्लोवनिजम) अकड़ना। The hysteric display of contortions and poses.

Clubbed-finger (क्लबड फिंगर) ऊंगली के कोमल ऊत्तक में सूजन। Swelling of the soft tissue at the extremities.

Clunes (क्लून्स) नितम्ब। The buttocks.

CM (सी.एम.) कल सुबह को। Cras mane, tomorrow morning.

CM (सी.एम.) सेन्टीमीटर। Centimeter.

CM² (सी एम स्क्वायर) वर्ग सेन्टीमीटर। Square centimeter.

CM³ (सी एम क्यूब) घन सेन्टीमीटर। Cubic centimeter.

C/min (सी/मिन) प्रतिमिनट संख्या। Counts per minute.

CMO (सी.एम.ओ.) मुख्य चिकित्सा अधिकारी। Chief medical officer.

CN (सी.एन.) कल रात को। Cras nocte, tomorrow night.

Cnemis (स्नेमिस) पैर का नीचे का भाग, टिबिया हड्डी। Lower leg, tibia bone.

Cnemitis (स्नेमाइटिस) टिबिया हड्डी में सूजन। Inflammation of the tibia.

Cnemoscoliosis (स्नेमोस्केलियोसिस) पैर का पार्श्व में झुकना। Bending the leg lateral side.

CNS (सी.एन.एस.) केन्द्रीय तंत्रिका तंत्र। Central nervous system.

CO (को) कार्बन मोनोक्सॉइड का प्रतीक। Symbol for carbon monoxide.

CO_2 (सीओटू) कार्बनडाइऑक्साइड Formula for carbon dioxide.

Coagulable (कोएगुलेबल) थक्का बनने की क्षमता। Capable of being clotting.

Coagulant (कोएगुलेन्ट) तरल पदार्थ को जमाना। Coagulation of a fluid.

Coagulometer (कोएगुलोमीटर) रक्त के जमने में लगे समय को मापने वाला यंत्र, मशीन। An apparatus for measuring the blood coagulation time.

Coagulopathy (कोएगुलोपैथी) रक्त के जमने में किसी भी तरह की गड़बड़ी। Any defect in blood clotting.

Coalescence (कोएलेसेन्स) दो से अधिक अंगों का मिलना। The union of 2 or more parts.

Coapt (कोएप्ट) पास-पास लाना। To bring together as in suturing the edges of a wound.

Coarctate (कोआर्कटेट) आपस में दबाना। To press together.

Coarctotomy (कोआर्कटोटॉमी) किसी आकृति का विभाजन करना। Cutting or division of a structure.

Coarse (कोआर्स) खर्खर। Gross, not fine.

Coat (कोट) झिल्ली। The membrane covering a part.

Cobalamin (कोबेलेमिन) विटामिन बी$_{12}$। The general term for compounds containing Vit B_{12}.

Coccobacillus (कॉकोबेसिलस) छोटा तथा मोटा जीवाणु। Short and thick bacterium.

Coccydynia (कॉक्सीजडानिया) कॉक्सिक्स में दर्द होना। Pain in the coccyx.

Coccygectomy (कॉक्सीजेक्टॉमी) कॉक्सिक्स को काटकर निकाल देना। Excision of the coccyx.

Coceal (कॉकल) गोलाणुओं द्वारा उत्पन्न। Pertaining to or caused by colei.

Coceoid (कॉकॉयड) गोलाणु से मिलता-जुलता। Resembling a coccus.

Cochin-leg (कोचिन-लेग) हाथी-पैर। Elephantiasis.

Cochlea (काक्लिया) कर्णावर्त, कान की मध्य का भाग। A spiral tube of ear filled with fluid.

Cochleariform (कॉक्लियरीफॉर्म) चम्मच की शक्ल का। Spoon-shaped.

Cochlitis (कॉक्लाइटिस) कॉक्लिया की सूजन। Inflammation of the cochlea.

Coctostabile (कॉक्टोस्टेबिल) गर्म करने पर भी कोई परिवर्तन नहीं होना। Incapable of being altered.

Cohabitation (कोहेवीटेशन) संभोग। Copulation.

Cohesion (कोहेसन) आकर्षण। The attraction of aggregation.

Cohesiveness (कोहेसिवनेस) जुड़े रहने की योग्यता। The ability of cohesia.

Coital (कॉयटल) लैंगिक संसर्ग से सम्बन्धित। Pertaining to the sexual intercourse.

Coitophobia (कॉयटोफोबिया) लैंगिक संसर्ग से डर। Morbid fear of sexual intercourse.

Coitus (कोइटस) संभोग, सहवास। Act of venery, coition.

Colacixe (कोलेयक्सी) बड़ी आँत का फैलना। The dilatation of the colon.

Colectasia (कोलेक्टेसिया) आँत का फूल जाना। Distension of the colon.

Colectomy (कोलेक्टॉमी) बड़ी आँत के भाग को काट कर निकाल देना। The excision of a portion of colon.

Colfixation (कोलफिक्सेशन) नीचे गिरे कोलन को ऊपर लटका कर सर्जरी द्वारा स्थिरीकरण करना। The fixation or suspension of the colon in the treatment of ptosis.

Colic (कोलिक) दर्द से पीड़ित। Pertaining to or affected by pain. Severe pain in abdomen caused by obstruction in intestines.

Colipuncture (कोलीपंक्चर) कोलन के फुलाव को कम करने के लिए सर्जरी द्वारा छोटा सा छेद बनाना। Surgical puncture of the colon to relieve distension.

Colocentesis (कोलोसेन्टेसिस) कोलन के फुलाव को कम करने के लिए सर्जरी द्वारा छोटा सा छेद बनाना। Surgical puncture of the colon to relieve distension.

Colitis (कोलाइटिस) बड़ी आंत में सूजन। Inflammation of large colon.

Colla (कोला) बहुवचन। Plural of collum.

Collagen (कोलेजन) श्वेत तन्तुओं की एक अघुलनशील प्रॉटीन जो त्वचा, कण्डरा, हड्डी, उपास्थि अन्य सभी संयोजी ऊतकों में पाई जाती है। An insoluble protein of white fiber found in skin, tendon, bone, cartilage, ligament and all other connective tissue.

Collagenitis (कोलेजेनाइटिस) कोलेजन में दर्द व सूजन होना। Inflammation of the cologen fibers.

Collagenolytic (कोलेजीनोलाइटिक) कोलेजन को घोल देने वाला। Dissolution of the collagen.

Collagenous (कोलेजीनस) कोलेजन उत्पन्न करने वाला। Producing or containing collagen.

Collapsing (कोलैप्सिंग) सदमें में आकर चित पड़ जाना कमजोर व्यक्ति का। The person suddenly falling into extreme prostration like shock.

Colliculus (कोलीक्यूलस) छोटा सा उभार। A small eminence.

Collilongus (कोलीलोन्गस) गर्दन की बड़ी पेशी। The long muscle of the neck.

Colliquative (कोलीक्यूएटीव) प्रचुर। Excessive.

Colloid cyst (कोलॉयड सिस्ट) थैली जो लसलसे तरल से भरी होती है। A sac containing a jelly like liquid.

Colloidal (कोलॉयडल) कोलॉयड से सम्बन्धित। Pertaining to or characteristic of a colloid.

Collopexia (कोलोपैक्सिया) गर्भाशयग्रीवा का स्थिरीकरण। Fixation of the cervix of the uterus.

Collum (कोलम) गर्दन। The neck.

Collunarium (कौलूनेरियम) नासा-धोवन। A nose-wash.

Collyrium (कोलीरियम) आँखों में डालने की दवा। A lotion for the eyes.

Coloboma (कोलोबोमा) मंत्रविदर। A fissure, especially the parts of the eye.

Colon (कोलन) बड़ी आँत, मलाशय। Large intestine, from the cecum to rectum.

Colonalgia (कोलोनल्जिया) कोलन में दर्द होना। Pain in the colon.

Colonic (कोलोनिक) कोलन सम्बन्धी। Relating to the colon.

Colonopathy (कोलोनोपैथी) कोलन का कोई भी रोग। Any disease of the colon.

Colonorrhagia (कोलोनोरेह्जिया) कोलन संरक्त का स्राव। Hemorrhage from the colon.

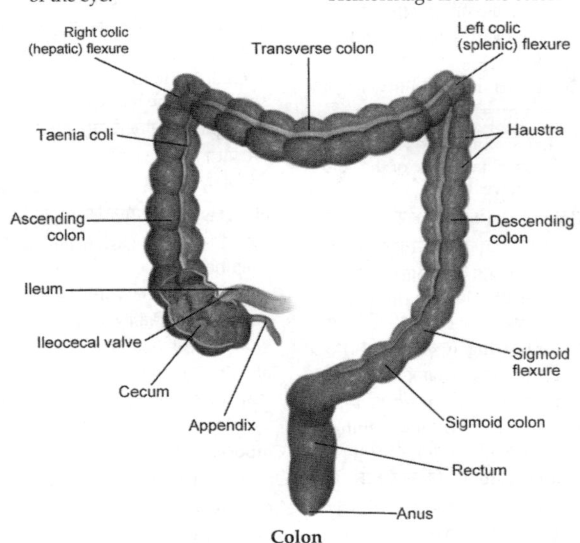

Colon

Colonorrhea (कोलोनोरिह्या) कोलन से पानी जैसा स्राव निकलना। Watery discharge from colon.

Colonoscopy (कोलोनोस्कोपी) कोलन का नेत्रों से परीक्षण करना। Visual examination of colon by colonoscopy.

Coloproctitis (कोलोप्रोक्टाइटिस) बड़ी आंत व मलाशय में जलन। Inflammation of the colon and rectum.

Coloptosis (कोलोप्टोसिस) कोलन का नीचे खिसक जाना। Downward displacement of the colon.

Colopuncture (कोलोपंक्चर) फुलाव को कम करने के लिए सर्जरी द्वारा कोलन में छेद करना। Surgical puncture of the colon to relieve distension.

Color gustation (कलर जस्टेशन) किसी वस्तु को चखने से उसके रंग का पता चल जाना। The sense of color of a thing, caused by tasting it.

Color hearing (कलर हीयरिंग) किसी वस्तु की आवाज सुन कर उसके रंग का पता चल जाना। The sense of color of a things caused by hearing its sound.

Colorectostomy (कोलोरेक्टोस्टॉमी) कोलन व मलाशय के बीच एक रास्ता बनाना। Formation of a passage between the colon and the rectum.

Colorrhaphy (कोलोरैह्फी) कोलन को टांका लगाना। Suture of the colon.

Colostrum (कोलस्ट्रम) माँ का पहला गाढ़ा पीला दूध। A thin, yellow fluid secreted by the breast.

Colotomy (कोलोटॉमी) बड़ी आंत को काटना। Cutting into colon.

Colovaginal (कोलोवैजाइनल) कोलन व योनि से सम्बन्धी। Pertaining to the colon.

Colovesical (कोलोवैसीकल) कोलन व मूत्राशय से सम्बन्धी। Pertaining to the colon and the bladder.

Colpalgia (कोलपलजिया) योनि में पीड़ा।

Pain in vagina.

Colpectasia (कोलपेक्टेसिया) योनि का फैल जाना। Distension of vagina.

Colpectomy (कोल्पेक्टॉमी) योनि को काटकर निकाल देना। Excision of vagina.

Colpitis (कोल्पाइटिस) योनि का प्रदाह। Inflammation of vagina.

Colpocele (कोल्पोसील) योनि में हर्निया। Hernia into vagina.

Colpocleisis (कोल्पोक्लीसिस) शल्य-क्रिया द्वारा योनि को बंद

कर देना। To close the vagina by surgery.

Colpo-colp (कोल्पो-कोल्प) योनि से सम्बन्धित एक उपसर्ग। A prefix pertaining to the vagina.

Colpocystotomy (कोल्पोसिस्टोटॉमी) योनि से होते हुए मूत्राशय में चीरा लगाना। To make an incision into the urinary bladder through the vagina.

Colpodynia (कोल्पोडाइनिया) योनि में दर्द होना। Pain in the vagina.

Colpopexy (कोल्पोपैक्सी) योनिस्थिरीकरण। Vaginofixation.

Colpoplasty (कोल्पोप्लास्टी) योनिकी प्लास्टिक सर्जरी। Plastic surgery of the vagina.

Colpoptosis (कोल्पोप्टोसिस) योनि भ्रंश। Prolapse of the vagina.

Colporrhagia (कोल्पोरेह्जिया) योनि से रक्त स्त्राव होना। Excessive discharge from the vagina or vaginal hemorrhage.

Colporrhaphy (कोल्पोरैह्फी) योनि की भित्ति को सीना। Suturing of the vagina.

Colporrhexis (कोल्पोरेह्क्सिस) योनि भित्ति का फट जाना। Rupture or laceration of the vagina.

Colpospasm (कोल्पोस्पाज्म) योनि की जकड़न। Spasm of the vagina.

Colpostenosis (कोल्पोस्टेनोसिस) योनि का छोटा होना। Narrowing of the vagina.

Colpotomy (कोल्पोटॉनी) योनि में चीरा लगाना। Any incision of the vagina.

Colpoxerosis (कोल्पोजिरोसिस) योनि का असामान्य तरीके से सूख जाना। Abnormal dryness of the vagina.

Coma (कोमा) गहन मूर्च्छा। A prolonged state of deep unconsciousness.

Coma Bacillus (कॉमा बेसीलस) हैजा फैलाने वाला जीवाणु। The Spirillum of asiatic cholera.

Comatose (कॉमाटोस) बेहोश। Affected with or in a condition of coma.

Combustible (कम्बस्टिबिल) जलाया जाने योग्य। Capable of burning.

Combustion (कम्बसन) जलना। The process of oxidation.

Comedo (कॉमेडो) मुहासा। Black head.

Comedogenic (कॉमेडोजेनिक) मुहासें पैदा करने वाला। Producing comedones.

Commensal (कॉमेनसल) अन्य प्रकार के जीवों के साथ रहने

तथा भोजन करने वाला प्राणी। Together of two or more dissimilar organisms.

Comminute (कमीन्यूट) किसी चीज को तोड़कर टुकड़े-टुकड़े कर देना। To break into pieces.

Comminution (कमीन्यूशन) किसी ठोस वस्तु के टूटकर छोटे-छोट टुकड़े हो जाना। Breaking of a solid thing into small pieces.

Commissural (कमीश्रल) किसी संयोजिका से सम्बन्धी। Pertaining to a commissure.

Commissure (कमीशर) संयोग। A Joining or uniting.

Commode (कमोड) मल-मूत्र पात्र। A receptacle for feces and urine.

Common Cold (कॉमन कोल्ड) जुकाम। A virus infection of the paper breathing organ.

Communicating (कमयूनिकेटिंग) संयोजी। Connecting.

Compact (कॉम्पैक्ट) गठीला। Having a dense structure.

Comparative (कम्पैरेटिव) तुलनात्मक। Relating to comparison.

Compatible (कॉमपैटिबिल) अनुकूल। Capable of existing together.

Compensation (कम्पनसेशन) हर्जाना। The state of counter balancing a defect of structure or function.

Complain (कम्पलेन) बीमारी, कष्ट। Any morbid state.

Complement (कोमप्लीमेन्ट) सहायक। Assisting each other.

Complex (कॉमप्लेक्स) उलझा हुआ। Complicated.

Complexion (कॉमप्लेक्शन) हाव-भाव, रंग-रूप। Color, texture general appearance of the face.

Component (कम्पोनेन्ट) घटक। Constituent.

Compos mentis (कोम्पस मेन्टिस) बुद्धिमान। Sound mind.

Comprehension (कॉमप्रिहेन्सन) ज्ञान, समझ। Mental grasp of meaning and relationship.

Compress (कम्प्रेस) दबाव, सेक। Folded cloth for local pressure and dressing the wounds.

Compression (कम्प्रेशन) आपस में दबाने की क्रिया, दबाव डालने वाला। The state of being compressed.

Compressor (कम्प्रेसर) दबाव डालने वाला। An instrument for compressing a vessel.

Concave (कौन्केव) अंदर की ओर घुसा हुआ। Having a depressed or hollowed surface.

Concavoconcave (कौन्केवोकौन्केव) दो विपरीत तलों में से प्रत्येक का खोखलापन होना। Concave on each of the two opposite surface.

Conceive (कन्सीव) गर्भवती होना, कोई विचार बनाना। To become pregnants to form an idea.

Concentric (कन्सैन्ट्रिक) एक केन्द्रिक। Having a common center.

Concept (कन्सैप्ट) दिमाग में किसी वस्तु के लिए बना विचार। An idea formed of a thing in the mind.

Concha (कौन्का) बाह्य कान या कर्णपाली। The external ear or the pinna.

Conchitis (कौन्काइटिस) शुक्तिका शोथ। Inflammation of the concha of the ear and nose. (The depression in the external ear and nose leading to its central opening).

Conchoidal (कौन्कॉयडल) खोली की शक्ल वाला। Having the shape of a small.

Conchoscope (कौन्कोस्कोप) नासिका-गुहा का परीक्षण करने वाला यंत्र। An instrument for examining the nasal cavity.

Conchotomy (कौन्कोटॉमी) किसी नासा-सूक्तिका में चीरा लगाना। Incision of a nasal concha.

Concoction (कौन्कोक्शन) पाचन-क्रिया। The digestive process.

Concomitant (कॉनकमीटैन्ट) इसी समय होने वाला। Occurring at the same time.

Concrete (कन्क्रीट) ठोस बना हुआ। Condensed hardened or solidified.

Condenser (कन्डैन्सर) गैसों तथा द्रवों को ठोस बनाने वाला उपकरण। A device for condensing gas or light.

Concretion (कान्क्रेशन) पथरी। A stone or calcules.

Condense (कन्डैन्स) अधिक गाढ़ा बनाना। To make more dense.

Condiment (कौण्डीमैन्ट) वह पदार्थ जो भोजन को स्वादिष्ट बनाता है। Substance who makes the food tasty.

Conduction (कन्डक्शन) चालन, संचार। The transmission of heat, light or sound waves through suitable media.

Conductivity (कन्डक्टीविटी) चालकता, संचारिता। The capacity for conduction.

Condylar (कौन्डाइलर) स्थूलक सम्बन्धी। Pertaining to conduction.

Condyle (कन्डाइल) कीली हड्डी के सिरे पर उभार, जिससे जोड़ बनता है।

(Gr kondylos, knuckle)

Pertaining to a condyle.

Condyloma (कौन्डाइलोमा) मांसगुल्स। Condylomata a cuminata; venerea warts; anal warts; anogenital warts.

Confinement (कन्फाइन्मैन्ट) प्रसूति काल। The period of child birth.

Conflict (कान्फ्लिक्ट) संघर्ष, दिमाग में दो अलग-अलग इच्छाओं का उठना। The arising of two opposite desires or emotions in the mind.

Confluence (कान्फ्लूएन्स) संगम। A flowing or running together.

Conformation (कन्फोरमेशन) प्राकृतिक आकार, बनावट। The natural shape.

Congenital (कान्जेनाइटल) जन्मजात, आनुवंशिक। Existing right from birth, heredity.

Congested (कनजैस्टेड) खून की अधिक मात्रा से युक्त। Containing an abnormal amount of blood.

Congestive (कन्जैस्टिव) रक्त की अधिकता से सम्बन्धी। Pertaining to congestion.

Conglobation (कौन्गलोबेशन) एक गोल पिण्ड में इकट्ठा होना। Aggregation into a rounded mass.

Coni (कोनाई) बहुवचन। Plural of conus.

Conical (कोनिकल) शंक्वाकार। Cone-shaped.

Conium (कोनियम) जहरीला पेड़ का रस। Poison hemlock.

Conjugate (कोन्ज्यूगेट) संयुग्म। Coupled.

Conjugation (कोन्ज्यूगेशन) संगम। A form of reproduction or cell division.

Conjunctiva (कन्जन्कटाइवा) आँखों की श्लैष्मा झिल्ली। The membrane that covers the eye ball and lines the inner surface of the eyelids.

Conjunctival (कन्जन्कटाइवल) नेत्रश्लेष्मा से सम्बन्धित। Relating to the conjunctiva.

Conjunctivitis (कन्जन्कटीवाइटिस) आँखों की श्लैष्मिक झिल्ली का प्रदाह। Inflammation of the conjunctiva.

Consanguinity (कौन्सेन्ग्यूइनिटी) खून का संबंध। Blood relationship.

Conscience (कौन्साइंस) विवेक। The intense sense of feeling.

Conservation (कन्जरवेशन) हानि होने, क्षति पहुँचने या सड़ने से बचाने के लिए परिरक्षित करना। Preservation from loss, injury or decay.

Consistency (कनसिस्टैन्सी) कठोरता। The density or hardness.

Constant (कौन्सटेन्ट) स्थिर, अपरिवर्तनशील। Not changing.

Constipate (कौन्सटीपेट) कब्ज पैदा करना। To cause constipation.

Constipation (कौन्सटीपेशन) कठिनाई से मल विसर्जित होना। Difficulty in defecation.

Constitution (कौन्सटीट्यूशन) शरीर का गठन एवं इसकी कार्य

सम्बन्धी आदतें। Make-up of the body and its functional habits.

Constricted (कौन्सट्रीक्टेड) सिकुड़ा हुआ। Drawn together in a part.

Constricture (कौन्स्ट्रीक्चर) सिकुड़ने, दबाव देने वाली पेशी। The contracting or compressing.

Constrigent (कौन्सट्रीजेन्ट) कब्जियत करने वाला पदार्थ। Any agent causing bowel obstruction.

Constructive (कौन्सट्रक्टीव) रचनात्मक। Productive.

Consumptive (कन्जम्पटिव) क्षय रोग। Wasting disease tuberculosis.

Contagion (कौन्टेजियोन) छूत से फैलने वाला रोगों का संचार। The communication of disease by contact.

Contagium (कौन्टेजियम) संक्रमण उत्पन्न करने वाला साधन। The agent causing infection.

Contaminant (कौन्टामिनेन्ट) प्रदूषित करना। To cause contamination.

Contamination (कौन्टामिनेशन) संदूषण, दूषण। The act of contaminating.

Contiguity (कौन्टीगुइटी) सम्पर्क। Contact.

Contorted (कॉनटोरटेड) मोड़ा हुआ। Twisted.

Contour (कॉनटूर) किसी भाग की बाह्य रूप रेखा। Outline of a part.

Contra (कॉन्ट्रा) विपरीत अथवा विरूद्ध को बताने वाला उपसर्ग। Prefix signifying opposition.

Contraception (कॉन्ट्रासेप्शन) गर्भनिरोध। Prevention of conception.

Contract (कॉन्ट्रेक्ट) सिकुड़ना। To shrink.

Contractile (कॉन्ट्रेक्टाइल) सिकुड़ने अथवा छोटे होने की क्षमता। Capability of conception.

Contracture (कॉन्ट्रेक्चर) स्थाई, कठोरता की अवस्था। A state of permanent rigidity.

Contuse (कॉन्ट्यूज) अन्दरूनी चोट मारना। To bruise.

Contusion (कॉन्टयूजन) एक प्रकार की रगड़न। A short of abrasion.

Concussion (कन्कसन) आघात। A violent shock or shaking.

Convalescent (कौन्वेलेसेन्ट) ऑपरेशन की समाप्ति के पश्चात पूर्ण स्वास्थ्य लाभ प्राप्त कर रहो हो।

The person recovering from an illness or operation.

Conversion (कन्वरजन) एक स्थिति से दूसरी स्थिति में आने की अवस्था रूपान्तरण।

Transformation of an embryo into a physical manifestation, transmutation.

Convex (कॉन्वैक्स) किनारों पर दबा हुआ लेकिन बीच में उभरा हुआ। Curved outward on the external surface.

Convexoconvex (कॉन्वैक्सोकॉनवेक्स) दोनों ओर से उभरा हुआ। Convex on both surfaces.

Convolute (कॉन्वोल्यूट) लपेटा हुआ। Rolled.

Convoluted (कॉन्वोल्यूटेड) एक भाग का दूसरे पर लिपट जाना। Rolled together with one part over the other.

Convulsion (कन्वलजन) अनैच्छिक पेशीय संकुचन बेहोशी एवं दौरा पड़ना। Involuntary muscle contraction and relaxations.

Coordination (कोऑर्डिनेशन) सामंजस्य। Harmonious action.

Cophosis (कोफोसिस) बहरापन। Loss of hearing.

Copiopia (कोपिओपीआ) आँखों की थकान। The fatigued condition of the eyes.

Copious (कोपियस) अत्यधिक। Excessive.

Copper (कोपर) ताम्बा। A reddish-brown metal.

Coprolalia (कोप्रोलेलिया) गंदी भाषा का प्रयोग करना। Filthy or obscene speech.

Coprolith (कोप्रोलिथ) मलपथरी। Hard fecal concretion in the intestine.

Coprology (कोप्रोलॉजी) मल का अध्ययन। Study of the feces.

Coprophilia (कोप्रोफिलिया) मल में असामान्य रूचि होना। Abnormal interest in feces.

Coprozoa (कोप्रोजोआ) आंत से बाहर मल में पाये जाने वाले एक कोशिकीय जीव। Protozoa found in the feces outside of the intestine.

Copulation (कौपुलेशन) संगम। Sexual intercourse.

Coracoid (कौराकोइड) कौए की चोंच जैसी। Shaped like a crow's beak.

Corclisis (कौरक्लाइसिस) पुतली का बंद होना। Closing of the pupil.

Cord (कॉर्ड) बन्धन। Ligature.

Cordate (कॉर्डेट) हृदय की आकृति का। Heart-shaped.

Cordial (कॉर्डियल) हृदय को उत्तेजित करने वाला। Stimulating the heart.

Corectasis, Corectasia (कौरेक्टेसिस, कौरेक्टेसिया) नेत्रपटल का फैल जाना। Dilation of the pupil.

Coremetry (कोरिमीट्री) आँख की पुतली को मापना। Measuring the pupil of the eyes.

Coreoplasty (कोरियोप्लास्टी) पुतली की प्लास्टिक सर्जरी करना। Plastic surgery of the pupil.

Corn (कोर्न) मस्सा। A horny hardness of the skin.

Cornea (कोर्निया) नेत्र पटल। The transparent coat of front part of eye ball.

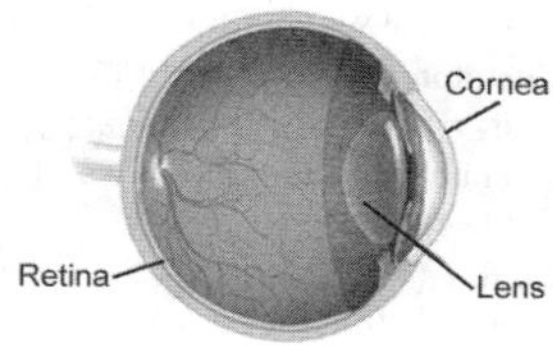

Corneous (कोर्नियस) नुकीला। Corniculata.

Corneum (कोर्नियम) बाहर की त्वचा की सबसे बाहर की परत। Stratum corneum epidermidis, the outmost layer of the epidermis.

Corniculate (कॉर्निकुलेट) जिसमें छोटे-छोटे सींग के समान उभार हो। Containing small horn shaped projections.

Cornification (कॉर्निफिकेशन) कठोर घृंगी पदार्थ में बदल जाना जैसे त्वचा का होता है। Conversion into hard horny material as that of the skin.

Cornified (कॉर्निफाइड) घृंगी ऊतक में परिवर्तित। Converted into horny tissue.

Corolla (कोरोला) फूल का अन्दरूनी आवरण। The intenal part of floral envelope of a flower.

Corona (कोरोना) शिखर। As of the height.

Coroner (कोरोनर) आकस्मिक मृत्यु के कारणों की जांच करने वाला अधिकारी। An officer who holds inquests on those dead from violence.

Corporis (कोरपोरिस) शरीर। The body.

Corpse (कोरप्स) निष्प्राण शरीर। A dead body.

Corpulency (कार्पुलैन्सी) मोटापा। Obesity.

Corpulent (कार्पुलैन्ट) मोटा व्यक्ति। Fatty person.

Corpus (कॉर्पस) किसी अंग का मुख्य भाग। Main part of an organ.

Corpuscle (कॉपुसल) एक छोटा गोल पिण्ड। A small rounded mass.

Correlation (कोरिलेशन) पारम्परिक सम्बन्ध। Interdependance.

Corroborant (कोरोबोरेन्ट) पौष्टिक अथवा बलवर्धक। A tonic invigorating remedy.

Corroding (कोरोडिंग) तीखा, तीखी। Eating away.

Corrugation (कोरूगेशन) झुर्री। Wrinkling.

Corrugator (कोरूगेटर) त्वचा को खींचने वाली पेशी जिससे त्वचा पर झुर्रियां पड़ जाती है। A muscle that wrinkles.

Cortical (कॉर्टिकल) किसी कोर्टेक्स से सम्बन्धित। Pertaining to a cortex.

Corticofugal (कॉटिकोफ्यूगल) बाहरी सतह से दूर जाने वाला। Passing away from the outer surface.

Coryza (कोराइजा) सर्दी-जुकाम। Acute rhinitis.

Cosmesis (कोस्मेसिस) रोगी के रंग-रूप को निखारने के लिए किया जाने वाला ऑपरेशन। An operation performed for the improvement of appearance of the patient.

Cosmetic (कोस्मेटिक) सुन्दर बनाने वाला पदार्थ। A beautifying substance.

Costa (कोस्टा) पसली। A rib.

Costalgia (कोस्टेल्जिया) पसली में दर्द होना। Pain in the rib.

Costectomy (कोस्टेक्टॉमी) किसी पसली को काट कर निकाल देना। Excision of a rib.

Costiform (कोस्टीफार्म) पसली के आकार का। Rib-shaped.

Costive (कोस्टीव) कब्ज करने वाली। Reluctant in speech or action, unforthcoming

Costocervical (कोस्टोसर्वाइकल) पसलियों एवं गर्दन से सम्बन्धित। Pertaining to the ribs and the neck.

Costoinferior (कोस्टोइनफिरीयर) नीचे की पसलियों से सम्बन्धित। Pertaining to the lower ribs.

Costophrenic (कोस्टोफ्रैनिक) पसलियों एवं मध्यपर से सम्बन्धित। Pertaining to the ribs and diaphragm.

Costotome (कोस्टोटोम) किसी पसली को काटने वाला चाकू। A knife for cutting through a rib of cartilage.

Cotton (कोटन) रूई। The seed-hair of many species of gossypium.

Cough (कफ) खांसी। A sudden noisy explosion of air from the lungs through glottis.

Countenance (काउंटेनेन्स) आकृति, मुखाकृति। Complexion, appearance.

Counter shock (काउन्टर शॉक) प्रति-आघात। An electric shock applied to the head to terminate a disturbance of its rhythm.

Counteract (काउन्टरैक्ट) किसी वस्तु के खिलाफ काम करना। To do against something.

Counteraction (काउन्टरैक्शन) रोकथाम। Contrary action.

Counterirritation (काउन्टरइर्रीटेशन) प्रतिक्षोभण। Irritation produced in one part of the body.

Coup (कूप) मुक्का, आघात। A blow, stroke.

Coup De souleil (कूप डी सोयली) लू लगना। Sun-stroke.

Courses (कोर्सज) माहवारी। Menses.

Cover glass (कवर-ग्लास) ढ़कना, ढ़क्कन। A thin glass over the plate, the object on a microscopic slice.

Cow-Pox (काऊ-पोक्स) छोटी माता, गोशीतला। Virus disease of the Cow.

Coxa (कोक्सा) कूल्हा अथवा कूल्हे का जोड़। Hip or hip joint.

Coxalgia (कोक्सैल्जिया) कूल्हें के जोड का दर्द। Pain in the hip joint.

Coxarthropathy (कोक्सारथ्रोपेथी) कूल्हें के जोड़ का कोई भी रोग। Any disease of the hip joint.

Coxitis (कोक्साइटिस) कूल्हें के जोड़ की सूजन। Inflammation of the hip-joint.

Crab (क्रेब) जांघ। The thigh.

Cradle (क्रेडल) पालना, झूला। A semicircle of thin wood, or strips of wood and wire.

Cramp (क्रेम्प) पेशियों का अचानक एवं प्रबल रूप से सिकुडना व दर्द करना। Sudden and violent contraction of the muscles.

Cranial (क्रेनियल) कपाल सम्बन्धी। Pertaining to the cranium.

Cranioaural (क्रेनियोऔरल) कपाल एवं कान से सम्बन्धी। Pertaining to the cranium and the ear.

Craniocele (क्रेनियोसील) मस्तिष्कहर्निया। Encephalocele.

Craniodidymus (क्रेनियाडाइडीमस) संयुक्त जुडवा बच्चे जिनके शरीर जुड़े होते हैं परन्तु सिर दो होते है। Conjoined twins with fused bodies but two heads.

Craniopagus (क्रेनियोपेगस) दो जुड़वा बच्चे जो सिर से जुड़े रहते है। Twins joined at the head.

Craniophor (क्रेनियोफोर) किसी खोपड़ी की माप लेते समय थामे रखने वाला एक उपकरण। An apparatus for holding a skull while taking its measurement.

Craniorachischisis (क्रेनियोरिचिइसचीसीस) खोपड़ी और रीढ का जन्मजात बिदर। Congenital fissure of the skull and spine.

Craniosclerosis (क्रेनियोस्कलेरोसिस) खोपड़ी की कठोरता। A hardening of the cranium.

Craniotabes (क्रेनियोटेब्स) खोपड़ी की हड्डी का पतला पड़ना। Rachitic thinning of the skull.

Cranium (क्रेनियम) खोपड़ी का वह भाग जिसके भीतर मस्तिष्क बंद

रहता है। The portion of the skull which encloses the brain.

Craniomalacia (क्रेनियोमैलेसिया) खोपड़ी की कोमलता। A softening of the skull.

Cras (क्रेस) कल। Tomorrow.

Crasis (क्रेसिस) खून की सामान्य दशा। Normal individual condition of the blood.

Crassamentum (क्रेसमेनटम) थक्का। A clot.

Crater (क्रेटर) कोटर। A sinus.

Crateriform (क्रेटेरीफॉर्म) कोटराकार। Shaped like a bowl.

Craving (क्रेविंग) लालसा। Earnest desire.

Crazy (क्रेजी) पागल। Mad.

Creaking (क्रेकिंग) चरमराहट। Grating sound.

Crease (क्रीज) सिकुड़न। A line made of folding.

Creatinemia (क्रिएटिनीमिया) खून में क्रिएटिन का अधिक मात्रा में पाया जाना। Excess of creatine in the blood.

Cremate (क्रेमेट) शव को जला देना। Burning of a dead body.

Crematorium (क्रेमेटोरियम) शवों को जलाने का स्थान। A place for burning the dead body.

Crena (क्रेना) दरार। A notch or cleft.

Creophagy, Creophagism (क्रियोफेजी, क्रियाफेजिज्म) मांस खाना। The eating of flesh.

Crepitant (क्रेपीटेन्ट) शुष्क एवं फटी हुई आवाज वाला। Having a dry and craig sound.

Crepitus (क्रेपीटस) चरचराहट। The peculiar rattle of pneumonia.

Crescent, Crescentic (क्रिसेन्ट, क्रिसेन्टिक) अर्द्धचन्द्राकार। Shaped like a new moon.

Crest (क्रैस्ट) उभरा हुआ भाग। Forming its principal border.

Cretinism (क्रिएटिनिज्म) बौनापन। A condition of arrested development due to insufficiency of the thyroid gland.

Crevice (क्रिविस) छोटी सी दरार। Small fissure.

Cribriform (क्रिब्रीफोर्म) चलणी के समान। Sieve like.

Cricoid (क्रिकॉयड) छल्ले जैसा। Ring-shaped.

Crik (क्रिक) कोई दर्दनाक तथा ऐंठन युक्त रोग। Any painful spasmodic affection.

Crinogenic (क्रायनोजेनिक) स्रावी। Causing secretion.

Crippled (क्रिपल्ड) विकलांग। Handicapped.

Crisis (क्राइसिस) संकटपूर्ण। The culmination of the symptoms of a disease, either for recovery or death.

Crista (क्रिस्टा) चोटी। A ridge.

Crotalus (क्रोटलस) रेंगने वाला सांप और उसका विष। A rattle snake and also its poison.

Croton (क्रोटन) जमालगोटा। A genus of trees furnishing cascarilla and croton oil.

Croup (क्रोप) स्वरयंत्र की अवरूद्धता के कारण होने वाली अविराम खांसी। Laryngeal obstruction due to inflammation of the larynx and trachea, with dyspnea and membranous deposit.

Crown (क्राऊन) किसी भी दाँत के ऊपर जैसी संरचना का शीर्ष भाग जो दाँत की सुरक्षा करे। The top portion of any organ like teeth.

Cruor (करूर) जमा हुआ खून। Coagulated blood.

Crus (क्रस) टांग जैसी बनावट का। The leg like-structure.

Crush (क्रस) कुचल देना। To make into small fragments.

Crusta (क्रस्टा) पपड़ी। A scab.

Cryalgesia (क्रायेल्जेसिया) ठण्डी वस्तु लग जाने के कारण दर्द होना। Pain from the application of cold.

Cryesthesia (क्रिस्थेसिया) अतिसंवेदनशीलता। Abnormal sensitiveness to cold.

Cryolysis (क्राइयोलाइसिस) ठण्ड से नष्ट कर देना। Destruction by cold.

Cryptogam (क्रिप्टोगम) ऐसे पौधे जिनमें फूल नहीं लगते। A flowerless plant.

Cryptopyic (क्रिप्टोपाइक) जिसके शरीर के भीतर ही भीतर पस पड़ गया हो। Having concealed suppuration.

Crystallization (क्रिस्टालाइजेशन) दानों का बनना। Formation of the crystals.

CS (सी.एस.) सिजेरियन सैक्सन। Cesarean section.

CSF (Cerebrospinal fluid) (सी. एस.एफ.) सेरीब्रोस्पाइनल फ्लूड की एक द्रव जो मस्तिष्क एंव सुशमारज्जु को चोट से बचाता है। A fluid protect the brain and spinal cord from injury.

CSF (सी.एस.एफ.) प्रमस्तिष्कमेरू-तरल। Cerebro spinal fluid.

Cubital (क्यूबिटल) अल्ना। Pertaining to the ulna or to the forearm.

Cuboid (क्यूबॉयड) घनाकार। Like a cube.

Cu-Cm (सीयू-सी-एम) घनसेन्टीमीटर। Cubic centimeter.

Cucumis sativus (कुकुमिस-स्टीवस) खीरा। Cucumber.

Cul-de-sac (कल-डे-सैक) अन्ध-थैली। A passage without an outlet.

Culicide (क्यूलीसाइड) मच्छरों को नष्ट करने वाला पदार्थ। An agent that kills mosquitoes.

Cuneiform (क्यूनीफॉर्म) फनाकार। Wedge-shaped.

Cuniculus (क्यूनीकुलस) खुजली पैदा करने वाले कीट द्वारा त्वचा में बना छिद्र। A burrow in the skin made by the itch mite.

Cunnilingus (क्यूनीलिन्गस) मुख एवं जीभ का प्रयोग करने से स्त्री में जनंनागों का उत्तेजित होना। Stimulation of the female genital organs by using the mouth and the tongue.

Cup (कप) प्याला। A cupping glass.

Curd (कर्ड) दही। The coagulum of milk.

Curet (क्यूरेट) खुरचना। Curetle.

Curettage (क्यूरेटेज) खुरचना। Curettement.

Curvature (करवेचर) टेढ़ापन। Bending.

Cusp (कूस्प) दन्ताग्र, नोक। The pointed crown of teeth.

Cuspid (कस्पीड) नुकीला। Furnished with a cusp.

Cutaneous (क्यूटेनियस) त्वचा सम्बन्धी। Pertaining to the skin.

Cuticle (क्यूटिकिल) बाहरी त्वचा। Outer skin.

Cutification (क्यूटिफिकेशन) चमड़ी का निर्माण। The formation of skin.

Cutis (क्यूटिस) त्वचा। The true skin.

CV (सी.वी.) कल शाम। Tomorrow evening.

Cyanemia (सायनीमिया) रक्त का नीला हो जाना। Blueness of the blood.

Cyanhidrosis (साइनहाइड्रोसिस) नीलापन के लिए हुए पसीने का निकलना। Exudation of bluish sweat.

Cyanopia (साइनोपिया) प्रत्येक वस्तु नीली दिखाई देना। Defective vision in with all the things.

Cyanosed (साइनोस्ड) नीलरोग से पीड़ित। Affected with cyanosis.

Cyanuria (साइनूरिया) नील मूत्र का विसर्जित होना। The excretion of blue urine.

Cyathus (साइथस) गिलास भर। A glass full.

Cyclitis (साइक्लाइटिस) पलकों की सूजन। Inflammation of a cilliary body.

Cycloid (साइक्लॉयड) किसी वृत्त से मिलता-जुलता। Resembling a circle.

Cyclopia (साइक्लोपिया) एक आँख का जन्मजात अभाव होने की दशा। The condition of the congenital absence of one eye.

Cyema (साइमा) गर्भ भ्रूण। The product of conception.

Cyetic (साइटिक) गर्भ सम्बन्धी। Relating to pregnancy.

Cylindreuria (सिलिण्डरूरिया) मूत्र में सिलिण्ड्रॉयड की विद्यमानता Presence of cylinderoids in the urine.

Cylindrical (सिलिण्ड्रीकल) बेलनाकार। Having a shape of a cylinder.

Cymbocephalic (सिम्बोसिफेलिक) नाव के आकार का सिर वाला। Having a boat-shaped head.

Cynobex (साइनोबेक्स) कुत्ते के भौंकने जैसी आवाज करने वाली सूखी खांसी। Dry barking cough.

Cynophobia (साइनोफोबिया) कुत्तों से डर। Morbid fear of dogs.

Cyophoria (सायोफोरिया) गर्भकाल। The period of pregnancy.

Cypriphobia (साइप्रीफोबिया) लैंगिक संसर्ग से बहुत डर लगना। A great dislike for fear of coitus.

Cyst (सिस्ट) पुष्क, पुटःकोशिका। A membranous sac or cavity of abnormal character in the body and are containing fluids.

Cystalgia (सिस्टेल्जिया) मूत्राशय में दर्द होना। Pain in the bladder.

Cystaptosis (सिस्टेप्टोसिस) मूत्राशय का फटना। A rupture of the bladder.

Cystatrophia (सिस्टेट्रोफिया) मूत्राशय का सूखना। Atrophy of the bladder.

Cystectasia (सिस्टेक्टेसिया) मूत्राशय का फूलना। Dilatation of the bladder.

Cystirrhagia (सिस्टेरिङ्जिया) मूत्राशय से रक्तस्राव होना। Hemorrhage from the bladder.

Cystocele (सिस्टोसील) योनि में मूत्राशय की बहिःसरग होना। A prolapse of the bladder into the vagina.

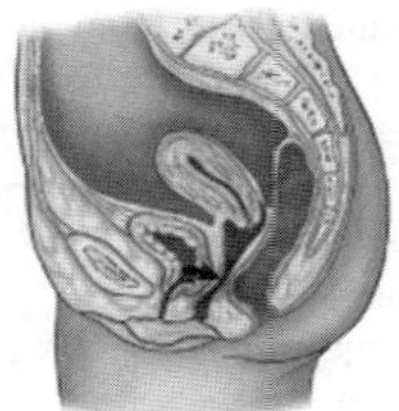

Cystoid (सिस्टॉड) पुटी जैसा। Resembling a cyst.

Cystolith (सिस्टोलिथ) मूत्र-पथरी। A urinary or vesical calculus.

Cystolithiasis (सिस्टोलिथिएसिस) मूत्राशय में पथरियों का बनना। Formation of stones in the urinary bladder.

Cystoplegia (सिस्टोप्लेजिया) मूत्राशय का पक्षाघात। Paralysis of the bladder.

Cystorrhaphy (सिस्टोरैह्फी) मूत्राशय को सीना। Suture of the urinary bladder.

Cystorrhea (सिस्टोरिह्या) मूत्राशय में श्लेष्मा का स्राव। Mucus discharge from the urinary bladder.

Cystorrhexis (सिस्टोरैह्क्सिस) मूत्राशय का फट जाना। Rupture of urinary bladder.

Cystospasm (सिस्टोस्पाजम) मूत्राशय का ऐंठन के साथ संकुचन। Spasmodic contractions of the urinary bladder.

Cystostomy (सिस्टोस्टॉमी) शल्य-क्रिया द्वारा मूत्राशय में छिद्र बनना। Surgical formation of an opening into the urinary bladder.

Cystoureterogram (सिस्टोयूरेट्रोग्राम) मूत्राशय एवं मूत्रनली का एक्स-रे चित्र। X-ray film of the urinary bladder and the ureter.

Cyte (साइट) एक प्रत्यय जिसका अर्थ कोशिका है। A suffix meaning cell.

Cytocidal (साइटोसिडल) कोशिका को मारने वाला। Causing the death of cell.

Cytocide (साइटोसाइड) कोशिका नाशक। An agent that is destructive to cell.

Cytogenesis (साइटोजेनेसिस) कोशिका का जनन। The development of cells.

Cytology (साइटोलॉजी) कोशिका की उत्पत्ति, उनकी संरचना व कार्य का अध्ययन। The study of the formation, structure and function of the cells.

Cytolysis (साइटोलाइसिस) जीवित कोशिकाओं का नष्ट होना। Destruction of living cells.

Cytometry (साइटोमीट्री) कोशिकाओं को गिनना एवं मापना। The counting and measuring of cells.

Cytopenia (साइटोपीनिया) रक्त में कोशिकाओं की कमी होना। Deficiency of cells in the blood.

Cytophagus (साइटोफेगस) कोशिकाओं को नष्ट करना। Destruction of cells.

Cytoplasm (साइटोप्लाज्मा) कोशिका-द्रव्य। The living material of the cell external to the nucleus.

Cytoskeleton (साइटोस्कैलेटन) किसी कोशिका की अन्दर की रचनात्मक ढांचा। The internal structural frame work of a cell.

Cytosome (साइटोसोम) केन्द्रक के अतिरिक्त कोशिका का भाग। The portion of a cell except its nucleus.

Cytostatic (साइटोस्टेटिक) कोशिकाओं की संख्या में ज्यादा होना एवं इनकी गुणन क्रिया को रोकने वाला। Preventing the growth and multiplication of cells.

Cytotechnology (साइटोटैक्नोलॉजी) विकृतियों का पता लगाने के लिए कोशिकाओं का सूक्ष्मदर्शीय परीक्षण करना। Microscopic examination of the cells to detect abnormalities.

Cytothesis (साइटोथेसिस) चोट खाई हुई कोशिकाओं की मरम्मत करना। Repair of the injured cells.

Cytotoxic (साइटोटोक्सीक) कोशिकाओं को विषाक्त करने वाला पदार्थ। Any substance which is toxic to cells.

Cytotoxicity (साइटोटॉक्सीसिटी) कोशिकाविशी होने की अवस्था। The state of being cytotoxic.

Cytotropic (साइटोट्रॉपिक) कोशिकाओं के प्रति आकर्षित होने वाला। Having attraction for cells.

Cytozoic (साइटोजोइक) किसी कोशिका के भीतर अथवा उससे संलग्न रहने वाला जैसे कुछ एककोशिकीय जन्तु। Living within or attached to a cell, as certain protozoa.

Cytozoon (साइटोजून) एक कोशिकीय जन्तु जो अन्तःकोशिका परजीवी की भांति एक कोशिका में रहता है। The protozon that lives as intracellular parasite.

Cyturia (साइटूरिया) मूत्र में किसी भी प्रकार की कोशिकाओं का पाया जाना। Presence of cells of any find in the urine.

D

D (डी) दशमलव के चिन्ह के रूप में प्रयुक्त किया जाने वाला। Symbol for decimal.

D & C (डी एण्ड सी) गर्भाशयग्रीवा का विस्फारण एवं आखुरण करना। Dilatation of the cervix and curettage of the uterus.

D & E (डी एण्ड इ) गर्भाशय का विस्फारण एवं शून्यीकरण। Dilatation and evacuation of uterus.

Dacnomania (डैक्नोमेनिया) हत्या करने का उन्माद। Mania for killing.

Dacryadenalgia (डैक्रीएडीनेल्जिया) अक्षु ग्रंथि में दर्द होना। Pain in a lacrimal gland.

Dacryagogatresia (डैक्रीएगोगेटेसिया) किसी आँसू की नली का बंद हो जाना। Occlusion of a tear duct.

Dacryagogue (डैक्रीएगोग) आँसू उत्पन्न करने वाला पदार्थ। An agent causing a flow of tears.

Dacrycystalgia (डैक्रीसिस्टैल्जिया) किसी अक्षु नली का दर्द। Pain in the lacrimal sac.

Dacryo, Docry (डैक्रियो, डैक्री) आँसुओं का संकेत देने वाले उपसर्ग। Prefixes indicating lacrimal gland.

Dacryocyst (डैक्रीयोसिस्ट) आँसू की थैली। The lacrimal sac.

Dacryocystectomy (डैक्रीयोसिस्टेक्टॉमी) अक्षुकोश की झिल्लीयों को काटकर अलग कर देना। Excision of the membranes of the lacrimal sac.

Dacryocystitis (डैक्रीयोसिस्टाइटिस) अक्षुकोश का प्रदाह। Inflammation of the lacrimal sac.

Dacryocystorhinostomy (डैक्रीयोसिस्टोराह्ईनोस्टॉमी) नाक की निकास नली को जोड़ने के लिये किया जाने वाला ऑपरेशन। To make a surgical connection between lacrimal sac and the nasal cavity.

Dacryocystotomy (डैक्रीयोसिस्टोटॉमी) अक्षुकोश में चीरा लगाना। Incision of the lacrimal sac.

Dacryolith (डैक्रीयोलिथ) अक्षुकोश में पथरी। Lacrimal calculus.

Dacryops (डैक्रीयोप्स) अक्षु नली से पस का निकलना। Discharge of pus from the lacrimal duct.

Dacryopyosis (डैक्रीयोपायोसिस) अक्षु उपकरण में पस का बनना। Formation of pus in the lacrimal apparatus.

Dacryostenosis (डैक्रीयोस्टेनोसिस) आँसू नली का तंग हो जाना। Norrowing of a lacrimal duct.

Dactyl (डैक्टाइल) हाथ या पैर की अंगुली। Digit.

Dactyledema (डैक्टाइलीडीमा) हाथ या पैर की उंगुली का सूजन। Edema of the fingers or toes.

Dactylian (डैक्टाइलियन) अंगुलियों के बीच चिपकाव पैदा हो जाना। Adhesion between the fingers or toes.

Dactylic (डैक्टाइलिक) अंगुली जैसी आकार का। Of the form of a digit.

Dactylitis (डैक्टाइलाटिस) अंगुलियों का सूजन। Inflammation of a fingers or toes.

Dactylography (डैक्टाइलोग्राफी) अंगुली की छाप का अध्ययन। The study of fingers print.

Dactylogryposis (डैक्टाइलोग्राइपोसिस) अंगुलियों का स्थायी रूप से संकुचन होना। Permanent contraction of the fingers.

Dactylomegaly (डैक्टाइलोमेगैली) अंगुलियों का अत्यधिक लम्बा हो जाना। Abormally large fingers or toes.

Dactylus (डैक्टाइलस) हाथ या पैर की एक अंगुली। A finger or a toe.

Daft (डैफ्ट) पागल। Insane.

Daltonism (डाल्टोनिज्म) रंग को पहचानने की अयोग्यता। Color blindness.

Damage (डैमेज) नुकसान। Loss.

Damp (डैम्प) नम। Moist.

Damp-proof (डैम्प-प्रूफ) सील-प्रतिरोधी। Resistant to damp.

Danders (डैन्डर्स) पपड़ियाँ। The skin particles of animals which may cause allergy when breathed.

Dandruff (डैण्ड्रफ) बालों की जड़ों तथा त्वचा पर जमने वाली पपड़ी। Cast of cells from the outer layer of skin mainly noted in the scalp.

Dandy fever (डैन्डी फिवर) डेंगू, हड्डी-तोड़ बुखार। Dengue.

Danielassen's disease (डैनीयलसन्स डिजिज) कुष्ठ रोग। Leprosy.

Dartos (डार्टोस) अण्डकोष की झिल्ली। The muscular contractile tissue under the skin of the scrotum.

Dactylolysis (डैक्टाइलोलाइसिस) अंगुलियों का नष्ट होना। Destruction of a digit as in leprosy.

Day blindness (डे-ब्लाइन्डनेस) दिन में दिखाई नहीं देना। Subnormal vision in the day light.

Dazzle (डेजल) तेज रोशनी से धुंधला दिखाई देना। Occurrence of dimness of vision in very bright light.

DDS (डी.डी.एस.) दन्त चिकित्सक। Doctor of dental surgery.

DDT (डी.डी.टी) कीटाणुनाशक घोल जिससे मच्छरों को मारा जाता है। Dichlorodipheny trichloro-ethane.

Deafness (डीफनैस) बहरापन। Complete or partial loss of ability to hear.

Death (डैथ) शरीर के सभी कार्यों का रूक जाना। Permanent cessation of all vital parts including that of brain.

Death rate (डैथ रेट) किसी क्षेत्र की प्रति 1000 आबादी में एक निर्दिष्ट समय में होने वाली मौतों की संख्या। Number of deaths per 1000 population in a given time.

Death rattle (डैथ रेटल) मरते हुए व्यक्ति के गले में से घर्घर आवाज सुनायी देना। A sound heard in the throat of the dying person caused by the accumulation of mucus.

Debilitant (डेबीलिटेन्ट) कमजोरी पैदा करने वाला। That which causes weakness.

Debility (डेबीलिटी) कमजोरी। Weakness.

Debridement (डेबराइडमैन्ट) मरे हुए ऊतक को अलग करना जब तक कि चारों ओर का स्वस्थ ऊतक दिखाई नहीं दे जाता। Removal of foreign matrial along with devitalized tissue.

Debrisoquin (डैबरीसोक्यूइन) खून की तीव्रता को रोकने वाली दवा। Antihypertensive drug.

Decameter (डेकामीटर) 10 मीटर। A measure of 10 meters.

Decapitation (डीकैपिटेशन) सिर को शरीर से अलग कर देना। Beheading.

Decaying (डीकेईंग) गलने-सड़ने लगना। Deteriorating.

Deceleration (डेसीलेरेशन) शीघ्रता में कमी आना। Decrease in rapidity.

Decibel (डेसीबल) ध्वनि की तीव्रता की इकाई। Unit of intensity of sound.

Decidua (डेसीडुआ) गर्भाशय की पतनशील झिल्ली जो प्रसव के साथ निकल जाती है, आंवल। The altered mucous member one of the pregnant uterus.

Deciduoma (डेसीड्यूमा) पतनिका के भग्नावशेष मिले रहते हैं। The intrauterine tumor.

Deciduous (डेसिडुअस) गिरने वाला। Falling off.

Deciduous teeth (डेसिडुअस टीथ) दूध के दाँत प्रत्येक जबड़े में

10 होते हैं। 6 महीने की आयु में प्रकट होते हैं तथा 6 वर्ष के अंत तक गिर जाते हैं। Primary dentition of 20 teeth that erupt between 6 months and 3 years.

Deciliter (डेसीलीटर) एक लीटर का दसवां भाग। 100 ml.

Decimeter (डेसीमीटर) एक मीटर का दसवां भाग। 1/10th of meter or 10 cm.

Decipara (डेसीपेरा) 10वीं बार गर्भवती होने वाली स्त्री। A woman pregnant for the 10th time.

Decline (डैक्लाइन) कम होना। Decrease.

Decoction (डिकोक्शन) वनस्पति-पदार्थों को पानी के साथ उबालकर बनाई गई तरल औषधि। A liquid medicinal preparation made by boiling vegetable substance with water.

Decompensation (डीकमपेनसेशन) क्षतिपूर्ति न कर सकना। A failure of compensation.

Decomposition (डिकम्पोजीशन) सड़ना-गलना। Decay, putrefaction.

Decompression illness (डिकम्प्रेशन इलनैस) उन व्यक्तियों में जिनका एकदम से वायुमण्डलीय दबाव के कम होने से वास्ता पड़ता है जैसे समुद्र के गोताखोर या वायुयान चालक में होने वाला एक रोग जिसमें खून एवं ऊतकों में नाइट्रोजन के बुलबुलों की विद्यमानता से हाथों, पैरों तथा पेट में दर्द होता है। Illness arising from rapid reduction of surrounding pressure as in sea divers suddenly coming to surface, symptoms are due to release of dissolved nitrogen.

Decongestant (डीकन्जैस्टैन्ट) शोथ को कम करने वाला। Reducing congestion or swelling.

Decortication (डीकोर्टीकेशन) किसी अंग के आवरण का शल्य-क्रिया द्वारा हटा देना। Surgical removal of the cortex or outer covering of an organ.

Decrudescence (डैक्रूडिसेन्स) किसी रोग के लक्षणों की गंभीरता में कमी होना। Decrease in the severity of the symptoms of a disease.

Decryohemorrhea (डैक्रीयोहीमोरिह्या) खून के साथ मिश्रित आँसुओं का बहना। Discharge of tears mixed with the blood.

Decubitus (डेक्यूबिटस) लेटे रहने की स्थिति। Position assumed in lying down.

Decubitus-ulcer (डेक्यूबिटस-अल्सर) शरीर के किसी भाग पर लगातार पड़ने वाला दबाव से

उत्पन्न जख्म जैसे–किसी बीमारी में लम्बे समय तक बिस्तर पर पड़े रहने से उत्पन्न पीठ का जख्म। Skin ulceration to prolonged pressure commonly over bony prominences.

Decussation (डेकूसेशन) दो रचनाओं का अंग्रेजी के अक्षर 'एक्स' के रूप में क्रॉस करना। A crossing of structures in the form of 'X'.

Dedentition (डीडैन्टीशन) दाँतों का अभाव। Loss of teeth.

Defecation (डीफीकेशन) मल त्यागना। To excrete the feces.

Deferences (डिफैरेन्स) दूर ले जाने वाला। Carrying away.

Defibrillation (डिफिब्रिलेशन) भौतिक साधन जैसे विद्युत स्तब्धता द्वारा रोकना अथवा हृदय के विकम्पन को औषधियों का प्रयोग करके। Stoppage of heart by drugs or electrical current.

Defibrination (डीफिब्रिनीशन) खून से फाइब्रिन हटा देना। Removal of fibrin from the blood.

Deficiency (डेफिसीयेन्सी) कमी होना। A lack or shortage.

Definition (डेफीनीशन) परिभाषित करना। The precise.

Definitive (डेफीनेटिव) निश्चित, अंतिम। Limiting the extent.

Defluxio (डिफ्लोक्सीओ) दस्त। Diarrhea.

Deformity (डिफोर्मिटी) पूर्व में सामान्य रूप से बने किसी भाग की आकृति में होने वाला परिवर्तन। An alteration in the natural form or alignment of an organ.

Degeneration (डिजेनेरेशन) किसी ऊतक या अंग का क्षय। Deterioration in a tissue or organ.

Deglutition (डेग्लूटिशन) निगलने की क्रिया। The act of swallowing.

Dehydration (डिहाइड्रेशन) किसी पदार्थ से पानी का अलग होना। Removal of water from a substance.

Delactation (डिलेक्टेशन) दूध छुड़ाना। The act of weaning.

Deleterios (डेलीटीरियस) हानिकारक, घातक। Harmful, injuries.

Deletion (डिलीशन) किसी गुणसूत्र से अनुवांशिक पदार्थ का निकलना। The loss of genetic material from one chromosomal.

Delirium (डेलीरियम) उन्माद। A condition of mental conversion and excitement marked by defective perception and belief in non-existence circumstances, usually illusions and hallucination.

Delivery (डिलीवरी) प्रसव, प्रसूति, बच्चा जनना। Child birth, parturition.

Delusion (डिल्यूजन) भ्रम। A false belief which cannot be altered by argument or reasoning.

Dement (डिमेन्ट) पागल। An insane person.

Dementia (डिमेनसिया) पागलपन। Mental.

Demineralization (डीमिनेरेलाइजेशन) खनिज लवणों की विशेषकर हड्डियों की हानि। Loss of mineral salts especially from the bones.

Demography (डिमोग्राफी) मानव आबादी का स्वास्थ्य रोग, जन्म, मृत्यु सम्बन्धी सांख्यिकीय अध्ययन। Statistical and quantitative study of characteristic of human population like- size, growth, age, density, sex.

Demonomania (डिमोनोमेनिया) खुद को भूत–प्रेत महसूस करने का पागलपन। A kind of madness in which the patient fancies himself a devil.

Demonophobia (डिमोनोफोबिया) भूत–प्रेत का डर। Morbid dread of the devil.

Demulcent (डीमलसेन्ट) शरीर के भाग को शांत करने वाला। Soothing the part of the body or softening the skin to which it is applied.

Demyelination (डीमाइलीनेशन) किसी तंत्रिका के माइलिन आवरण का नष्ट होना। Destruction of removal of myelin sheath of a nerve.

Denaturation (डिनेचुरेशन) किसी पदार्थ की सामान्य प्रकृति में परिवर्तन होना। A change in the usual nature of substance.

Denatured (डीनेचर्ड) विकृतिकरण द्वारा परिवर्तित। Changed by denaturation.

Dendrite (डेण्ड्राइट) पार्श्वतन्तु। A branched protoplasmic process of a neurons that conducts impulses to cell body.

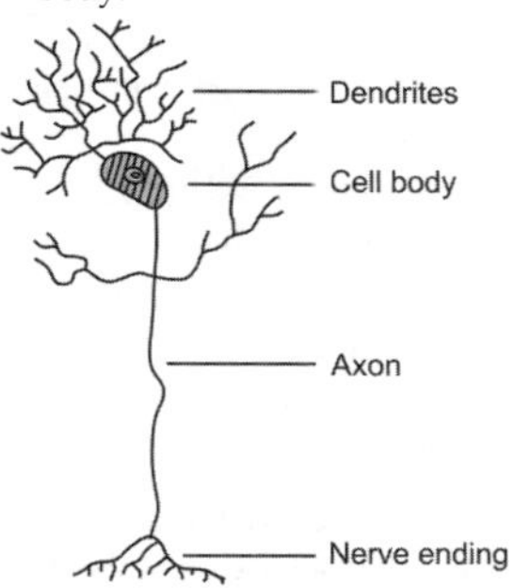

Dendritic (डेन्ड्राइटिक) वृक्ष की आकृति जैसा। Tree like in shape.

Dengue (डेन्गू) हड्डी-तोड़ बुखार। Break bone-fever.

Densimeter (डेन्सिमीटर) किसी पदार्थ के घनत्व का पता लगाने वाला यंत्र। An instrument for measuring density.

Densitometry (डेनसाइटोमेट्री) किसी पदार्थ के घनत्व का पता लगाना। Determination of the density of a substance.

Dental arch (डैन्टल आर्क) दाँतों की काटने एवं चबाने वाली सतहों से बनने वाला चाप। The arch formed by the cutting and chewing surface.

Dental plaque (डैन्टल प्लाक) दाँतों पर लगा रहने वाला मुखीय सूक्ष्मजीवों एवं उनके उत्पादों का एक चिपचिपा पिण्ड। Tenacious mass of oral microorganism and their products adhering on the teeth.

Dental pulp (डैन्टल पल्प) रक्त कोशिकाओं एवं तंत्रिकाओं के जाल सहित संयोजी ऊतक जो दाँत तथा इसकी जडों के भीतर केन्द्रीय स्थान में स्थित रहता है। The connective tissue along with the network of blood capillaries and the nerves occupying the central space in the tooth and its roots.

Dentin (डैन्टिन) दाँत का मुख्य पदार्थ जो मज्जा गुहा को चारों ओर से घेरे होता है अथवा दाँतों को बनाने वाला एक विशेष कठोर पदार्थ। The body structure of the teeth.

Dentinogenesis (डैन्टिनोजेनेसिस) दन्त विकास में दन्त धातु का बनना। Formation of dentin in the development of a tooth.

Dentinogenesis imperfecta (डैन्टिनोजेनेसिस इम्पर्फेक्टा) एक आनुवांशिक रोग जिसमें किसी दाँत के दन्त धातु का अपूर्ण निर्माण होता है। A hereditary condition in which there is imperfect formation of the dentin of a tooth.

Denture (डेन्चर) नकली दाँत। A set of artificial teeth.

Deodorant (डियोडोरेन्ट) दुर्गन्ध दूर करने वाला पदार्थ। Preparation which masks or diminishes any unpleasant odor.

Depersonalization (डीपर्सोनेलाइजेशन) अवैयक्तिकीकरण। A state in which a person loses the feeling of his own identify in relation to others in his family.

Depilation (डेपिलेशन) बालों की सफाई। The process of removing the hair.

Depletion (डेप्लीशन) शरीर से खून, तरल आदि पदार्थों को बाहर निकालना। Removal of the substance such as blood, fluid, etc.

Depolarization (डीपोलेराइजेशन) ध्रुवता में कमी होना अथवा उसका नष्ट हो जाना। Reduction in or destruction of polarity.

Depressant (डिप्रेसैन्ट) शरीर के किसी कार्य को कम करने वाला पदार्थ। An agent diminishing a body function.

Depression (डिप्रेशन) हताशा, अवसाद। A hollow or lowered part.

Depuration (डिपयूरेशन) शुद्धिकरण की एक प्रक्रिया। Cleansing process.

Dermatitis (डर्माटाइटिस) त्वचा की सूजन। Inflammation of the skin.

Dermatoglyphics (डर्माटोग्लाइफिक्स) अंगुली चिन्ह-विज्ञान। Study of lines of hand and feet for drawing inference about one's susceptibility to disease.

Dermatome (डर्मेटोम) चर्म-उच्छेदक। Area of skin innervated by one segment of spinal cord.

Dermatomyositis (डर्मेटोमायोसाइटिस) त्वचा एवं पेशियों की सूजन। Inflammation of the skin and the muscles.

Dermatophobia (डर्मेटोफोबिया) चर्म रोग के होने का अत्यन्त भय। Abnormal fear of having a skin disease.

Dermatophyte (डर्मेटोफाइट) एक कवक परजीवी जो त्वचा पर वृद्धि करता है। A fungus parasite which grows on the skin.

Dermatophytosis (डर्मेटोफाइटोसिस) हाथ-पैरों की त्वचा का विशेषकर पैरों की अंगुलियों के बीच में होने वाला कवक संक्रमण। Athlete's foot. A fungus infection of the skin of the hands and feet especially between the toes.

Dermatoplastic (डर्मेटोप्लास्टिक) त्वचा निरोपण से सम्बन्धित। Pertaining to the skin grafting.

Dermatorrhagia (डर्मेटोरेह्जिया) त्वचा से खून का बाहर निकलना। Hemorrhage from the skin.

Dermis (डर्मिस) वास्तविक त्वचा। The true skin or corium.

Dermoid (डर्मायड) त्वचा के समान। Like the skin.

Dermoid cyst (डर्मायड सिस्ट) डिम्बग्रंथि अथवा फेफड़ों में अथवा खोपड़ी पर होने वाला एक सुद्म पुटीच अबुर्द जिसमें बाल, दाँत या त्वचा पाई जाती है। A benign cystic tumor occurring in the ovary or lungs or the skull, etc. in which hair, teeth or the skin are found.

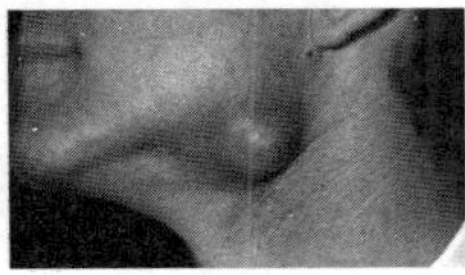

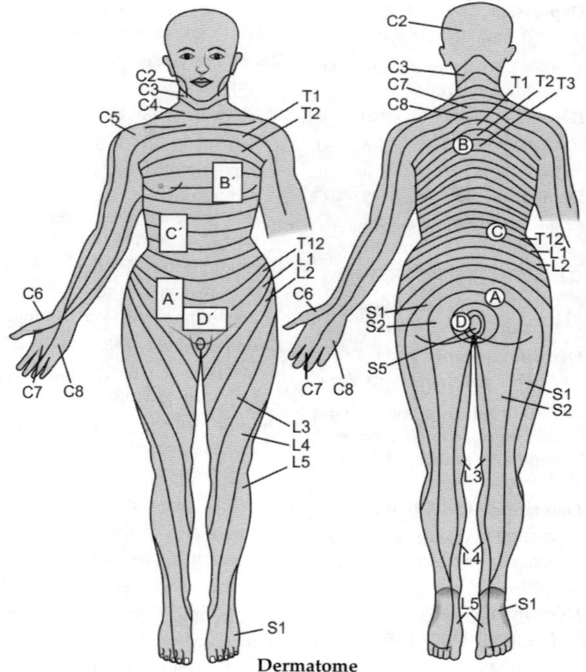

Dermatome

Desalination (डीसैलाइनेशन)

किसी पदार्थ जैसे समुद्र के पानी से आंशिक या पूर्ण रूप से लवणों का अलग हो जाना। Partial or complete removal of salts from a substance as from sea water.

Desaturation (डीसैचुरेशन)

विसंतृप्तीकरण। The out or the result of making something loss completely saturated.

Descemet's membrane

(डेस्सीमेट्स मेम्ब्रेन) स्वच्छमण्डल की अंतःकला परत तथा मुख्य

अस्तर के बीच स्थित एक पतली झिल्ली। A fine membrane situated between the endothelial layer of the cornea and the substantia propria.

Desensitization (डीसेन्सीटाइजेशन) सुग्राहीकारक पदार्थ। Prevention of anaphylaxis usually by administering repeated small doses of the drugs causing anaphylaxis.

Desicant (डैसिकैन्ट) खुष्की लाने वाला। Causing dryness.

Desiccation (डैसिकेशन) सुखाने की क्रिया। The process of drying up.

Desmitis (डेस्माइटिस) किसी स्नायु की सूजन। Inflammation of a ligament.

Desmorrhexis (डेस्मोरेह्क्सिस) किसी स्नायु का फट जाना। Rupture of a ligament.

Desquamation (डेस्क्आमेशन) खाल उतरना। Shedding off the epidermis.

Destructive (डेस्ट्रक्टीव) विनाशकारी। Causing ruin.

Detachment (डिटैचमेन्ट) अलग करना। The act of separating or detaching.

Detector (डिटैक्टर) किसी वस्तु की विद्यमानता का पता लगाने वाला उपकरण, उदाहरण के तौर पर झूठ बोलने का पता लगाने वाला उपकरण। An apparatus for determining the presence of something, e.g. lie-detector.

Detergent (डिटर्जेन्ट) शोधक, अपमर्जिक। A cleaning agent.

Deterioration (डीटेरियोरेशन) शारीरिक एवं मानसिक क्रियाओं का धीरे-धीरे कम होते जाना। Slow impairment of the physical and mental function.

Determination (डीटरमीनेशन) दिशा निर्धारण। Establishing the nature or process identify of a substance, organism or event.

Detonation (डीटोनेशन) विस्फोट, धमाका। A violent noise caused by an explosive.

Detoxify (डिटॉक्सीफाई) किसी पदार्थ के विषैले गुण को अलग करना। The removal of toxic quality of a substance to treat toxic overdose of a dry alcohol.

Detrition (डेट्रीशन) शरीर के किसी भाग का जैसे दाँतों का रगड़ से क्षय होना। The wearing away of a part of the body as of the teeth by friction.

Detritus (डेट्राइटस) कंकड, अपरद। Degenerative matter produced by disintigration.

Detrusor (डेट्रूसर) शरीर का वह भाग जो नीचे को धकेलता है जैसे कोई पेशी, निस्सारिका। The part of the body which pushes down, e.g. a muscle.

Detumescence (डीटुमिसेन्स) किसी सूजन का घटना। Subsidence of a swelling.

Deuteranopia (डयूटिरेनोप्या) वर्णान्धता जिसमें हरे रंग का बोध नहीं होता। Color blindness in which green color is not perceived.

Deviant (डेविएन्ट) सामान्य से विच. लित हो जाने वाला। One who turns aside from the normal.

Deviation (डेविएशन) सामान्य से विचलित होना। Departure from normal.

Devitalization (डीवाइटलाइजेशन) जीवन समाप्त हो जाना। Destruction of vitality or life.

Devolution (डीवोल्यूशन) प्रति विकास। The reverse of evolution.

Dextrality (डैक्सट्रालिटी) दांये हाथ से कार्य करना या लिखना। Right handedness.

Dextrocardia (डैक्सट्रोकार्डिया) हृदय का शरीर के दायीं ओर स्थित रहना। Location of the heart on the right side of the body.

Dextropedal (डेक्सट्रोपेडल) दायें पैर सम्बन्धी। Related to right foot.

Dextrophobia (डैक्सट्रोफोबिया) शरीर के दायीं ओर विद्यमान वस्तुओं का रोगोत्पादक भय। Morbid fear of or aversion to the objects on the right side of the body.

Dextroposition (डैक्सट्रोपोजीशन) दाईं ओर को विस्थापन। Displacement to the right side.

Dextrose (डेक्सट्रोज) द्राक्ष-शर्करा। A sugar of glucose group.

Dextroversion (डेक्सट्रोवरजन) दक्षिणवर्तन। A turning to the right.

Diabetes (डायबिटीज) ऐसा रोग जिसमें अत्यधिक मूत्र विसर्जित होना। A disease characterized by excessive of urine.

Diabetic (डायाबिटीक) मधुमेह से सम्बन्धित। Pertaining to diabetes.

Diabetogenous (डायाबिटोजीनस) मधुमेह रोग उत्पन्न करने वाला। Caused by diabetes.

Diacele (डायासेली) तृतीय मस्तिष्क गह्वर। The third cavity of the brain.

Diadelphic (डाइडेल्फिक) वह स्त्री जिसके दो गर्भाशय होते है। Having double uterus.

Diadochokinesia (डायाडोचोकिनेजिया) शीघ्र पर्यायगति। The normal power of alternately bringing a limb into opposite position.

Diagnosis (डायग्नोसिस) रोग निदान। The act of distinguishing disease by symptoms.

Dialators (डाइलेटर्स) फैलाने वाला। A thing that dilates something like a tube or cavity in the body.

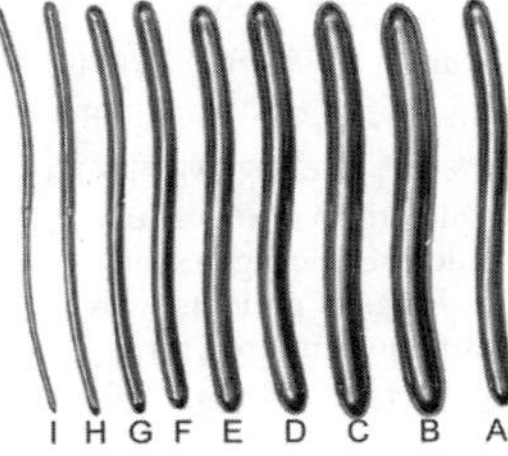

Dialysate (डायलायसेट) विलगित। Any product taken from a solution by dialysis.

Dialysis (डायलायसिस) विलगत। A separation of parts in general, the separation of crystalline from colloid substance by means of a porous diaphragm.

Diameter (डायमीटर) व्यास। A straight line passing through the center of a body.

Diapedesis (डायपेडेसिस) खून वाहिनियों की भित्तियों से श्वेत अणुओं का पारगमन। The passage of blood cells through the vessels wall into the tissues.

Diaphanography (डायाफैनोग्राफी) पारप्रदीपन के द्वारा शरीर के किसी भाग का विशेष रूप से स्तन का कैंसर के लिए परीक्षण करना। Examination of a body part by transillumination, especially of the breast for the detection of cancer.

Diaphanoscope (डायाफैनोस्कोप) शरीर की किसी गुहा का पार-प्रदीपन करने वाला यंत्र। An instrument for transillumination of a body cavity.

Diaphoresis (डायाफोरेसिस) अत्यधिक पसीना आना। Profuse sweating.

Diaphoretic (डायाफोरेटिक) वह वस्तु जिससे अधिक पसीना आता है। Agents that profuse sweating.

Diaphragm (डायाफ्राम) वक्ष-गुहा का उदर-गुहा से अलग करने वाला पेशीकलामय विभाजन, मध्य पर।
The musculomentor anus partition separating the thoracic cavity from the abdominal cavity.

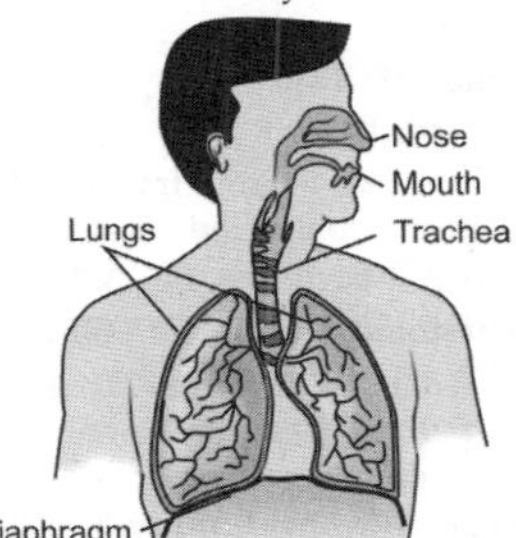

Diaphysis (डायाफाइसिस) किसी लम्बी हड्डी का माण्ड।
The shaft of a long bone.

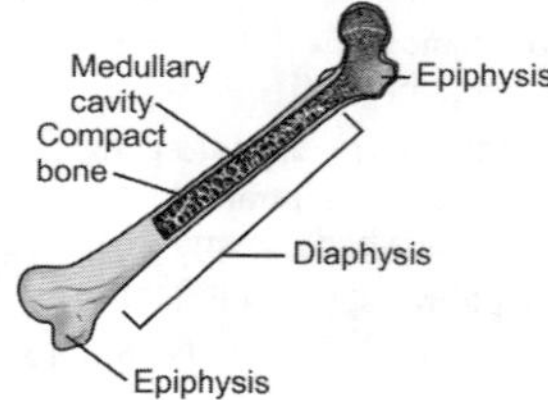

Diapyesis (डायापाइसिस) पस पड़ जाना। Suppuration.

Diarrhea (डायरिह्या) दस्त लगना। Frequent passage of loose or watery motions.

Diascope (डायास्कोप) साफ काँच की एक प्लेट। A glass plate held against the skin for examining superficial lesions blanch but not hemorrhagic lesions.

Diastasis (डायसटेसिस) अनुशिथिलता। A separation of bones without fracture relaxation period of cardiac cycle, as opposed to systole.

Diastolic pressure (डायस्टोलिक प्रेशर) निम्न रक्तचाप। The period of least pressure in the arterial vescular system.

Diathermy (डायथर्मी) शरीर की गहरी स्नायुओं में गर्मी पैदा करने के लिए प्रयुक्त विद्युत धारा का प्रयोग। The passage of a high frequency electric current through the tissue whereby heat is produced.

Diatomic (डायटोमिक) ऐसे यौगिक को निर्दिष्ट करने वाला जिसके एक अणु में दो परमाणु होते हैं। One group of unicellular microscopic algae seen in lungs of patients with antemortem drowning.

Diaxon (डायग्जोन) एक तंत्रिका-कोषिका जिसमें दो अक्षतन्तु होते हैं। A neuron having two axons.

Diazoreaction (डायजोरियेक्षन) यक्ष्मा तथा आंत्रिक ज्वर के निदानार्थ की जाने वाली मूत्र जांच। The urinary test for phthisis and typhoid fever.

Dichotomy (डायकोटॉमी) दो भागों में विभाजित करना। Difurcable of a vein dividing two parts.

Dicoria (डायकोरिया) प्रत्येक आँख में दो पुतलियों का होना। Presence of double pupil in each eye.

Dicrotic (डायक्रोटिक) द्वि नाड़ी स्पन्द से सम्बन्धित। Pertaining to a double pulse or having a double beat.

Dicrotic notch (डाइक्रोटिक नौच) किसी नाड़ी रेखांकन में अवरोही भुजा पर स्थित एक दाँत। In a pulse training a notch on the testing limb.

Didactylous (डाइडैक्टाइलस) जन्मजात एक हाथ या पैर में केवल दो अंगुलियों वाला।

Having only two digits in one hand or foot congenitally.

Didelphia (डाइडेल्फिया) दो गर्भाशय से युक्त होने की दशा। The condition of having a double uterus.

Didymitis (डीडाइमाटिस) शुक्रग्रन्थि में सूजन। Inflammation of testicle.

Didymodynia (डीडाइमोडाइनिया) शुक्रग्रन्थि में दर्द होना। Pain in a testis.

Diebus alternis (डाइबस-अल्टरनिस) एक दिन छोड़कर। Every other day.

Diencephalon (डाएनसिफैलॉन) अन्तर्मस्तिष्क। The middle brain including the thalaming and the third ventricle.

Diet (डाइट) भोजन, आहार। Food substances normally consumed in the course of living.

Dietetics (डाइटेटिक्स) भोजन अथवा इसके नियमन से सम्बन्धित। Pertaining to diet or its regulation.

Dietis crisis (डाइटिस क्राइसिस) चलायमान गुर्द के मामले में जब गुर्दा हिलता-डुलता है तो मूत्रनली में ऐंठन आ जाना। (Renal colic from partial obstruction of ureter.

Dietitian (डाइटीशियन) आहार विज्ञानी।

A person experienced in field of nutrition and dietetic advice.

Differential (डिफरेन्सीयल) सापेक्ष रक्त गणना। Determination of number of each variety of leukocytes in one micro liter of blood. (*i*) **Blood count** (ब्लड काउन्ट) रक्त कण

Diffraction (डिफरेक्शन) प्रकाश किरणों को उसके घटकों में तोड़ना। The deflection of a ray of light on passing through a small opening.

Diffusion (डिफ्यूजन) वह क्रिया जिसके द्वारा बहुत-सी गैसें एक-दूसरे में घुसकर घुल-मिल जाती हैं। A process by which various gases intermingle as a result of natural movement in the particles and molecule.

Digestion (डायजेशन) पाचन। The conversion of food into proper condition to supplied nourishment for the body.

Digestive system (डायजेस्टीव सिस्टम) पाचन तंत्र, आमाषय से गुर्दा तक का भाग। The abdominal organs which digest the food and absorb it.

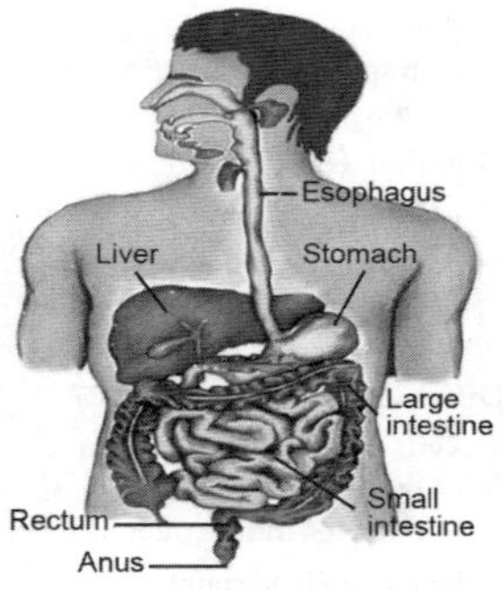

Digit (डिजिट) हाथ या पैर की एक अंगुली। A finger or toe.

Digitalis (डिजिटेलिस) नागफली का रस, हृदय रोगों की एक मूल औषधि। The botanical name or the fox glove, a basic drug for use in certain heart disease.

Diglossia (डाइग्लोसिया) दो भागों में बंटी हुई जीभ। Bifid tongue.

Dilatation (डाइलेटेशन) फैलाव। The act of spreading or expanding in all direction dilatation.

Dilatation and Evacuation (डाइलेशन एण्ड एवाकुएशन) चिमटियों का प्रयोग करके गर्भधारण में उत्पादों को निकाल देना। Dilatation of the cervix and removal of the early product of conception.

Dilatation and Curettage (D and C) (डाइलेशन एण्ड क्यूरेटेज) विस्फाटक द्वारा गर्भाशय ग्रीवा को फैलाना तथा गर्भाशय की भीतर की दीवार को खुरेदना। Dilatation of the cervix and curettment of the endometrium.

Diluent (डाइलुएण्ट) घोल हल्का करने वाला। Diluting the solution.

Dimetria (डाइमीट्रिया) दो गर्भाशय होने की अवस्था। A condition of having double uterus.

Dimorphism (डाइमोर्फिज्म) दो रूपों में स्थित रहने का गुण। The quality of existing in two forms.

Dimorphous (डाइमोर्फस) दो भिन्न रूपों में उत्पन्न होने वाला। Occurring in two different forms.

Dimple sign (डिम्पल साइन) झुर्री। Usually circular and small in the chin, cheek sacral region.

Dinomania (डिनोमेनिया) नाचने का पागलपन। Dancing mania.

Dinus (डिनस) चक्कर। Vertigo.

Diphallus (डाइफेलस) पूर्ण अथवा अपूर्ण शिश्न। Complete or incomplete double penis or clitoris.

Diphasic (डाइफेजिक) दो प्रावस्थाओं में उत्पन्न होने वाला। Occurring in or having two phases.

Diphonia (डाइफोनिया) बोलने में एक साथ दो भिन्न स्वर ध्वनियों का उत्पन्न होना। Simultaneous production of two different voice tones in speaking.

Diphtheria (डिफ्थीरिया) कॉनीबैक्टीरिया डिफ्थीरिया नामक जीवाणु द्वारा बच्चों में होने वाला तीव्र संक्रामक रोग। Acute infections disease characterized by fever sore throat, cervical lymph adenopathy formation of gray pseudomembrane at the site of infection.

Diphtheroid (डिफ्थेरॉयड) डिफ्थीरिया को उत्पन्न करने वाला जीव। Resembling diphtheria or diphtheria bacillus.

Diplegia (डाइप्लेजिया) शरीर के दोनों ओर के समान भागों का पक्षाघात।

Paralysis of the leg and hand of one side.

Diplocoria (डिप्लोकोरिया) एक आँख में दो पुतलियों का होना। Double pupil in an eye.

Diploe (डिप्लोइ) कपाल-पटों के मध्य कोशिकीय अस्थि ऊतक। The cellular boney tissue between the cranial tables.

Diploidy (डिप्लॉयडी) द्विगुणित होने की अवस्था। The state of being diploid.

Diplomyelia (डिप्लोमाइलिया) सुषुम्ना की सहज दो भागों में विभाजित होने की अवस्था। A congenital doubling of the spinal cord.

Diplopia (डिप्लोपिया) दोहरा दिखाई देना। Double vision.

Dipsesis (डिपसेसिस) अत्यधिक प्यास लगना। Abnormal or excessive thirst.

Dipsomania (डिप्सोमेनिया) शराब के लिए पागलपन। Mania for alcohol.

Direct light reflex (डाइरैक्ट लाइट रिफ्लैक्स) पुतली के ऊपर रोशनी डालने से तुरन्त ही इसका सिकुड़ जाना। Immediate constriction of the pupil on throwing light over it.

Disc, Disk (डिस्क) एक चपटी, वृत्ताकार तश्तरीनुमा संरचना। A flat circular, plate like structure.

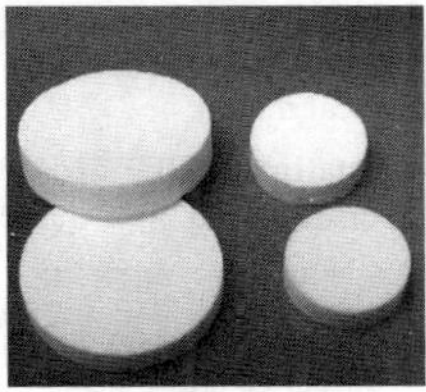

Discitis (डिस्साइटिस) चक्रिका का शोथ। Inflammation of the disk.

Discoloration (डिस्कलेरेशन) मलिनीकरण। The act of staining.

Discrete (डिस्क्रीट) पृथक। Separate.

Discus (डिस्कस) बिम्ब। A disk.

Disease (डिजीज) शरीर के किसी अंग में कोई भी अवरोध।

Literally the lack of ease or illness.

Disengagement (डिसएन्गेजमैन्ट) भ्रूण के सिर का माँ की श्रोणी के भीतर से बाहर को निकल आना। The evergence of the head of the fetus from within the pelvis of the mother.

Disharmony (डिसहार्मोनी) सामंजस्य का अभाव। Lack of coordination.

Disinfectant (डिसइनफेक्टैन्ट) सूक्ष्मजीवों को नष्ट करना भौतिक उपायों द्वारा। Destruction of disease producing microorganism or their toxins or vectors by chemical or physical means.

Disinfestation (डिसइन्फैस्टेशन) रोग उत्पन्न करने वाले परजीवियों एवं कीटाणुओं को मारने की क्रिया। The process of killing the parasites and insects causing diseases.

Disintegration (डिसिन्टिग्रेशन) किसी पदार्थ का उसके अवयवों में विघटित हो जाना। The breaking down of a substance into its constituents.

Dislocation (डिस्लोकेशन) विस्थापन। The displacement of organ or articular surface.

Disorientation (डिसओरियेन्टेशन) स्थिति भ्रांति। Loss of orientation.

Dispensary (डिस्पैन्सरी) औषधालय। The place for dispensing the medicines and treatment.

Dispensatory (डिस्पैन्सेटरी) ऐसी पुस्तक जिसमें औषधियों का उनके निर्माण एवं प्रयोगों का वर्णन होता है।

A book which describes the medicines, their preparations and their use.

Dispense (डिस्पैन्स) नुस्खा तैयार करना एवं इसे रोगी को देना। To prepare a prescription and to hand over it to the patient, suspension of very fine particles in a liquid.

Dispersion (डिस्पर्सन) छितराने की क्रिया। The process of scattering.

Dispersonalization (डिस्पर्सनेलाइजेशन) एक मानसिक रोग जिसमें रोगी अपने व्यक्तित्व या अंगो के अस्तित्व को अस्वीकार करता है। A mental disease in which the patient denies the existence of his or her personality or body parts.

Displacement (डिसप्लेस्मैन्ट) किसी सामान्य स्थिति अथवा स्थान से हटकर असामान्य स्थिति। Removal form the normal position or place to an abnormal position or place.

Disposition (डिस्पोजिशन) एक स्वभाविक प्रवृत्ति जो किसी रोग को ग्रहण करने की ओर प्रवृत्त होने से प्रकट हो सकती है। Individual aptitude, behavior as sum total of such evident characteristics.

Dissect (डिस्सैक्ट) शरीर रचना सम्बन्धी अध्ययन करने के लिए शव के ऊतकों एवं भागों को काटना। To split to go into detail, to separate various parts of cadaver.

Dissection (डिस्सैक्शन) विच्छेदन। The cutting part of body parts for study.

Disseminated (डिस्सेमिनेटेड) काफी बड़े क्षेत्र में फैला हुआ जिसे विशेषकर रोग उत्पन्न करने वाले जीवों के लिए प्रयोग किया जाता है। Scattered or widely distributed.

Dissipation (डिस्सीपेशन) किसी पदार्थ का फैलाव। Dispersion of matter.

Dissociation (डिस्सोसियेशन) वियोजन। Separation of part of a compound.

Dissolution (डिस्सोलयूशन) ऐसी क्रिया जिसमें एक पदार्थ दूसरे में घुल मिल जाता है। Breaking up the integrity of anatomical entity.

Dissolve (डिस्सोल्व) विलय करना। Dispersion of a solid within a liquid.

Distal (डिस्टल) दूरस्थ, केन्द्र से दूर। Away from the center, peripheral.

Distance (डिस्टेन्स) दूरी। The measure of space between two objects.

Distend (डिस्टैण्ड) फैलाना। To stretch out or to inflate.

Distensibility (डिस्टैन्सीबिलिटी) फूलने योग्य होने का गुण। Properly of being distensible.

Distillate (डिस्टीलेट) आसवन का कोई उत्पाद। A product of distillation.

Distillation (डिस्टीलेशन) वाष्पन-क्रिया द्वारा किसी तरल पदार्थ का संचयन करना। Vaporization, then condensing a liquid.

Distoma (डिस्टोमा) दो मुँह वाला कृमि। A genus of trematode worms having two mouths.

Distomiasis (डिस्टोमियेसिस) द्विमुखकृमिरोग। The presence of distoma in the body.

Distortion (डिस्टोरशन) विरूपन। Change from regular to irregular.

Distractibility (डिस्ट्रेक्टीविलिटी) ध्यानान्तरण। Inability to focus ones attention or mental wandering.

Distress (डिस्ट्रेस) कष्ट। Physical or mental trouble.

Distribution (डिस्ट्रीब्यूशन) वितरण। The layout pattern or spreading. Supply of nerve blood vessels.

Diuresis (डायूरेसिस) अधिक पेशाब आना। Excretion of urine.

Diuretics (डायूरेटिक्स) वह औषधि जिससे पेशाब अधिक आता है। Drugs causing secretion of urine.

Diurnal (डायूरेनल) दिवाकाल सम्बन्धी। Happening in the daytime.

Divergence (डायवर्जेन्स) किसी सामान्य बिन्दु से दूर जाना। The moving away from a common point.

Diverticular (डाइवर्टिकुलर) अंधवर्ध से सम्बन्धित। Pertaining to or resembling a diverticulum.

Diverticulum (डाइवर्टिकुलम) छेद, अंधनली। A pouch or sac protruding from the wall of a tube or a hollow organ.

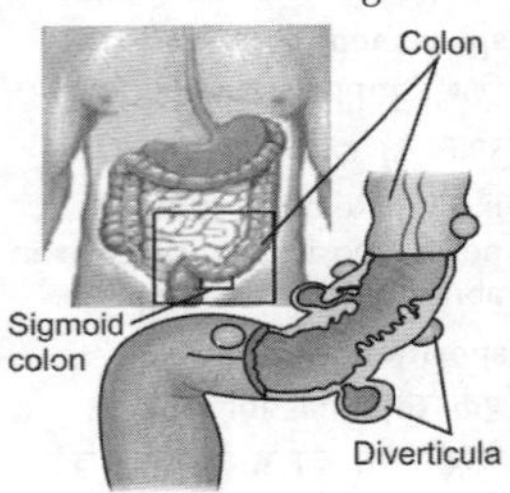

Division (डिवीजन) भाग, विभाजन। Separation.

Divulsion (डाइवल्शन) ताकत लगाकर दूर को खींचना। A pulling apart by force.

Dizziness (डिजीनेस) चक्कर। Vertigo.

Docche (डूश) औषधि युक्त ठण्डे एवं गर्म पानी की एक धार। A steam of fluid director against the body externally or into a body cavity.

Doctor (डॉक्टर) चिकित्सक। A licensed medical practitioner.

Doctrine (डॉक्ट्राइन) सिद्धांतों की शिक्षा पद्धति। The system of the principles tought.

Dolichocephalic (डोलिकोसिफैलिक) लम्बे सिर वाला। Long headed.

Dolichomorphic (डोलिकोमॉर्फिक) लम्बे, पतले शरीर वाला। Having a long, thin body.

Dolor (डॉलर) दर्द, पीड़ा। Pain.

Dolorimeter (डोलोरीमीटर) दर्द के अंश को डोल में मापने वाला यंत्र। An instrument for measuring the degree of pain in dols.

Dominance (डोमीनैन्स) प्रधानता। Supermacy or ascendancy.

Donor (डोनर) दाता। An individual from whom blood, tissue or an organ taken for transplantation.

Doping (डोपिंग) किसी औषधि या अन्य पदार्थ का किसी व्यक्ति में, विशेष रूप से कार्य में सुध ाार लाने के लिए किसी खिलाड़ी में प्रयोग करना। In sports, medicines use of drugs to improve sports performance commonly androgenic anabolic steroids.

Dormancy (डोर्मेन्सी) प्रसुप्तावस्था। Sleeping stage.

Dormant (डोर्मेंट) सोया हुआ। Sleeping.

Dorsad (डोर्साड) पीठ की ओर। Towards the back.

Dorsal (डोरसल) पृष्ठस्थ। Pertaining to the back or the posterior part of an organ.

Dorsalgia (डोर्सेल्जिया) पीठ में दर्द। Pain in the back.

Dorsi (डोर्सी) पीठ या पीछे की ओर संकेत करने वाले उपसर्ग। Prefixes indicating back.

Dorsiflexion (डोर्सीफ्लेक्शन) पीछे की ओर मुड़ना। Bending backward.

Dorsolateral (डोर्सोलेट्रल) पार्श्व एवं पीठ से सम्बन्धित। Pertaining to the back and the side.

Dosage (डोजेज) मात्रा-निर्धारण। The determination of the proper remedy.

Dose (डोज) मात्रा। The quantity of medicines taken at a time.

Dosimeter (डोसीमीटर) एक्स-रे की निकासी को मापने वाला। An instrument for measuring the X-ray output.

Dotage (डॉटेज) बुढ़ापा। Senility.

Dracontiasis (ड्राकोनटेएसिस) नारू रोग। Infestation with dracunculus, medinensis.

Draft (ड्राफ्ट) बौना। An abnormally under developed person.

Drain (ड्रेन) नाली, नली। A passage or charme of exist for discharge from an abscess, etc.

Drainage (ड्रेनेज) निकास। The gradual removal of the contents of a suppurating cavity.

Drastic (ड्रासटिक) बहुत तेजी से असर करने वाला। Acting strongly.

Draught (ड्रौट) पेय। A drink.

Drawsheet (ड्रॉ-शीट) रोगी के नीचे बिस्तर पर बिछा देने वाला चादर। A sheet stretched across the bed under the patient.

Drawsiness (ड्राउजिनेस) उनींदापन। The state of being sleepy.

Dresser (ड्रेसर) मरहम पट्टी करने वाला। The person who dresses the wounds.

Dressing (ड्रेसिंग) रोगग्रस्त स्थान को ढकना। Covering, protecting or supporting the diseased part.

Drift (ड्रिफ्ट) किसी बाह्य बल के कारण होने वाली गति जो अक्सर उद्देश्यहीन होती है। Movement due to an external force which is often aimless.

Drill (ड्रिल) छेद करने का वेधनी। A boring tool.

Drip (ड्रिप) किसी तरल पदार्थ औषधि को धीरे-धीरे बूंद-बूंद करके शरीर में पहुंचाना। The administration of a liquid medicine slowly drop by drop.

Droplet infection (ड्रॉपलेट-इन्फैक्शन) सूक्ष्म संक्रमित कणों के द्वारा फैलना। Spreading of infection by fine infected particle.

Dropsy (ड्रॉप्सी) ऊतकों में तरल पदार्थ का संचित हो जाना जिससे शोफ उत्पन्न हो जाता है। Accumulation of fluid in the tissue causing edema.

Drowning (ड्राउनिंग) डूब जाना। Asphyxiation due to immersion in liquid.

Drug abuse (ड्रग एब्यूज) किसी औषधि का खुद ही अधिक प्रयोग करना। Overuse or misuse of a drug by self-administration.

Drug addiction (ड्रग एडिक्शन) अधिक मात्रा में औषधि का प्रयोग करने से होने वाली दशा। A condition caused by excessive or continued use of a drug.

Drum (ड्रम) कान का पर्दा। The membrane tympanic.

Drunkenness (ड्रन्केननैस) शराब के नशे में धुत रहना। Alcoholic intoxication.

Ducrey's bacillus (डूक्रेज बेसिलस) दण्डाकार जीवाणु जो जोड़ों में पाये जाते है, ग्राम-ऋण दण्डाणु। Gram -ve rod shaped organism.

Duct (डक्ट) नलिका, वाहिनी। A tube giving exists to secretion of a gland or conducting any fluid.

Ductal (डक्टल) किसी वाहिनी से सम्बन्धित।
Pertaining to a duct.

Ductile (डक्टाइल) बिना टूटे हुए लम्बे होने की क्षमता रखना। Capable of being elongated without breaking.

Ductule (डक्ट्यूल) बहुत छोटी नली। A very small duct.

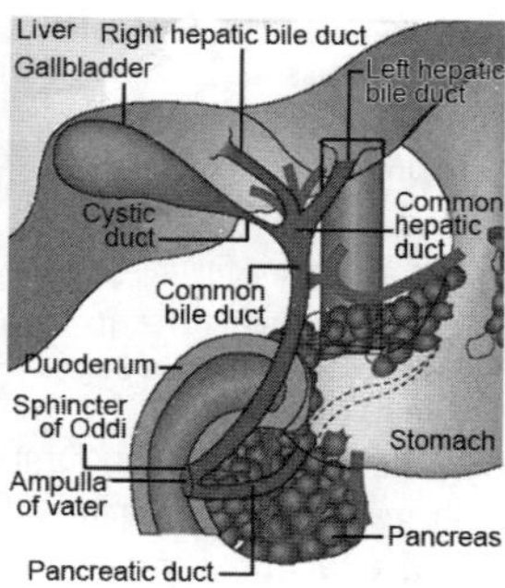

Duct

Dullard (डलार्ड) मुर्ख मनुष्य। A stupid person.

Dumbness (डम्बनेस) गूंगापन। Muteness.

Dumping syndrome (डम्पिंग सिण्ड्रोम) एक संलक्षण जिसमें खाना खाने के पश्चात् पसीना आता है तथा आमाशय को काटकर निकाल देने के फलस्वरूप उसके भीतर स्थित पदार्थो में एकदम से छोटी आँत में पहुँच जाने के कारण होता है। Dumping to stomach contents into the intestine manifesting with weakness and sweating soon after food in patient of gastrojejunostomy.

Dupuytren's contracture (डयूपुइट्रेन्स कॉन्ट्रैक्चर) अंगूठे वाली अंगुली का स्थायी रूप से हथेली की ओर मुड़ जाना। Contraction of the palmer aponeurosis.

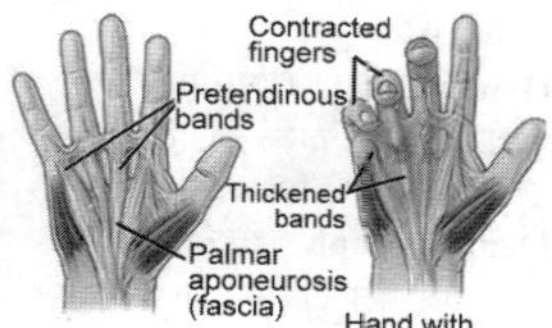

Duramater (डयूरामैटर) मस्तिष्क की बाहरी झिल्ली। The tough fibrous semi-transparent outer membrane lining the skull and covering the brain.

Duritis (डयूराइटिस) मस्तिष्क की बाहरी झिल्ली में सूजन। Inflammation of the dura.

Duskinesia (डस्काइनेसिया) ऐच्छिक गति की शक्ति में अवरोध उत्पन्न हो जाना। Impairment of the power of voluntary movement.

DVM (डी.वी.एम.) पशु रोग चिकित्सक।

Doctor of veterinary medicine.

DVT (डी.वी.टी.) गहन शिरा घनास्रता।

Deep vein thrombosis.

Dyad (डायड) जोडा।

Pair.

Dye (डाई) रंजक। A stain or coloring matter.

Dynamia (डायनेमिया) प्राण-शक्ति। Vital strength or energy.

Dynamic (डायनेमिक) गतिशील। Pertaining to or manifesting force.

Dynamogenic (डायनेमोजेनिक) शक्ति पैदा करने वाला। Generating force.

Dynamograph (डाइनैमोग्राफ) पेशीय बल का अभिलेखन करने वाला उपकरण। An apparatus for recording the muscular strength.

Dyne (डाइन) बल की दशमलव मापन विधि की इकाई, एक ग्राम वजन को एक सेकण्ड में एक सेमी तक सरकाने में लगने वाला बल। Force needed for importing acceleration of one cm in 1 sec to a 1 gm mass.

Dysacusis (डिएसकुसिस) सुनने में कठिनाई होना। Difficulty in hearing.

Dysarthria (डिसार्थिया) कठिन एवं वेष युक्त बोली। Difficult and defective speech.

Dysbasia (डिसबेसिया) विशेषकर केन्द्रीय तन्त्रिका तंत्र के रोग के कारण चलने में कठिनाई होना। Difficulty in walking especially due to the disease of the CNS.

Dyscalculia (डिस्केल्कुलिया) मस्तिष्क के रोग के कारण गणित के प्रश्नों को हल करने में असमर्थ। Inability to solve the mathematical problems due to brain disease.

Dyscoia (डिस्कोया) बहरापन। Deafness.

Dysentery (डिसेन्ट्री) ऐसा रोग जिसमें आंत की विशेषकर कॉलन की सुजन हो जाती है। Inflammation of the mucosal lining of the GIT.

Dysesthesia (डिसेस्थीसिया) किसी भी प्रकार के संवेद विशेषकर स्पर्श संवेद में बाधा उत्पन्न हो जाना। Impairment of any sense specially of touch.

Dysgammaglobulinemia (डिस्गामाग्लोबुलिनीमिया) रक्त में इम्युनोगलोबुलिन की सान्द्रता में विषमता जो जन्मजात हो सकता है। Disproportion in the concentration of immunoglobulins in the blood which may be congenital.

Dysgenesis (डिस्जेनेसिस) विशेषकर भ्रुण में होने वाला कवकास। Maldevelopment specially of the embryo.

Dysgeusia (डिस्गीयुसिया) स्वाद की अनुभुति में अवरोध उत्पन्न हो जाना। Impairment of the sense of taste.

Dysgraphia (डिसग्राफिया) लिखते समय हाथ कांपना। Writer's cramps.

Dyshidrosis (डिस्हाइड्रोसिस) हाथ व पैर में पसीने के कारण होने वाली तकलीफ, छोटी फुंसियां, फोड़ा। Disorder of sweating recurrent vesicular eruption on the limbs with intense itching.

Dyslexia (डिस्लैक्सिया) केन्द्रीय तंत्रिका तंत्र में कोई व्रेष उत्पन्न हो जाने के कारण लिखी हुई भाषा की व्याख्या करने में असमर्थ। Inability to interpret the written language due to a defect in the central nervous system.

Dyslogia (डिस्लोजिया) मानसिक विकारों के कारण विचारों को अभिव्यक्त करने में कठिनाई। Difficulty in expressing the ideas due to mental disorder.

Dysmaturity (डिस्मैच्युरिटी) भ्रूण का अपनी गर्भावस्था आयु की अपेक्षा छोटा। The condition of the fetus of being small or immature for its gestational age.

Dysmelia (डिस्मेलिया) अधिक भुजाओं में जन्मजात विकृति होना।

Congenital deformity of a limb or limbs.

Dysmenorrhea (डिस्मेनोरिह्या) मासिक धर्म के साथ दर्द होना कष्टार्तव। Pain during menstruation.

Dysmetria (डिस्मैट्रिया) पेशीय गति या किसी कार्य की गति को नियंत्रित करने में अक्षमता। Inablity to control the speed of muscular movement or of an act.

Dysopia (डिसोपिया) दोषपूर्ण दृष्टि होना। Defective or painful vision.

Dysorexia (डिसोरेक्सिया) अस्वभाविक भूख लगना। Abnormal hunger.

Dysosmia (डिसोस्मिया) सूंघने में किसी प्रकार की अस्वभाविकता होना। Perverted sense of smell.

Dysostosis (डिसोस्टोसिस) दोषयुक्त अस्थिभवन। Defective ossification.

Dyspareunia (डिसपैरीयूनिया) लैंगिक संसर्ग काल में योनि में दर्द होना। Occurrence of pain in the vagina during sexual intercourse.

Dyspepsia (डिस्पैप्सिया) पाचन क्रिया में अवरोध उत्पन्न हो जाना जिसकी खाना खाने के बाद अधिजठर प्रदेश में कष्ट होना विशेष्टता होती है, अग्निमांद्य या दुश्पचन। Impairment in the process of digestion which is characterized by discomfort in the epigastric region after meals.

Dysphagia (डिस्फजिया) निगलने में कठिनाई। Difficulty in swallowing.

Dysphasia (डिस्फेजिया) मस्तिष्क में क्षति होने के कारण बोलने में बाधा उत्पन्न होना। Impairment of speech due to lesion in the brain.

Dysphoria (डिस्फोरिया) बिना कारण उदासीनता एवं बेचैनी रहना। Depression and restlessness without any cause.

Dysplasia (डिस्प्लेसिया) ऊतकों के विकास में असामान्यता। Abnormality in the development of tissue.

Dyspnea (डिसनिया) सांस फूलना। Labored or difficult breathing.

Dyspragia (डिस्प्रेगिया) किसी भी कार्य को करने में दर्द होना। Pain or difficulty in performing any function.

Dyssomnia (डिस्सोम्निया) निद्रा में विघ्न पड़ना। Disturbance in sleep.

Dysstasia (डिस्सटेसिया) खड़े होने में कठिनाई। Difficulty in standing.

Dystaxia (डिस्टैक्सिया) ऐच्छिक गतियों को नियंत्रण में करने में कठिनाई उत्पन्न होना। Difficulty in controlling the voluntary movements.

Dystocia (डिस्टोसिया) कष्ट के साथ प्रसव होना। Difficult labor or child birth.

Dystonia (डिस्टोनिया) विकृत पेशीय तान। Pertaining to dystonia.

Dystopia (डिस्टोपिया) किसी अंग का विस्थापन हो जाना। Malposition displacement of any organ.

Dystopic (डिस्टोपिक) अपने स्थान पर न रहने वाला। Not in place.

Dystrophia, Dystrophy (डिस्ट्रॉफिया, डिस्ट्रॉफी) दोषयुक्त पोषण। Any disorder caused by defective nutrition or metabolism.

Dysuria (डिस्यूरिया) कठिनाई में मूत्र त्याग होना। Painful micturation.

Dyszoospermia (डिस्जूस्पर्मिया) शुक्राणुओं का अपूर्ण निर्माण। Imperfect formation of spermatozoa.

E

Ear (इयर) कान। Organ of hearing.

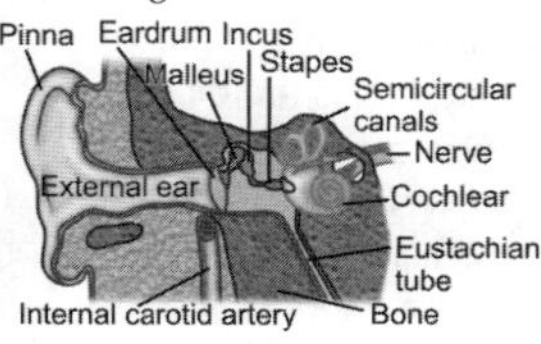

Ear-lobe (इयर-लोब) कर्णपाली का निचला मांसल भाग बाह्य श्रवणीय नली में। The lower fleshy part of the auricle device for plugging.

Ear-plug (इयर-प्लग) अवरोध उत्पन्न करके कान में ध्वनि के प्रवेश को रोकने वाला एक उपकरण। The external auditory canal, thereby preventing access of sound to internal ear.

Earache (इयरऐक) कान का दर्द। Pain in the ear.

Eardrum (इयरड्रम) मध्यवर्ग-गुहा। The cavity of the middle ear.

Earwax (इयरवैक्स) कान का मैल। Cerumen.

Eburnation (एबरनेषन) हड्डी का एक ठोस एवं कठोर हाथी दांत के समान पिण्ड में बदल जाना। Conversion of bone into a dense and hard, ivory like mass.

Ecchondroma (इकॉण्ड्रोना) उपास्थि-ऊतक का बाहर की ओर बढ़ना। A cartilaginous tumor.

Eccrine (एक्राइन) बाह्यस्रावी। Pertaining to secretion especially of the sweat glands.

Echinococcus (इकिनोकोकस) एक प्रकार का फीताकृमि जो मनुष्य में रोग उत्पन्न करता है। A type of tapeworm which causes disease in man.

Echo (इको) गूंज, प्रतिध्वनि। Repetition of sound caused by reflection of sound waves.

Echocardiogram (इकोकार्डियोग्राम) इकोकार्डियोग्राफी द्वारा उत्पन्न रेखाचित्रित अभिलेख। The graphic record produced by echocardiography.

Echocardiography (इकोकार्डियोग्राफी) अल्ट्रासाउण्ड का प्रयोग करके हृदय की आँतरिक रचनाओं को दृष्टिगत करना। To visualize the internal cardiac structures by the use of ultrasound.

Echokinesia (इकोकाइनेसिया) किसी दूसरे व्यक्ति के हाव-भावों को

अनैच्छिक रूप से बार-बार दुहराना। Involuntary repetition of the gestures of another person.

Echopraxia (इकोप्रेक्सिया) दूसरे के कामों की नकल करना। To copy the action of others.

Echo virus (इको वाइरस) श्लेष्मज्वराणु। A virus related to influenza which causes obscure types of infection.

Eclampsia (एकलैम्पसिया) गर्भक्षेप। Puerperal convection.

Eclecticsm (एकलैक्टिसिज्म) चिकित्सा की एक प्राचीन पद्धति जिसमें मुख्यतया वानस्पतिक औषधियों द्वारा रोगों की अपेक्षा व्यक्तिगत चिन्हों एवं लक्षणों की चिकित्सा की जाती है। Medicine where treatment is dependent upon individual signs and symptoms rather than the disease as a whole.

Ecocide (इकोसाइड) स्वेच्छा से पर्यावरण से कुछ भाग को नष्ट कर देना। To destroy some portion of the environment willingly.

Ecological (इकोलॉजीकल) पारिस्थितिक। Pertaining to ecology.

Ecology (इकोलॉजी) प्राणियों के जीवन इतिहास एवं वातावरण से उनके सम्बन्धों का अध्ययन करना। Study of the life history of the organisms and their environment.

Ecostate (इकोस्टेट) पसलियों से हीन। Without ribs.

Ectasia (एक्टेसिया) विस्फारण। Dilation of a tubular structure.

Ectasis (एकटेसिस) किसी अंग-विशेष का असाधारण रूप से फैल जाना। An abnormal distension of a part.

Ecthyma (इकथेमा) पस भरी फुंसियों से युक्त उद्‌भेद। An eruption of large, round pustules, quite distinct from each other.

Ectocervix (एक्टोसर्विक्स) बहिजरायुग्रीवा, योनि में स्थित रहने वाला भाग। The portion of the canal of the uterine cervix.

Ectoderm (एक्टोडर्म) बहिष्चर्म, विकसित भ्रूण के तीन कोषिकीय स्तरों में से सबसे बाहर का स्तर। The external primitive layer of the embryo.

Ectomelia (एक्टोमीलिया) भुजाओं की लम्बी हड्डियों का जन्मजात अल्प विकसन। Congenital hypoplasia or aplasia of the long bones of the limbs.

Ectomorph (एक्टोमोर्फ) कमजोर। Linear slender body builds with poor musculature.

Ectoparasite (एकटोपेरासाइट) बाह्य परजीवी। Parasite living an outer surface of body.

Ectopia (एक्टोपिया) अस्थानता। Malposition or displacement.

Ectopic (एक्टोपिक) असामान्य स्थिति में स्थापित। Relating to ectopia, located in an abnormal position.

Ectopic pregnancy (एक्टोपिक प्रेग्नैन्सी) निशेचित डिम्ब का गर्भाशय के बाहर, सामान्यतया डिम्ब वाहिनी में आरोपित हो जाना। Extrauterine gestation.

Ectopic rhythm (एक्टोपिक रिद्म) कोई भी असामान्य अथवा अनियमित हृदय-ताल। Any abnormal or irregular cardiac rhythm.

Ectoplasm (एक्टोप्लाज्म) किसी कोशिका जीवद्रव्य का सबसे बाहरी स्तर। The outermost layer of cell protoplasm.

Ectostosis (एक्टोस्टोसिस) पर्यास्थिकला या पैरीऑस्टियम के नीचे हड्डी का बनना। Formation of bone beneath periosteum.

Ectothrix (एक्टोथ्रिक्स) ऐसा कवक जैसे–माइक्रोस्पोरम जो बालों के कॉण्डों के ऊपर आरथ्रोस्पोरों को उत्पन्न करता है। Fungus growing on hair shafts.

Ectozoa (एक्टोजोआ) जूं। External parasites.

Ectozoon (एक्टोजोन) बहिःपरजीवी। Parasite living another animal.

Eczema (एक्जिमा) दाद। A chronic skin condition of allergic origin.

ED (ई.डी.) प्रभावी मात्रा। Effective dose.

EDD (ई.डी.डी.) प्रसव की संभावित तिथि। Expected date of delivery.

Edema (एडेमा) पानी वाली सूजन। Tissue swelling due to retained fluid.

Edentia (इडैन्टिया) दाँतों का अभाव। Absence of teeth.

Edge (ऐज) किनारा। A margin or border.

Effacement (एफैसमेन्ट) प्रसव के दौरान भ्रूण का मार्ग बनाने के लिए गर्भाशय ग्रीवा का विस्फारित हो जाना। The dilation of the cervix during labor to permit the passage of the fetus.

Effect (इफैक्ट) प्रभाव। The result or consequence of an action.

Effector (इफैक्टर) वह पेशी जो तंत्रिका आवेगों की प्रत्यक्ष अनुक्रिया में संकुचित होती है। A motor or secretory nerve ending in a muscle, gland or organ.

Efferent (इफैरेन्ट) केन्द्र से बाहर की ओर ले जाने वाला। Conveying from a center.

Effervescence (इफरवेसेन्स) किसी द्रव की सतह पर गैस के बुलबुले बनना। Formation of gas bubbles on the surface of a liquid.

Effleurage (इफल्यूरेज) मालिश करते समय थपथपाना। The stroking in massage.

Effluent (एफ्लुएन्ट) बहाने वाला। Flowing out.

Effusion (इफ्यूजन) बहाव। Escape of fluid lair into a cavity.

Egesta (एजेस्टा) मल। The excrement of the body.

Ego (इगो) अहम्। The conscious sense of the self.

Egoism (इगोइज्म) दूसरों का नुकसान कराके अपने फायदे को खोजना। An inflated estimate of one's value or effectiveness.

Egomania (इगोमैनिया) आत्म-सम्मान एवं स्वार्थ के लिए पागलपन। Mania for self-estimate and self-interest.

Ejaculation (इजाकुलेशन) जोर से अचानक बाहर को निकल जाना विशेषतया पुरूष मूत्रमार्ग से वीर्य का निकलना। Ejection of seminal fluid from male urethra.

Ejection fraction (इजैक्षन फ्रैक्षन) प्रंकुचन के दौरान वेन्ट्रिकल द्वारा फेंके गए रक्त की प्रतिशतता जो 60 से 70% तक होती है। The percentage of blood ejection from the ventricle during systole which is 60 to 70%.

Elastic (इलास्टिक) लचीला। Endowed with elasticity.

Elasticity (इलास्टीसिटी) लचीलापन। The quality of returning to its original size after stretching.

Elastometer (इलास्टोमीटर) लचीलेपन को मापने वाला उपकरण। A device for measuring the elasticity.

Elastometry (एलास्टोमीट्री) ऊतकों के लचीलेपन को मापना। The measurement of elasticity of the tissue.

Elastorrhexis (इलास्टोरेह्क्सिस) इलास्टिक ऊतक का फट जाना। Rupture of the elastic tissue.

Elation (एलेशन) खुशी में झूम जाना। Joyful emotion.

Elbow (एल्बो) ऊपरी बाहु एवं अग्रबाहु के बीच का जोड़ कोहनी। The joint between the upper arm and the forearm.

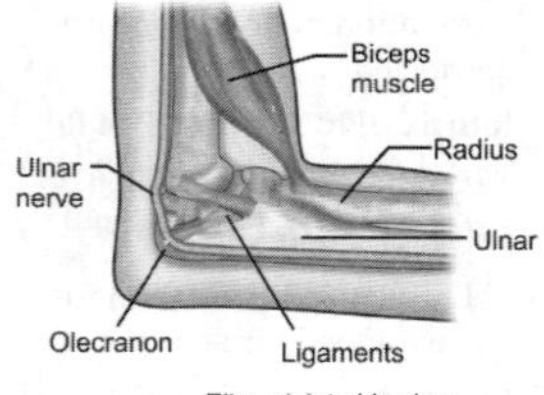

Elbow joint-side view

Elcosis (एल्कोसिस) बदबूदार घाव। Fetid ulceration.

Elective therapy (इलैक्टिव थेरैपी) शल्य-क्रिया सम्बन्धी चिकित्सा जिसकी तुरन्त आवश्यकता नहीं होती बल्कि यह रोगी की सुविधानुसार की जा सकती है। A planned convenient therapy operation.

Electric-shok (इलैक्ट्रिक-शॉक) विद्युत स्पर्श से बेहोशी हो जाना। Tissue injury from passage of electricity.

Electro-occulogram (इलैक्ट्रो-ओक्यूलोग्राम) विद्युत-नेत्र लेख। Graphic record of eye position and movement.

Electroanalgesia (इलैक्ट्रोएनलजेसिया) विद्युत का प्रयोग करके दर्द में आराम पहुंचाना। To cause relief from pain by using electricity.

Electrocardiogram (इलैक्ट्रोकार्डियोग्राम) विद्युत-यंत्र द्वारा लिया गया हृदय आवेगों का अनुरेखन या रेखा चित्र। A tracing of the cardiac impulse by an electrical instrument.

Electrocardiograph (इलैक्ट्रोकार्डियोग्राफ) हृदय पेशी के कार्य में होने वाले वैद्युत परिवर्तनों को रिकार्ड करने वाला उपकरण। An apparatus for recording the electrical variations in the action of cardiac muscle.

Electrocautery (इलैक्ट्रोकॉटरी) एक होल्डर में फिट हुए प्लेटिनम के तार को विद्युत-धारा से गर्म करके ऊतकों का दहन करना। The direct or alternating current is passed through a resistant metal wire electrode, generating heat.

Electrocoagulation (इलैक्ट्रोकौगुलेशन) विद्युत-धारा द्वारा ऊतक का स्कन्दन करना। Coagulation of tissue by means of an electric current.

Electroconvulsive therapy (इलैक्ट्रोकनवल्सिव थिरैपी) विद्युत द्वारा दौरे उत्पन्न करके किसी विशिष्ट मानसिक रोग की चिकित्सा करना। Treatment of some specific mental disease by inducing convulsions by means of electricity.

Electrode (इलैक्ट्रोड) विद्युतचालक। That part of any electric apparatus designed to be applied to the body.

Electrodesiccation (इलैक्ट्रोडेसीकेशन) छोटी-उच्च-बारम्बारता की विद्युत-धारा द्वारा निर्जलीकरण उत्पन्न होने से ऊतक का नष्ट होना। A technique of electric diathermy.

Electrodialysis (इलैक्ट्रोडायालाइसिस) किसी विलयन में जिसमें इलैक्ट्रोलाइट एवं कोलाइड दोनों होते हैं,

विद्युत-धारा प्रवाहित करके इलैक्ट्रोलाइटों को कोलाइडों से पृथक करने की एक विधि। A method of separating electrolytes from colloids by passing current through the solution.

Electrodynamometer (इलैक्ट्रोडाइनैमोमीटर) किसी विद्युत धारा की शक्ति मापने का यंत्र। An instrument to measure the strength of an electric current.

Electroencephalogram (इलैक्ट्रोएन्सीफैलोग्राम) विद्युत मस्तिष्क लेख। A training of an electroencephalograph.

Electroencephalograph (इलैक्ट्रोएन्सीफैलोग्राफ) विद्युत मस्तिष्क लेखन में प्रयोग किया जाने वाला यंत्र। An instrument used in electro-encephalograph.

Electrogoniometer (इलैक्ट्रोगोनियोमीटर) संधियों के कोणों एवं उनके गति करने के फैलाव को मापने वाला एक विद्युत उपकरण। An electrical apparatus for measuring angles of joints and their range of movements.

Electrolysis (इलैक्ट्रोलाइसिस) विद्युत-अपघटन। Dissolution of a compound body by electricity.

Electrolyte (इलैक्ट्रोलाइट) विद्युत-अपघट्य। A compound capable of resolution by electrolysis.

Electrometer (इलैक्ट्रोमीटर) विद्युत की तीव्रता को मापने वाला यंत्र। An instrument for determining electric intensity.

Electromotive-force (EMF) (इलैक्ट्रोमोटिव फोर्स ई.एम.एफ.) विद्युत को एक स्थान से दूसरे स्थान तक प्रवाहित करने वाली शक्ति जिससे एक विद्युत-धारा उत्पन्न होती है। The difference in potential that causes the flow of electricity. It is measured in volts.

Electromyogram (इलैक्ट्रोमायोग्राम) विद्युतपेशी लेख। The graphical representation produced by an electromyograph.

Electromyography (इलैक्ट्रोमायोग्राफी) किसी कंकालीय पेशी का विद्युतपेशीलेख लेकर उसका अध्ययन करना। Preparation, study and interpretation of electromyograms.

Electronics (इलैक्ट्रोनिक्स) विद्युत उपकरणों का विज्ञान। The science of the electrical equipment.

Electrophoresis (इलैक्ट्रोफोरेसिस) विद्युतीकरण संचलन। The movement of charged colloidal particles as a result of changes in electric potential.

Electrophysiology (इलैक्ट्रोफिजियोलॉजी) विद्युत शरीर क्रिया विज्ञान। The study of electrical phenomena in living tissues.

Electroretinogram (इलैक्ट्रोरेटिनोग्राम) प्रकाश उद्दीपन द्वारा उत्पन्न रेटिना की विद्युत-सक्रियता का लेख प्रमाण। A record of the electricals activity of the retina produced by light stimulation.

Electrostatic (इलैक्ट्रोस्टेटिक) स्थिर विद्युत से सम्बन्धित। Pertaining to the static electricity.

Electrotherapeutics (इलैक्ट्रोथिरापूटिक्स) विद्युत द्वारा रोगों की चिकित्सा। Treatment of the diseases by electricity.

Electrotoma (इलैक्ट्रोटोम) शल्य-क्रिया में प्रयोग में लाया जाने वाला एक विद्युत दहन उपकरण। An electrocautery device used in surgery.

Element (एलीमैन्ट) किसी वस्तु के प्राथमिक घटकों में से एक अवयव। A substance that cannot be further broken down to substances different from it, e.g. Carbon, Sodium, calcium, etc.

Elephantiasis (एलीफैन्टियेसिस) हाथी-पांव। Hypertrophy of skin and subcutanecus tissues due to lymphatic stasis.

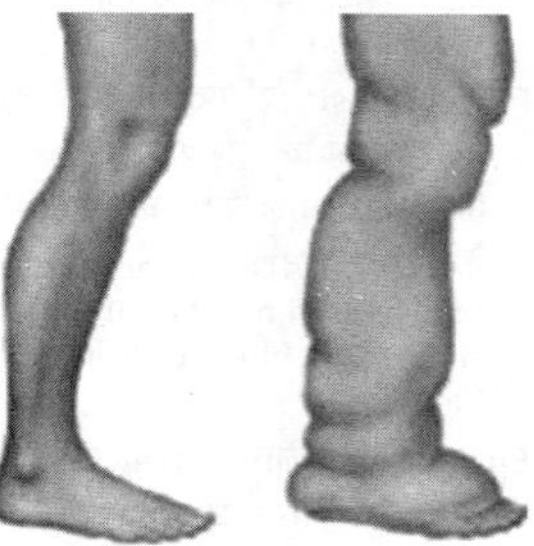

Healthy leg Elephantiasis

Elevator (एलिवेटर) ऊतकों को ऊपर उठाने वाला यंत्र जैसे दबी हुई हड्डी। An instrument for raising the tissues as the depressed bone or the roots of the teeth.

Eliminate (एलिमिनेट) बाहर निकाल देना। To expel.

Elimination (एलिमिनेशन) बाहर निकालने की क्रिया। The act of expulsion.

Elinquid (इलिनक्यूइड) गूंगा। Mute.

Elixir (इलिक्जिर) जलअक्सीर, सुरस। Sweatened hydroalcoholic liquid.

Ellipsoid (एलिप्सॉयड) आगे-पीछे से पतला तथा बीच में मोटा। Spindle-shaped, fusiform, tapering at both ends.

Elliptocyte (एलिप्टोसाइट) अण्डाकार लाल रक्त कोशिका। Oval-shaped red blood cell.

Elliptocytosis (एलिप्टोसाइटोसिस) रक्त में अधिक संख्याओं में अण्डाकार लाल रक्त कोशिकाओं के होने की दशा। Condition of increased number of oval-shaped red blood cells in the blood.

Elongation (एलोन्गेशन) फैलाने की क्रिया उस रोगी से सम्बन्धित जो बिना इजाजत अस्पताल से जाने की तैयारी में है। The act of extending pertaining to the patient who is ready to go away from the hospital without permission.

Elutriation (इल्यूट्रीएशन) धोकर अलग करने की क्रिया। Process of separating by washing.

Emaciation (एमेसिएशन) अत्यधिक दुबला पतला होना। The condition of being extremely lean.

Emasculation (इमैस्कुलेशन) डिम्बग्रंथियों को काटकर हटा देना। Excision of testicles or ovaries.

Embalming (इमबैलमिंग) मृत शरीर को सड़ने से बचाने के लिए उसके भीतर एवं बाहर पूतिरोधी तथा रक्षक पदार्थो का प्रयोग करना। Use to out sepsis and preservatives to prevent premature biodegradation of dead body.

Embolectomy (एमबोलेक्टॉमी) अन्तःशल्य को निकालकर हटा देना। Removal of an embolus.

Embolism (एमबोलिज्म) किसी रक्त वाहिनी में रक्त का थक्का। Obstruction of a blood vessel by a blood clot or foreign substance.

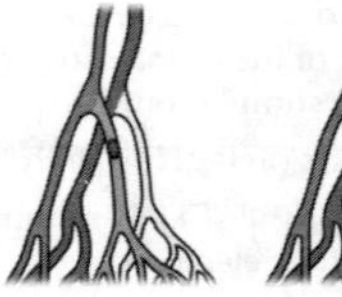

Embolus (एमबोलस) जमा हुआ रक्त। A blood clot or other body occluding blood vessels.

Embryo (एम्ब्रियो) गर्भावस्था के दूसरे सप्ताह से लेकर 8 वें सप्ताह तक का विकसित होता हुआ गर्भित डिम्ब। The early stage of the fetus.

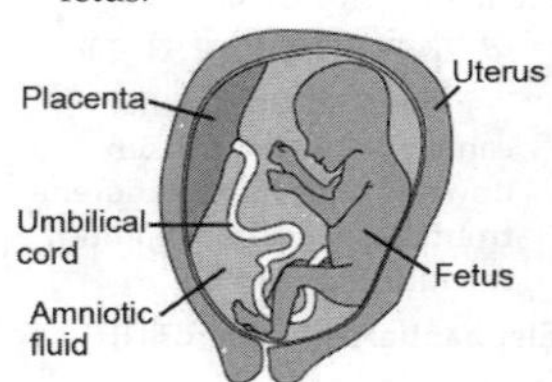

Embryocidal (एम्ब्रियोसाइडल) कोई भी वस्तु जो भ्रूण को मार देती है। Anything that kills an embryo.

Embryoctony (एम्ब्रियोक्टॉनी) गर्भाशय में स्थित जीवित भ्रूण को नष्ट कर देना। To destory the living embryo or fetus in the uterus.

Embryogeny (एम्ब्रियोजेनी) भ्रूण की वृद्धि एवं विकास। The growth and development of an embryo.

Embryology (एम्ब्रियोलॉजी) भ्रूण की रचना तथा विकास सम्बन्धी रचना। The science of embryonic evolution.

Emesis (इमेसिस) वमन। Vomiting or the cut of vomiting.

Emetic (इमेटिक) वमनकारी। Medicine or substance that produces vomiting.

Emigration (इमिग्रेशन) शोध की प्रक्रिया में श्वेत रक्त कोशिकाओं का सूक्ष्म रक्त वाहिनियों की दीवारों से होकर गुजरना। Passage of WBC through walls of capillaries.

Eminence (इमिनैन्स) उभार। A protuberance or process.

Emissary (एमिसरी) निकास। Outlet.

Emission (एमिसन) स्वप्नदोष। An ejaculation or sending forth.

Emmetropia (इमेट्रोपिया) सामान्य दृष्टि। The condition of being without ametropia.

Emmetropic (इमेट्रोपिक) सामान्य दृष्टि से सम्बन्धित। Normal vision.

Emolleint (इमोलिएन्ट) ऊतकों को कोमलता प्रदान करने वाला पदार्थ। An agent which softens tissues.

Emotion (इमोशन) भावावेग, एक मानसिक अवस्था जैसे–भय, घृणा, प्रेम, क्रोध, दुःख। A mental state or feeling such as fear, hate, grief, joy, with some changes in cardiorespiratory function.

Emotivity (इमोटीविटी) आवेश-अनुक्रिया के लिए किसी व्यक्ति की क्षमता। The capability of a person for emotional response.

Emphysema (एम्फायसिमा) वातास्फीति। Pathological distension of tissue by air gas.

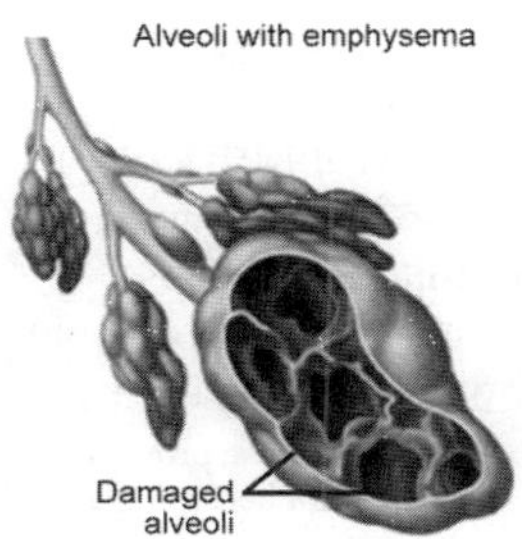

Empiric (एम्पीरिक) अनुभव पर आधारित चिकित्सक। A medical practitioner based on experience, quack.

Empirical (एम्पीरिकल) प्रयोगसिद्ध। Relying on a derived from an observation.

Emprosthotonos (एम्प्रोस्थोटोनोस) ऐसी ऐंठन जिसमें शरीर आगे की ओर झुक जाता है। The spasm in which the body is bent forward.

Emptysis (एम्पटाइसिस) बलगम में खून आना। Hemoptysis.

Empyema (एम्पाइमा) फुफ्फुसावरण में मवाद का इकट्ठा हो जाना। Accumulation of pus in a cavity or body, especially the chest.

Empyesis (एम्पायेसिस) पीबदार फुंसी। Any pustular eruption.

Empyocele (एम्पायोसील) जलवृषण या हाइड्रोसील में पस पड़ जाना। Formation of pus in a hydrocele.

Emulgent (एमलजेन्ट) बाहर निकालने वाला। Draining out.

Emulsification (एमलसिफिकेशन) पायसीकरण, वसा के बड़े कणों को एकरूप से वितरित छोटे कणों में तोड़ देना। The process of making or of becoming an emulsion.

Emulsion (इमल्सन) ऐसा द्रव जिसमें किसी तैलीय पदार्थ के बारीक कण निलम्बित रहते हैं। A liquid with fine particles of an oily substance suspended in it.

Enamel (इनैमल) दांतों पर सफेद चमकदार पत्थर। The exterior coating of the teeth.

Enanthem, Enanthema (एननथेम, एननथेमा) श्लेश्मिक कला पर विस्फोट। Eruption on the mucous membrane.

Enantiopathy (इनैनटियोपैथी) एक रोग की चिकित्सा दूसरा रोग उत्पन्न करके करना। Treatment of one disease by producing another disease.

Encephalalgia (एनसिफैलेल्जिया) सिर में बहुत तेज दर्द होना। Cephalalgia, deep seated pain in the head.

Encephalitis (एनसिफैलाइटिस) मस्तिष्क शोथ। Inflammation of the brain.

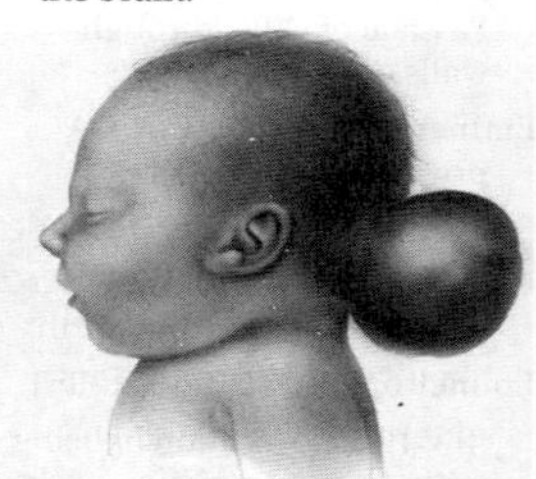

Encephalocele (एनसिफैलोसील) कपाल में स्थित किसी फटन या दरार से होकर मस्तिष्क के पदार्थ का बाहर निकलना। Hernia of the brain, protrusion of the brain substance through a cranial fissure.

Encephalogram (एनसिफैलोग्राम) मस्तिष्क की एक्स-रे फिल्म। X-ray film of the brain.

Encephalomalacia (एनसिफैलोमैलेसिया) मस्तिष्क का मुलायम हो जाना। Softening of the brain.

Encephalomeningocele (एनसिफैलोमैनिन्गोसील) मस्तिष्क आवरणों एवं मस्तिष्क पदार्थ का कपाल में स्थित किसी दरार से होकर बाहर निकल आना। Protrusion of the meninges and the brain substance through a fissure in the cranium.

Encephalomyelitis (एनसिफैलोमायलाइटिस) मस्तिष्क एवं सुषुम्ना का शोध। Inflammation of the brain and the spinal cord.

Encephalopathy (एनिसिफैलोपैथी) मस्तिष्क का कोई भी रोग। Any disease of the brain.

Encephalotome (एनसिफैलोटोम) मस्तिष्क में चीरा लगाने वाला यंत्र। An instrument for incision the brain.

Encondroma (एनकॉण्ड्रोमा) ऐसे स्थान पर जहां पर उपास्थि नहीं होती, उत्पन्न होने वाला एक सुक्ष्म उपास्थि अर्बुद। A cartilaginous tumor.

Encopresis (एनकोप्रेसिस) निरंकुशपुरीशता। Involuntary passage of the feces.

Endarterectomy (इण्डार्टेरेक्टॉमी) किसी धमनी के सबसे भीतर के स्तर को शल्यक्रिया द्वारा काटकर अलग कर देना। Surgical removal of the innermost coat of an artery.

Endarteritis (एण्डार्टीराइटेस) किसी धमनी के सबसे भीतरी स्तर का शोथ। Inflammation of the innermost coat of an artery.

Endemic (एन्डेमिक) किसी विशेष आबादी में उत्पन्न होने वाला कोई रोग जिसकी मृत्यु दर कम होती है जैसे–खसरा। A disease occurring in a particular population but has low mortality rate as measles.

Endermic (एण्डर्मिक) त्वचा द्वारा दी जाने वाली। Introduced through the skin by abrading surface.

Endocarditis (एण्डोकार्डाइटिस) हृदयावरक झिल्ली का प्रदाह। Inflammation of the lining membrane of the heart.

Endocervicitis (एण्डोसर्विसाइटिस) अन्त-गर्भाशय ग्रीवा शोथ।

Inflammation of mucus lining of endocervix.

Endocrine Gland (एण्डोक्राइन गलैण्ड) अन्तःस्रावी ग्रंथि जो एक आन्तरिक स्राव जैसे हॉर्मोन को उत्पन्न करती है और उसे रक्त अथवा लसीका में छोड़ती है। Glands secrete directly into blood steam.

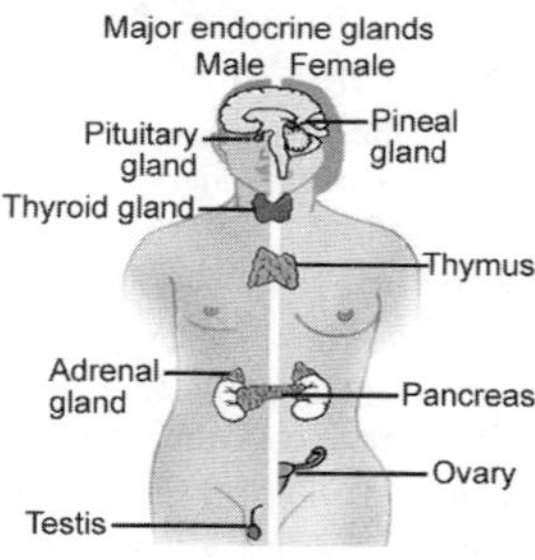

Endocytosis (एण्डोसाइटोसिस) किसी कोशिका की अपनी भित्ति के अन्तर्वेशन द्वारा बाह्य पदार्थ का भक्षण करने की विधि। A method of ingestion of a foreign substance by a cell.

Endoderm (एण्डोडर्म) किसी भ्रूण की कोशिकाओं की भीतरी परत। Inner layer of cells of an embryo.

Endodontics (एण्डोडोन्टिक्स) दन्तमूल तथा आसपास के चारों ओर के ऊतकों के रोगों के कारणों, निदान, रोकथाम एवं चिकित्सा से होता है। A branch of dentistry concerned diagnosis, treatment and prevention of disease of dental pulp and its surrounding tissue.

Endogenous, Endogenic (एण्डोजीनस, एण्डोजेनिक) जीव के भीतर उत्पन्न होने वाला। Produced in the organism.

Endolymph (एण्डोलिम्फ) कान के अंदर का तरल पदार्थ। Fluid in the inner ear.

Endometriosis (एण्डोमीट्रियोसिस) अन्तर्गर्भाशय कला ऊतक का गर्भाशय गुहा से बाहर उत्पन्न होना। Proliferation of endometrium at ectopic site.

Endometritis (एण्डोमैट्राइटिस) अन्तर्गर्भाशय कला का शोथ। Inflammation of the endometrium.

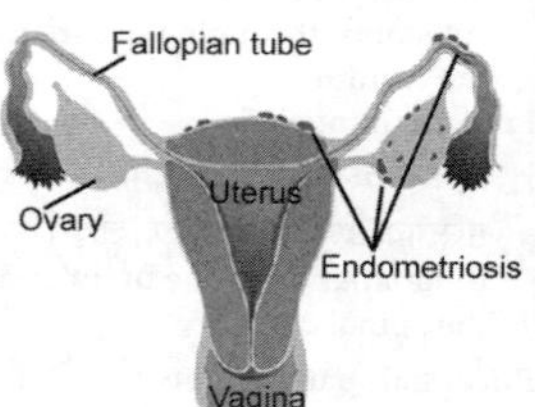

Endomorph (एण्डोमॉर्फ) ऐसा व्यक्ति जिसका शारीरिक गठन इस प्रकार का होता है जिसमें अन्तर्जनस्तर-ऊतकों की प्रधानता होती है और सम्पूर्ण शरीर

मुलायम एवं गोलाई लिये हुए होता है। Body build characterized by predominance of tissues derived from endoderm.

Endoneurium (एण्डोन्यूरियम) किसी परिसरीय तंत्रिका में इसके तन्तुओं को अलग करने वाला संयोजी ऊतक का आच्छद। A connective tissue sheath in a peripheral nerve, separating its fibers.

Endopelvic (एण्डोपैल्विक) श्रोणी के भीतर स्थित। Situated within the pelvis.

Endophthalmitis (एण्डोफ्थैल्माइटिस) आँख का अन्दरूनी प्रदाह। Inflammation within substance of eye.

Endorgan (एण्डऑर्गन) किसी संवेदी तंत्रिका तंतु का अंतिम चौड़ा भाग। The terminal explained portion of a sensory nerve fiber.

Endosalpingitis (एण्डोसैल्पिन्जाइटिस) डिम्ब-वाहिनियों को आश्रित करने वाली श्लैश्मिक झिल्ली की सूजन। Inflammation of the mucous membrane lining of the fallopian tube.

Endoscope (एण्डोस्कोप) शरीर में स्थित किसी प्राकृतिक छिद्र या द्वार द्वारा निरीक्षण करने के लिए प्रयोग में आने वाला एक यंत्र। A device containing optical system for observing or conducting surgery in hollow structure like abdomen pelvis.

Endoscopy (एण्डोस्कोपी) अन्तःदर्शन। Examination of the body cavities with the endoscope.

Endosis (एण्डोसिस) बुखार उतरना। Infermission of fever.

Endosteitis (एण्डोस्टाइटिस) अन्तस्थि का शोथ। Inflammation of the endosteum of medullary cavity.

Endotheliocytosis (एण्डोथीलियोसाइटोसिस) अन्तःकला कोशिकाओं का असामान्य रूप से संख्या में बढ़ जाना। An abnormal cavity in the endothelial cells.

Endothelioma (एण्डोथीलियोमा) रक्त-वाहिनियों को आस्तरित करने वाली अन्तःकला का दुर्दम अबुर्द। Malignant tumor of the endothelium lining of the blood vessels.

Endotheliosis (एण्डोथीलियोसिस) अन्तःकला कोशिकाओं का वृद्धि करना। Growth of endothelial cells.

Endothrix (एण्डोथ्रिक्स) रोम काण्ड के भीतर पनपने वाला कोई भी कवक। Fungus growth within hair.

Endotoxemia (एण्डोटॉक्सिमिया) रक्त अन्तर्जीवविषों की विद्यमानता से उत्पन्न होने वाला विषरक्तता। Toxemia due to presence of endotoxin in blood.

Endotoxin (एण्डोटॉक्सिन) जीवाणु के शरीर के भीतर बंद रहता है और जीवाणु टुटने पर ही मुक्त होता है। Bacterial toxin released after death of bacteria.

Endotracheal (एण्डोट्रेकियल) श्वासप्रणाल के अंदर। Within the trachea.

Endplate (एण्डप्लेट) किसी तंत्रिका तन्तु का किसी पेशी कोशिका पर समाप्त होने वाला अंतिम चपटा एवं वृत्ताकार फैला हुआ भाग। The terminal end of nerve fiber to a muscle.

End Product (एण्ड-प्रोडक्ट) प्रतिक्रिया का एक श्रृंखला के अंत में बचा हुआ अंतिम पदार्थ। The finding product of a chemical metabolic process.

Enema (एनीमा) मलाषय में किसी तरल को प्रविष्ट करना। Introduction of a fluid into the rectum.

Energetics (एनर्जेटिक्स) शक्ति का वैज्ञानिक अध्ययन। Scientific study of the energy.

Energy (एनर्जी) कार्य करने की क्षमता। Power, the ability to do work.

Enervate (एर्नवेट) शक्तिहीन करना। To weaken.

Engagement (एन्गेजमैंट) प्रस्तुति करने वाले भाग का उर्ध्व तंग श्रोणी मार्ग में प्रवेश कर जाना। The entrance of the fetal head or the part being presented into the superior pelvic narrow passage.

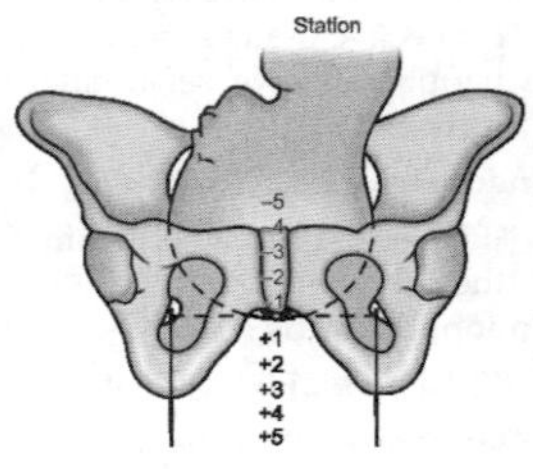

Engorgement (एनगोर्जमैंट) द्रवों से फुलाव, अतिरक्तता। Hyperemia, congestion of blood vessels.

Engram (एनग्राम) अनुभव द्वारा छोड़ा गया कुछ अंश, छाप, निशान। A trace in the protoplasm of the cells of the nervous system left by a stimulus or experience.

Enology, Oenology (एनोलॉजी) शराब का वैज्ञानिक अध्ययन। Scientific study of the wine.

Enophthalmos (एनोफ्थैलमोस) नेत्रगोलक का नेत्रगुछा के भीतर धंस जाना। Recession of the eyeball into the orbit.

Ensiform (एन्सिफोर्म) तलवार के आकार की रचना। Sword-shaped.

Enstrophe (एन्सट्रोफ) भीतर की ओर घूम जाना। Inversion or a turning inward.

Enteralgia (एन्टेरेल्जिया) आँत में दर्द होना। Pain in the intestine.

Enterelcosis (एन्टेरेलकोसिस) आँत में जख्म बन जाना। Ulceration of the intestine.

Enteric-Coated (एन्ट्रिक-कोटेड) किसी विशेष यौगिक की तह चढ़ी हुई गोली। Tablet or capsule coated with special coating that only dissolves in intestine.

Enteritis (एन्टेराइटिस) आँतों में विशेषकर छोटी आँत में सूजन। Inflammation of the intestine especially the small intestine.

Enterobiasis (एन्टेरोबिएसिस) सूत्रकृमियों के कारण होने वाली बीमारी। Infestation with pinworm.

Enteroclysis (एन्टीरोक्लाइसिस) आँत में किसी तरल का इन्जैक्शन लगाना। Injection of a liquid into the intestine.

Enterococus (एन्टीरोकोकस) मानव आँत में रहने वाला कोई भी स्ट्रेप्टोकोकस। Any streptococcus of the human intestine.

Enterocolities (एन्टीरोलाइटिस) छोटी आँत एवं कोलन का शोथ। Inflammation of the small intestine and the colon.

Enterocolostomy (एन्टीरोकोलोस्टॉमी) शल्य क्रिया द्वारा छोटी आँत को कोलन से जोड़ना। To join the small intestine to the colon by surgery.

Enterocystoplasty (एन्टीरोसिस्टोप्लास्टी) आँत को किसी भाग का प्रयोग करके प्लास्टिक सर्जरी द्वारा मूत्राशय को बढ़ाना। Use of a portion of small intestine to enlarge the bladder.

Enteroenterostomy (एन्टीरोएन्टेरोस्टॉमी) आँत के दो खण्डों के बीच जो लगातार नहीं होते, शल्यक्रिया द्वारा सम्बन्ध स्थापित करना। Establishing communication between two intestinal segments that are not continuous.

Enterogastrone (एन्टीरोगैस्ट्रोन) ड्योडिनम का एक हॉर्मोन जो आमाशय की गतिशीलता एवं उसके स्राव को कम करता है और इस प्रकार भोजन को आमाशय से ड्योडिनम में मुक्त होने को नियंत्रित करता है। A hormone secreted by intestinal mucosa that control the intestinal gastric emptying. Fat stimulation its secretion.

Enterolith (एन्टीरोलिथ) आँत में पथरी। Stone in the intestine.

Enteromegalla, Enteromegaly (एन्टीरोमेगेलिया, एन्टीरोमेगैली) आँत का बढ़ जाना। Enlargement of the intestines.

Enteron (एण्टेरोन) पाचन नली। The alimentary canal.

Enteropathogen (एन्टीरोपैथोजन) आँत के रोग को उत्पन्न करने वाला कोई भी सूक्ष्मजीव। Any microorganism producing intestinal disease.

Enteropexy (एन्टीरोपैक्सी) शल्यक्रिया द्वारा आंत को उदर-भित्ति से स्थिर कर देना। Fixation of the intestine to the abdominal wall by surgery.

Enterovirus (एन्टेरोवाइरस) आंत्रविषाणु। The intestinal virus.

Enterozoon (एन्टेरोजोन) आँतों के अन्दर रहने वाला परजीवी। An instestinal parasite.

Entoderm (एन्टोडर्म) अन्तष्चर्म। The simple cell layer lining the cavity of the primitive intestine.

Entomology (एन्टोमोलॉजी) जीव-विज्ञान की वह शाखा जिसका सम्बन्ध कीड़ों के अध्ययन से होता है। The branch of biology which is concerned with the study of insects.

Entopic (एन्टोपिक) आँख के भीतर से सम्बन्धित। Pertaining to the inferior of the eye.

Entropion (एन्ट्ररोपियोन) अंदर की ओर बट जाना। The rolling in or the turning inward, as of the margin of an eyelid.

Enucleate (एन्यूक्लिएट) पूर्णतया बाहर निकाल लेना जैसे—नेत्र गोलक को उसकी नेत्र-गुहा से बाहर निकाल लेना। To take out as a whole as the eyeball from its orbit.

Enuresis (एन्यूरेसिस) असंयत मूत्रता। Involuntary urination or incontinence of urine.

Envenomation (एन्वीनोमेशन) डंक मारने से विष का शरीर में प्रवेश करना। Entrance of poison into the body through a bite or sting.

Enzyme (एन्जाइम) पाचन रस। Substance created by living cells, whose presence aids no other process within the body or speeds it to completion.

Eosin (इयोसिन) आकारिकी में प्रयुक्त की जाने वाली एक गुलाबी रंग की छान। A rose colored stain or dye used in histology.

Eosinophil (इयोसिनोफिल) एक कणिकीय श्वेत रक्त कोशिका जिसमें दो खण्ड वाला एक केन्द्रक होता है, दोनों खण्ड क्रोमैटिन के एक धागे से जुड़े

होते हैं। Cell having an affinity for eosin.

Eosinophillia (इओसिनोफीलिया) रक्त में अत्यधिक संख्या में इओसिनोफिलों का पाया जाना। Presence of a large number of eosinophils in the blood.

Ependyma (इपेन्डाइमा) मस्तिष्क एवं मेरूदण्ड की झिल्ली। Membrane lining the cerebral ventricles and central canal of the spinal cord.

Ependymitis (इपेन्डाइमाइटिस) आन्तरीय कला-शोध। Inflammation of ependyma.

Ephebiatrics (इफीबियाट्रिक्स) चिकित्सा-शास्त्र की वह शाखा जिसमें युवा व्यक्तियों के रोगों का अध्ययन किया जाता है। A branch of medicine dealing with the study of the disease of adolescents.

Ephebology (एफीबोलॉजी) यौवन विज्ञान। Study of puberty and its changes.

Epiblepharon (इपिब्लेफेरोन) निचली पलक के किनारे के आर-पार गुजरती है जिससे पलक के बाल भीतर की ओर आँख के विरूद्ध दब जाते है। A fold of skin passing across lids so that eyelashes are pressed against eye.

Epicanthus (इपिकैन्थस) त्वचा की एक लम्बरूप तह जो नाक के दोनों ओर होती है तथा भीतरी नेत्र कोण एवं मांसांकुर को ढके होती है। A vertical fold of skin on either side of the nose covering the inner cantharis and caruncle.

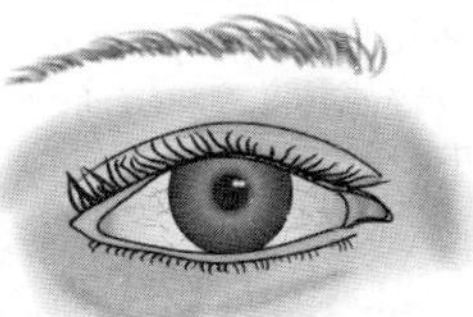

Internal epicanthus

Epicondyle (इपिकॉण्डाइल) किसी हड्डी पर जोड़ बनाने वाले सिरे पर स्थूलक के ऊपर स्थित एक उभार। An eminence upon a bone, at its articular end above a condyle.

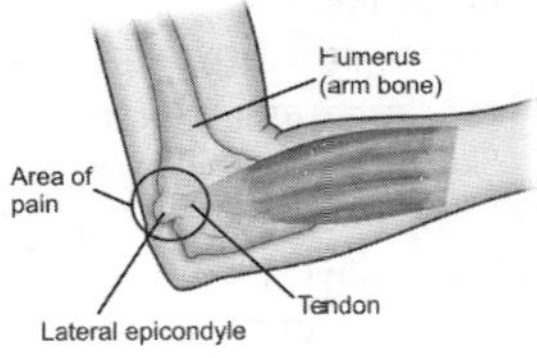

Epicyte (एपिसाइट) कोशिका कला। Cell membrane.

Epidemic (इपिडेमिक) ऐसा रोग जो शीघ्रता से फैलता है तथा एक ही क्षेत्र के बहुत से लोगों पर एक साथ आक्रमण करता है। A disease spreading rapidly and attacking a large number of people in a region.

Epidemiology (इपिडेमियोलॉजी) जानपदिक रोगों का वैज्ञानिक अध्ययन। Scientific study of the epidemic diseases.

Epidermis (इपिडर्मिस) त्वचा की रक्त वाहिनियों से रहित बाह्य परत। An outer nonvascular layer of the skin.

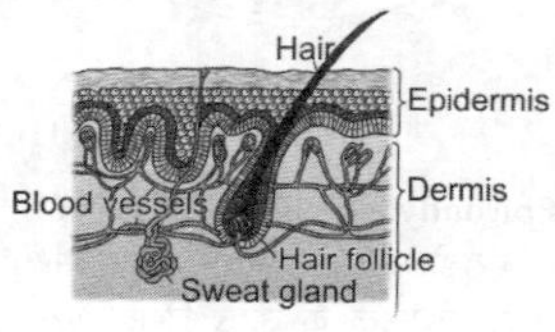

Epidermization (इपिडर्माइजेशन) त्वचा निरोपण। Skin-grafting.

Epidermomycosis (इपिडर्मोमाइकोसिस) किसी कवक द्वारा उत्पन्न त्वचा का रोग। Skin disease caused by a fungus.

Epidermophyton (इपिडर्मोफाइटोन) कवकों का एक वंश जो त्वचा एवं नाखूनों को आक्रमित करता है, बालों को नहीं। A genus of fungic attacks the skin and the nails but not the hair.

Epididymis (इपिडीडिमिस) प्रत्येक शुक्रग्रंथि के पिछले किनारे से संलग्न, लम्बी रस्सी के समान एक संरचना। An elongated, cord-like structure attached to the posterior border of each testis.

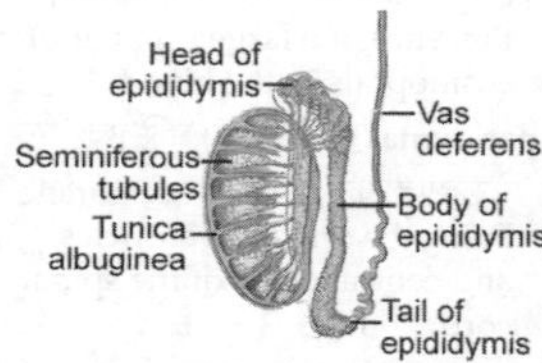

Epididymitis (इपिडीडिमाइटिस) अधिवृषण का शोथ। Inflammation of the epididymics.

Epididymo-orchitis (इपिडीडायमो-ओरचाइटिस) अधिवृषण-वृषणशोथ। Inflammation of the epididymis.

Epidural (इपिड्यूरल) ड्यूरा मेटर के ऊपर स्थित। Situated upon the duramater.

Epigastric Reflex (इपिगैस्ट्रिक-रिफ्लेक्स) अधिजठरीय प्रदेश की त्वचा को खरोंचने पर रैक्टस एब्डोमिनिस पेशी में ऊपरी भाग में संकुचन होना। Contraction of the upper portion of the rectus abdominis muscle on scratching the skin of the epigastric region.

Epigastrium (एपिगैस्ट्रियम) उदर का ऊपरी एवं बीच का

उरपत्रक के आसपास का भाग। The upper-middle part of the abdomen about the xiphisternum.

Epiglottis (इपिग्लोटिस) पतली ढ़क्कन के समान उपास्थि की एक संरचना जो निगलते समय स्वरयंत्र के द्वार को ढ़क लेती है और इस प्रकार भोजन को वायु मार्ग में जाने से रोकती है। Leaf-shaped flat membrane covering entrance of larynx during swallowing.

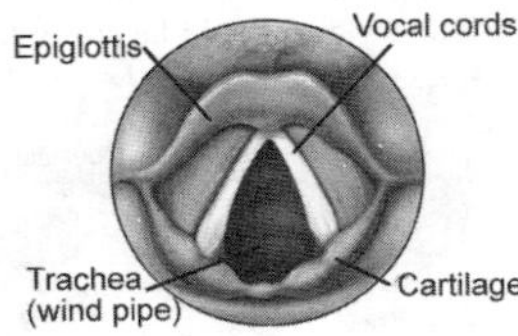

Epiglottitis (इपिग्लोटाइटिस) उपकण्ठ प्रदाह। Inflammation of epiglottis.

Epilate (एपिलेट) जड़ से बालों को अलग करना। To extract hair by the roots.

Epilation (एपिलेशन) बालों का जड़ से अलग होना। Removed of the hair by roots.

Epilepsy (एपिलेप्सी) मिर्गी। Recurrent, paroxymal electrical dysfunction of brain characterized by altered consciousness and motor phenomena.

Epileptic (एपिलेप्टिक) मिर्गी रोग से पीड़ित व्यक्ति। Concerning epilepsy.

Epileptiform (इपिलेप्टीफोर्म) अपस्मार या मिर्गी के समान। Like epilepsy.

Epimenorrhagia (इपिमेनोरैह्जिया) मासिक धर्म का बार-बार एवं अधिकता से होना। Menstruration occurring frequently and excessively.

Epimorphosis (इपिमोर्फोसिस) किसी जीव के किसी भाग की कटी हुई सतह पर वृद्धि होने से उसका पुनर्जन्म होना। The regeneration of a part of an organism by growth at the cut surface.

Epimysium (इपिमाइसियम) कंकाल पेशी के सबसे बाहर चारों ओर से घेरे रहने वाला संयोजी ऊतक का आवरण। An outermost connective tissue sheath surrounding a skeletal muscle.

Epinephrine (इपिनेफ्रीन) एड्रीनलीन। Adrenaline hormone secreted by the adrenal medulla, which is a potent synthesized from phenylalanine having ionotropic, bronchodilator and sympathomimetic effects.

Epinephritis (इपिनेफ्राइटिस) एड्रीनल ग्रन्थि का शोध। Inflammation of the adrenal gland.

Epineurium (इपिन्यूरियम) किसी तंत्रिका संयोजी ऊतक का आच्छद। The connective tissue sheath of a nerve.

Epiphora (इपिफोरा) आँसुओं के अत्यधिक मात्रा में उत्पन्न होना। Overflow of tears due to excess secretion of tears or to obstruction of the lacrimal duct.

Epiphysis (इपिफाइसिस) किसी लम्बी हड्डी का सिरा जो काण्ड की अपेक्षा चौड़ा होता है तथा काण्ड से एक उपास्थि-चक्र द्वारा पृथक रहता है। The end of a long bone which is wider than the shaft and separated from it by a cartilaginous disk.

Epiphysitis (इपिफाइजाइटिस) अधिवर्ध को किसी लम्बी हड्डी के काण्ड से जोड़ने वाली उपास्थि का शोथ। Inflammation of an epiphysis, or of the cartilage joining the epiphysis to the shaft of a long bone.

Epiplocele (इपिप्लोसील) हर्निया जिसमें वपा या औमेन्टम होता है। Hernia containing omentum.

Epiploic (इपिप्लोइक) वपा से सम्बन्धित ।Pertaining to the omentum.

Epipygus (इपिपाइगस) नितम्बों से जुड़ी रहने वाली एक अतिरिक्त भुजा। An extra limb attached to the buttocks.

Episcleral (इपिस्क्लेरल) अधिष्वेतपटल सम्बन्धी। Overlying sclera of eye.

Episioplasty (इपिजियोप्लास्टी) भग की प्लास्टिक सर्जरी करना। Plastic surgery of the vulva.

Episiotomy (इपिजियोटॉमी) प्रसव को आसान बनाने एवं मूलाधार को फटने से रोकने के लिए प्रसव की द्वितीय अवस्था के अंत में मूलाधार एवं योनि में एक चीरा लगाना भगच्छेन। Incision of perineum to facillitate delivery and avoid laceration.

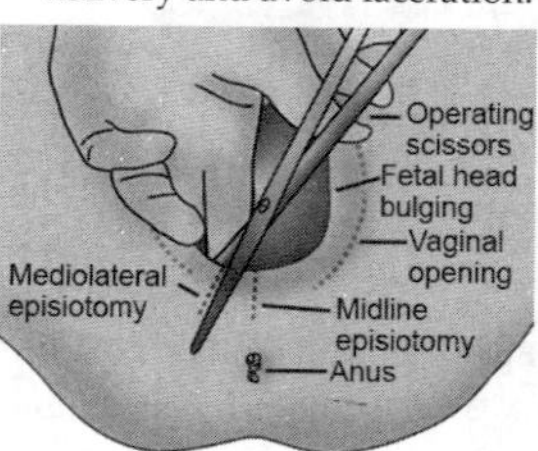

Epispadias (एपिस्पेडियास) अधिमूत्रमार्ग। A urethral opening on the dorsum of the penis.

Hypospadias

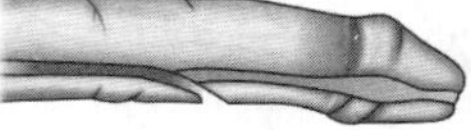

Epispadias

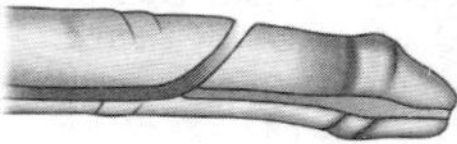

Episplenitis (एपिस्पेनाइटिस) प्लीहासम्पुट शोथ। Inflammation of the capsule of the spleen.

Epistasis (इपिस्टेसिस) किसी भी स्राव का रूक जाना। Suppression of any discharge.

Epistaxis (इपिस्टैक्सिस) नाक से खून बहना। Nose bleeding.

Epithelial (इपिथीलियल) उपकलापरक। Pertaining to or composed of epithelium.

Epithelioid (इपीथीलियॉड) उपकला से मिलता-जुलता। Resembling epithelium.

Epithelioma (इपीथीलियोमा) दुर्दम उपकलाबुद। A malignant tumor of the epithelium.

Epizootic (इपीजोटिक) पशुओं को होने वाला एक महामारी रोग। Widespread disease among animals.

Eponychium (एपोनीकियम) भ्रूण की घृंगी बाह्य त्वचा जिससे नाखून का विकास होता है। The horny epidermis of the fetus from which the nail develops.

Epoophorectomy (इपूफोरेक्टॉमी) शल्यक्रिया द्वारा पराडिम्बग्रंथि को अलग कर देना। Surgical removal of the parduarium

Equation (इक्वेशन) दो भागों के बीच समानता की एक अभिव्यक्ति। An expression of equality between two parts.

Equatorial (इक्वेटोरियल) किसी मध्यरेखा से सन्बन्धित। Pertaining to an equator.

Equilibrating (इक्वीलिब्रेटिंग) संतुलन को बनाये रखने वाला। Maintaining equilibrium.

Equilibrium (इक्वीलिब्रिम) संतुलन। A state of balance.

Equine (इक्वाइन) घोड़े से सम्बन्धित। Pertaining to or derived from the horse.

Equipotential (इक्वीपोटेन्शियल) बराबर शक्ति वाले। Having the equal strength.

Equitoxic (इक्वीटॉक्सिक) बराबर की विषाक्तता वाला। Having an equivalent toxicity.

Eradication (इरेडीकेशन) उन्मूलन। Extirpation.

Erben's reflex (एरबेन्स रिफ्लैक्स) सिर एवं धड़ को बलपूर्वक आगे की ओर मोड़ने पर नाड़ी गति का धीमा हो जाना। Slowing of the pulse rate on bending the head and the trunk forward forcibly.

Erb's Paralysis (एर्ब्स पैरालाइसिस) पांचवी और छठी मेरूदण्डीय तंत्रिकाओं के ग्रैव-मूलों के ग्रस्त हो जाने पर कंधे एवं ऊपरी बाहु की पेशियों का पक्षाघात हो जाना। Paralysis of muscles supplied by C5 and C6.

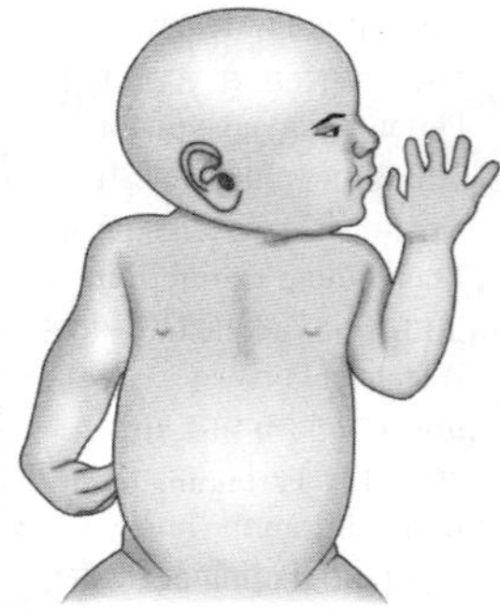

Erectile tissue (इरेक्टाइलटिषू) वाहिकायम ऊतक जो रक्त से भर जाने पर उच्छत हो जाता है। The vascular tissue which filled with blood, becomes erect or rigid as the clitoris, penis or nipples.

Erection (इरेक्शन) उत्थान। The state achieved when erectile tissue is hyperaemic.

Erethism (एरीथज्म) उद्दीपनों के प्रति अत्यधिक संवेदनशीलता। Excess sensibility to stimuli.

Ergasthenia (एर्गोस्थीनिया) अत्यधिक कार्य करने में कमजोरी हो जाना। Weakness due to overwork.

Ergocalciferol (एर्गोकैल्सीफेरोल) विटामिन डी-2। Vitamin D2.

Ergometer (एर्गोमीटर) किसी व्यक्ति द्वारा किए गए कार्य की मात्रा को मापने वाला उपकरण। An apparatus for measuring amount of work performed.

Ergophobia (एर्गोफोबिया) काम करने का रोगात्पादक भय। Morbid fear of working.

Ergotism (एर्गोटिज्म) अर्गटात्यय। Ill effects produced by ergot.

Erosion (इरोजन) कटाव। Intersection. The process of eroding.

Erotology (इरोटोलॉजी) प्रेमविज्ञान। The study of love and its manifestations.

Erotomania (इरोटोमैनिया) कामोन्माद। Exaggerated sexual behavior.

Erotophobia (इरोटोफोबिया) यौन प्रेम का रोगोत्पादक भय। Morbid fear of sexual love.

Erratic (ऐराटिक) भ्रमण करने वाला। Eccentric.

Eructation (एरक्टेशन) मुख द्वारा आमाशय से वायु का बाहर निकलना जिसमें अक्सर एक विशिष्ट प्रकार की ध्वनि निकलती है। Ejection of wind from the stomach through the mouth, usually with a characteristic sound.

Eruption (इरप्शन) फुन्सी, दाना। A discoloration or breaking act of pimples on the skin.

Erysipelas (एरिसिपेलास) स्ट्रैप्टोकोकस पायोजीनस के संक्रमण द्वारा उत्पन्न त्वचा

एवं अवत्वक् ऊतकों का एक सांसर्गिक रोग जिसमें त्वचा सूज जाती है, लाल हो जाती है तथा ज्वर आता है एवं अन्य सार्वदैहिक लक्षण उत्पन्न हो जाते हैं। Inflammatory cutaneous desease characterized by extreme redness.

Erysipeloid (एरिसिपेलॉयड) विसर्प से मिलता-जुलता। Resembling erysipelas.

Erythema (इरीदीमा) कोशिकाओं का रक्ताधिक्य होने के कारण त्वचा का असामान्य रूप से लाल हो जाना। Abnormal redness of the skin due to congestion of the blood capillaries.

Erythroblast (इरिथ्रोब्लास्ट) लाल रक्तकणों को जन्म देने वाली कोशिका। Of red blood corpuscles.

Erythroblastosis fetalis (इरिथ्रोब्लास्टोसिस फीटालिस) गर्भ लोहितकोशिका-प्रसूमयता। A pathological condition in the newborn child due to a difference of child's and the mother's blood.

Erythrocyanosis (इरिथ्रोसायनोसिस) ठण्ड के कारण विशेषकर स्त्रियों में त्वचा का नीला पड़ जाना। Bluish discoloration of the skin occurring especially in females due to cold.

Erythrocyte (इरिथ्रोसाइट) केन्द्रक रहित लाल रक्त कोशिका अथवा कणिका जिसमें हिमोग्लाबिन होता है। Non-nucleated blood cell or corpuscle containing hemoglobin.

Erythrocythemia (इरिथ्रोसाइथीमिया) रक्त में लाल रक्त कोशिकाओं की संख्या बढ़ जाना। An increase in the number of red blood cells in the blood.

Erythrocytosis (इरिथ्रोसाइटोसिस) लोहित-कोशिकाओं का अत्यधिक बढ़ना। Over production of red cells.

Erythroderma (इरिथ्रोडर्मा) शरीर के बहुत से स्थानों में असामान्य रूप से त्वचा का लाल हो जाना। Abnormal redness of the skin over widespread areas of the body.

Erythrodontia (इरिथ्रोडोन्शिया) दाँतों की लाल-ब्राउन वर्ण-कला। Reddish-brown pigmentation of the teeth.

Erythroid (इरिथ्रॉयड) लाल रंग वाला। Producing red blood cells.

Erythromelagia (इरिथ्रोमलेजिया) बाहयांगों का एक दर्दनाक रोग जिसमें रोगग्रस्त भाग बैंगनी रंग के हो जाते हैं। Burning and throbbing affect that come and go.

Erythrophage (इरिथ्रोफेज) लाल रक्त कणों का शोषण करने वाला। Phagocyte absorbing hemoglobin.

Erythrophile (इरिथ्रोफाइल) ऐसी वस्तु जो शीघ्र ही लाल रंग से अभिरंजित कर देती है। An agent that readily stains red.

Erythropoiesis (इरिथ्रोपॉयसिस) लाल रक्त कोशिकाओं का बनना। The formation of red blood cells.

Erythropsia (इरिथ्रोप्सिया) ऐसी दशा जिसमें वस्तुएं लाल दिखाई देती है। The condition in which the things appear to be red.

Esculent (एस्कलेन्ट) खाने योग्य। Fit the eaten, eatable, edible.

Esophagalgia (इसोफेगेल्जिया) ग्रासनली में दर्द होना। Pain in the esophagus.

Esophagectasia, Esophagectasis (इसोफेगेक्टेसिया, इसोफेगेक्टेसिस) ग्रासनली का चौड़ा होना। Dilation of the esophagus.

Esophagismus (इसोफेगिस्मस) ग्रासनली में ऐंठन होना। Spasm of the esophagus.

Esophagodynia (इसोफेगोडाइनिया) ग्रासनली में दर्द होना। Pain in the esophagus.

Esophagoenterostomy (इसोफेगोएन्ट्रौस्टॉमी) अमाशय को शल्यक्रिया द्वारा काटकर निकाल देने के पश्चात् ग्रासनली एवं आँत में सम्बन्ध स्थापित करना। To make a connection between the esophagus and the intestine after excision of the stomach.

Esophagomalacia (इसोफैगोमैलेसिया) ग्रास नली की दीवारों का मुलायम हो जाना। Softening of the walls of the esophagus.

Esophagomyotomy (इसोफैगोमायोटॉमी) ग्रास नली के पेशीय स्तर में शल्यक्रिया द्वारा चीरा लगाना। To make a surgical incision into the muscular coat of the esophagus.

Esophagoplication (इसोफेगोप्लीकेशन) ग्रासनली की दीवारों को भीतर की ओर मोड़कर इसके विस्फारण को कम करना। Reduction of esophageal dilatation by infolding its walls.

Esophagotomy (इसोफैगोटॉमी) शल्यक्रिया द्वारा ग्रासनली में चीरा लगाना। To make an incision into the esophagus by surgery.

Esophagus (इसोफेगस) ग्रसनी से आमाशय तक फैला लगभग 9 इंच लम्बा एक पेशीकलामय नाल जो निगले हुए भोजन को मुख से आमाशय में पहुँचाता है।

The musculomembranous tube extending from pharynx to stomach.

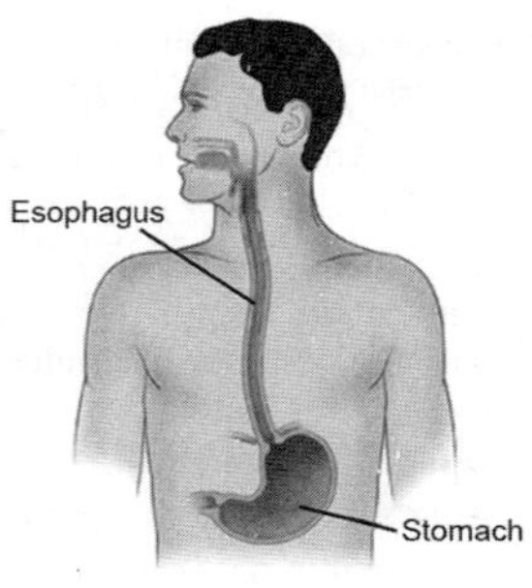

Esophoria (इसोफोरिया) किसी आँख का अंदर की ओर घूम जाना। Tending of the visual lines inward.

ESR (इ.एस.आर.) लोहित कोशिका अवसादन दर।

Erythrocyte sedimentation rate.

Essence (एसेन्स) किसी औषधि का निकाला गया सार।

The extracted qualities of a drug.

Essential (एसेन्शियल) आवश्यक। Necessary.

Ester (ईस्टर) किसी कार्बनिक अम्ल के किसी एल्कोहॉल के साथ संयुक्त होने से बना एक यौगिक जिसमें पानी निकल जाता है। Compound formed by organic acid with alcohol.

Esthesia (एस्थीसिया) संवेदना। Sensation.

Esthesiometer (एस्थीसियोमीटर) संवेदनामापी। A device for measuring tactile sensibility.

Esthetics (एस्थेटिक्स) सौंदर्यकला विज्ञान। The branch of philosophy dealing with beauty.

Estival (एस्टिवल) ग्रीष्म ऋतु से सम्बन्धित। Pertaining to or occurring in summer.

Estradiol (इेस्ट्राडियोल) डिम्ब ग्रंथि द्वारा उत्पन्न स्टैरॉयड जिसमें ईस्ट्रोजन के गुण होते हैं। A steroid produced by the ovary and having the qualities of estrogen.

Estrogen (ईस्ट्रोजन) डिम्ब ग्रंथि द्वारा उत्पन्न एक नारी लिंग हार्मोन जो द्वितीयक लैंगिक विशिष्टताओं के विकसित होने के प्रति उत्तरदायी होता है। $C_{18}H_{22}O_2$, Natural estrogenic hormones less active than estradiol but more active than estriol.

Estrone (ईस्ट्रोन) गर्भवती स्त्री के मूत्र मे पाया जाने वाला ईस्ट्रोजन उत्पन्न करने वाला एक हार्मोन। An estrogenic hormone found in the urine of a pregnant woman.

Estrus (ईस्ट्रस) कामोन्माद। Sexual desire.

Ethambutol (ईथामब्यूटोल) ऐलोपैथिक चिकित्सा में प्रयुक्त की जाने वाली एक जीवन रक्षक औषधि। Synthetic tuberular drug.

Etherization (ईथेराइजेशन) ईथर के प्रयोग से असंवेदनता उत्पन्न करना या बेहोशी लाना। To induce anesthesia by using ether.

Ethics (इथिक्स) आचार-संहिता। A system of morals.

Ethnobiology (एथनोबायोलॉजी) बहुत सी जातियों के जैवीय लक्षणों का अध्ययन। Study of the biological characteristics of various races.

Ethnocentrism (इथनोसेन्ट्रिज्म) रोगी की हालत पर ध्यान देने की अपेक्षा उसकी देखभाल करने वाले को अधिक महत्त्व देना। To give more importance to the caretaker rather than considering the patients condition.

Ethnology (एथनोलॉजी) मानव-जाति विज्ञान। The science dealing with different races of men.

Ethology (इथोलॉजी) जन्तु-व्यवहार विज्ञान। The scientific study of animal behavior.

Ethopharmacology (इथोफार्मकोलॉजी) व्यवहार पर औषधि प्रभावों का अध्ययन। The study of drug effects on behavior.

Etiology (इटियोलॉजी) रोगों के कारणों का अध्ययन। The study of the cause of disease.

Etiotropic (इटियोट्रॉपिक) किसी रोग के कारण को दूर करने वाली औषधि। The drug or treatment removing the cause of a disease.

Eubiotics (यूबायोटिक्स) स्वास्थ्य-विज्ञान। The science of healthy and hygienic living.

Eucapnia (यूकेप्निया) रक्त में कार्बन-डाइऑक्साइड की सामान्य मात्रा का पाया जाना। Presence of normal amount of carbon dioxide in the blood.

Eucholia (यूकोलिया) बाइल की सामान्य दशा। Normal condition of the bile.

Eucrasia (यूक्रेसिया) सामान्य स्वास्थ्यावस्था। Condition of normal health.

Eudiaphoresis (यूडिएफोरेसिस) पसीने का सामान्य रूप से निकलना।

Normal secretion of perspiration.

Eudiometer (यूडियोमीटर) वायु की शुद्धता की जाँच करने एवं गैसों का विष्लेशण करने वाला एक यंत्र। An instrument for testing the purity of air and making analysis of the gases.

Eudipsia (यूडिप्सिया) सामान्य प्यास लगना। Normal thirst.

Eugenics (यूजेनिक्स) सुजनन विज्ञान। The science dealing with genetic and prenatal influence that affects the expression of certain characteristic in offsprings.

Eunuch (यूनक) नामर्द। A castrated male.

Euphonia (यूफोनिया) सामान्य स्पष्ट ध्वनि वाला होना। The condition of having a normal clear voice.

Euphoria (यूफोरिया) सुखाभास, स्वास्थ्यचिंतन। A sense of health, a sense of well-being.

Euploidy (यूप्लॉयडी) गुणसूत्रों के पूरे सैटों में युक्त होने की अवस्था। The condition of having complete sets of chromosomes.

Euryopic (यूरियोपिक) चौड़ी आँखों वाला। Wide-eyed.

Eustachian tube (यूस्टेचियन ट्यूब) मध्यकर्ण से लेकर ग्रसनी तक फैली 3 से 4 सेमी लम्बी श्रवण-नली। The auditory canal 3 to 4 cm long extending from the middle ear to the pharynx.

Eutectic (यूटेक्टिक) आसानी से पिघला हुआ। Easily melted.

Euthanasia (यूथैनेसिया) वेदना रहित मृत्यु। An easy or painless death.

Euthenics (यूथेनिक्स) मानव-सुपरिस्थितिकी। The science of improvement of population through modification of environment.

Euthyroid (यूथाइरॉयड) सामान्य रूप से कार्य करने वाली थॉइरायड ग्रंथि।

Thyroid gland with normal function.

Evacuate (इवाकुएट) खाली करना या दस्त लाना। To empty or to purgate.

Evaluation (इवैल्यूएशन) खोज या जाँच। Assessment.

Evanescent (इवानेसेन्ट) क्षण जीवी। Of short duration.

Evaporation (इवापोरेशन) द्रव अवस्था से वाष्प में बदलना। Change from liquid form to vapor.

Evenomation (इवीनोमेशन) साँप अथवा किसी कीड़े के काटने से पीड़ित व्यक्ति से उसके जहर को निकाल देना।

Removal of venom from the victim of a snake or insect bite.

Eventration (इवेन्ट्रेशन) उदरीय भित्ति में स्थित छिद्र से होकर आँतों का बाहर निकल आना। Protrusion of the intestines through an opening in the abdominal wall

Eversion (इवर्जन) बाहर की ओर मुड़ जाना Turning outward.

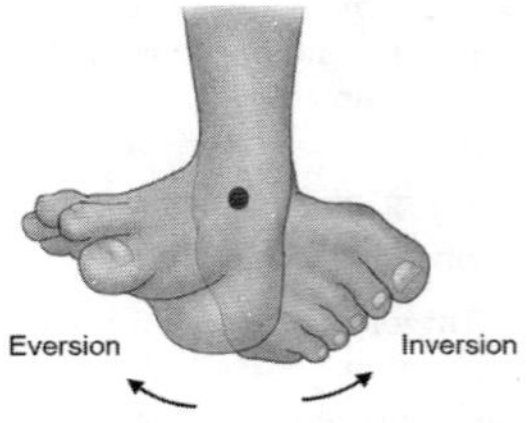

Evisceration (इविसिरेशन) आँतरिक अंगों को धक्का देकर बाहर निकाल देना। Pushing out of the internal organs.

Evocation (इवोकेशन) स्मृति के आधार पर अथवा कल्पना द्वारा किसी नई वस्तु का निर्माण करना। To create a new thing on the basis of memory or by imagination.

Exacerbation (एक्सेसर्बेशन) किसी रोग की तीव्रता में वृद्धि होना। In the severity of a disease.

Exanthem (एक्जेन्थेम) त्वचा का कोई भी विस्फोट जिसके साथ सूजन होती है और बुखार भी आ जाता है जैसे–खसरा में होता है। Any eruption of the skin accompanied by inflammation with pyrexia, e.g. measles.

Excavator (एक्सकेवेटर) हड्डी को अलग करने वाला चम्मच के आकार का एक यंत्र। A Spoon-shaped instrument for removing the tissue or bone.

Exchange Transfusion (एक्सचेंज ट्रान्सफ्यूजन) रक्त को बार-बार थोड़ी-थोड़ी मात्रा में निकालना एवं उसके स्थान पर नया रक्त चढ़ाना। Transfection and withdrawal of small amount of blood until blood volume is entirely replaced.

Excipient (एक्सीपिएन्ट) किसी औषधि के साथ मिलाया जाने वाला कोई भी निष्क्रिय पदार्थ जो उस औषधि को उचित कठोरता एवं आकृति प्रदान करता है। Any inert substance added to a drug to give suitable consistency or form to the drug.

Excise (एक्साइज) अलग कर देना। To cut out or remove surgically.

Excitability (एक्साइटेबिलिटी) उद्दीप्यता। Irritability.

Excitation (एक्साइटेशन) उत्तेजित होने की क्रिया। The act of stimulation.

Exclusion (एक्सक्लूजन) दूर करना। Elimination.

Excoriated (एक्सकोरियेटेड) छिली हुई त्वचा। Abraded skin.

Excoriation (एक्सकोरियेशन) त्वचा का छिलना। Abrasion of the skin.

Exenteration (एक्सेन्टेरेशन) आशय-निष्कासन। Evisceration.

Exercise (एक्सरसाइज) पेशियों को क्रियाशील बनाना अथवा स्वास्थ्य सुधारना। Bodily exertion or performance of the muscular activity for the improvement of health or correction of physical deformity.

Exeresis (एक्सेरेसिस) शल्यक्रिया द्वारा काटकर अलग कर देना। Excision or surgical removal.

Exertion (एक्जुर्शन) परिश्रम। Labor.

Exflagellation (एक्सफ्लेजीलेशन) मच्छर के आमाशय में मलेरिया परजीवी प्लाज्मोडियम में किसी लघुयुग्मक-जनक से कशाभ रूपी लघुयुग्मकों का बनना।

The formation of microgametes from microgametocytes occurs in plasmodia in the stomach of mosquito.

Exfoliation (एक्सफोलिएशन) मृत ऊतक का परतों के रूप में गिरना, पपड़ियाँ उतरना। The falling off in layers of the dead tissue.

Exhaustion (एग्जाशन) अत्यधिक थकान, हवा खींचने की क्रिया। The state of being extremely tired the act of drawing off the air.

Exhibitionism (एग्जीविषनिज्म) किसी भी प्रकार से, अधिकतर जननांगों का अनावरण करके विपरीत लिंग के व्यक्ति का ध्यान अपनी ओर आकर्षित करने की प्रवृति, प्रदर्शनीयता। Tendency to attract attention to one by any means.

Exhumation (एक्सह्यूमेशन) दफनाने के बाद कब्र से मृत शरीर को निकाल देना। Removal of a dead body from the grave after it has been buried.

Exitus (एक्जिटस) मृत्यु। Death.

Exocrine (एक्सोक्राइन) बहिःस्रावी, किसी वाहिनी के द्वारा बाहर की ओर स्रावित करने वाली ग्रंथि। The gland secreting externally through a duct.

Exodontology (एक्सोडोन्टोलॉजी) दन्त-चिकित्सा की वह शाखा जिसका सम्बन्ध दांत निकालने से होता है। Branch of dentistry concerned with extraction of teeth.

Exomphalos (एक्सोम्फैलोस) नाभि-हर्निया। Umbilical hernia.

Exophoria (एक्सोफोरिया) दृष्टि-अक्ष का बाहर की ओर झुक जाना। Deviation of the visual axis outwards.

Exophthalmia (एक्जोपथैल्मिया) नेत्रगोलक का नेत्र गुहा से बाहर निकल आना। Exophthalmos.

Protrusion of the eyeball from its orbit.

Exophthalmos (एक्जोफ्थैल्मोस) नेत्रगोलक का नेत्र गुहा से बाहर निकल आना। Exophthalmia.

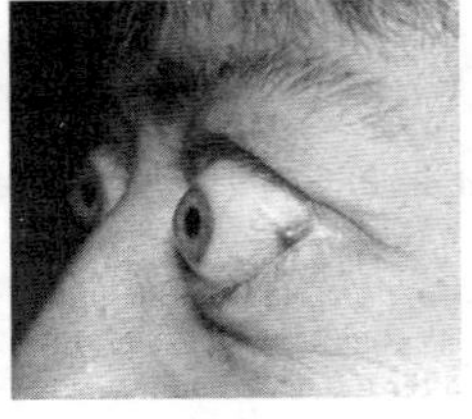

Exoplasm (एक्सोप्लाज्म) बहिःपरासरण। The outer protoplasm of a cell.

Exostosis (एक्सोस्टोसिस) हड्डी का एक सुदम अबुर्द। An unnatural growth from a bone.

Exotic (एक्जोटिक) विदेशों में उत्पन्न होने वाला। Foreign.

Exotoxin (एक्जोटॉक्सिन) बहिर्जीवविष। Toxins produced by microorganism to surrounding medium.

Exotropia (एक्सोट्रोपिया) टेढ़ा-मेढ़ा दिखाई देना, नेत्र बहिर्विचलन। Divergent squint.

Expectoration (एक्सपैक्टोरेशन) बलगम, कफ। Discharge of mucus with coughing.

Expiration (एक्सपाइरेशन) श्वास छोड़ना, मृत्यु। Expelling of breath from the lungs, death.

Explode (एक्सप्लोड) फट जाना। To burst out.

Exposure (एक्सपोजर) नग्न करने की क्रिया, अनावरण। To make somebody naked.

Expulsion (एक्सपलसन) निकालने की क्रिया। The act of expelling.

Exsangvination (एक्ससैनग्वीनेशन) बाह्य रक्त स्राव के कारण होने वाली रक्त की अत्यधिक हानि। Heavy loss of blood due to internal or external hemorrhage.

Extension (एक्सटेन्सन) प्रसार, फैलाव। Straightening, as an aron.

Extinguish (एक्सटिंग्विष) नष्ट कर देना। To abolish.

Extracapsular (एक्ट्राकैप्सुलर) आँख के लैन्स के कैप्सूल के बाहर स्थित अथवा उत्पन्न होने वाला। Outside the capsule.

Extracorporeal (एक्सट्राकार्पोरियल) शरीर के बाहर स्थित अथवा उत्पन्न होने वाला। Situated or occurring outside the body.

Extract (एक्सट्रैक्ट) निष्कर्ष, सार। The condensed active principle of a drug.

Extradural (एक्सट्राड्यूरल) दृढ़तानिका के बाहर। Outside the dura mater.

Extramural (एक्सट्राम्यूरल) किसी अंग की दीवार के बाहर स्थित

अथवा उत्पन्न होने वाला। Situated or occurring outside the wall of an organ.

Extrasensory (एक्ट्रासैन्सरी) पांच संवेंदों पर निर्भर न रहने वाला बोध जैसे विचारों का स्थानान्तरण होना। Perception not depending on the five senses, such as transference of thoughts.

Extrasystole (एक्सट्रासिस्टोल) अतिरिक्त प्रकुचन। Premature beats in the pulse rhythm.

Extravasation (एक्सट्रावेसेशन) रिसाव, परिस्राव। Fluid escaping from vessel.

Extremity (एक्सट्रीमिटी) बाह्यांग। The outer part of the body, as hand, foot, etc.

Extropion (एक्ट्रोपियोन) शरीर के किसी भाग जैसे आँख की पलक का बाहर को उलट जाना। Eversion of eyelid margin.

Extroversion (एक्सट्रोवर्जन) अंदर से बाहर को उलट जाना। The condition of being turned inside out.

Extrovert (एक्सट्रोवर्ट) वह व्यक्ति जो बाह्य वस्तु एवं कार्यों में रूचि रखता है। Thinking of outward things.

Extrusion (एक्सट्रजन) असामान्य बाह्य स्थिति को ग्रहण करना। A pushing or forcing out of a normal position.

Extubation (एक्सट्यूवेशन) किसी नली को निकाल देना। Removal of a tube.

Exuberant (एक्सूबीरेन्ट) उत्पादन में अत्यधिक, प्रसन्न। Excessive in production, happy.

Eye (आई) आँख।

The organ of sight, vision.

Eye bank (आई बैंक) नेत्र बैंक। An organization that collects

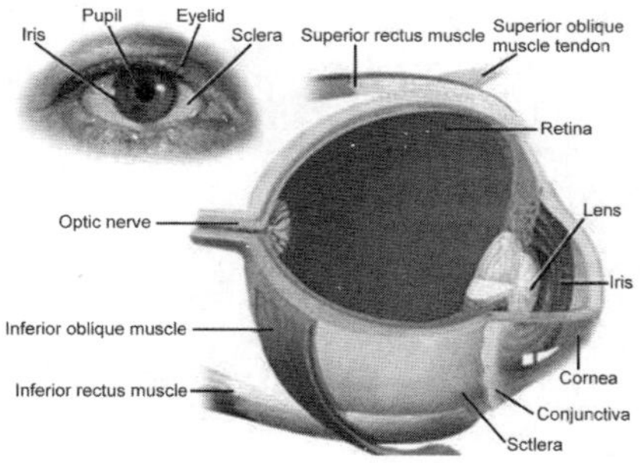

corneas and stores them for transplantation.

Eyeglass (आईग्लास) दोषयुक्त दृष्टि को ठीक करने के लिए प्रयोग में लाया जाने वाला काँच का एक लैंस। A glass lens used to correct the defective vision.

Eyelash (आईलैश) आँख की पलक के किनारे पर उगने वाला एक बाल। A hair growing on the margin of an eyelid.

Eyelid (आईलिड) आँख की पलक। One of the two movable protective folds covering the anterior surface of the eyeball.

Eyesight (आईसाइ) दृष्टि। Vision.

Eye strain (आई स्ट्रेन) अत्यधिक प्रयोग करने से अथवा दोषयुक्ति दृष्टि होने से उत्पन्न होने वाली आँख की थकान। Tiredness of the eye due to overuse or from defective vision.

F

Fabrication (फेब्रीकेशन) इस प्रकार झूठ बोलना कि वह सही प्रतीत होता है। To tell a lie in such a way as it seems true.

Face (फेस) चेहरा, ललाट। Front part of the human head, from the head to chin.

Facet (फेसेट) फलक। A small smooth area on a bone or hard surface.

Facetectomy (फेस्टेक्टॉमी) किसी कषेरूका के जोड़ बनाने वाले फलक को शल्यक्रिया द्वारा काटकर अलग कर देना। Excision of the arteriolar facet of a vertebra.

Facia (फेशिया) बन्धन, डोरी। A connective tissue sheath consisting of fibrous tissue and fact which unite the skin to the underlying tissues.

Facial Center (फेसियल सेन्टर) आनन केन्द्र। Brain center responsible for facial movement.

Facial Spasm (फेसियल स्पाज्म) चेहरे की ऐंठन अथवा अकड़न। Involuntary contraction of muscles supplied by facial nerve.

Facies (फेशीज) मुखाकृति, चेहरा। The expression or appearance of face.

Factitious (फेक्टीशियस) नकली, बनावटी। Unnatural, self-induced.

Factitious disorders (फेक्टीशियस डिसार्डर) ऐसे रोग जो वास्तविक नहीं होते बल्कि केवल अस्पताल में ठहरने के लिए उन्हें कृत्रिम रूप से पैदा किया जाता है। A condition in which a person without a malingering, motive, acts as if they have an illness by deliberately producing, feigning or exaggerating symptoms purely to attain a patient's role.

Factor (फेक्टर) कारण। One of the contributing causes in any action.

Facultative (फेक्लटेटिव) विकल्पजीवी। Having the power of living under different conditions.

Faculty (फेकल्टी) क्षमता, योग्यता। Any specific power or function.

Fahrenheit (फारेनहाइट) एक तापमान मापने का पैमाना जिस पर पानी के जमने का बिन्दु 32° एवं उबलने का बिन्दु 212° चिंहित रहता है। A temperature scale with freezing point of water at 32° and boiling point at 212° Point.

Failure (फेल्योर) असफलता। Inability to function or perform satisfactorily.

Falciform (फेलसीफार्म) हंसियाकार। Sickle-shaped.

Falciform ligament (फेल्सीफार्म लिंगामैन्ट) दात्राकार बंधन। The triangular, ligament attached to sides of the sacrum and coccyx by its base.

Falciform Process (फेल्सीफार्म प्रोसेस) प्रमस्तिष्क दात्र। That portion of falciform ligament along the inner margin of ramus of ischium.

Fallopian tube (फेलोपियन ट्यूब) डिम्बबाही नलिका। One of the two tubes opening out the upper part of the uterus.

False-negative (फाल्स-नेगेटिव) एक परीक्षण जिससे पता चलता है कि जिस रोग की जाँच की गई है वह विद्यमान नहीं है जबकि वास्तव में वह होता है। A test indicating that the disease is not present when actually it is present.

False-positive (फाल्स-पॉजिटिव) एक परीक्षण जिससे पता चलता है कि जिस रोग की जांच की गई है वह विद्यमान है जबकि वास्तव में वह नहीं होता। A test indicating that the disease is present when in fact it is not.

False ribs (फाल्स रिब्स) नीचे की पाँच पसलियाँ। The five inferior ribs.

Falx (फॉक्स) कोई भी हंसियाकार रचना। Any-sickle-shaped structure.

Fames (फेम्स) भूख। Hunger.

Familial (फेमिलीयल) परिवारिक सम्बन्धी। Pertaining to the family.

Family (फेमिली) परिवार। A group of individuals descending from a common ancestor.

Family Planning (फेमिली प्लानिंग) परिवार कल्याण। Planning and spacing of child birth according to wishes of the couple rather than by chance.

Fantasy (फेन्टेसी) स्वप्न लेना। Day dreaming.

Farad (फेराड) विद्युत-क्षमता की एक इकाई। A unit of electric capacity.

Faradism (फेराडिज्म) विद्युत-रूप। The form of electricity furnished by a faradic machine.

Farmer's Lung (फार्मर्स लंग) यह रोगोत्पादक सूक्ष्मजीव एक्जिनोमाइसीटीज से युक्त फफूंदार सूखी घास, भूसे या अनाज से उत्पन्न धूल को सांस के साथ अंदर खींच लेने उत्पन्न से किसानों में देखा जाने वाला एलर्जीजन्य वायुकोश्ठिका शोध

है। Hypersensitive alveolitis on exposure to moldy hay.

Farsightedness (फारसाइटेडनैस) दूर की वस्तुओं को साफ-साफ देखने की क्षमता परन्तु पास की वस्तुऐं दिखाई न देना। Hyperopia or hypermetropia ability to see the distant objects clearly but not the near objects.

Fascicle (फेशिकिल) गुच्छा। A small bundle of fibers.

Fasciculation (फेशीकुलेशन) पूलिकाओं या गुच्छों का बनना। Formation of bundle of fibers.

Fasciculus (फेशीकुलस) गुच्छा। A little bundle of fibers.

Fasciectomy (फेशिएक्टॉमी) प्रावरणी के किसी टुकड़े को काट कर निकाल देना। Excision of a piece of fascia.

Fascitis (फेशियाइटिस) किसी प्रावरणी का शोध। Inflammation of a fascia.

Fastigium (फेस्टीजियम) चरम सीमा। The highest point; the most posterior portion of fourth ventricle in brain.

Fasting (फास्टिंग) उपवास करना, भूखा रहना। Staying without food.

Fat (फेट) वसा। Adipose tissue of body serving as energy reserve providing fat soluble vitamin.

Fatigue (फटीग) थकान। Feeling of tiredness resulting from continuing activity.

Fattly acids (फेटी एसिड्स) वसाम्ल। Any acid derived from fats.

Fauces (फोसेस) गले एवं ग्रसनी के बीच का संकीर्ण पथ। The constricted passage to the pharynx.

Favism (फेविज्म) दाद का एक रूप जो कुछ फलियां खाने से प्रकट होता है। A condition caused in some by eating certain beans, or inhalation of pollen or its flowers, characterized by fever, headache, abdominal pain, severe amenia, prostration and coma.

Favus (फेवस) त्वचा का एक कवक रोग जिसमें त्वचा पर मक्खी के छत्ते के समान पिण्ड बन जाते है जिनमें खुजली आती है। A fungus disease of the skin characterized by honeycomb-like masses accompanied.

Fear (फियर) डर। Emotional reaction to external or internal threat, a feature of depression.

Febrile (फेब्राइल) ज्वर से पीड़ित। Pertaining to a fever.

Feculent (फेक्यूलेन्ट) दुर्गन्धयुक्त या बदबूदार। Having sediment, foul.

Fecundation (फीकन्डेशन) निषेचन अथवा गर्भाधान। Fertilization or impregnation.

Fecundity (फीकान्डिटी) संतान उत्पन्न करने की क्षमता। Ability to produce offspring.

Feedback (फीड्बेक) प्रतिक्रिया, प्रतिपुष्टि। Information about reactions to a product, a persons performance a task which is used as a basis for improvement.

Feeder (फीडर) भोजन कराने वाला। One who feeds or gives food.

Feeding (फीडिंग) भोजन करना। Taking or giving a food.

Fehling's solution (फेहलिंग्स सॉल्यूशन) एक क्षारीय, ताँबे से युक्त घोल जो मूत्र में शुगर की विद्यमानता का पता लगाने एवं उसकी प्रतिशतता को निश्चित करने के लिये प्रयोग में लाया जाता है। An alkaline, copper containing solution used for detecting the presence and determining the percentage of sugar in the urine.

Felon (फेलन) अंगुलेबेढा। Very painful tumor found on the finger's or toes.

Felty's Syndrome (फेल्टी सिन्ड्रोम) यकृत-वृद्धि। Enlargement of liver.

Female (फिमेल) औरत। A woman, which produces offspring.

Feminization (फेमिनाइजेशन) पुरूष में सामान्य अथवा विकृतिजन्य द्वितीयक स्त्री लैंगिक लक्षणों का विकसित होना।

Femur (फीमर) जाँघ की लम्बी हड्डी जो ऊपर कूल्हे की हड्डी से तथा नीचे टिबिया एवं पटेला से जुड़ी होती है। The longest and largest bone of the body extending from pelvis to knee.

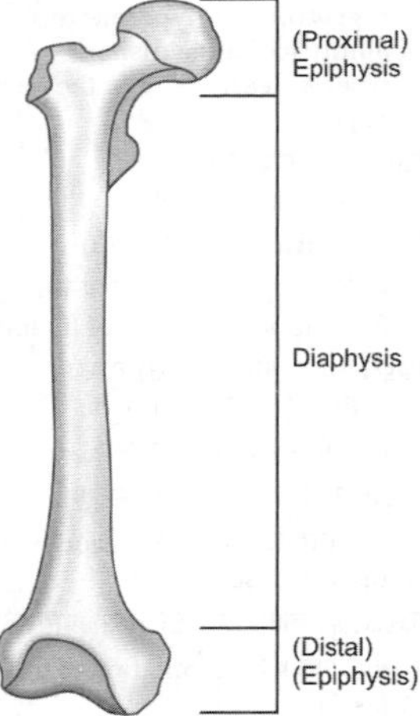

Fenestra (फेनेस्ट्रा) छिद्र। A window-like opening.

Fennel (फेनेल) सौंफ। The seeds are aromatic and carminative.

Feral (फीरल) घातक। Deadly.

Fern (फर्न) एक प्रकार का पौधा जिसमें कभी फूल नहीं लगता। A flowerless plant.

Ferritin (फेरीटिन) लोहे का वह रूप जिसमें वह शरीर के ऊतकों में

जमा होता है। The form of iron in which it is deposited in the body tissues.

Ferrokinetics (फेरोकाइनेटिक्स) लोहे के अवशोषण, उपयोग, संचय एवं उत्सर्जन का अध्ययन। Study of the absorption, utilization, storage and excretion of iron.

Ferrous (फेरस) लौह युक्त। Pertaining to or containing iron.

Ferrule (फेरूल) पट्टी या छल्ला। A band or ring of metal applied to the end of the root or crown of a tooth in order to strengthen it.

Fertilization (फर्टीलाइजेशन) गर्भाधान,निषेचन। The impregnation of an ovum by a spermatozoon.

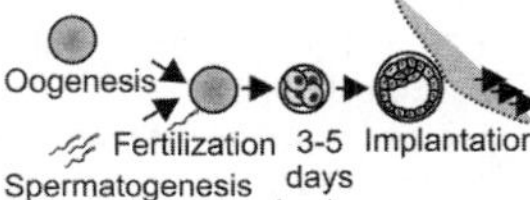

Fervescence (फरवेशेनस) अतिज्वरता। Fever.

Festers (फेसटर्स) घाव। Ulcers.

Festinant (फेसटिनेन्ट) तेज। Quick, rapid.

Feticide (फेटीसाइड) भ्रूण का नष्ट होना। The destruction of the fetus.

Fetoscope (फिटोस्कोप) भ्रूण दर्शन। A fiberoptic endoscope used in fetoscopy.

Fetotoxin (फिटोटौक्सिन) कोई भी वस्तु जो भ्रूण के लिये विषाक्त होती है। Anything that is toxic to the fetus.

Fetus (फीटस) गर्भाधान के पश्चात् से लेकर जन्म तक गर्भाशय में विकसित होता हुआ बच्चा, इस समय से पूर्व यह एम्ब्रियो कहलाता है। Child *in utero* from fertilization to birth.

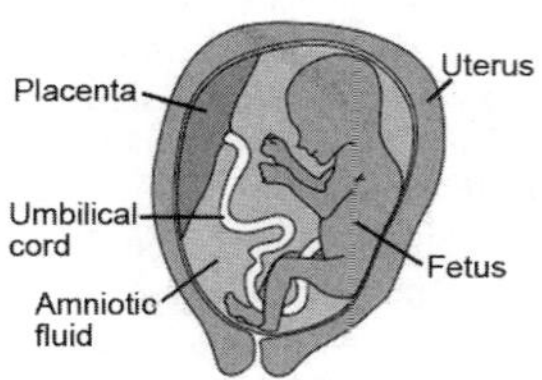

Fiber (फाइबर) रेशा, सूत्र। A filament.

Fibril (फाइब्रिल) एक छोटा तन्तु। A small fiber or filament.

Fibrillation (फिब्रिलेशन) सूत्रों या सूक्ष्म तन्तुओं का बनना। Spontaneous contraction of individual muscle fibers.

Fibrin (फाइब्रिन) रक्त जमाने वाला एक वर्णहीन तरल पदार्थ। A whitish portion from the blood and the serous fluid of the body.

Fibrination (फाइब्रिनेशन) रक्त में फाइब्रिन पदार्थ बढ़ना। The blood fibrin.

Fibrinogen (फाइब्रिनोजन) प्लाज्मा में विद्यमान एक प्रोटीन जो कैल्सियम आयनों की उपस्थिति में थ्रॉम्बिन की क्रिया से फाइब्रिन में परिवर्तित हो जाती है जो रक्त को जमाने में आवश्यक होती है।
A coagulation protein of plasma that is precursor of fibrin.

Fibrinogenolysis (फाइब्रिनोजीनोलाइसिस) रक्त में फाइब्रिनोजन का विघटन। Decomposition or dissolution of fibrinogen in the blood.

Fibrinogenopenia (फाइब्रिनोजीनोपीनिया) रक्त में फाइब्रीनोजन की कमी जो अधिकतर यकृत विमर के कारण होती है।
Reduction in blood fibrinogen.

Fibrinoid (फाइब्रिनॉयड) फाइब्रिन के समान। Resembling fibrin.

Fibrinolysis (फाइब्रिनोलाइसिस) फाइब्रिनोलाइसिन द्वारा फाइब्रिन का घुल जाना। Dissolution of fibrin by enzymatic Rxn (fibrinolysis).

Fibrinosis (फाइब्रिनोसिस) रक्त में फाइब्रिन का अधिक पाया जाना। Presence of fibrin in the blood in excess.

Fibroadenoma (फाइब्रोएडीनोमा) तन्त्वबुद। Adenoma with fibrous tissue stroma.

Fibrocartilage (फाइब्रोकार्टिलेज) एक प्रकार की उपास्थि जिसमें आधात्री या आधारक में सफेद। Cartilage containing fibrous tissue.

Fibrocyst (फाइब्रोसिस्ट) एक तन्तुमय अबुर्द जिसमें पुटीय ह्रास हो जाता है। A cystic fibroma.

Fibroid (फाइब्रॉयड) एक अबुर्द जिसमें तन्तुमय ऊतक होता है। Fibromyoma of uterus which may grow inwards or outwards to become subperitoneal.

Fibroma (फाइब्रोमा) संयोजी ऊतक का बना एक अबुर्द।
A tumor composed of fibrous or connective tissue.

Fibromatosis (फाइब्रोमेटोसिस) एक ही समय में बहुत से तन्तु अबुर्दों का उत्पन्न होना।
Fibrosis occurrence of many fibromas at a time.

Fibromyositis (फाइब्रोमायोसाइटिस) तन्तुपेशीय ऊतक का शोध।
Inflammation of the fibromuscular tissue.

Fibromyxoma (फाइब्रोमीक्सोमा) श्लेष्मतन्तु। A mucous and fibrous tissue.

Fibrosarcoma (फाइब्रोसार्कोमा) एक सार्कोमा जिसमें तन्तु-ऊतक होता

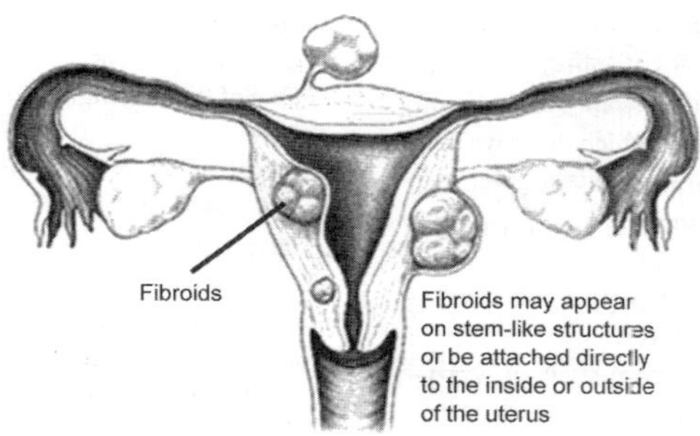

Fibroid

है। A sarcoma containing fibrous tissue.

Fibrosis (फाइब्रोसिस) असामान्य रूप से तन्तु-ऊतक का बनना। Formation of abnormal fibrous tissue.

Fibula (फिब्यूला) पिण्डली की बाहरी लम्बी हड्डी। One of the longest and thinnest bones of the body.

Field (फिल्ड) क्षेत्र। A specific area in relation to an object.

Filament (फिलामैन्ट) बारीक धागे के समान रचना। A fine thread-like structure or membrane.

Filaria (फाइलेरिया) सूत्रवत्-कृमि। Parasitic thread-like worm found mainly in the tropics and subtropics.

Filariasis (फाइलेरियासिस) नारू-रोग। Infestation with filaria.

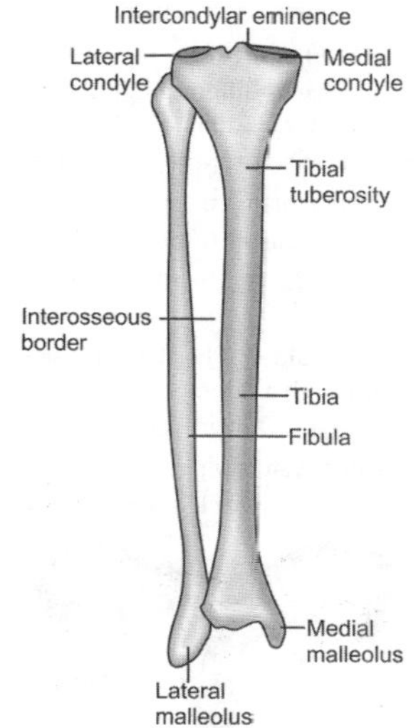

Fibula

Filaricidal (फाइलेरिसाइडल) फाइलेरिया कृमियों को नष्ट करने वाले से सम्बन्धित। Pertaining to that which destroys filariac.

Filliform (फिलीफोर्म) लम्बा धागे के समान। Long thread-like, filamentous.

Film (फिल्म) एक पतली परत। A thin layer.

Filter (फिल्टर) किसी भी छिद्रयुक्त पदार्थ से होकर जो किसी निश्चित परिमाण, से बड़े कणों को गुजरने से रोकता है, किसी द्रव को गुजारना।
Device for filtering light, liquid, radiation, etc.

Filtrate (फिल्ट्रेट) निस्यंदक से होकर गुजरने वाला द्रव। The liquid which passes through a filter.

Filum (फाइलम) एक धागे के समान संरचना।
The fluid that has been passed through a filter.

Fimbriate (फिम्ब्रियेट) अंगुली के समान प्रक्षेपण या उभार वाला। Having finger like-projections.

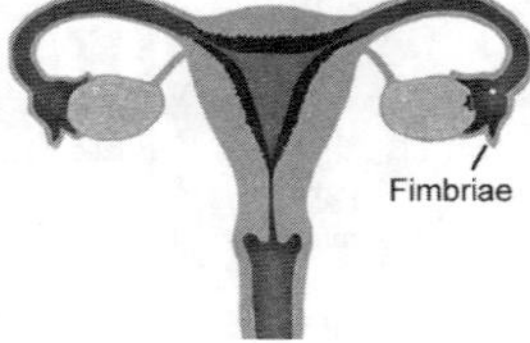

Finger (फिंगर) हाथ की पाँच अंगुलियों में से एक।
One of the five digits of the hand.

Fingerprint (फिंगर प्रिन्ट) अंगुली छाप जिसका किसी व्यक्ति की पहचान करने में उपयोग होता है।
The impression made by cutaneous ridge of the fleshy distal portion of a finger which is used for identification.

First-aid (फर्स्ट ऐड) प्राथमिक चिकित्सा। Primary help or immediate assistance given in the case of injury or sudden illness.

First cranial nerve (फर्स्ट क्रेनियल नर्व) घ्राण तंत्रिका। The olfactory nerve.

Fission (फिशन) विखण्डन।
Spliting into two or more parts, a method of asexual reproduction in bacteria, protozoa and other lower forms of life.

Fissiparous (फिशिपेरस) विखण्डन द्वारा सन्तानोत्पत्ति करने वाला। Reproducing by fission.

Fissure (फिशुर) दरार। Cleft, a fissure.

Fistula (फिस्टुला) नासूर।
An abnormal communication between two body surfaces or cavities.

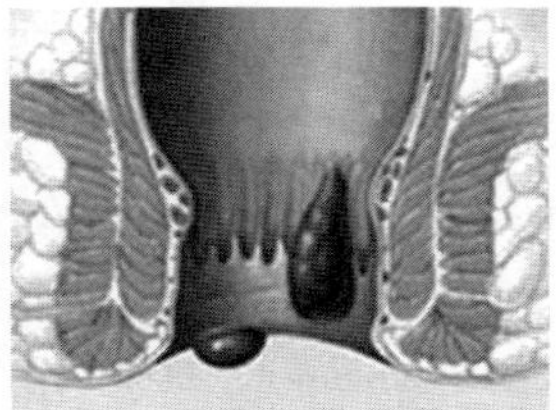

Fistula

Flacid (फ्लेसिड) ढीला-ढाला, पिलपिला, पेशीय तान की कमी वाला, कमजोर या मुलायम। Relaxed, flabby, having deficient muscular tone, weak or soft.

Flagellate (फ्लैजिलेट) एक या अधिक कशाभों से युक्त। Having one or more flagella.

Flagellation (फ्लैजिलेशन) थपथपा कर मालिश करना। Massage by stroke.

Flagellum (फ्लैजिलम) एककोषिकीय जन्तु की बाह्य सतह से उत्पन्न होने वाला लम्बा बाल के समान एवं हिलने-डुलने वाला उपांग। A long hair-like moving appendage arising from the external surface of a bacterium or a protozoon.

Flange (फ्लैन्ज) निकला हुआ किनारा। A projecting edge or rim.

Flank (फ्लैंक) पसलियों एवं इलियम हड्डी के ऊपरी किनारों के बीच स्थित शरीर का पार्श्वीय भाग। The side of the body between the ribs and the upper border of the illium.

Flap (फ्लैप) पल्ला। A loose, partly detached portion of skin and tissues.

Flare (फ्लेयर) वाहिका प्रेरक प्रतिक्रिया के कारण त्वचा पर किसी नुकीले यंत्र से खींचकर बनाई रेखा के चारों ओर फैली हुई लाली। A diffuse redness of the skin extending beyond the local reaction of the application of an irritant.

Flash-point (फ्लैश-पाइन्ट) वह तापमान जिस पर कोई पदार्थ एकदम से स्वतः जल जाता है और लपटे निकलने लगती है। The temperature at which a substance bursts into flame spontaneously.

Flat Foot (फ्लैट फूट) ऐसा रोग जिसमें पाँव चाप चपटा हो जाता है। The condition in which the arch of the foot becomes flattened.

Flatness (फ्लेटनैस) समतलता। The state of being flat.

Flatulence (फ्लेटुलैन्स) अमाशय एवं आँत में अत्यधिक गैस बनना। Formation of gas in excess in the stomach and intestine.

Flatus (फ्लेटस) पाचन नली में स्थित गैस आंत्र वायु। Gas in the digestive tract.

Flatus tube (फ्लेटस ट्यूब) आंत्रवायु नली। A rectal tube which is pushed to facilitate expulsion of gas.

Flavism (फ्लेविज्म) बालों का पीलापन। Paleness of hair.

Flesh (फ्लेश) मांस। A soft tissue of the body.

Flex (फ्लैक्स) झुकाना, मोड़ना। To bend.

Flexibility (फ्लेक्सीबिलिटी) लचीलापन। Capability of bending without breaking.

Flexion (फ्लैसन) मोड़, नमन। The process of flexing or bending.

Flexor (फ्लैसर) आकुंचर, आकोचक। A muscle and contraction flexes or bend. A part or joints.

Flicker (फिलकर) फड़फड़ाना, झिलमिलाना। To quiver, flutter.

Floaters (फ्लोटर्स) नजर के सामने तैरती चीजें। Floating bodies in the vitreous humor which are visible to the person.

Floating ribs (फ्लोटिंग रिब्स) 11वीं तथा 12वीं पसलियाँ जो स्टर्नम से जुड़कर जोड़ नहीं बनाती। 11th and 12th ribs which do not articulate with the sternum.

Flocculation (फ्लोकुलेशन) किसी घोल में छितरे बारीक कणों का आपस में एकत्रित होकर बड़े पिण्ड बन जाना जो अक्सर नम्न नेत्रों से दिखाई दे जाती है। The gathering together of fine dispersed particles in a solution larger visible particles.

Flocculus (फ्लोकुलस) गुच्छा। A small tuft of wool like-fibers.

Flooding (फ्लाडिंग) प्रचुर रक्त स्राव। Profuse flow of blood, especially from the uterus.

Flora (फ्लोरा) सूक्ष्मजीवाणु। The collective plant organisms of particular region.

Florid (फ्लोरिड) चमकते हुए लाल रंग का। Shining of a bright red color.

Floumeter (फ्लोमीटर) द्रवों अथवा गैसों के बहने की गति को मापने वाला उपकरण। An apparatus of measuring the rate of flow of liquids or gases.

Fluctuation (फ्लकचुएशन) घटना-बढ़ना, परिवर्तन। Variation, change.

Fluent (फ्लुएन्ट) बहता हुआ। Flowing.

Fluidram (फ्लयूड्राम) चाय के चम्मच के बराबर का माप। A unit of liquid capacity equal to 1/8 fluid ounce.

Fluor (फ्लेयार) स्राव। A secretion or discharge.

Fluorescent (फ्लूयोरेसेन्ट) किसी प्रकार के प्रकाश विकिरण जैसे अल्ट्रावायलेट किरणों के प्रति आवृत होने पर प्रकाश फैलना। Emitting light or shining when exposed to other light rays.

Fluorescence (फ्लूयोरेसेन्स) किसी पदार्थ का किसी प्रकार के प्रकाश विकिरण जैसेः अल्ट्रावायलेट किरणों के प्रति अनावृत्त होने पर प्रकाश फेंकने का गुण, प्रतिदीप्ति। The power of body to change wave-rate of light passing through it.

Fluoridation (फ्लूयोरिडेशन) दाँत में कीड़ा लगने को रोकने के लिए जल आपूर्ति में फ्लूयोराइड को मिलाना। The addition of fluoride to a water supply in order to prevent the dental caries.

Fluoride (फ्लूयोराइड) जल में पाया जाने वाला नमक। A salt sometimes present in water.

Fluoroscope (फ्लूयोरोस्कोप) प्रतिदीप्ति दर्शन। The process of examining the tissues by a fluoroscope.

Flurometer (फ्लूयोरोमीटर) एक्स-रे द्वारा उत्पन्न विकिरण की मात्रा को मापने वाला एक उपकरण। An apparatus for measuring the amount of radiation produced by X-rays.

Flurosis (फ्लूयोरोसिस) पीने के पानी में अत्यधिक फ्लूयोराइड होना। Chronic fluorine poisoning causing motting of tooth enamel, and hyperlucency of bone.

Flutter (फलट्र) फड़फड़ हट, स्फुरण। Agitation or tremulousness especially of heart, twitching.

Flux (फ्लक्स) अत्यधिक, स्राव होने की अवस्था। An excessive flow of any of the body excretion.

FM (एफ.एम.) एक मिक्श्चर बनाओ। इसे नुस्खा लिखने में प्रयोग में लाया जाता है। Let a mixture be made. It is used in prescription writing.

Foam (फोम) झाग। Collection of small bubbles on the surface of a liquid.

Focus (फोकस) केन्द्र। Center.

Fog (फौग) कुहरा। Mist.

Fogging (फौगिंग) दृस्टिवैषम्य में अपवर्ती त्रुटि का पता लगाने की एक विधि। A method of determining the refractive error in astigmatism.

Foil (फॉयल) किसी धातु की बहुत ही पतली एवं लचीली चादर। Very thin and flexible sheet of a metal.

Fold (फोल्ड) परत, तह। A thin recurved margin or doubling back.

Foliaceous (फोलिएसीयस) किसी पत्ती से सम्बन्धित अथवा उससे मिलता-जुलता। Foliate, pertaining to or resembling a leaf.

Follicle (फॉलिकिल) एक छोटा स्रावी कोश या छोटी गुहा। A small secretory sac, cavity or gland.

Follicle-stimulating-hormone (फॉलिकिल स्टिमुलैटिंग हार्मोन) अग्र पीयूश ग्रंथि से उत्पन्न होने वाला एक हार्मोन जो डिम्ब ग्रंथि में कूप की वृद्धि को एवं शुक्रग्रंथि में शुक्रजनन को उत्तेजित करता है। A hormone produced by the anterior pituitary gland which stimulates the growth of the follicle in the ovary and spermatogenesis in the testis.

Folliculitis (फॉलिकुलाइटिस) पुटक अथवा पुटकों का शोध जैसे दाढ़ी का दाद। Inflammation of a follicle or follicles, e.g. ringworm of the beard.

Folliculosis (फॉलिकुलोसिस) लसीका पुटकों का अत्यधिक विकसित होना। Excessive development of the lymph follicles.

Fomentation (फोमेन्टेशन) सिकाई, सेंक। External application of hot, a warm application.

Fomes (फोम्स) संक्रामक पदार्थ, छूत की बीमारी के कीटाणु फैलाने वाले पदार्थ। A porous substance, absorbing and transmitting the contagion of disease.

Fontanel (फोन्टानेल) कलान्तराल या करोटि।
Aperture in the infant.

Fontanelle (फोन्टेनेली) अन्तराल। Skull at the function of the suture.

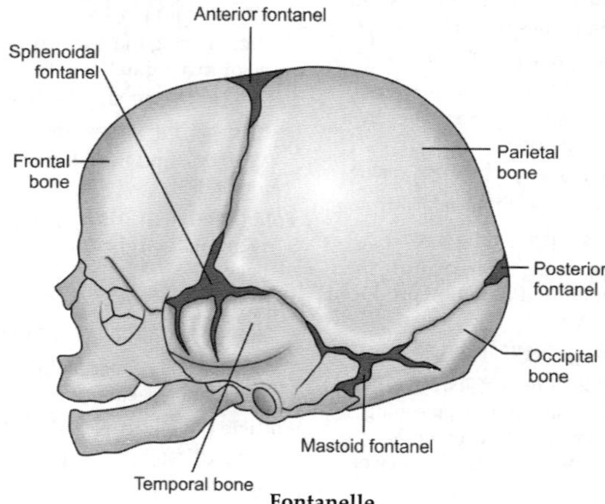

Fontanelle

Food-poisoning (फूड-पॉइजनिंग) विषैले पदार्थों से युक्त भोजन को ग्रहण करने से उत्पन्न दशा। A condition resulting from ingestion of food containing poisonous substances.

Foot-pound (फूट-पौण्ड) एक पौण्ड वजन को एक फुट ऊपर उठाने के लिए आवश्यक शक्ति की मात्रा। The amount of energy necessary to lift one pound weight to a vertical.

Foot-print (फूट-प्रिन्ट) पांव की छाप विशेषकर स्याही लगाकर ली गई छाप जो शिशुओं को पहचानने में काम आती है। An impression of the foot, especially an ink impression used for identification of the infants.

Foot Drop (फूट ड्राप) टांग के निचले भाग की अग्र पेशियों की कमजोरी जो लम्बे समय तक लगातार विशेषकर बेहोशी की हालत में बिस्तर पर लेटा रहा हो। Plants flexion of the foot from weakness or paralysis of the anterior muscle of the lower leg which may occur in a patient lying on bed continuously for a long time, especially if comatose.

Forage (फोरेंज) 1. घोड़े तथा मवेशियों का खाना। 2. विद्युत-दहन द्वारा बढ़ी हुई पुरःस्थ या प्रोस्टेट ग्रंथि में से होकर एक नाली बनाना। 1. Food for horses and cattles. 2. To create a channel through an enlarged prostate gland by means of an electric coutery.

Foramen (फोरामैन) एक द्वार, छिद्र। An opening, orifice or hole.

Force (फोर्स) ताकत। Strength, power.

Forceps (फोर्सेप्स) चिमटी, दो ब्लेडों वाला एक यंत्र जिसमें एक हैण्डिल होता है जो ऑपरेशन के दौरान ऊतकों को दबाने अथवा पकड़ने सिलाई करने वाली सूई को पकड़ने के काम आता है। A two bladed instrument with a handle used for compressing or grasping tissues.

Forcipate (फोर्सिपेट) चिमटी के आकार का। Shaped like a forceps.

Forearm (फोरआर्म) बांह का कोहनी एवं कलाई के बीच का भाग। Part of the arm between the elbow and the wrist.

Forensic (फोरेन्सिक) न्याय सम्बन्धी। Pertaining to or applied in legal proceedings.

Foreskin (फोरस्किन) शिष्नमुण्डच्छद, अग्रच्छद। The prepuce, a fold of skin over the glans—penis.

Forewaters (फोरवाटर्स) गर्भाशय-ग्रंथियों से उत्पन्न होने वाला एक पतला श्लेष्मा स्राव जो गर्भावस्था में योनि से बाहर निकलता

है। A thin mucus secretion discharged from the vagina during pregnancy produced by the uterine glands.

Forget's Sign (फेगेट्स साइन) बढ़े हुए तापमान की अपेक्षा नाड़ी गति का धीमा होना जैसा कि टायफॉयड ज्वर में देखा जाता है। Slowness of the pulse rate that would be expected the elevated temperature, as seen in typhoid fever.

Fork (फोर्क) अपने सिरे पर दो या अधिक भुजाओं से युक्त एक यंत्र। An instrument two or more prongs at the end.

Formation (फोर्मेशन) रचना, निर्माण। A structure, shape or figure.

Forme fruste (फोर्मे फ्रूस्टे) अपूर्ण रूप। Incomplete or atypical form of a disease.

Formication (फोर्मिकेशन) ऐसी अनुभूति होना जैसे छोटे-छोटे कीड़े शरीर पर रेंग रहे हो। A sensation as of small insects creeping upon the body.

Fornication (फोर्निकेशन) अविवाहितों के मध्य लैंगिक सम्भोग। The sexual intercourse between unmarried persons.

Fornix (फोर्निक्स) एक मेहराव की शक्ल की संरचना। An arch-shaped structure or voult-like space formed by such a structure.

Fortify (फोर्टीफाइ) ताकतवर बनाना। To strengthen.

Fossa (फोसा) हल्का दबा हुआ स्थान। A hollow or slightly depressed area.

Fossette (फोसेट) एक छोटा गड्ढ़ा। A small depression.

Foulage (फोलेज) पेशियों की मालिश में उन्हें गूंथना एवं दबाना। Kneading and pressing in massage of the muscles.

Fovea (फोविया) प्यालेनुमा गड्ढ़ा, लघु कोटर। A small cup-shaped pit.

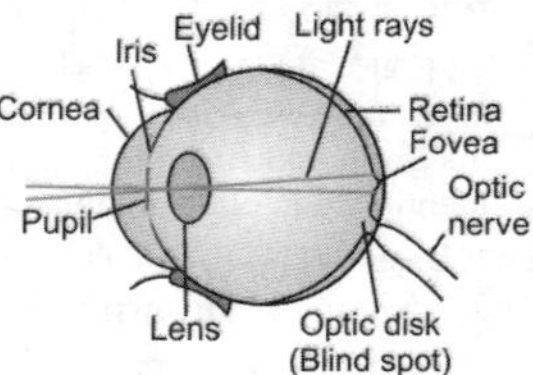

Foveated (फोविएटेड) विवरित। Pitted.

Foveation (फोविएशन) त्वचा पर गर्तो या छोटे-छोटे गड्ढों का बन जाना जैसे चेचक में होता है। Formation of pits on the skin as in smallpox.

Fractionation (फ्रैक्शनेशन) किसी पदार्थ अथवा मिक्श्चर के घटकों का पृथक होना। The separation of components of a substance or mixture.

Fracture (फ्रैक्चर) हड्डी का टूटना। The breaking of a bone.

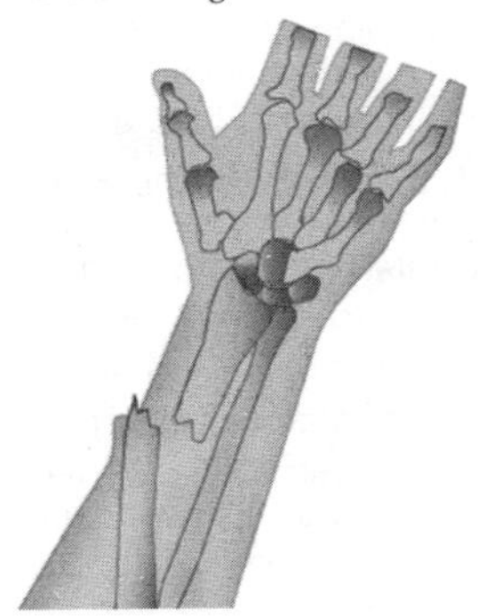

Fragilitas (फ्रेजिलिटास) भुरभुरापन। Brittleness.

Fragility (फ्रेजिलिटी) टूट जाने के लिए तत्परता। Readiness to be broken.

Fragmentation (फ्रेगमेन्टेशन) छोटे-छोटे टुकड़ों में बांट देना। A subdivision into fragments.

Frambesia (फ्रेमबेसिया) थाज। Yaws.

Fratricide (फ्रेट्रीसाइड) किसी व्यक्ति के भाई अथवा बहिन का कत्ल कर देना। Murder of one's brother or sister.

Freckle (फ्रेकिल) चकत्ता। Lentigo.

Freezing (फ्रीजिंग) हिमीकरण, गर्मी निकल जाने से द्रव से ठोस अवस्था में पहुँच जाने वाला। Passing from liquid to solid state due to loss of heat.

Fremitus (फ्रेमिटस) कम्पन्न जिसका ज्ञान परिस्पर्शन। Vibration which is perceptible by palpation or auscultation.

Frenectomy (फ्रनेक्टॉमी) बंध को शल्यक्रिया द्वारा काट कर अलग कर देना। Excision of a frenum.

Frenkle's-Exercise (फ्रेंकल एक्सरसाइज) फ्रेंकल व्यायाम। Exercises for tabes or salis to teach muscle and joints sense.

Frenulum-lingual (फ्रेनुलम लिंगुल) जिह्वा बंध। A fold of mucous membrane that extends from floor of mouth to the inferior surface of tongue along midline.

Frenzy (फ्रेन्जी) गुस्से से भरा हुआ। Violent mania.

Friable (फ्रियाबिल) आसानी से टूटना। Easily broken or pulverized.

Friction (फ्रिक्शन) रगड़। The act of rubbing.

Friction-rub (फ्रिक्शन-रब) दो सूखी सतहों के रगड़ने से उत्पन्न सुनाई देने वाली ध्वनि। The sound heard when two dry surfaces are rubbed together.

Fright (फ्राइट) डर। Fear.

Frigid (फ्रिजिड) ठण्डा। Cold.

Frigidity (फ्रिजिडिटी) 1. उदासी 2. किसी स्त्री को उत्तेजित करने पर भी उसमें लैंगिक इच्छा का जाग्रत न होना। Literally coldness, especially lack of normal sexual desire.

Frigolabile (फ्राइगोलेबाइल) ठण्ड से आसानी से नष्ट हो जाने वाला। Easily destroyed by cold.

Frigorific (फ्राइगोरीफिक) ठण्डक पैदा करने वाला। Producing coldness.

Frigostabile (फ्राइगोस्टेबिल) ठण्ड से नष्ट न हो सकने वाला। Incapable to be destroyed by cold.

Frog-belly (फ्रोग-बेलि) बच्चों का पेट अफरा जाना। Tympany of a child's belly.

Frog-face (फ्रोग-फेस) दादुराननन। A Distoration of the face from a swelling or tumor.

Frohlich's-syndrome (फ्रोहलिक्स सिण्ड्रोम) बच्चों में उत्पन्न होने वाला एक रोग जिसमें बच्चे बौने रह जाते हैं, उनमें मोटापा आ जाता है, उनका लैंगिक विकास नहीं होता। Obesity, hypogonadism, due to hypothalamic disturbance.

Frolement (फ्रोलमेन्ट) हथेली से हल्की-हल्की मालिश करना। Light friction or massage with the palm of the hand.

Frons (फ्रोन्स) माथा, ललाट। The forehead.

Frost (फ्रोस्ट) पाला, तुशार। Frozen dew or vapor.

Frost-itch (फ्रोस्ट-इच) ठण्ड से खुजली होना। Itching caused by cold.

Frostbite (फ्रोस्टबाइट) अत्यधिक ठण्ड के कारण खुले रहने वाले भागों जैसे–कान, नाक, गला, हाथ-पैरों की अंगुलियों आदि में क्षति पहुँचाना। Freezing and death of a body part due to cold exposure.

Frottage (फ्रोटेज) उसे रगड़ने पर लैंगिक इच्छा का जाग्रत होना। Arousal of sexual desire by pressing or rubbing against one of the opposite sex. Massage by rubbing.

Frozen-section (फ्रोजन-सैक्शन) किसी जमे हुए ऊतक नमूने से एक पतला टुकड़ा काटना। The cutting of a thin piece of tissue from a frozen specimen.

Fructose (फ्रक्टोस) फलशर्करा। The fruit sugar.

Fructosemia (फ्रक्टोसीमिया) रक्त में फलशर्करा का पाया जाना। Presence of fructose in the blood.

Frustration (फ्रस्ट्रेशन) इच्छित वस्तु प्राप्त न होना। Disappointment.

Fugitive (फ्यूगिटिव) भ्रमणकारी। Wandering.

Fugue (फ्यूग) सच्चाई से भागने की कोशिश। An attempt to escape from reality.

Fulguration (फ्लगुरेशन) विद्युत द्वारा ऊतकों का नष्ट होना। Destruction of tissue by electricity.

Full-term (फुल-टर्म) परिपक्व, गर्भावस्था के 38 सप्ताह पूर्ण होने के पश्चात् जन्म लेने वाला शिशु। In Obstetric, child born between 38–41 weeks of gestation.

Fulminant (फूलमिनेन्ट) अचानक गंभीरता के साथ घटने वाला। Occurring with sudden severity.

Fumigation (फ्यूमिगेशन) धूमनकारी पदार्थ का उपयोग करना। Exposure to disinfectant vapors.

Functional-disease (फन्कशनल-डिजीज) क्रियात्मक रोग। Emotional response to physical disease, taking the form of conversion or hysterical response.

Fundoplication (फण्डोप्लीकेशन) शल्य-क्रिया द्वारा आमाशय के फण्डस में खुलने वाले छिद्र के परिमाण को कम करना और पहले से अलग किये गये ग्रासनली के सिरे को। Surgical reduction in size of opening into fundus of stomach used in treating reflux esophagitis.

Fundus (फण्डस) किसी अंग की तली पैंदी अथवा उसका आधार। The bottom or base of any organ.

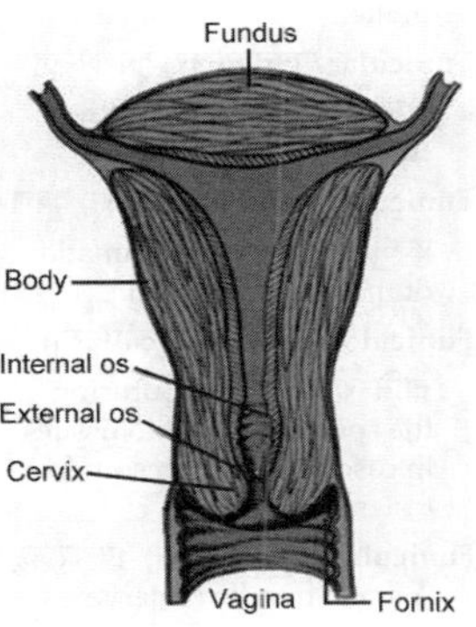

Funduscopy (फण्डस्कोपी) दृष्टिपटलपेशी द्वारा नेत्र-बुध्न का परीक्षण करना। Ophthalmoscopy, examination of the fundus of the eye with ophthalmoscope.

Fungal (फन्गल) किसी कवक से सम्बन्धित अथवा उसके द्वारा उत्पन्न। Pertaining to or caused by a fungus.

Fungicidal (फन्जिसाइडल) कवकनाशक। Denoting a fungicide.

Fungiform (फन्गीफोर्म) छत्रक से मिलता-जुलता। Resembling to the form of a mushroom or fungus.

Fungus (फंगस) फफूंद, फंगस। A vegetable cellular organism that subsists on organic matter.

Funicular (फनिक्यूलर) वृषणरज्जु सम्बन्धी। Pertaining to the funiculus.

Funiculitis (फनिक्यूलाइटिस) वृषण-रज्जु का शोध। Inflammation of the spermatic cord.

Funiculopexy (फनिक्यूलोपेक्सी) नाभि रज्जु बन्धन। Suturing the spermatic cord to tissues in cases of under descended testes.

Funiculus (फनिकयूलस) वृषणरज्जु। A small bundle of nerve fiber enclosed in a sheath of connective tissue.

Funiform (फ्यूनिफार्म) रज्जू जैसा। Cord-like.

Funnel-chest (फ्यूनेल-चेस्ट) कीपवक्ष। Sternal depression resembling funnel.

Furcula (फरक्यूला) भ्रूण की ग्रसनी का उभार। A forked elevation in the floor of the embryonic pharynx.

Furor (फरोर) पागलपन, गुस्सा। Madness, frenzy.

Furrow (फरोव) खांच, तह। Crease, foldor sulcus.

Furunculoid (फरनक्यूलोइड) पनसिका, फुंसी रोग। The systemic condition favoring boil-formation.

Furunculus (फरनक्यूलस) फुंसी। A furuncle.

G

Gadus callarias (गॉडस कैलेरीयस) कॉड मछली। Cod fish.

Gag (गैग) मुँह खुला रखने के लिए दाँतों के बीच रखा जाने वाला उपकरण, मुखरोधनी। A device for placing between the teeth to prevent closure of the jaws during surgery.

Gain (गेन) सुधार, बढ़ोतरी। Improvement, increasement.

Gait (गेट) चाल, चलने का ढंग। The mode of manner of walking.

Gait ataxic (गेट एटेक्सिक) लड़खड़ाते हुए चलना, गिरने को तैयार रहना। Difficulty in carrying out a movement with impaired muscular strength.

Gait cerebellar (गेट सेरेबेल्लर) लड़खड़ाती, टेढी-मेढी चाल। Etymology: L, cerebellun, small brain onorse, gete a way.

Gait cow (गेट कॉऊ) लहराते हुए चाल। घुटने के अंदर मुडे के कारण । A swaying movement due to knock-knee.

Gait equine (गेट इंक्विन) अश्व-चाल, क्रॉस लेग चाल। The center is a controlled three-beat gait that usually is a bit faster the average trot, but slower than the gallop.

Galactic (गैलेक्टिक) दुग्ध-प्रवाह से सम्बन्धित। Pertaining to flow of milk.

Galactocele (गैलेक्टिोसील) ऐसा जलवृषण या हाइड्रोसील जिसमें दुधिया तरल भरा होता है। A hydrocele filled with a milky fluid.

Galactometer (गैलेक्टोमीटर) दुग्ध. मापी, लैक्टोमीटर। Glucometer device for measuring the specific gravity of milk.

Galactorrhea (गैलेक्टोरिह्या) बच्चे को दूग्ध पिलाना छुड़ाने के पश्चात् होने वाला अत्यधिक दुग्ध प्रवाह। Excessive or continuous flow of milk after cessation of breastfeeding.

Galactose (गैलेक्टोज) दुग्ध शर्करा। A crystalline sugar obtained by the action of dilute acids on lactose.

Galactosemia (गैलेक्टोसीमिया) दुग्ध में शर्करा की अत्यधिक बढ़ी हुई मात्रा। Excess of galactose in the milk.

Galactosis (गैलेक्टोसिस) दुग्ध स्रावण। Secretion of milk.

Galactosuria (गैलेक्टोसूरिया) मूत्र में गैलेक्टोज का पाया जाना। Presence of galactose in the urine.

Galactotoxism (गैलेक्टोटॉक्सिज्म) दुग्ध विषाक्तता। Milk poisoning.

Galaxia (गैलेक्सिया) वक्ष-नली। The thoracic duct.

Gall (गाल) पित्त। Bile.

Gallbladder (गालब्लैडर) पित्ताशय, पित्तकोश। The pear-shaped reservoir for the bile on the under surface of the liver.

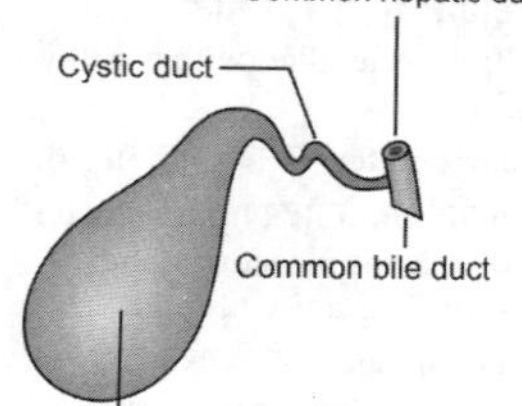

Gallon (गैलेन) तरल माप की एक ईकाई जो 4 क्वार्टस के बराबर होती है। A unit of liquid measure which is equal to 4 quarters.

Gallstone (गालस्टोन) पित्ताशय अथवा पित्त-वाहिनी में बनने वाली पथरी। A calculus formed in the gallbladder or bile duct.

Galvanic (गैल्वेनिक) सीधी विद्युत धारा से सम्बन्धित। Pertaining to galvanism.

Galvanocautery (गैल्वेनोकॉटरी) विद्युत-दहन। Electrocautery.

Galvanometer (गैल्वेनोमीटर) विद्युत्धारामापी। An instrument for measuring an electric current.

Galvanoscope (गैल्वेनोस्कोप) विद्युत् धारादर्शी। An instrument for revealing a galvanic current.

Galvanosurgery (गैल्वेनोसर्जरी) शल्यक्रिया में विद्युत धारा का प्रयोग। Use of galvanic current in surgery.

Gamete (गैमेट) युग्मक, डिम्ब। A sexual reproductive cell.

Gametic (गैमेटिक) युग्मक सम्बन्धी। Pertaining to gametes.

Gametocide (गैमेटोसाइड) युग्मकनाशी, जन्तुनाशी। An agent destructive to gamete especially the malarial gametocyte.

Gametogenesis (गैमेटोजेनेसिस) युग्मकजनन। Formation and development of gametes.

Gametogony (गैमेटोगोनी) युग्मकों द्वारा जनन। Reproduction by means of gametes.

Gammaglobulin (गामाग्लोब्यूलिन) रक्तसीरम में एक पौष्टिक पदार्थ जिसका सम्बन्ध रोगक्षमता से होता है। A protein substance in blood serum concerned with immunity against disease.

Gamma rays (गामा रेज) गामा किरणें। Non-charged hard X-rays.

Gammation (गैमेशन) कलिकोत्पादन द्वारा कोशिका विभाजन। Cell division by budding.

Gamogenesis (गैमोजेनेसिस) लैंगिक जनन। Sexual reproduction.

Gamopathy (गैमोपेथी) ऐसा रोग जिसमें रक्त के सीरम में इम्यूनोग्लोबिन बढ़ जाता है। A disease in which there is an increase of immunoglobin in the blood serum.

Gamophobia (गैमोफोबिया) शादी का रोगोत्पादक भय। Morbid fear of marriage.

Gangliated (गैंग्लिएटेड) गण्डिकाओं या गैंग्लियानों से युक्त। Having ganglia.

Gangliocyte (गैंग्लियोसाइट) एक गण्डिका कोशिका। A ganglion cell.

Ganglioma (गैंग्लियोमा) लसीका ऊतक का अबुर्द अथवा लसीका ग्रंथि की सूजन। Tumor of lymphoid tissue or a swelling of a lymphatic gland.

Ganglion (गैंग्लियोन) गण्डिका, कण्डरापुटी गुच्छिका, तंत्रिका-उपकेन्द्र। A collection of nerves fibers forming a subsidiary nerve center within the main nerve system.

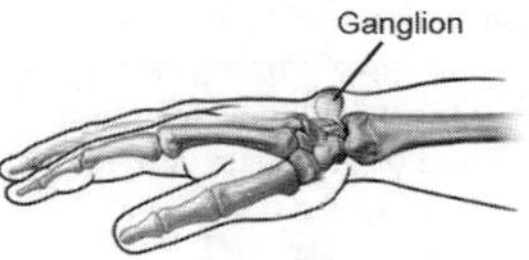

(*i*) **Carotid G** (केरोटिड गैंग्लियोन।) निचले हिस्से में एक गुफाओं वाला साईनस। One in the lower part of cavernous sinus. (*ii*) **Chorionic G** (कोरियोनिक गैंग्लियोन) अपरा के जरायुज अंकुरों से उत्पन्न होने वाले गोनेडोट्रॉपिन। Produced by chorionic villi of placenta. (*iii*) **Hepatic G** (हिपेटिक गैंग्लियोन) यकृत-गण्डिका। One around the hepatic artery.

Ganglioneuroma (गैंग्लियोन्यूरोमा) एक सुदम अबुर्द जो तंत्रिका तंतुओं एवं परिपक्व गण्डिका कोशिकाओं का बना होता है। A benign tumor consisted of the nerve fibers and mature ganglion cells.

Ganglionic (गैंग्लियोनिक) किसी गण्डिका से सम्बन्धित अथवा उसकी प्रकृति वाला। Pertaining to or nature of a ganglion.

Ganglionostomy (गैंग्लियोनोस्टॉमी) किसी साधारण सी गण्डिका में चिरा लगाना। To make an incision into a simple ganglion.

Gangrene (गैंग्रीन) ऊतक का गल जाना, विगलन, कोथ। Mortification or death of a part of the tissue of the body.

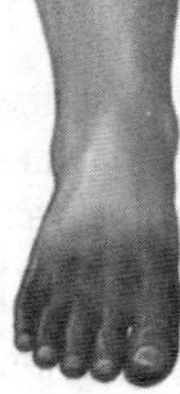

(*i*) **Diabetic G.** (डायबिटीक गैंग्रीन) मधुमेही कोथ। A complication of diabetes.

(*ii*) **Dry G.** (ड्राई गैंग्रीन) शुष्क कोथ। Occurs when the drainage of blood from the affected part is inadequate.

Gangrenous (गैंग्रीनस) कोथ सम्बन्धी। Relating to death of tissue due to obstructed blood circulation.

Garlic (गार्लिक) लहसुन। *Allium sativum,* it is medicinal plant.

Gaseous (गैसियस) गैस की प्रकृति वाला। Nature like gas.

Gasoline (गैसोलीन) पेट्रोल। A distillation product of petroleum.

Gasometric (गैसोमेट्रिक) गैसों की माप से सम्बन्धित। Pertaining to measurement of gas.

Gastrectomy (गैस्ट्रेक्टॉमी) अमाशय के किसी भाग को अथवा सम्पूर्ण अमाशय को शल्य-क्रिया द्वारा काटकर अलग करना। Excision of a part or the whole stomach.

Gastric digestion (गैस्ट्रिक डॉयजेशन) अमाशयिक पाचन। Digestion in the stomach by the enzymes of gastric juices.

Gastric juice (गैस्ट्रिक जूस) पाचक रस, जठर रस। The gastric fluid, almost colorless liquid secreted by the glands in the lining of the stomach.

Gastric lavage (गैस्ट्रिक लैवाज) अमाशय की धुलाई करना, अमाशय प्रक्षालन। To wash out the stomach.

Gastric ulcer (गैस्ट्रिक अल्सर) अमाशय में स्थित व्रण, जठर व्रण। An ulcer present in the stomach.

Gastrin (गैस्ट्रिन) पाचक रस से पैदा करने वाला एक हॉर्मोन। A hormone secreted by the gastric mucosa on entry of the food.

Gastritis (गैस्ट्राइटिस) जठरशोध। Inflammation of the mucous membranes of the stomach.

(*i*) **Atrophic g** (एट्रोफिक गैस्ट्राइटिस) शोशी जठरशोध। A chronic form with atrophy of the mucous membrane.

(*ii*) **Toxic g** (टॉक्सिक गैस्ट्राइटिस) किसी विष की क्रिया से जठरष्लेमकला का शोथ। Inflammation of the gastric mucosa caused by the action of poison or corrosive substance.

Gastrobrosis (गैस्ट्रोब्रोसिस) अमाशय में छिद्र होना। Perforation of the stomach.

Gastrocnemius (गेस्ट्रोक्निमाइस) उपरिस्थ-पिण्डिका। The leg, two headed muscle of the calf.

Gastrocolitis (गैस्ट्रोकोलाइटिस) अमाशय एवं कोलन का शोथ। Inflammation of stomach.

Gastrocolostomy (गैस्ट्रोकोलोस्टॉमी) अमाशय एवं कोलन के बीच मार्ग बनना।

To make a passage between the stomach and the colon.

Gastroduodenoscopy (गैस्ट्रोड्योडीनोस्कोपी) एण्डोस्कोप का प्रयोग करके अमाशय का नेत्र परीक्षण करना। Visual examination of the stomach and duodenum by using an endoscope.

Gastroenteritis (गैस्ट्रोएन्टेराइटिस) अमाशय एवं आंत्र का शोथ, जठरान्तशोथ। Inflammation of the stomach and intestine.

Gastroenterology (गैस्ट्रोएन्टेरोलॉजी) अमाशय एवं आँतों का वैज्ञानिक अध्ययन। Study of the stomach and intestines and their disease.

Gastroenterostomy (गैस्ट्रोएन्ट्रोस्टॉमी) शल्य-क्रिया द्वारा अमाशय एवं छोटी आँत के बीच मार्ग बनाना।
To make a passage between the stomach and intestine by surgery.

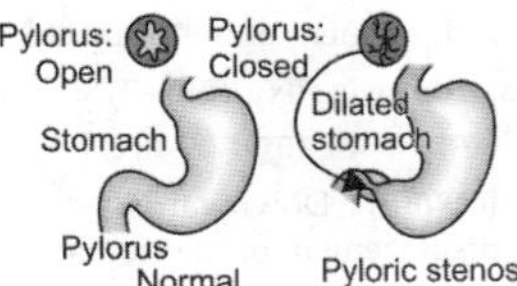

Gastroepiploic (गैस्ट्रोइपिप्लोइक) अमाशय एवं वृहद वपा से सम्बन्धित।
Pertaining to the stomach and the greater omentum.

Gastroesophageal (गैस्ट्रोऐसोफेगियल) अमाशय एवं ग्रासनली का शोथ।
Inflammation of the stomach and the esophagus.

Gastrofiberscope (गैस्ट्रोफाइबरस्कोप) अमाशय का नेत्र-परीक्षण करने के लिए प्रयोग में लाया जाने वाला फाइबरस्कोप।
A fiberscope for visual examination of the stomach.

Gastrojejunostomy (गैस्ट्रोजेजुनॉस्टामी) अमाशय एवं जेजुनम के बीच एक मार्ग बनाना।
To make a passage between the stomach and jejunum.

Gastrolith (गैस्ट्रोलिथ) अमाशय में विद्यमान पथरी।
A callus in the stomach.

Gastrolysis (गैस्ट्रोलाइसिस) जठरलयन। Surgical division of epigastric adhesions.

Gastromegaly (गैस्ट्रोमेगैली) अमाशय का बढ़ जाना। Enlargement of the stomach.

Gastroptosis (गैस्ट्रोप्टोसिस) अमाशय का नीचे की ओर विस्थापन। Downwards displacement of the stomach.

Gastroreflex (गैस्ट्रोरिफलेक्स) जठरबृहदांत्र-प्रतिवर्ष। Peristaltic wave in colon induced by entrance of food into stomach.

Gastrorrhagia (गैस्ट्रोरैह्जिया) अमाशय से रक्तस्राव होना। Hemorrhage from the stomach.

Gastrorrhaphy (गैस्ट्रोरैह्फी) अमाशय की सिलाई करना। Suture of the stomach.

Gastrospasm (गैस्ट्रोस्पाज्म) अमाशय में ऐंठन आ जाना। Spasm of the stomach.

Gastrostomy (गैस्ट्रोस्टॉमी) अमाशय में एक कृत्रिम छिद्र बनाना। To make an artificial opening into the stomach.

Gastrotome (गैस्ट्रोटोम) अमाशय छेदक। An instrument to perform gastrotomy.

Gauntlet (गौउंटलेट) दस्ताने के समान हाथ एवं अंगुलियों को ढ़कने वाली एक पट्टी। A bandage covering the hand and fingers like a glove.

Gel (जेल) किसी ठोस पदार्थ को लप्सी में बदलना, जेली बनाना। To convert a solid into a jelly.

Gelatin (जिलेटिन) श्लेषा, शिलिष, सरेस। A protein containing glue like substance obtained by boiling bones, skin and other tissue.

Gelatiniferous (जिलेटिनीफेरस) जिलेटिन उत्पन्न करने वाला। Producing gelatin.

Gelatinous (जिलेटिनस) जिलेटिन से युक्त अथवा चटनी के समान, लेसदार। Containing gelatin or jellylike.

Geminate (जोमिनेट) जोड़ो में उत्पन्न होने वाला। Occurring in pairs.

Gemination (जेमिनेशन) जोड़ों में विकसित होना। Development in pairs.

Gender (जैन्डर) किसी व्यक्ति का लिंग। The sex of an individual.

Gene (जीन) गुणसूत्र के अन्तर्गत विद्यमान वंश परम्परा को निर्धारित करने वाली इकाई, पित्तैक। A factor in the chromosome responsible for transmission of hereditary characteristics.

General (जनरल) सामान्य, साधारण। Pertaining to the whole body.

Generate (जेनेरेट) उत्पन्न करना, जन्म देना। To produce.

Generation (जेनेरेशन) सन्तानोत्पति की क्रिया, जनन, पीढ़ी। The process of reproduction.

Generic (जेनेरिक) किसी जीनस या वंश से सम्बन्धित, सामान्य, स्पष्ट। Pertaining to a genus general distinctive.

Genesis (जेनेसिस) प्रजनन, जनन, उत्पत्ति। The act of getting an origin or beginning process.

Genetics (जेनेटिक्स) आनुवंशिकी। Study of the role played by nuclear and extranuclear cellular structures in human avoid.

Genetotrophic (जेनेटोट्रॉफिक) आनुवांशिकी एवं पोषण सम्बन्धि। Pertaining to the genetics and the nutrition.

Genial (जेनियल) ठुड्डी सम्बन्धी। Pertaining to the chin.

Genioplasty (जेनियोप्लास्टी) ठुड्डी अथवा गाल की प्लास्टिक सर्जरी द्वारा मरम्मत करना। Repair of the chin or the cheek by plastic surgery.

Genital (जेनाइटल) जननांगों से सम्बन्धित। Pertaining to the sex organs.

Genitalia (जेनाइटेलिया) जननांग। Reproductive organs.

Genitourinary (जेनाइटोयूरीनरी) जननांगों एवं मुत्रांगों से सम्बन्धित। Pertaining to the genital and the urinary organ.

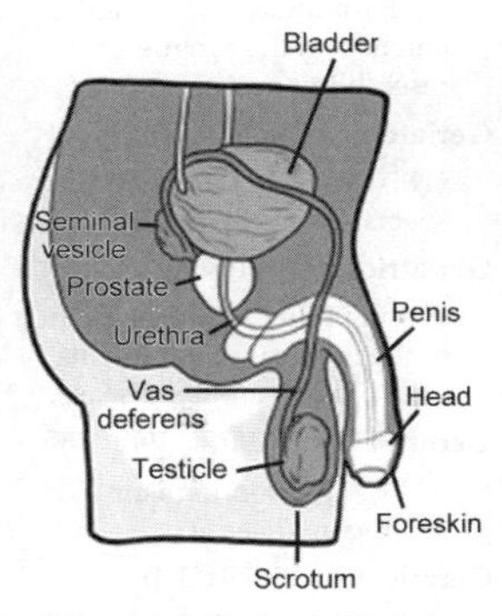

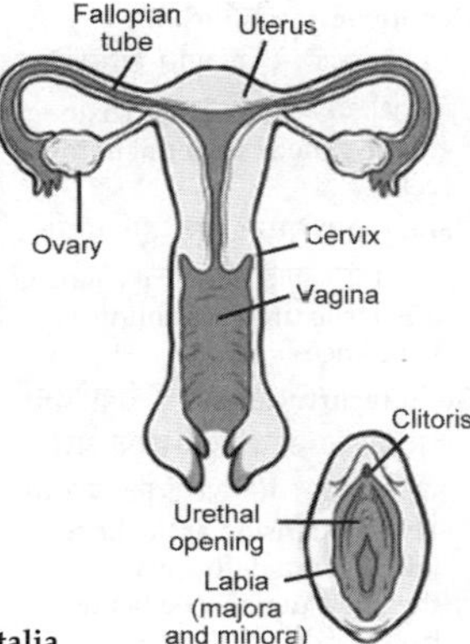

Genitalia

Genitourinary system (जेनाइटोयूरीनरी सिस्टम) वह संस्थान अथवा तंत्र जो मूत्र निर्माण एवं उसकी उत्सर्जन सम्बन्धी अंगों तथा जननांगों से मिलकर बनता है। The system consisting of the organ concerning the formation and excretion of the urine and the genital organ.

Genius (जीनियस) विशेष बुद्धि वाला अथवा अपूर्व बुद्धि का मनुष्य। The person having special intellectual power.

Genome (जीनोम) गुणसूत्रों या क्रोमोसोमों के अगुणित सैट में आनुवंशिक कारकों का पूरा सैट। The complete set of hereditary factor contained in the haploid set of chromosomes.

Genotoxic (जीनोटॉक्सिक) कोशिकाओं में विद्यमान आनुवंशिक पदार्थ के लिए विषैला। Toxic to the genetic material in the cells.

Genu (जीनू) घुटना, मुड़े हुए घुटने के समान कोई भी रचना। Knee, any structure resembling a bent knee.

Genu recurvatum (जीनू रीकर्वेटम) घुटनो का अन्दर की तरफ धस जाना, घुटने पर अत्यधिक प्रसार। Hyperextension at the knee joints, it is a deformity of the knee joints, knee bends backwards.

Genu varum (जीनू वेरम) इस अवस्था में टाँगे बाहर की ओर धनुष के आकार में मुड़ जाती है। Bowing of the lower leg in relation to the thigh—like a bow. Legs are bent outwards.

Genual (जेनुअल) घुटने से सम्बन्धित। Pertaining to the knee.

Genus (जीनस) वंश, जीवविज्ञान में जाति एवं कुल के बीच का विभाजन। In biology the division between the species and the family.

Geographical tongue (जियोग्राफिकल टंग) जिह्वा पर सतह के उखड़ने से बने चकते जो नक्शों के समान प्रतीत होते हैं। Formation of denuded patches on the tongue resembling maps.

Geriatrician (जेरीयाट्रिसिन) जराचिकित्सक। One who specializes in geriatrics.

Geriatrics (जेरीयाट्रिक्स) जराचिकित्साविज्ञान। The branch of the medical science deals with old age and its disease.

Germ (जर्म) रोगोत्पादक एक सूक्ष्म जीव। A microorganism producing disease.

Germicidal (जर्मीसाइडल) रोगोत्पादक सूक्ष्मजीवों को मारने वाला, रोगाणुनाशक। Destroying the disease producing microorganism germicide.

Germinal Epithelium (जर्मिनल इपिथीलियम) भ्रूण के जननांगी कटक की सतह को ढकने वाली उपकला।
The epithelium that covers the surface of the genital ridge of an embryo.

Germination (जर्मिनेशन) 1. गर्भित डिम्ब अथवा अण्डाणु का भ्रूण में विकसित होना 2. किसी पौधे के बीजों का उगना, अंकुरण।
1. Development of a fertilized ovum into an embryo. 2. The sprouting of the seeds of a plant.

Germinative (जर्मिनेटिव) अंकुरण अथवा किसी जनन-कोशिका से सम्बन्धित। Pertaining to germination or to a reproductive cell.

Germinoma (जर्मिनोमा) शुक्र ग्रन्थि अथवा डिम्ब ग्रन्थि में स्थित जनन-कोशिकाओं का एक अबुर्द। A tumor of the reproductive cells in the testis or ovary.

Geroderma (जीरोडर्मा) झुर्रीदार त्वचा। Appearance of senility brought about by premature loss of hair wrinkling of skin general body atrophy.

Gerontophilia (जीरोन्टोफीलिया) बूढ़े लोगों से स्नेह।
Fondness or love for old.

Gestagen (जेस्टेजन) प्रोजेस्टेरोन के प्रभावों को उत्पन्न करने वाला। Producing the effects of progesterone.

Gestation (जेस्टेशन) डिम्ब अथवा अण्डाणु के गर्भाधान के समय से लेकर बच्चे के जन्म लेने तक का काल, सगर्भता। The period from the time of fertilization of the ovum until birth of the child. (*i*) **Plural gestation** (पिल्यूरल जेस्टेशन) ऐसी सगर्भता जिसमें एक से अधिक भ्रूण होते है। Gestation in which there is more than one embryo.
(*ii*) **Secondary gestation** (सेकण्डरी जेस्टेशन) ऐसी सगर्भता जिसमें डिम्ब अपने आरोपण के प्रारम्भिक स्थान से अलग होकर नये स्थान पर विकसित होता है। Gestation in which the ovum become dislodged from its original place of implantation and continues to develop in a new situation.

Gesture (जेस्चर) किसी विचार, राय या मनोभाव को अभिव्यक्त करने वाली कोई भी चेष्टा संकेत। Any movement expressing an idea opinion or emotion.

Ghon's focus (घोन फोकस) प्रारम्भिक फुफ्फुसक्षय। Primary complex.

Giant cell (जीयान्ट सैल) एक वृहत कोशिका जिसमें कई केन्द्रक

होते हैं जो कई कोशिकाओं के बने प्रतीत होते हैं परन्तु उनकी कोई स्पष्ट रेखा नहीं होती। A large cell with several nuclei appearing to be made up of many cells but not clearly outlined.

Giardia (जियार्डिया) एक कशाभ युक्त जीव जो मनुष्य की छोटी आँत में श्लेष्मिक झिल्ली से लगे रहते हैं। A flagellated protozoa inhabiting intestinal mucosa.

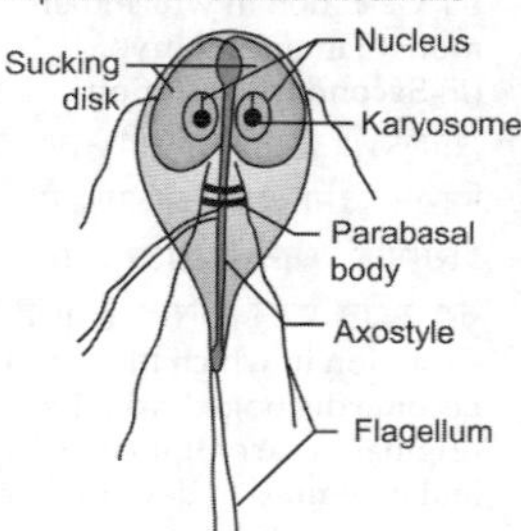

Giardiasis (जियार्डिएसिस) जियार्डिया लैम्बलिया के संक्रमण से उत्पन्न रोग। Infection caused of *Giardia lamblia.*

Gibbous (गिब्बस) कुबड़ा व्यक्ति। Person having humpback.

Gibbus (गिब्बस) कूबड़। Hump.

Giddiness (गिडीनैस) चक्कर आना। Dizziness—the state of being inconstant or unstable.

Gigantism (जाइजैन्टिज्म) महाकायता। An abnormal overgrowth especially in height.

Gigantomastia (जिगैन्टोमैस्टिया) स्तन का अत्यधिक बढ़ जाना। Extreme enlargement of the breast approximately 3% of the total body weight.

Gingiva (जिन्जाइवा) मसूड़ा। Gum.

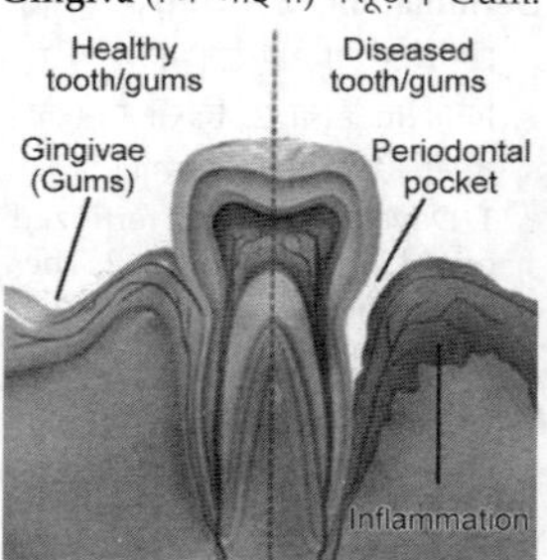

Gingival (जिन्जाइवल) मसूड़ा सम्बन्धी। Pertaining to the gum.

Gingivectomy (जिन्जीवेक्टॉमी) मसूड़े के रोगग्रस्त भाग को शल्य-क्रिया द्वारा काट कर अलग करना, मसूड़ोछेदन। Excision of the diseased protein of gum.

Gingivitis (जिन्जीवाइटिस) मसूड़ाशोथ। Inflammation of the gums.

Gingivoglossitis (जिन्जाइवोग्लोसाइटिस) मसूड़ों एवं

जिह्वा का शोथ। Inflammation of the gum and tongue.

Girdle (गर्डिल) कोई भी वस्तु जो शरीर को चारों ओर से घेरे होती है। Anything encircling. Any body structure.

(*i*) **Pelvic girdle** (पैल्विक गर्डिल) श्रोणि करधनी, श्रोणि मेखला, क्षोणिवलय। Also called bony pelvis. A bony of cartilaginous structure in vertebrates to attach and support the hind limbs fins.

(*ii*) **Shoulder girdle** (शोल्डर गर्डिल), कंधे करधनी स्कन्धमेखला। The shoulder girdle formed by the set of bones which connect the arm to the axial skeleton on each side consist of two clavicles and scapula.

Glabella (ग्लेबेला) दोनों भौं के बीच वाला स्थान। The small space between the eyebrows.

Glabrate (ग्लेब्रेट) गंजा, चिकना। Bald, smooth.

Glacial (ग्लेसियस) बर्फ के समान। Like ice.

Gland (ग्लैण्ड) ग्रन्थि, झिल्ली। A soft body, the function of which is to secrete some fluids and call hormones.
Types of glands:

(*i*) **Bartholin gland** (बार्थोलिन ग्लैण्ड) योनिकपाट ग्रन्थि। The vulvovaginal gland

(*ii*) **Cardiac gland** (कार्डियक ग्लैण्ड) हृदय ग्रन्थि। A coiled

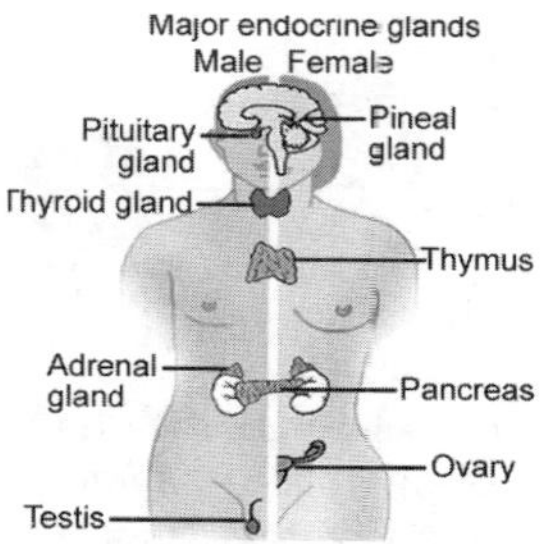

tubular gland located in the cardiac region of the stomach

(*iii*) **Ceruminous gland** (सेरूमिनस ग्लैण्ड) कर्णमल छोड़ने वाली ग्रन्थियां। Glands secreting the cerumen of the ears. (*iv*) **Lacrimal gland** (लेक्रिमल ग्लैण्ड) अश्रु-ग्रन्थि। A compound gland in the upper and outer part of orbit that secretes tears.

(*v*) **Lingual gland** (लिंगुअल ग्लैण्ड) जिह्वा-गलगण्ड। A tumor of thyroid tissue involving the embryonic rudiment at the base of the tongue.

(*vi*) **Mammary gland** (मेमैरी ग्लैण्ड) स्तन ग्रन्थि। The milk secreting organ. (*vii*) **Pineal gland** (पिनीयल ग्लैण्ड) पिनियल ग्रन्थि। The pineal body.

(*viii*) **Pituitary gland** (पिट्यूटरी ग्लैण्ड) पीयूष ग्रन्थि। A term for the hypophysis of the brain.

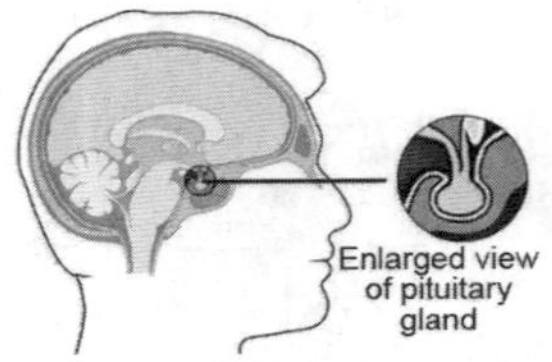

(*ix*) **Salivary gland** (सैलाइवरी ग्लैण्ड) लार ग्रन्थि, तीन पैरोटिड, सबलिंगुअल एवं सबमैण्डिबुलर लार ग्रंथी। The three parotid, sublingual and submandibular salivary gland.

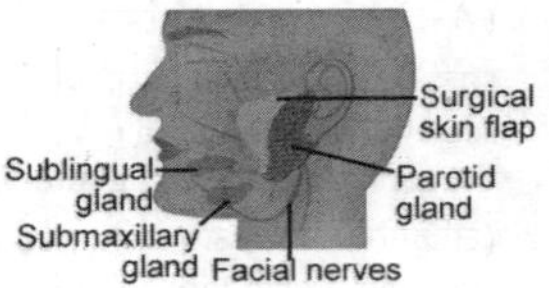

(*x*) **Sebaceous gland** (सिबेसियस ग्लैण्ड) वसा ग्रन्थियां। The glands of the skin secreting sebum.

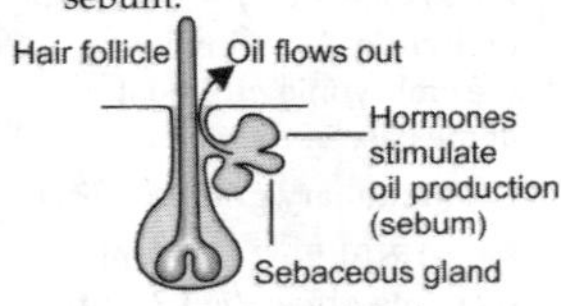

(*xi*) **Serous gland** (सेरोउस ग्लैण्ड) सीरम ग्रन्थियाँ। Gland secreting a thin water fluid.

Glander (ग्लैण्डर) घोड़े तथा खच्चरों को होने वाला एक संक्रमण रोग। A contagious febrile ulcerative disease communicable of horses.

Glandula (ग्लैण्डुला) एक छोटी ग्रन्थि। A small gland.

Glans (ग्लैन्स) एक गोल पिण्ड, मुण्ड। A rounded mass or gland-like structure.

Glanular (ग्लैनुलर) शिश्न मुण्ड अथवा भगशिश्निका मुण्ड से सम्बन्धित। Pertaining to the gland penis or top of the glans clitoridis.

Glare (ग्लेयर) बहुत तेज चमकती रोशनी, चौंध। Strong bright light.

Glassitis (ग्लोसाइटिस) जिह्वाशोथ। Inflammation of the tongue.

Glassodynia (ग्लोसोडाइनिया) जीभ में दर्द होना। Pain in the tongue.

Glassograph (ग्लोसोग्राफ) जिह्वालेख। An instrument for showing the movement of the tongue in speaking.

Glassopharyngeal (ग्लासोफेरेन्जियल) जिह्वा एवं ग्रसनी से सम्बन्धित। Pertaining to the tongue and the pharynx.

Glassoplegia (ग्लोसोप्लेजिया) जिह्वा का पक्षाघात। Paralysis of the tongue.

Glaucoma (ग्लोकोमा) आँखों का एक रोग जिसमें दृष्टि धुंधली पड़ जाती है, अंधिमंथ। A hardening of the eyeball due to interference with normal circulation of the eye fluids.

Gleet (ग्लीट) जीर्ण मूत्रमार्गशोध में मूत्रमार्ग से निकलने वाला श्लेष्मिक अथवा सपूय स्राव। A mucous of purulent discharge from the urethra in chronic urethritis.

Glenoid (ग्लीनॉयड) असंगर्त, कूपास, गर्तवत। Pitlike shallow resembling a socket.

Glenoid cavity (ग्लीनॉयड कैविटी) असंगर्त गुहा। A shallow depression on a bone into which another bone fits to form a joint. A fossa in the head of the scapula for the humerus.

Glenoid fossa (ग्लीनॉयड फोसा) असंगर्त खात। A depression in the temporal bone receiving the condyle of the lower jaw.

Glia (ग्लीया) तन्त्रिका-बंध। Neuroglia.

Gliadin (ग्लीयाडिन) गेहूं में स्थित एक प्रोटीन जिसमें विषैला कारक होता है। A water insoluble protein present in the gluten of wheat.

Gliocytoma (ग्लियोसाइटोमा) तंत्रिकाबंध कोशिका का एक अबुर्द। A neuroglial cell tumor.

Glioma (ग्लियोमा) तंत्रिकाबन्धाबुर्द। A sarcoma of neurological origin.

Gliomatous (ग्लियोमेटस) तंत्रिकाबंधबुर्द से पीड़ित। Suffering from glioma.

Gliomotosis (ग्लियोमोटोसिस) तंत्रिका बंधाबुर्द का बनना। Formation of glioma.

Globlet cell (गोब्लेट सैल्स) चषक कोशिकाऐं। Cup like cells in the intestinal epithelium

Globulin (ग्लोबुलिन) रक्त गोलिकायें। A group of proteins found in animal tissue which differs from the albumins in the heat.

Globulin antihemophilic (Antihemophilic globulin) (ग्लोबुलिन एन्टीहीमोफिलिक) अनुवांशिक रक्त-स्कंदन। Genetics bleeding disorder.

Globulinuria (ग्लोबुलिनूरिया) मूत्र में ग्लोबुलिन का पाया जाना। Presence of globulin in the urine.

Globus (ग्लोबस) गोलाकार रचना। A spherical structure.

Globus hystericus (ग्लोबस हिस्टीरिकस) हिस्टीरिकस रोग के दौरान गले में एक तरफ अण्डे जैसी संरचना हो जाना। The feeling of a lump in the throat, during hysteria.

Glomangioma (ग्लोमेन्जियोमा) कोशिका गुच्छाबुर्द, वाहिका गुच्छाबुर्द। A benign tumor developing from an enteric venous glomus of skin.

Glomectomy (ग्लोमेक्टॉमी) शल्यक्रिया द्वारा किसी वाहिकागुच्छ को काटकर निकाल देना। Removal of a glomus by surgery.

Glomeruli (ग्लोमेरूलाई) ग्लोमेरूलस का बहुवचन। Plural of glomerulus.

Glomerulitis (ग्लोमेरूलाइटिस) वृक्कीय कोशिकागुच्छों की सूजन। Inflammation of the renal glomeruli.

Glomerulonephritis (ग्लोमेरूलोनेफ्राइटिस) वृक्कशोध के साथ वृक्कीय कोशिकागुच्छों एवं वृक्कीय नलिकाओं का शोथ, स्तवक वृक्कशोध। Nephritis with inflammation and degeneration of the renal glomeruli and the renal tubular.

Glomerulopathy (ग्लोमेरूलोपैथी) वृक्क के कोशिकागुच्छ का कोई भी रोग। Any disease of the glomerulus of the kidney

Glomerulosclerosis (ग्लोमेरूलोस्क्लेरोसिस) वृक्कीय कोषिकागुच्छों की तन्तुमयता। Fibrosis of the renal glomeruli.

Glomoid (ग्लोमॉयड) वाहिकागुच्छ के समान दिखाई देने वाला। Resembling a glomus.

Glomus (ग्लोमस) सीधी शिराओं से जुड़ी रहने वाली सूक्ष्म धमनिकाओं से बना एक छोटा, गोल पिण्ड जिसमें बहुत से तंत्रिका तन्तु होते हैं। A small round most made up of tiny black vessels and found in stroma containing many nerve fibers.

Glossa (ग्लोसा) जिह्वा। The tongue.

Glottis (ग्लॉटिस) कण्ठद्वार, श्वासनली का मुख। The opening into the windpipe at the larynx.

Glucagon (ग्लूकेगोन) एक पॉलीपेप्टाइड हार्मोन जो रक्त में ग्लूकोज की सान्द्रता को बढ़ा देता है और अल्पग्लूकोजरक्तता की अनुक्रिया में अग्नाशय के लैंगरहैन्स की द्वीपसमूहों की एल्फा कोशिकाओं से स्रावित होता है। Polypeptide hormone secreted by alfa cells of pancreas that raises blood sugar and relaxes smooth muscles of GI tract.

Glucocorticoid (ग्लूकोकार्टिकॉयड) एड्रीनल ग्रन्थि के कॉर्टेक्स से स्रावित होने वाले कॉर्टिकोस्टैरॉयड हार्मोनों के समूहों में से एक जिसका सम्बन्ध कार्बोहाइड्रेट एवं प्रोटीन चपापचय से होता है। A class of adrenal hormones that are released in response to stress and effect carbohydrate and protein metabolism.

Glucogenesis (ग्लूकोजेनेसिस) ग्लाइकोजन से ग्लूकोज का बनना। Formation of glucose from glycogen.

Glucogenic (ग्लूकोजेनिक) ग्लूकोज उत्पन्न करने वाला। Producing glucose.

Glucose (ग्लूकोज) यह कार्बोहाइड्रेट चपापचय का अन्तिम उत्पाद होता है और शरीर की शक्ति के लिए मुख्य स्रोत होता है। अधिक ग्लूकोज ग्लाइकोजन में परिवर्तित होकर यकृत एवं पेशियों में जमा होता है। It is the end product of carbohydrate metabolism and is the chief source of energy for the body excess of glucose which is stored in the liver and muscles for the use when needed.

Glucose tolerance test (ग्लूकोज टोलेरैन्स टैस्ट) रोगी की शुगर का चयापचय करने की क्षमता का पता लगाने के लिए किए जाने वाला एक परिक्षण। A test by which the ability of the patient to metabolize sugar is determined.

Glucoside (ग्लूकोसाइड) शरीर में शर्करा का पाया जाना। A body containing glucose.

Glucosuria (ग्लूकोसूरिया) मूत्र में अनियमित ग्लूकोज का पाया जाना। Presence of abnormal glucose in the urine.

Glutamine (ग्लूटामिन) एक शाक्-मिश्रण। A vegetable compound.

Gluteal (ग्लूटियल) नितम्बों से सम्बन्धित। Pertaining to the buttocks.

Gluten (ग्लूटेन) गेहूँ तथा अन्य अनाजों में पाई जाने वाली एक प्रोटीन। A protein of wheat and other grains.

Gluteus maximus (ग्लूतियस मेक्सिमस) कूल्हे की बड़ी पेशी। A giant muscle of the hip.

Glutinous (ग्लूटिनस) चिपकने वाला। Adhesive sticky.

Glycemia (ग्लाइसीमिया) रक्त में शुगर या ग्लूकोज की विद्यमानता। Glycosemia; Presence of sugar or glucose in the blood.

Glycerin (ग्लिसरिन) तेल से निकाला हुआ एक सत्त्व। The chemical of the alcohol group.

Glycogen (ग्लाइकोजन) काइर्बोहाइड्रेट पाचन एवं अवषोशण के पश्चात् भविष्य में शुगर में परिवर्तन होने एवं पेशीय कार्य करने में प्रयुक्त होने के लिए अथवा ऊष्मा को मुक्त करने के लिए यकृत या पेशियों में जमा हो जाता है। The storage form of carbohydrate in the body like liver and muscle.

Glycogenase (ग्लोइकोजिनेस) ग्लाइकोजन का जल अपघटन करने वाला एक एन्जाइम जिसमें डैक्सट्रोज बनता है। An enzyme which hydrolyzes the glycogen by which dextrose is formed.

Glycogenesis (ग्लाइकोजेनेसिस) ग्लूकोज से ग्लाइकोजन का बनना। The formation of glycogen from glucose.

Glycogenetic (ग्लाइकोजेनेटिक) ग्लाइकोजन के बनने से सम्बन्धित। Pertaining to the formation of glycogen.

Glycogenolysis (ग्लाइकोजीनोलाइसिस) शरीर के ऊतकों में ग्लाइकोजन का ग्लूकोज में परिवर्तित होना। Conversion of glycogen into glucose in the tissue of the body.

Glycogen storage disease (ग्लाइकोजन स्टोरेज डिज़ीज) कोई भी रोग जिसमें असामान्य रूप से यकृत में ग्लाइकोजन संचित हो जाता है। Any disease character is by abnormal storage of glycogen in the liver.

Glycogeusia (ग्लाइकोग्यूसिया) मुख में मीठा स्वाद मालूम होना। A sweet taste in the mouth.

Glycoptyalism (ग्लाइकोटायलिज्म) थूक में ग्लूकोज पाया जाना। Glycosialia; presence of glucose in the saliva.

Glycorrhachia (ग्लाइकोरैह्किया) प्रमस्तिष्क मेरू-द्रव में शुगर का पाया जाना। Presence of sugar in the cerebrospinal fluid.

Glycoside (ग्लाइकोसाइड) मधुमेय। Natural substance compared of a sugar another compound.

Glycosuria (ग्लाइकोसूरिया) मूत्र में ग्लूकोज का पाया जाना। Presence of glucose in the urine

Gnashing (नैशिंग) दाँत पीसना। The grinding of the teeth together.

Gnat (नैट) डाँस, मच्छर। The insects smaller than mosquitoes.

Gnathalgia (नैथेल्जिया) जबड़े में दर्द होना। Pain in the jaw.

Gnathion (नैथियोन) ठुड्डी के बीच का एंव सबसे नीचे का बिन्दु। The middle and the lowest point.

Gnathitis (ग्नैथाइटिस) जबड़े का शोध। Inflammation of the jaw.

Goiter (ग्वॉयटर) गलगण्ड, घेंघा। An enlargement of thyroid gland (*i*) **Adenomatous goiter** (एडिनोमेटस-ग्वॉयटर) ग्रन्थ्यबुर्दी गलगण्ड। Thyroid enlargement due to adenoma.

(*ii*) **Colloid goiter** (कोलॉइउ ग्वॉयटर) कलिल गलगण्ड, कोलाइड गलगण्ड। Thyromegaly with great increase in follicular contents. (*iii*) **Cystic goiter** (सिस्टिक ग्वॉयटर) पुटीय गलगण्ड। One due to the presence of one or more cysts within the glioma. (*iv*) **Exophthalmic goiter** (जियोप्थेल्मिक ग्वॉयटर) नेत्रोत्सेधी गलगण्ड। Goiter exophthalmos and cardiac palpitation Basedow's disease.

Gold (गोल्ड) स्वर्ण, सोना। A yellow metallic element.

Gonad (गोनाड) जननग्रन्थि, जननद, जननपिण्ड। A generic term referring to male and female sex glands.

Gonadal dysgensis (गोनाडल-डिस्जेनेसिस) टरनर रोग। Turner's syndrome.

Gonadotrophic (गोनाडोट्रॉफिक) जननग्रन्थियों को उत्तेजित करने वाला। Stimulation of the gonads.

Gonadotropin (गोनाडोट्रॉपिन) एक जननग्रन्थि उद्दीपक हार्मोन, जननग्रन्थिपोषी। A gonad stimulation hormone (*i*) **Anterior pituitary gonadotropin** (एन्टीरियर पिट्यूटरी गोनाडोट्रॉपिन) अग्र पीयूष ग्रन्थि से उत्पन्न होने वाले दो हार्मोन पुटक उद्दीपक हार्मोन एवं ल्यूटिनीकारी हार्मोन। Two hormones, follicle stimulating hormone and luteinizing hormone produced by the anterior pituitary gland.

Goniometer (गोनियोमीटर) किसी जोड़ की गतियों एवं इसके कोणों को मापने वाला उपकरण। An apparatus for measuring the movement and angles of a joint.

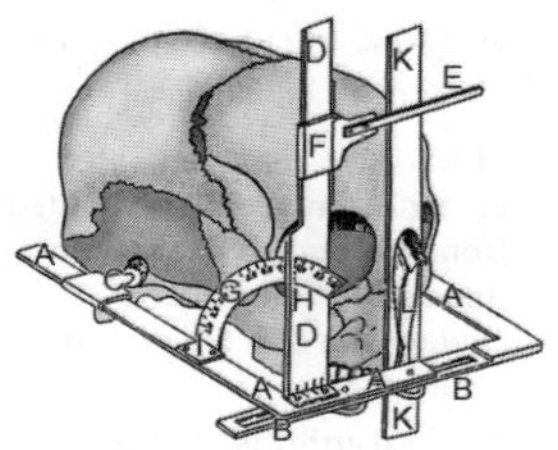

Gonioscopy (गोनियोस्कोपी) नेत्र के अग्रज कक्ष के कोण का निरीक्षण करने वाला यंत्र। An instrument used for inspecting the angle of the anterior chamber of the eye.

Goniotomy (गोनियोटॉमी) अधिमन्ध के उपचारार्थ किया जाने वाला आँख का ऑपरेशन, नेत्रकोणछेदन। Operation for glaucoma.

Gonococcal (गोनोकॉकल) गोनोकॉकस नामक जीवाणुओं से सम्बन्धित अथवा उनके द्वारा उत्पन्न। Pertaining to or caused by gonococci.

Gonococcus (गोनोकॉकस) नाइसीरिया गोनोरीह् जाति का गोनोरिह्या या सूजाक उत्पन्न करने वाला जीवाणु। *Neisseria gonorrhoeae* causative organism of gonorrhea.

Gonorrhea (गोनोरिह्या) गोनोकॉकस नामक जीवाणुओं का संक्रमण जो लैंगिक सम्पर्क द्वारा एक व्यक्ति से दूसरे व्यक्ति में संचारित होते हैं। इसमें पुरूष में मूत्रमार्गशोथ हो जाता है। Infection of the bacteria gonococci transmitted from one person to another through sexual contacts characterized in the male by urethritis.

Gonorrheal arthritis (गोनोरिह्यल आर्थराइटिस) सूजाक से किसी जोड़ में सूजन हो जाना। Inflammation of a joint due to gonorrhea.

Goodells sign (गुडेल्स साइन) गर्भावस्था में गर्भाशयग्रीवा का मुलायम हो जाना। Softening of the cervix during pregnancy.

Goose flesh (गूज फ्लेश) ठण्ड, स्तब्धता अथवा भय से होने वाले त्वचा रोम का खड़े हो जाना, वलयी रोम। Transient roughness of skin contraction of arrector pili muscles as a reaction to cold or shock.

Gorget (गॉर्जेट) एक चौड़ी नालीदार रचना से युक्त। यंत्र जो चाकू के बिन्दू के आघात से कोमल ऊतकों की रक्षा करने के लिए प्रयोग में लाया जाता है। An instrument widely grooved used to protect the soft issue from injury on point of the knife.

Gossypol (गॉजीपॉल) कपास के बीजों में पाया जाने वाला रासायनिक पदार्थ। A toxic chemical of cotton seed.

Gouge (गूज) हड्डी या किसी कठोर ऊतक को काटने के लिये प्रयुक्त किये जाने वाला यंत्र। An instrument with a grooved blade for cutting away a bone or hard tissue.

Gout (गाउट) गठिया, रक्त में यूरिक अम्ल के अत्यधिक हो जाने के कारण जोड़ों में सूजन आ जाना। A disease associated inflammation of joints swelling uric acid in the blood.

Gouty (गाउटी) गठिया की प्रकृति का अथवा उससे सम्बन्धित। Nature of or pertaining to gout.

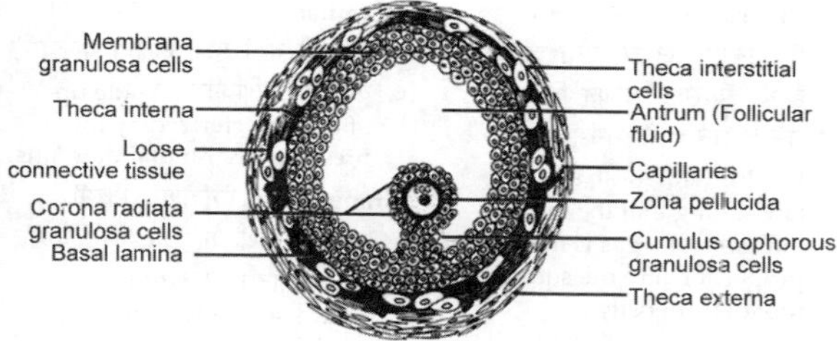

Graafian follicle

Graafian follicle (ग्राफियन फॉलिकिल) ग्राफी पुटक, क्षुद्र कोश। Minute vesicles in the stoma of an ovary each containing a simple ovum.

Gracile (ग्रेसाइल) दुर्बल, पतला, नाजुक। Slender, thin, delicate.

Gracilis (ग्रेसाइलिस) तनुपेशी। The rectus internus femoris muscle.

Gradient (ग्रेडिएन्ट) एक आनुपातिक उतार-चढ़ाव, प्रवणता, क्रमिकता। A proportional rise and fall.

Grading (ग्रेडिंग) क्रमनिर्धारण, श्रेणीकरण। To arrange in order.

Graft (ग्राफ्ट) कोई भी ऊतक अथवा अंग जिसका आरोपण अथवा प्रत्यारोपण किया जाना है, निरोपण, पैबन्द। Transplanted tissue in part of body for repair of a defect.

Graft allogeneic (ग्राफ्ट एलोजैनिक) समनिरोप। Allograft or homograft, involving transplantation cells organ and tissues from individuals of the same species.

Graft autogenous (ग्रॉफ्ट ऑटोजीनस) रोगी के अपने शरीर से लिया गया भाग का निरोप। Graft of tissues cells taken from the patient's own body.

Graft cadaver (ग्रॉफ्ट काडडेवर) मृत्यु के तुरन्त बाद शव से प्राप्त निरोप-ऊतक जैसे त्वचा, अस्थि और कॉर्निया आदि भाग को किसी और के प्रयोग (use) में लेना। Grafting tissue such as skin, bone and cornea, etc. taken from the dead body immediately after death a live human.

Grafting (ग्राफ्टिंग) किसी ऊतक या अंग का आरोपण या प्रतिरोपण करना। To implanting or transplanting of a tissue or an organ.

Graham's law (ग्राहम्स लॉ) एक नियम जिससे पता चलता है कि किसी गैस का विसरण उसके घनत्व के वर्गमूल के विपरीतानुपाती होता है। A law stating that the rate of diffusion of a gas is inversely proportional to the square root of its density.

Grain (ग्रेन) एक बीज विशेषकर अनाज के पौधे का बीज या अनाज का दाना। A seed especially of a cereal plant.

Gram (ग्राम) समतुल्य 1000 mg. A unit of weight of metric system equal to 1000 mg.

Gram method (ग्राम मेथड) जीवाणुओं को स्टेन करने की पद्धति, जीवाणुओं को अभिरंजित करने की विधि। A method of staining bacteria.

Grandiose (ग्रैण्डियोज) मनोरोग चिकित्सा में, किसी व्यक्ति के अपने को अधिक धनवान, योग्य एवं महत्त्वपूर्ण समझने से सम्बन्धित। In psychiatry pertaining to one's exaggerated concept of being more wealthy, important and capable.

Grand mal (ग्रेन्ड मल) महामिर्गी, दुर्दम अपस्मार। Major of generalized epilepsy.

Granular (ग्रेनुलर) कणिकाओं या दाने से बना हुआ अथवा दानेदार, कणीय, कणिकीय। Made up of or characterized by the presence of granular of grains.

Granulation (ग्रेनुलेशन) किसी कठोर पदार्थ का छोटे-छोटे कणों में विभाजन। The division of a hard substance into small particles.

Granule (ग्रेन्यूल) एक छोटा दाने के समान पिण्ड। A small grain-like body.

Granulocyte (ग्रेनुलोसाइट) एक कणिकीय श्वेत रक्त कोशिका जैसे इओसिनोफिल या बेसोफिल आदि, कणिका कोशिका। A granular white blood cells such as eosinophil or basophil, etc.

Granulocytopenia (ग्रेनुलोसाइटोपीनिया) रक्त में कणिकीय श्वेत रक्त कोशिकाओं का असामान्य रूप से घट जाना, कणिका कोशिका अल्पता। Reduction of granulocyte in the blood abnormally.

Granulocytopoietic (ग्रेनुलोसाइटोपॉयटिक) कणिकीय श्वेत रक्त कोशिकाओं के बनने से सम्बन्धित। Pertaining to the formation of granulocytes.

Granulocytosis (ग्रेनुलोसाइटोसिस) रक्त में कणिकीय श्वेत रक्त

कोशिकाओं का बढ़ जाना। Excess of granulocytes in the blood.

Granuloma (ग्रेन्यूलोमा) कणिकागुल्म। A tumor or growth formed of the granulation tissue (*i*) **Dental granuloma** (डैन्टल ग्रेन्यूलोमा) किसी दाँत की जड़ पर उत्पन्न होने वाला कणिका गुल्म। A granuloma developing at the root of a tooth. (*ii*) **Infectious granuloma** (इन्फैक्शियस ग्रेन्यूलोमा) कुछ विशिष्ट संक्रामक रोग जैसे क्षय रोग, सिफिलिस तथा कवक संक्रमण आदि में बनने वाला कणिकागुल्म। Granuloma formed in some specific infectious disease such as tuberculosis syphilis and fungus infection, etc. (*iii*) **Inguinal granuloma** (इन्गुवाइनल ग्रेन्यूलोमा) वंक्षण कणिकागुल्म। Ulcerating granuloma of the pudenda granuloma venereum. (*iv*) **Lipoid granuloma** (लाइपॉयड ग्रेन्यूलोमा) ऐसा कणिकागुल्म जिसमें वसीय ऊतक अथवा कोलेस्ट्रॉल होता है। Granuloma containing fatty tissue or cholesterol.

Granulomatosis (ग्रैन्यूलोमेटोसिस) बहुत से कणिकागुल्मों का बनना। To formation of multiple granulomas.

Granuloplasm (ग्रेन्यूलोप्लाज्म) दानेदार कोशिकाद्रव्य। Granular cytoplasm.

Granulopoiesis (ग्रेन्यूलोपॉयसिस) कणिका कोशिका उत्पत्ति। Granulocytopoiesis.

Granulosa (ग्रेन्यूलोसा) डिम्बग्रन्थि के ग्राफी पुटक के विधानया वेष्टन में कोशिकाओं को एक परत। A layer of cells in the theca of the Graafian follicle of the ovary.

Granulosis (ग्रेन्यूलोसिस) कणिकाओं का बनना। The formation of granules.

Graphesthesia (ग्रेफेस्थीसिया) छूकर त्वचा पर अनुरेखित अथवा लिखित रेखाओं, चिन्हो, संख्याओं या शब्दों को पहचानने की क्षमता। Ability to recognize the lines, symbols, numbers, or words traced or written on the skin by touching.

Grapho (ग्रैफो) उपसर्ग जिसका अर्थ लिखना होता है। Prefix meaning to write.

Graphorrhea (ग्रैफोरिह्या) अर्थहीन शब्दों का लिखना। The writing of meaningless words.

Graphospasm (ग्रैफोस्पाज्म) लिखते समय हाथ का काँपना। Writer's cramp.

Grasp (ग्रास्प) पकड़ना, गहरी पकड़। To hold.

Grattage (ग्रेटेज) रोग उत्पन्न करने वाली अतिवृद्धि को ब्रुश से रगड़ कर अथवा खुरच कर अलग कर देना। Removal of a disease producing outgrowth by rubbing with a brush or by scratching.

Grave (ग्रेव) गम्भीर, खतरनाक। Serious, dangerous.

Grave disease (ग्रेव डिज़ीज) नेत्रोत्सेधी गलगण्ड। Exophthalmic goiter.

Gravel (ग्रेविल) बहुत छोटी-छोटी पथरियाँ जो कणों के रूप में बनती है। Very small calculi occurring in the form of particles.

Gravid (ग्रेविड) गर्भवती, सगर्भा। Pregnant.

Gravidity (ग्रेवीडीटी) किसी स्त्री की कुल गर्भावस्थाओं की संख्या। The total number of pregnancies.

Gravimetric (ग्रेवीमेट्रिक) वजन की माप से सम्बन्धित। Pertaining to the measurement by weight.

Gravitation (ग्रेवीटेशन) पृथ्वी से दूर स्थित वस्तुओं के लिए पृथ्वी द्वारा उत्पन्न आकर्षण, गुरूत्वाकार्षण। The attraction of the earth for the objects which are at a distance from it.

Gravity (ग्रेविटी) पृथ्वी से दूर स्थित वस्तुओं पर लगने वाली पृथ्वी द्वारा उत्पन्न आकर्षण की शक्ति या बल, गुरूत्व। The force of attraction of the earth on the objects which are at a distance from it.

Gray (ग्रे) धूसर, भूरा। A color between white and black.

Gray matter (ग्रे मैटर) मस्तिष्क का बाह्य एवं सुषुम्ना रज्जु का भीतरी धूसर द्रव्य। The term applied to the outer gray portion of the brain and the inner gray portion of the spinal cord.

Graze (ग्रेज) हल्का-सा छिल जाना। Slight abrasion.

Grinder's disease (ग्राइन्डर्स) धूल से श्वसन द्वारा उत्पन्न फेफड़ों का रोग। Chronic lung disease due to dust inhalation.

Gripes (ग्राइप्स) आँतों में रूक-रूक कर उठने वाला बहुत तेज दर्द। Colic intermittent severe pain in the intestine.

Grit (ग्रिट) मिट्टी, धूल या बालू के छोटे-छोटे कण, केकड़ी। Small particles of mud, dust or sand.

Grittines (ग्रिटीनैस) किरकिरापन। The quality of being gritty.

Groan (ग्रोन) कराहना। To make the sound expressing grief or pain.

Groin (ग्रोइन) पेट और जांघ के बीच में स्थित दबा हुआ भाग। To suppressed part between the abdomen and the thighs.

Groove (ग्रूव) एक लम्बा तंग स्थान, खातिक। Long narrow channel.

Ground itch (ग्राउण्ड इच) पैर के तलुवे में होने वाला शोथ जो एक प्रकार अंकुश कृमि के लार्वा के तलवे में घुसने से उत्पन्न होता है। Skin inflammation in foot due to invasion by larva of hookworm.

Grouping (ग्रुपिंग) समूह, वर्ग, समुच्चय। A number of similar objects or structures considered together.

Growing pain (ग्रोविंग पेन) वर्धिश्णु दर्द, योवन-कालिक अंगपीड़ा। Pain in the musculoskeletal system in growing children.

Growth (ग्रोथ) वृद्धि, शारीरिक व मानसिक वृद्धि। The progressive increase in size or development both physical/mental in a living thing.

Gruel (ग्रुअल) जल में उबला हुआ कोई भी अनाज। Grains boiled in water.

Gubernaculum dentis (ग्यूबर्नाकुलम-डेंटिस) दंत संयोजी रज्जु। A connective tissue band uniting the tooth sac and gums.

Gubernaculum testis (ग्यूबर्नाकुलम टेस्टीस) वृषण विस्थापन, वृषणनिदेशक रज्जु। It is the guiding structure for the descend of the testis into the scrotum through inguinal canal.

Gubernaculums (ग्यूब्रेनेकुलम) रज्जु-बन्ध, निदेषक। A fibrous cord connecting two structures.

Guide (गाइड) किसी व्यक्ति की हाथ की गति का अथवा हाथ में पकड़े यन्त्र का मार्गदर्शन करने वाला उपकरण। An apparatus directing the motion of one's hand or of an instrument one's hands.

Guide wire (गाइडवार) एक तार या स्प्रिंग जो किसी मूत्राशल्याका या अन्य यन्त्र के स्थापन के लिए मार्गदर्शक के रूप में प्रयोग में लाया जाता है। A wire or spring used as a guide for placement of a catheter or other instrument.

Guillotine (गिलोटीन) टॉन्सिल या काकलक को काटकर अलग कर देने वाला एक यन्त्र। An instrument for excising a tonsil or the uvula.

Guilt (गिल्ट) दोष, अपराध। Feeling grief for doings what is thought to be wrong.

Guinea pig (ग्वाइनिया पिग) परीक्षण के उद्देश्य से प्रयोगशाला में काम आने वाला कुतर कर खाने वाला एक छोटा जन्तु। A small rodent in the laboratory for experimental purpose.

Guinea worm (ग्वाइनिया वर्म) नहरूआ, नहरवा, गिनीकृमि।

Nematode parasite of tropic responsible for dracunculiasis *Dracunculus medinensis.*

Gullet (गलेट) ग्रासनली। The esophagus.

Gum (गम) एक मांसल पदार्थ जो दाँतो की ग्रीवाओं को चारों ओर से घेरे होता है तथा मेक्जिला एवं मैन्डिबल के दन्तउलूखल प्रवर्धो को ढके होता है, मसूड़ा। The fleshy tissue covering the alveolar process of jaw.

Gumma (गम्मा) ऊतकों का एक कणिकागुल्मीय अबुर्द जो अधिकतर यकृत में बनता है परन्तु अन्य अंगों जैसे मस्तिष्क हृदय, शुक्रग्रन्थि, हड्डी तथा त्वचा में भी बन सकता है। A granulomatous tumor of the tissue most frequently occurring in the liver but may occur in other organ such as the brain, heart, testis, bone, and skin.

Gummy (गम्मी) मसूड़े, गोंद अथवा गम्मा से मिलता-जुलता। Resembling gum or gumma.

Gurney (गर्नी) रोगियों को लाने-ले जाने के लिए अस्पताल में प्रयोग में लाया जाने वाला पहियेदार पलंग। A wheeled cot used in hospital for transporting the patients.

Gustatory (गस्टेटरी) स्वाद के ज्ञान से सम्बन्धित। Pertaining to sense of taste.

Gustometry (गस्टोमीट्री) स्वाद ज्ञान की तीव्रता को मापना। Measurement of the sense of taste.

Gut (गट) आँत। The intestine or the bowel.

Gutta (गट्टा) एक बूँद। A drop.

Gutta-percha (गटा-पर्चा) कुछ पौधों के दूध को सुखा या जमाकर प्राप्त होने वाला एक प्रकार का भूरापन लिए हुए लचीला पदार्थ जिसका दन्त-चिकित्सा में दाँतों को जोड़ने के लिए एवं विकलांगोपचार में स्प्लिन्ट या कुशा में प्रयोग किया जाता है। A kind of greyish flexible substance obtained by dryness or coagulating the milk of certain tree used as a dental cement in dentistry and in splints in orthopedics.

Guttering (गटरिंग) हड्डी का खाँचा। Groove in bone.

Guttur (गट्टर) गला। The throat.

Gymnophobia (जिम्नोफोबिया) नग्न शरीर को देखने का रोगोत्पादक भय। Morbid of seeing a naked body.

Gynandroid (गाइनैड्रॉयड) एक उभयलिंगी अथवा स्त्री कूट-उभयलिंगी। A hermaphrodite or a female pseudohermaphrodite.

Gynatresia (गाइनेट्रेसिया) योनि का बन्द रहना। Closure of the vagina.

Gynecic (गाइनीकिक) स्त्री सम्बन्धी। Pertaining to the woman.

Gynecoid (गाइनीकॉयड) स्त्री के समान। Woman-like.

Gynecology (गाइनीकोलॉजी) स्तनों सहित स्त्री जननांगी रोगों का अध्ययन, स्त्रीरोगविज्ञान। The study of the disease of the female genital organs including the breasts.

Gynecomastia (गाइनीकामैस्टिया) पुरूष में स्तन-ग्रन्थियों का अत्यधिक बढ़ जाना जिनसे कभी-कभी दूध भी निकलने लगता है। Abnormally enlarged mammary glands in the male sometimes secreting milk.

Gynephobia (गाइनीफोबिया) स्त्रियों से अत्यधिक घृणा होना या स्त्रियों का रोगोत्पादक भय। Abnormal aversion to women or morbid fear of women.

Gynocogenic (गइनीकोजोनिक) स्त्री के विशिष्ट लक्षणों को उत्पन्न करने वाला। Producing female characteristic.

Gypsum (जिप्सम) जलयोजित कैल्सियम सल्फेट का एक प्राकृतिक रूप जिसे 130° से. तक गर्म करने पर जलीय अंश निकल जाता है और प्लास्टर ऑफ पेरिस बन जाता है। A natural form of hydrated calcium sulfate which on heating to 130 °C loses its water content and becomes plaster of paris.

Gyroma (गाइरोमा) डिम्बग्रन्थि का एक अबुर्द जो एक संवलित पिण्ड का बना होता है। An ovarian tumor consisting of a convoluted mass.

Gyrospasm (गाइरोस्पाज्म) सिर को घुमा देने वाली सिर की ऐंठन। Rotatory spasm of the head.

Gyrus (गाइरस) प्रमस्तिष्क-कॉर्टेक्स के बहुत से संवलनों या लहरिकाओं में से एक जो पिछली नालियों तथा गहरी नालियों द्वारा अलग-अलग होते है, कर्णक। One of the many convolution of the cerebral cortex separated by shallow grooves and the deeper groover (*i*) **Frontal Gyrus** (फ्रॉन्टल गाइरस) ललाट कर्णक। The convolution of the frontal lobe.

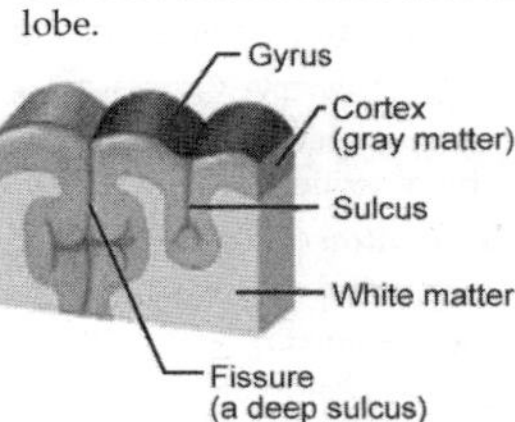

H

H (एच) हाइड्रोजन का रासायनिक प्रतीक। Chemical symbol for Hydrogen.

Habena (हैबेना) पट्टी, पट्टिका, फ्रीनम अथवा बंध। A bondage, a frenum or restricting fibrous bond.

Habenula (हैबेनुला) 1. लघुबंध अथवा चाबुक के समान रचना। 2. मस्तिष्क की पीनियल ग्रन्थि से जुड़ी रहने वाली एक डंठल। 1. A frenum of whiplike structure. 2. A peduncle or stalk attached in the pineal gland of the brain.

Habenular (हैबेनुलर) पीनियल ग्रन्थि के डंठल से सम्बन्धित। Pertaining to the stalk of the pineal gland.

Habit (हैबिट) वह क्रिया जिसके बार-बार उत्पन्न होने की विशिष्टता होती है, अभ्यास, आदत। The action which is characterized by repetition.

Habituation (हैबिचुएशन) अभ्यस्तता। The state of being accustomed.

Hacking (हैकिंग) रह-रहकर या रूक-रूक कर होने वाला। Short and interrupted.

Hacking cough (हैकिंग कफ) रूक-रूक कर उठने वाली खांसी। The interrupted cough.

Hair (हेयर) केरेटिन की बनी धागे के समान एक रचना जो त्वचा में दबे हुए अंकुरक से उत्पन्न होती है, कोश, बाल, रोम। A threadlike structure compared of keratin developing from the papilla embedded in the dermis.

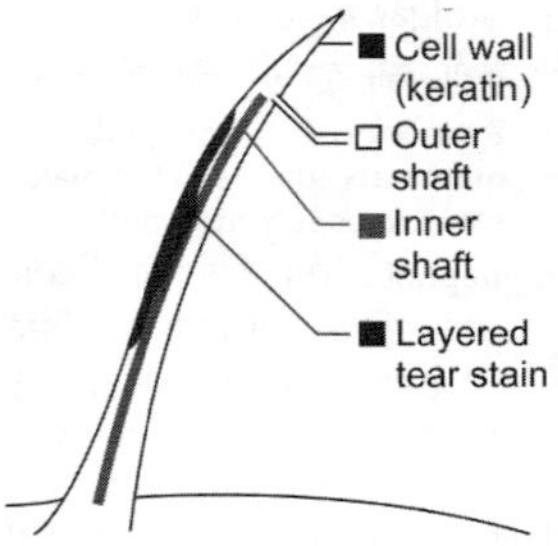

Hair bulb (हेयर बल्ब) रोम मूल का निचला चौड़ा भाग, रोम कन्द। The lower expanded portion of a hair root.

Hair follicle (हेयर फॉलिकिल) रोमकूप, लोपकूप, रोमपुटक, केशपुटक। A recess lodging the root of a hair or resembling hair.

Hairy (हेयरी) बालों का अथवा बालों के समान। Resembling hair.

Halitosis (हैलिटोसिस) बदबूदार सांस। Bad breath.

Halitus (हैलिटस) निकाली गई सांस। The expired breath.

Half life (हॉफ-लाईफ) किसी विकिरणशील या रेडियोएक्टिव पदार्थ के आधे केन्द्रकों का विकिरण सक्रिय गलन से अपनी सक्रियता खोने में लगने वाला समय। Time taken for half the nuclear of a radioactive.

Hallucal (हैलूकल) पैर के अंगूठे से सम्बन्धी। Pertaining to the hallux.

Hallucination (हेलुसिनेशन) विभ्रम, दृष्टिभ्रम, वहम जैसे–दृष्टि, ध्वनि, स्वाद। A false perception or image about sight round smell taste or touch.
(*i*) **Auditory hallucination** (ऑडिटरी हेलुसिनेशन) ध्वनियों का मिथ्या बोध या विभ्रम होना, श्रवण विभ्रम। False perception of sound. (*ii*) **Olfactory hallucination** (ऑलफैक्टरी हेलुसिनेशन) गन्ध का मिथ्या बोध, घ्राणविभ्रम। False perception of smell. (*iii*) **Gustatory hallucination** (गेस्टेटरी हेलुसिनेशन) किसी वस्तु के स्वाद का पता चलना जो वास्तव में नहीं होती, स्वाद विभ्रम। Perception of taste of something which is actually not present. (*iv*) **Tactile hallucination** (टैक्टाइल हैलुसिनेशन) किसी वस्तु से स्पर्श किए जाने का मिथ्या बोध, स्पर्श विभ्रम। False perception of touching something.

Hallucinogen (हैलुसिनोजन) विभ्रम उत्पन्न करने वाला कारक, विभ्रमजनक। An agent producing hallucinations.

Hallucinogenesis (हैलुसिनोजेनेसिस) विभ्रम की उत्पत्ति होना। Production of hallucination.

Hallucinosis (हैलुसिनोसिस) विभ्रम से ग्रस्त होने की अवस्था जैसे तीव्र एल्कॉहली विभ्रम जिसमें भय या चिंता तथा श्रवण विभ्रम होते हैं, विभ्रमता। The state of being affected with hallucination acute iconic hallucination marked by fear or anxiety and auditory hallucinations.

Hallux (हैलक्स) पैर का अंगूठा, पादांगुष्ठ। The great toe.

Hallux valgus (हैलक्स वेल्गास) अन्य अंगुलियों की ओर को विस्थापित पैर का अंगुठा, पादांगुष्ठ बर्हिनति। The great toe displaced.

Halo (हैलो) 1. दृष्टि पटलदर्शी द्वारा नेत्र परीक्षण करने पर पीत बिन्दू

के चारों ओर दिखाई देने वाला छल्ला या घेरा। 2. किसी चमकती हुई वस्तु अथवा प्रकाश के चारों ओर बनने वाला प्रकाश या रंग का एक वृत। 1. A ring seen surrounding the macula lutea in ophthalmoscopic examination 2. A circle of light or color surrounding a shining body or light.

Halogen (हैलोजन) एक अधाटिवक तत्व जो हाइड्रोजन से संयुक्त होकर अम्ल तथा धातु से मिलकर लवण बनाता है जैसे क्लोरीन, ब्रोमीन। A nonmetallic element which combines with the hydrogen to form acids and with the metal form salts, e.g. chlorine, bromine.

Haloid (हैलॉयड) लवण अथवा हैलोजन के समान। Resembling salt or a halogen.

Halophile (हैलोफिल) गाढ़े नमक के घोल में वृद्धि करने वाला एक जीव। The organism which grows in concentrated salt solution.

Halsted's operation (हालस्टेड्स ऑपरेशन) वंक्षण हर्निया में किया जाने वाला ऑपरेशन, स्तन कैंसर में किया जाने वाला ऑपरेशन। An operation for inguinal hernia operation for breast cancer.

Halsted's suture (हालस्टेड्स स्यूचर) आँतों के जख्मों में थोडी-थोड़ी दूर पर लगे टांके। The interrupted suture for the intestinal wounds.

Hamartoma (हैमार्टोमा) प्रभावित भाग में सामान्य रूप से स्थित परिपक्व कोशिकाओं एवं ऊतकों की एक अतिवृद्धि से उत्पन्न होने वाला एक सुदम अबुर्द। A tumor resulting from an overgrowth of nature cells and tissue normally present in the affected part.

Hamate (हैमेट) अंकुश-युक्त। Hooked.

Hammer (हैमर) ठोकने के काम आने वाला एक यंत्र जिसमें एक सिर होता है जो एक हैण्डिल से जुड़ा होता है, हथौड़ा। An instrument with the head attached for to a handle for striking blows.

Hammer finger (हैमर फिंगर) हाथ की अंगुली की दूरस्थ सन्धि की एक विकृति जिसमें वह आंकुचित हो जाती है जिससे वह हथौड़े के समान प्रतीत होती है। Mallet finger a deformity of the distal joint of a finger in which it is fixed so that it looks like a hammer.

Hamstring (हैम्सट्रिंग) जानुपृष्ठ-अवकाश की अभिमध्य एवं पार्श्वीय सीमाएँ बनाने वाली कण्डराओं में

से एक। One of the tendons making the boundaries of the popliteal space medially one laterally.

Hamular (हैमुलर) अंकुशवत्, अंकुशाभ। Hook-shaped.

Hand (हैण्ड) हस्त, हाथ। Manus; the distal portion of the superior limb, comprising of carpus, metacarpus and digits. (*i*) **Ape hand** (एपी हैण्ड) ऐसा हाथ जिसमें अंगूठा स्थायी रूप से प्रसारित हो जाता है। The hand in which the thumb is permanently extended. (*ii*) **Cleft hand** (क्लैफ्ट हैण्ड) हाथ की ऐसी विकृति जिसमें अंगुलियों के बीच का विभाजन फैलकर करभ या हथेली तक पहुँच जाता है। A deformity of the hand in which the division between the ringer extends into the metacarpus or palm.

Handedness (हैण्डेडनेस) दूसरे की अपेक्षा एक ओर के हाथ का प्रयोग करने की प्रवृति। The tendency to use the hand of one side in preference to the other.

Handicap (हैण्डीकैप) जन्मजात अथवा उपार्जित कोई भी शारीरिक अथवा मानसिक दोष जो किसी व्यक्ति के सामान्य जीवन व्यतीत करने में बाधा उत्पन्न करता है। Congenital or acquired any physical or mental defect preventive person from leading a normal life.

Hangnail (हैंगनेल) नाखून की जड़ से उखड़ा मांस, छिलौरी। A narrow strip of skin partly detached the nail fold.

Hangover (हैंगओवर) नशेड़ियों में पाई जाने वाली घबराहट, थकान, बेचैनी आदि। Headache, depression, fatigue and irritability present sometimes often consumption of alcohol or CNS depressant.

Haphalgesia (हैफेल्जेसिया) वस्तुओं को छूने पर दर्द होना, वस्तुस्पर्श भीति। Pain on touching the objects.

Haphephobia (हैफीफोबिया) अन्य व्यक्ति से छू जाने का रोगोत्पादक भय। Morbid fear of being touched by another person.

Haplodont (हैप्लोडोन्ट) कटकों से रहित दाँतों वाला अथवा जिसके दन्त शीर्ष पर गुलिकाएँ नहीं होती। Having teeth without ridges or tubercles on the crcwn.

Haploid (हैप्लोयड) शुक्राणु या अंडाणु में गुणसूत्रों की संख्या को दर्शाना। Denoting the number of chromosomes in sperm or ova.

Hapten (हैप्टेन) अपूर्ण प्रतिजनन। Incomplete or partial antigen.

Haptices (हैप्टिक्स) स्पर्श-ज्ञान का विज्ञान। The science of the sense of touch.

Haptic hallucination (हेप्टिक हेलुसिनेशन) स्पर्श किये जाने, तापमान अथवा वेदना का विभ्रम। False perception of being touched or of the temperature or pain.

Haptometer (हैप्टोमीटर) स्पर्श-ज्ञान की तीव्रता को मापने वाला उपकरण। An apparatus for measuring the acuteness of sense of touch.

Hard (हार्ड) दृढ़, कठोर। Firm rigid.

Hardiness (हार्डीनैस) साहस। Boldness.

Hardness (हार्डनैस) जल का खनिज लवणों विशेषकर कैल्सियम एवं मैग्नीसियम लवणों से युक्त होने का गुण। The quality of water containing mineral substances especially the calcium and magnesium salts.

Harelip (हेयरलिप) दोनों होंठ प्रमुखतया ऊपर वाले होठ का जन्म से ही खण्डित रहना। A cleft in the upper lip due to faulty fusion of medium nasal process and the lateral maxillary process.

Harelip suture (हेयरलिप स्यूचर) शल्य-क्रिया द्वारा कटे हुए होंठों पर लगाए गए टांके जो संख्या में 8 होते हैं। A twisted figure of eight suture used in surgical correction of harelip.

Harpoon (हार्पून) एक यंत्र जिसके सिरे पर एक हूक होता है जो ऊतक के छोटे टुकड़े जैसे पेशी का परीक्षण हेतु प्राप्त करने के लिए प्रयोग में लाया जाता है। An instrument with a hook at its end used for obtaining a small piece of tissue such as muscle for examination.

Hartmann's solution (हार्टमैन्स सोल्यूशन) 0.6 ग्राम सोडियम क्लोराइड, 0.08 ग्राम पोटेशियम क्लोराइड, 0.02 ग्राम कैल्सियम क्लोराइड तथा 0.31 ग्राम सोडियम लैक्टेट को पानी में घोलकर पानी सहित 100 मि.ली. तक बनाया गया एक निर्जीवाणुक घोल जो निर्जलीकरण की चिकित्सा में इन्जैक्शन द्वारा प्रयोग में लाया जाता है। A solution of 0.6 gm NaCl, 0.03 gm KCl, 0.02 gm $CaCl_2$ and 0.3 gm sodium lactate in 100 ml of water used for fluid and electrolyte replacement.

Haversian (हैवर्शियन) हैवरप्रणीत, हैवर के सिद्धान्तों पर आधारित। Relation to the various osseous structures described by Clopton Havers.

Hashish (हशीश) पोश्त, भांग। An extract from flower stalk and leaves of *Cannabis sativa* smoked or chewed for its euphoric effect.

Haunch (हौन्च) कुल्हे एवं नितम्ब। The hips and the buttocks.

Haustra (होस्ट्रा) बड़ी आँत या कोलन के लघुकोशों से युक्त कोष्ठ, आवलियाँ। The socculate pouches of the colon.

Haustus (होस्टस) औषधि की एक घूँट। A draught of medicine.

Haversian canals (हैवर्शियन कैनाल्स) अस्थि-ऊतक में पाई जाने वाली छोटी-छोटी रक्तधर, नलिकाएँ, हैवर्शियन नलिकाएँ। Minute vascular canals found in the osseous tissue.

Hay fever (हे फीवर) परागकणों के सांस के साथ खिंचकर अन्दर पहुँचने से उत्पन्न एलर्जीजनक रोग होता है। पराग ज्वर। Allergic rhinitis usually caused by airborne pollens fungal spores.

Hb (एचबी) हीमोग्लोबिन। Hemoglobin.

HDL (एचडीएल) अधिक घनत्व वाली लाइपोप्रोटीन। High density lipoprotein.

Head (हैड) सिर, शीर्ष, मुण्ड, सर। The upper part of the body containing brain; caput.

Headache (हैडेक) सिर दर्द जो तीव्र अथवा जीर्ण हो सकता है, शिरोवेदना। Pain in the head which may be acute and chronic. (*i*) **Coital headache** (कॉयटल हैडेक) लैंगिक संसर्ग (सम्भोग) के दौरान अथवा कामोत्तेजना के चरमोत्कर्ष पर पहुँचने के तुरन्त बाद अचानक सिर में होने वाला दर्द। Headache occurring suddenly during sexual intercourse or just after orgasm. (*ii*) **Exertional headache** (एग्जर्शनल हैडेक) कठोर शारीरिक कार्य करने के पश्चात् सिर में कुछ देर के लिए होने वाला तेज दर्द। An acute headache of short duration occurring after doing strenuous physical work. (*iii*) **Histamine headache** (हिस्टामीन हैडेक) एलर्जी में हिस्टामीन के द्वारा पाया मेटर एवं डयूरा मेटर की धमनियों के चौड़ा होने तथा फैलने से ठप-ठप करता हुआ सिर का दर्द। A throbbing pain due to dilatation and stretching of the pial and dural arteries caused by histamine allergy. (*iv*) **Ocular headache** (ऑकुलर हैडेक) दृष्टि दोषों के कारण, ग्लोकोमा में अथवा नेत्र के विभिन्न भागों के शोध में होने वाला सिर में दर्द। Headache occurring due to across of refraction glaucoma or inflammation of the different parts of the eye. (*v*) **Post-traumatic headache** (पोस्टट्रॉमेटिक हैडेक) सिर में

चोट लगने के पश्चात् होने वाला सिर दर्द। Headache occurring following by head injury.

Heal (हील) रोग मुक्ति दिलाना अथवा स्वस्थ बनाना, विरोहण। To cure or make healthy.

Healing (हीलिंग) शारीरिक अथवा मानसिक सामान्य अवस्था की पुनःप्राप्ति। रोगमुक्त करना, विरोहण। Restoration to normal, mental or physical state.

Health (हैल्थ) शारीरिक, मानसिक एवं सामाजिक कुशलता की अवस्था, स्वास्थ्य। The condition of physical, mental and social well-being.

Health screening (हैल्थ स्क्रीनिंग) जन-स्वास्थ्य परीक्षा। Public health examination.

Hear (हीयर) कानों के द्वारा ध्वनियों का अनुभव करना या सुनना। To perceive sounds by the ear or to listen.

Hearing aid (हीयरींग ऐड) बहरे व्यक्तियों द्वारा सुनने के लिए प्रयोग में लाया जाने वाला एक उपकरण जो आवाज को बढ़ा देता है। An apparatus for amplifying the sound used for hearing by the deaf persons.

Hearing loss (हीयरींग लौस) आंशिक अथवा पूर्ण बधिरता (बहरापन)। Partial or complete deafness.

Heart (हार्ट) हृद, हृदय, दिल। An organ keeping up the circulation of blood. (*i*) **Abdominal heart** (एब्डोमिनल हार्ट) उदर-गुहा में विस्थापित हृदय। A heart which is displaced into the abdominal cavity. (*ii*) **Athlete's heart** (एथलेट्स हार्ट) लम्बे समय तक व्यायाम होते रहने के परिणामस्वरूप खिलाड़ियों का बढ़ा हुआ हृदय। Enlarge heart of the athlete's a result of prolonged exercise. (*iii*) **Dilated heart** (डाइलेटेड हार्ट) हृदय की भित्तियों के फैलने से बड़ा हुआ हृदय। Enlarged heart due to stretching of its walls. (*iv*) **Tobacco heart** (टुबैको हार्ट) ऐसा हृदय जिसमें अत्यधिक तम्बाकू का प्रयोग करने से अनियमित हृदय स्पन्दन होते है। The heart showing irregular heartbeats due to excessive use of tobacco.

Heart failure (हार्ट फेल्योर) हृद्य स्पन्दन का रूक जाना। Cessation of the heart beat.

Heart lung machine (हार्ट-लंग मशीन) हृदय एवं फेफड़ों के कार्यों

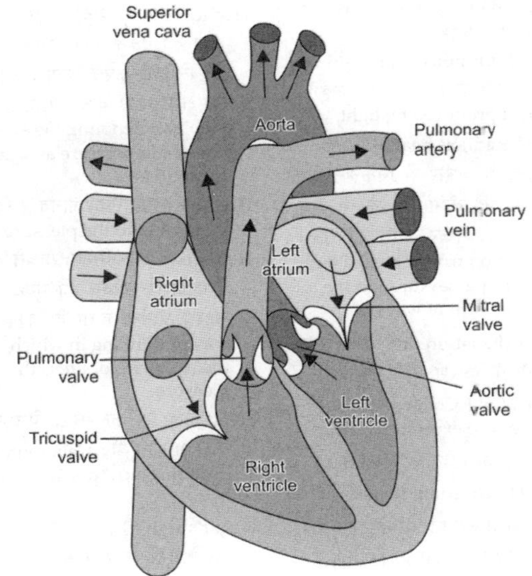

Heart

को कायम रखने के लिए एक उपकरण जबकि उनमें से एक अथवा दोनों उचित रूप से कार्य करने के लिए निष्फल हो जाते हैं। A device for maintaining the function at the heart and lungs while either or both fail to function properly.

Heart rate (हार्ट रेट) प्रति मिनट हृदयस्पंदों की संख्या। The number of the beats of the heart per minute.

Heat (हीट) 1. तापमान बढ़ने की अनुभूति। 2. वह शक्ति जो तापमान बढ़ाती है। 1. The sensation of an increase in temperature 2. The energy which increase the temperature. (*i*) **Latent heat** (लेटेन्ट हीट) किसी दिए हुए तापमान पर ठोस को द्रव या द्रव को गैस में परिवर्तित करने के लिए आवश्यक ऊष्मा। Heat required to convert solid into liquid or liquid into gas at a given temperature.

(*ii*) **Luminous heat** (ल्यूमिनस हीट) प्रकाश द्वारा उत्पन्न ऊष्मा। Heat produced by light.

(*iii*) **Radiant heat** (रेडियन्ट हीट) गर्म शरीर से निकलने वाली ऊष्मा जो तरंगों के रूप में वायु से होकर गुजर जाती है। Heat given off from a heated body which passes through the air in the form of waves.

Heat exhaustion (हिट एग्जॉशन) गर्मी के कारण भारी कमजोरी आ जाना। Collapses due to excessive exposure to heat.

Heat stable (हीट स्टैबिल) ताप स्थिर। Resistant to heat .

Heat stroke (हीट स्ट्रोक) ऊष्माघात, तापाघात। Final stage in heat exhaustion.

Heave (हीव) आह भरना, क्षेप। To sigh.

Heberden's nodes (हैबरडैन्स नोड्स) अस्थिर संधिशोध में हाथ की अँगुलियों की अन्तिम अँगुल्यस्थियों की बड़ी हुई गुलिकाएँ। Enlarged tubercles of the last phalanges of the fingers seen in osteoarthritis.

Hebetude (हेबेट्यूड) सुस्ती छाई रहनी या भावशून्यता। Dullness or apathy.

Hectic (हैक्टिक) आदी, अभयस्त, शाम को बढ़ने वाले तापमान को निर्दिष्ट करने वाला जैसा कि क्षयरोग में देखा जाता है। Habitual denoting the evening rise of temperature as seen in tuberculosis.

Hedonic (हीडोनिक) आनंद सम्बन्धी। Pertaining to the pleasure.

Hedonism (हीडोनिज्म) सोचने का ढंग जिसमें जीवन का मुख्य उद्देश्य आनन्द होता है। The way of thinking in which the main aim of life is the pleasure.

Heel (हील) पैर का सबसे पिछला गोल भाग, एड़ी। Calx round posterior most portion of the foot.

Hegar's sign (हैगर्स साइन) प्रारम्भिगर्भा अवस्था में गर्भाशयग्रीवा का अत्यधिक कोमल हो जाना। Marked softening of the uterine cervix in early pregnancy.

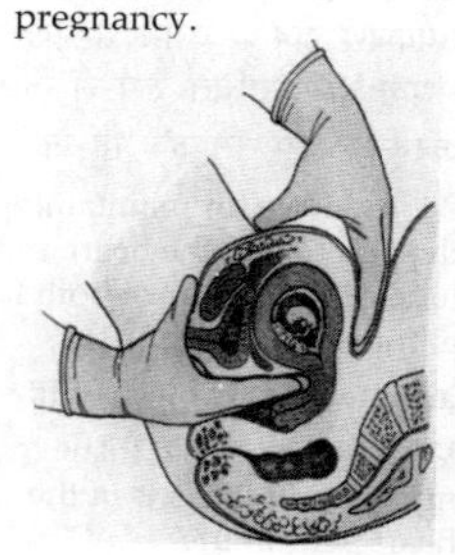

Height (हाइट) ऊँचाई लम्बवत माप। Vertical measurement.

Heimlich sign (हिमलिक साइन) किसी व्यक्ति द्वारा दम घुटने का संकेत देने के लिए हाथ के अंगूठे तथा तर्जनी ऊंगली से गले को पकड़ लेना। Grasping one's throat with the thumb and index finger to signal choking.

Helcoid (हैल्कॉयड) व्रण या जख्म के समान, व्रणभ। Like an ulcer.

Heli (o) [हैली (ओ)] सूर्य का संकेत देने वाला एक उपसर्ग। A prefix indicating sun.

Helical (हैलीकल) किसी कर्णकुण्डलिनी से सम्बन्धी, कर्ण कुण्डलिनी के आकार का। Pertaining to helix shaped, like a helix

Helicine (हैलीसीन) पेंचदार या घुमावदार, सर्पिल, किसी कर्णकुण्डलिनी अथवा कुण्डली से सम्बन्धित। Spiral pertaining to a helix or coil.

Helicoid (हैलीकॉयड) किसी कर्णकुण डलिनी से मिलता-जुलता अथवा पेंचदार। Resembling a halix or spiral.

Heliophobia (हीलियोफोबिया) सूरज की किरणों का डर, सूर्यरश्मिभीति। A morbid fear of sunlight.

Heliotherapy (हीलियोथिरैपी) सूर्य के प्रकाश द्वारा रोगों की चिकित्सा करना, सूर्यरश्मिचिकित्सा। Treatment of the disease by sunlight.

Helium (हीलियम) वायुमण्डल में बहुत सूक्ष्म मात्रा में विद्यमान एक गैस। A gas present in the atmosphere in very minute quantity.

Helix (हैलिक्स) 1. कर्णपाली का ऊपरी एवं पश्च स्वतन्त्र किनारा, कर्णकुण्डलिनी। 2. चक्करदार संरचना। 1. The superior and posterior free margin of the pinna of the ear. 2. A coiled structure.

Helminth (हैल्मिन्थ) कीड़े के समान जन्तु। Worm like animal.

Helminthemesis (हैल्मिन्थइमेसिस) कीड़ों की उल्टी होना, कृमिवमन। Vomiting of worms.

Helminthiasis (हैल्मिन्थिएसिस) आँतों में कृमियों का होना। The condition of having intestinal worm.

Helminthoma (हैल्मिन्थोमा) परजीवीय कृमियों द्वारा बना अबुर्द। A tumor formed by parasitic worms.

Helmintic (हैल्मिन्टिक) परजीवीय कृमियों से सम्बन्धित अथवा उनसे पीड़ित। Pertaining to or infected from parasitic worms.

Helotomy (हीलोटॉमी) किसी हीलोमा या ठेंठ को काट कर

अलग कर देना। Excision of a heloma.

Hema (हीमे) रक्त को संकेत करने वाला एक उपसर्ग। A prefix indicating blood.

Hemafecia (हीमोफीसिया) रक्त से युक्त मल। Feces containing blood.

Hemagglutination (हीमेग्लुटिनेशन) लाल रक्त कोशिकाओं का गुच्छों के रूप में एकत्रित हो जाना, लोहितकोशिका समूहन। Clustering of red blood cells.

Hemagogue (हीमेगौग) रक्तस्राव विशेषकर मस्तिष्क रक्तस्राव को बढ़ाने वाला कारक, रक्तस्रावी। An agent increasing the blood flow especially the menstrual flow.

Hemangiectasis (हीमैन्जिएक्टेसिस) रक्त वाहिनियों का विस्फारण (चौड़ा हो जाना), रक्तवाहिका विस्फार। Dilation of the blood vessels.

Hemangioma (हीमैन्जियोमा) विस्फारित रक्त वाहिनियों से बने हुए सुक्ष्म अबुर्द, रक्तवाहिकाबुर्द। A benign tumor made up of dilated blood vessels.

Hemarthrosis (हीमार्थ्रोसिस) किसी जोड़ में खून का रिसाव होना, रक्तसंधि। Effusion of blood from a joint.

Hematin (हीमैटिन) हीमोग्लोबिन अणु का प्रोटीन रहित भाग, रक्तरंजक। The non-protein of the hemoglobin molecule.

Hematinic (हीमैटिनिक) रक्त में हीमोग्लोबिन स्तर एवं लाल रक्त कोशिकाओं की संख्या बढ़ाने वाला, रक्त वर्धक। An agent increasing the hemoglobin level and the number of red blood cells in the blood.

Hematobillia (हीमैटोबीलिया) पित्त अथवा पित्त वाहिनियों में रक्त का पाया जाना। Presence of blood in the bile or ducts.

Hematobium (हीमैटोबियम) रक्त में रहने वाला एक परजीवी। A parasite living in the blood.

Hematochezia (हीमैटोकेजिया) रक्त से युक्त मल का विसर्जित होना। Excretion of the stools containing blood.

Hematochyluria (हीमैटोकाइलूरिया) रक्त से युक्त एवं काइल या वसा लसीका का पाया जाना। Presence of blood and chyle in the urine.

Hematocrit (हीमैटोक्रिट) रक्त में लाल रक्त कोशिकाओं की आयतन, प्रतिशतता। Red blood cells volume in blood, percentage.

Hematoid (हीमैटॉयड) रक्त से मिलता-जुलता रक्ताभ, खून जैसा। Resembling blood.

Hematologist (हीमैटोलॉजिस्ट) रक्त-विज्ञान विशेषज्ञ। Specialist in hematology.

Hematoma (हीमैटोमा) रक्तगुल्म या रक्तबुर्द। Localized collection of blood.

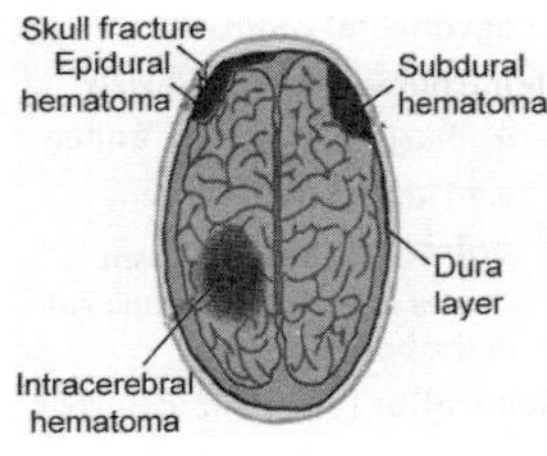

Hematomediastinum (हीमैटोमीडियास्टाइनम) मध्यस्थानिका में खून का रिसाव होना। Effusion of blood in the mediastinum.

Hematometra (हीमैटोमीट्रा) गर्भाशय में आतर्व रक्त का संचित होना, रक्तगर्भाशय। Accumulation of menstrual blood in the uterus.

Hematomphalocele (हीमैटोम्फैलोसील) ऐसा नाभि हर्निया जिसमें रक्त होता है। An umbilical hernia containing blood.

Hematomyelitis (हीमैटोमायलाइटिस) रक्त के रिसाव के साथ सुषुम्ना रज्जु का शोथ। Inflammation in the spinal cord due to effusion of blood.

Hematopenia (हीमैटोपीनिया) रक्त की कमी होना। Deficiency of blood.

Hematophagous (हीमैटोफेगस) रक्त पर जीवित रहने वाला, खून पीने वाला। Living on blood, blood drinker.

Hematoporphyrinuria (हीमैटोपोरफाइरीन्यूरीया) मूत्र में हीमैटोपोरफाइरीन का पाया जाना। Finding of hematoporphyrine in the urine.

Hematopostema (हीमैटोपोस्टीम) ऐसा फोड़ा जिसमें खून होता है। An abscess containing of blood.

Hematorrhachis (हीमैटोरेह्चिस) सुषुम्ना रज्जु में रक्तस्राव होना। Hemorrhage into the spinal cord.

Hematoscheocele (हीमैटोस्कियोसील) वृषण में रक्त का संचित हो जाना। Accumulation of blood in the scrotum.

Hematosteon (हीमैटोस्टीयोन) किसी अस्थि की मज्जागुहा में रक्तस्राव होना। Hemorrhage into the medullary cavity of bone.

Hematuria (हीमैटूरिया) मूत्र के साथ रक्त का निकलना। Passage of blood in urine.

Heme (हीम) हीमोग्लोबिन अणु का लौह युक्त एवं प्रोटीन रहित भाग जो अपने ऑक्सीजन-वाहन गुणों

के लिए उत्तरदायी होता है। An iron containing protein free portion of the hemoglobin molecule responsible for its oxygen carrying propertiers.

Hemeralopia (हीमेरेलोपिया) दिवान्धता, दिन में दिखाई न देना। Day blindness.

Hemiageusia (हेमीएगयूसिया) जिह्वा के एक ओर स्वाद का पता न चलना। Loss of sense of taste on one side of the tongue.

Hemialgia (हेमीएल्जिया) शरीर के आधे भाग में दर्द होना। Pain in one half of the body

Hemianacusia (हेमीएनेकुसिया) एक कान में बहरापन। Deafness in one ear.

Hemianesthesia (हेमीएनीस्थीसिया) शरीर के एक ओर असंवेदना, पक्ष असंवेदनता अर्थात् अनुभूति होने का अभाव। Anesthesia, i.e. loss of sensation on one side of the body.

Hemianopia (हेमीएनोपिया) दृष्टिदोष-विशेष, जिसमें आधा ही दिखाई देता है, अर्धदृष्टिता। Blindness of one half of the visual field.

Hemiballismus (हेमीबेलिज्मस) अर्धांग-उद्वेष्टलास्य। Involuntary chorea like movements one side of the body only.

Hemicastration (हेमीकेस्ट्रेशन) किसी एक शुक्रग्रन्थि या डिम्बग्रन्थि को निकाल देना। The removal of one testicle or ovary.

Hemicentrum (हेमीसेन्ट्रम) किसी कशेरूका-काय का कोइ भी आधा पार्शिव भाग। Either lateral half of vertebral-centrum.

Hemichorea (हेमीकोरिया) शरीर के केवल एक पार्श्व को प्रभावित करने वाला कोरिया रोग, अर्धांगलास्य। Hemiballism chorea affecting only one side of the body.

Hemicolitis (हेमीकोलाइटिस) शरीर पर एक ओर बालों का भूरा हो जाना। Grayness of the hair on one side of the body.

Hemicrania (हेमीक्रेनिया) खोपड़ी के केवल आधे भाग का जन्म से विकास होना। Congenital development of only one half of the skull.

Hemidiaphoresis (हेमीडायाफोरेसिस) शरीर के एक ओर पसीना आना। Sweating on one side of the body.

Hemidrosis (हेमीड्रोसिस) खून मिला पसीना निकलना। Secretion of sweat containing blood.

Hemiectromelia (हेमीएक्ट्रोमीलिया) शरीर के एक ओर कुरूप भुजाओं का पाया जाना। Deformed extremities on one side of the body.

Hemiepilepsy (हेमीएपीलेप्सी) शरीर के आधे पार्शिव भाग को रोगग्रस्त करने वाला अपस्मार। Epilepsy effecting one lateral half of the body.

Hemiglossitis (हेमीग्लोसाइटिस) जिह्वा के आधे भाग का शोथ। Inflammation of one half of the tongue.

Hemihyperesthesia (हेमीहाइपरीस्थीसिया) शरीर के एक ओर संवेदनशीलता का बढ़ जाना। Increased sensitiveness of one side of the body.

Hemihypertonia (हेमीहाइपरटोनिया) शरीर के एक ओर पेशी तान का बढ़ जाना। Increased muscle tone on one side of the body.

Hemihypoplasia (हेमीहाइपोप्लेसिया) शरीर अथवा किसी अंग के आधे भाग का अल्प विकास होना। Decreased development of one half of the body of an organ.

Hemimelus (हेमीमीलस) किसी भुजा के दूरस्थ सम्पूर्ण आधे अथवा इसके कुछ भाग अभाव से युक्त भ्रूण। A fetus with absence of all or a part of the distal half of a limb.

Heminephrectomy (हेमीनेफ्रेक्टॉमी) किसी गुर्दे के एक भाग को शल्य-क्रिया द्वार काटकर निकाल देना। Excision of a portion of a kidney.

Hemioplagia (हेमियोपैल्जिया) सिर के एक ओर तथा उस ओर की आँख में दर्द होना। Pain in one side of the head and the eye of that side.

Hemiplegia (हेमीप्लेजिया) शरीर के पार्श्व का पक्षाघात। Paralysis of one half of body

(*i*) **Cerebral hemiplegia** (सेरीब्रल हेमीप्लेजिया) मस्तिष्क विक्षति के कारण होने वाला एक ओर का पक्षाघात। Hemiplegia caused by brain lesion.

Hemispasm (हेमीस्पाज्म) शरीर अथवा चेहरे के केवल एक ओर आकर्ष या ऐंठन हो जाना, पक्षाकर्ष। Spasm of only one side of the body or face.

Hemisphere (हेमीस्फीयर) किसी गोलाकार रचना का आधा भाग जैसे प्रमस्तिष्कगोलार्द्ध या अनुमस्तिष्कगोलार्द्ध। Either half of the cerebrum or cerebellum.

Hemithorax (हेमीथोरैक्स) छाती का आधाभाग। One half of the chest.

Hemitremor (हेमीट्रेमर) शरीर के एक पार्श्वीय अर्द्धभाग में कम्पन होना। Tremor present in one lateral half of the body.

Hemivertebra (हेमीवर्टीब्रा) किसी कशेरूका के एक पार्श्वीय अर्द्ध भाग का जन्मजात अभाव

अथवा उसका अपूर्ण विकास। Congenital absence or failure of development of half of vertebra.

Hemo (हीमो) एक उपसर्ग जिसका अर्थ रक्त होता है। A prefix meaning blood.

Hemoagglutination (हेमोएग्लुटिनेशन) लाल रक्त कोशिकाओं का गुच्छा के रूप में एकत्रित होना। The clustering of red blood cells.

Hemoagglutinin (हीमोएग्लुटिनिन) लाल रक्त कोशिकाओं को गुच्छों में एकत्रित करने वाली समूहिका। An agglutinin clustering the red blood cells.

Hemobilia (हीमोबीलिया) पित्त अथवा पित्त वाहिनियों में रक्त का पाया जाना। Presence of blood in the bile of bile ducts

Hemobilinuria (हीमोबिलीन्यूरिया) रक्त एवं मूत्र में यूरोबिलिन का पाया जाना। Presence of urobilin in the blood and urine.

Hemochromatosis (हीमोक्रोमेटोसिस) लोह चयापचय का एक विकार जिसमें ऊतकों में अधिक लोहा जमा हो जाता है साथ ही यकृत बढ़ जाता है तथा त्वचा में कॉसे के रंग की वर्णकता हो जाती है और मधुमेह हो जाता है। A disorder of iron metabolism in which the iron is deposited in the tissue in excess with the enlargement of the liver and the bronze skin pigmentation and diabetes mellitus.

Hemoconcentration (हीमोकन्सन्ट्रेशन) रक्त के तरल भाग के घट जाने के फलस्वरूप लाल रक्त कोशिकाओं का अपेक्षाकृत संख्या में बढ़ जाना, रक्तसांद्रता। A relative increase in the number of RBC as result of decrease in the fluid portion of the blood.

Hemocytoblast (हीमोसाइटोब्लास्ट) अस्थि मज्जा में पाई जाने वाली भ्रूणीय कोशिका जिससे सभी रक्त कोशिकाओं का बनना समझा जाता है। The embryonic cell found in the bone marrow from which all the blood cells are thought to be formed.

Hemocytogenesis (हीमोसाइटोजेनेसिस) रक्त कणिका का बनना। Hematopoiesis.

Hemocytology (हीमोसाइटोलॉजी) रक्त कोशिकाओं की संरचना एवं उनके कार्यो का अध्ययन। The study of the structure and function of the blood cells.

Hemocytotripsis (हीमोसाइटोट्रिप्सिस) अत्यधिक दबाव से लाल रक्त कोशिकाओं का नष्ट होना। Destruction of red blood cells by extreme pressure.

Hemodialysis (हीमोडायालाइसिस) रक्त में स्थित कुछ रासायनिक पदार्थों को अर्धपारगम्य झिल्ली से विसरित होने की दरों में अंतर होने के कारण, रक्त को अर्धपारगम्य झिल्ली से बनी नलियों से गुजार कर, इन पदार्थों को रक्त से अलग करना, रक्त-अपोहन। Removal of certain chemical substances from the blood by passing it through the tubes mode of semipermeable membrane due to difference in rates of their diffusion through the semipermeable membranes.

Hemodialyzer (हीमोडायालाइजर) रक्त-अपोहन के लिए प्रयोग में लाया जाने वाला एक उपकरण। An apparatus used for performing hemodialysis.

Hemodilution (हीमोडाइल्यूशन) रक्त के तरल भाग का बढ़ जाना जिससे रक्त में लाल रक्त कोशिकाओं की सांद्रता घट जाती है, रक्ततनुता। An increase in the fluid portion of the blood so that the concentration of RBC is reduced.

Hemodynamics (हीमोडायनामिक्स) रक्तसंचार प्रकरण, रक्तसंचार-विज्ञान। Study of blood circulation.

Hemoflagellate (हीमोफ्लैजीलेट) परजीवी की भांति रक्त में रहने वाली कोई भी कशाभी एककोशिकीय जन्तु जैसे–ट्रिपेनोसोमा, लीषमैनिया। Any flagellate protozoan of the blood, e.g. *Trypanosoma leishmania*.

Hemogglutinative (हीमोग्लुटीनेटिव) लाल रक्त कोशिकाओं का समूह करने वाला। Causing agglutination of the red blood cells.

Hemoglobin (हीमोग्लोबिन) अस्थि मज्जा में बनने वाला लाल रक्त कोशिका का लोहयुक्त एवं ऑक्सीजन वाहक वर्णक जिसके कारण रक्त का रंग लाल होता है। The iron containing and oxygen carrying pigment of the RBC formed in the bone marrow which gives red color to the blood.

Hemoglobinemia (हीमोग्लोबिनीमिया) रक्त की प्लाज्मा में हीमोग्लोबिन का पाया जाना, हीमोग्लोबिनरक्तता। Presence of hemoglobin in the blood plasma.

Hemoglobinolysis (हीमोग्लोबिनोलाइसिस) हीमोग्लोबिन का विघटन होना। Disintegration of hemoglobin.

Hemoglobinometer (हीमोग्लोबिनोमीटर) रक्त में

हीमोग्लोबिन की मात्रा का पता लगाने वाला यंत्र। Apparatus for estimating blood Hb.

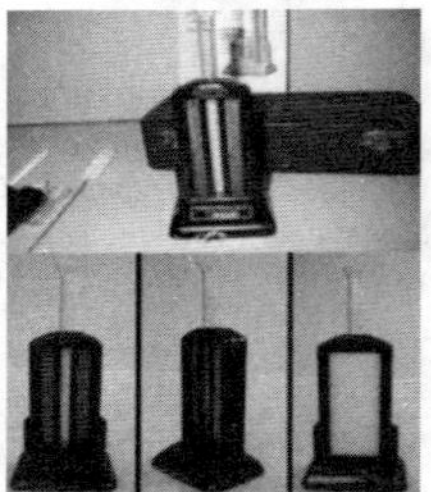

Hemoglobinuria (हीमोग्लोबिनूरिया) लाल रक्त कोशिकाओं से मुक्त हिमोग्लोबिन का मूत्र में पाया जाना। Presence of the hemoglobin in the urine.

Hemogram (हीमोग्राम) रक्तणुवीक्षण, रक्ताणुचित्र। Differential blood count.

Hemolith (हीमोलिथ) किसी रक्त वाहिनी की दीवार में स्थित एक पथरी।
A calculus in the wall of a blood vessels.

Hemolysin (हीमोलाइसिन) रक्त-अपघटन करने वाला कारक।

An agent causing hemolysis.

Hemolysis (हीमोलाइसिस) लाल रक्त कोशिकाओं का टूटना, रक्त-अपघटन।

Destruction of RBC.

Hemolyze (हीमोलाइज़) लाल रक्त कोशिकाओं को तोड़ना। To produce hemolysis.

Hemopathy (हीमोपैथी) रक्त का कोई भी रोग। Any disease of the blood.

Hemoperfusion (हीमोपरफ्यूजन) रक्त से विषैले पदार्थों को अलग करने के लिए रक्त को अधिशोषी सामग्री जैसे सक्रियत चारकोल से होकर गुजरना। To pass the blood through absorptive material such as activated charcoal to remove toxic substances from the blood.

Hemopericardium (हीमोपैरीकार्डियम) पेरिकार्डियम आवरण में रक्त का एकत्रित होना, रक्तहृदयावरण, रक्तवरिहृद्।

Accumulation of blood in the pericardial sac.

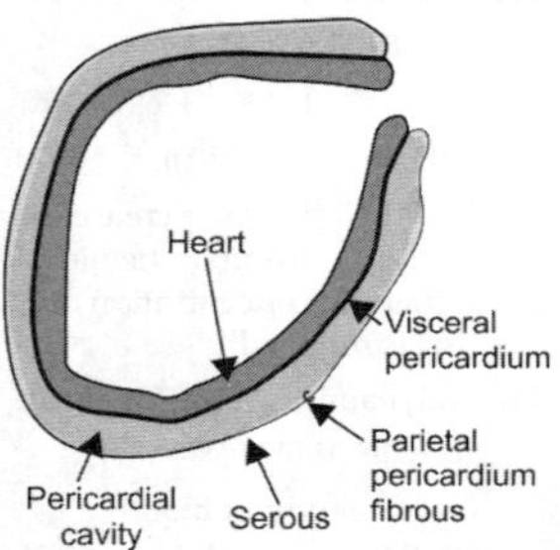

Hemoperitoneum (हीमोपैरीटोनियम) पैरीटोनियम गुहा में रक्त का संचित हो जाना, रक्तपर्युदर्या। Accumulation of blood in the peritoneal cavity

Hemophilia (हीमोफिलिया) एक आनुवंशिक रक्तस्रावी रोग जिसमें किसी रक्त स्कन्दन कारक की कमी होने से रक्त जमने में निष्फल हो जाता है और असामान्य रक्तस्राव होने लगता है तथा जोड़ों में सूजन हो जाती है। A hereditary hemorrhages disease in which blood fails to clot due to deficiency of a blood coagulation factor and abnormal bleeding occurs with swelling of the joints.

Hemophiliac (हीमोफीलिएक) हीमोफिलिया रोग से ग्रस्त व्यक्ति। The person affected with hemophilia.

Hemophthalmia (हीमोफ्थेल्मिया) आँख के भीतर रक्त का रिसाव होना, रक्त नेत्र। Effusion of blood within the eye.

Hemopneumopericardium (हीमोन्यूमोपैरीकार्डियम) हृदयावरण गुहा में रक्त एवं वायु का पाया जाना। Presence of blood and air in the pericardial cavity.

Hemopneumothorax (हीमोन्यूमोथौरैक्स) फुफुसावरणी गुहा में रक्त एवं वायु का पाया जाना, रक्त-वातवक्षा। Blood and air in the pleural cavity.

Hemopoisis (हीमोपोयसिस) रक्त बनाने वाला, रक्तोत्पादक, रक्तजनक। Formation of blood cells.

Hemoprotein (हीमोप्रोटीन) रक्त वर्णक हीम के साथ संयुक्त कोई भी प्रोटीन। Any protein combined with the blood pigmented (Hem) iron.

Hemoptysis (हीमोप्टाइसिस) खून का थूकना अथवा खून मिले हुए बलगम का निकलना, रक्त निष्ठवन। Spitting of blood or expectoration of blood mixed sputum.

Hemorrhage (हीमोरेह्ज) रक्त वाहिनियों से रक्त की मुक्ति, रक्तस्राव, खून बहना। Escape of blood from the blood vessel; bleeding. (*i*) **Antepartum hemorrhage** (एन्टीपार्टम हीमोरेह्ज) प्रसव से पूर्व होने वाला रक्तस्राव। Bleeding occurring before the onset of labor. (*ii*) **Cerebral hemorrhage** (सेरीब्रल हीमोरेह्ज) प्रमस्तिष्कीय रक्तस्राव। Hemorrhage occurring into the cerebrum. (*iii*) **Uterine hemorrhage** (यूटेराइन हीमोरेह्ज) गर्भाशय-गुहा में होने वाला रक्तस्राव। Bleeding occurring in the uterine cavity.

(*iv*) **Postpartum hemorrhage** (पोस्टपार्टम हीमोरेह्ज) बच्चे के जन्म के पश्चात् गर्भाशय से होने वाला रक्तस्राव प्रसवोत्तर रक्तस्राव। Bleeding from the uterus occurring after child birth.

Hemorrhagenic (हीमोरेह्जेनिक) रक्तस्राव उत्पन्न करने वाला। Causing hemorrhage.

Hemorrhoid (हीमोरॉह्यड) गुदा-मलाशय क्षेत्र में विस्फारित एवं ऐंठी हुई अर्श-शिराओं का। Pile a mass of the dilated and tortuous hemorrhoid veins in the anorectal region.

Hemorrhoidectomy (हीमोरॉह्यडेक्टॉमी) अर्शों को शल्यक्रिया द्वारा काट कर अलग करना। Excision of hemorrhoids.

Hemosalpinx (हीमोसैलपिंक्स) डिम्ब वाहिनियों में रक्त संचित हो जाना। Bleeding into fallopian tubes.

Hemosialemesis (हीमोसियालेमेसिस) थूक के साथ मिश्रित रक्त की उल्टी होना। Vomiting of blood mixed with saliva.

Hemosiderin (हीमोसाइडेरिन) लाल रक्त कोशिकाओं के टूटने से निकलने वाले हीमोग्लोबिन से उत्पन्न होने वाला एक लोह-युक्त वर्णक। An iron containing pigment produced from the hemoglobin from disintegration of the red blood cells.

Hemosiderosis (हिमोसाइडेरोसिस) हीमोसाइडेरिन का विशेषकर यकृत एवं प्लीहा में जमा होना जो ऐसे रोगों में जमा होता है जिनमें लाल रक्त कोशिकाएँ नष्ट होती है, जैसे–रक्तसंलायी अरक्तता। Deposition of hemosiderin especially in the liver and spleen which occur in the disease marked by red cell destruction such as hemolytic anemia.

Hemostasis (हीमोस्टेसिस) रक्तस्राव का रूक जाना। Arrest of bleeding.

Hemotemesis (हीमैटेमेसिस) रक्त वमन, खून की उल्टी होना। Vomiting of blood.

Hemothorax (हीमोथौरेक्स) फुफ्फुसावरणी गुहा में रक्त का संचित हो जाना, रक्तवक्ष। Accustomization of blood in the pleural cavity.

Hemotropic (हीमोट्रॉपिक) रक्त अथवा रक्त कोशिकाओं की ओर आकर्षित होने वाला। Attracted towards the blood or blood cells.

Hemotympanum (हीमोटिम्पैनम) मध्य कर्ण में रक्तस्राव होना। Hemorrhage into the middle ear.

Hemozoic (हीमोजुइक) रक्त में विद्यमान परजीवीय एककोशिकीय जन्तु। Hemotozoic parasitic protozoa in the blood.

Hepatic (हिपैटिक) यकृत सम्बन्धी। Pertaining to the liver.

Hepatic coma (हिपैटिक कॉमा) यकृत की निष्फलता के कारण होने वाली मूर्च्छा। Coma due to liver failure.

Hepatic duct (हिपैटिक डक्ट) यकृत नली, पित्त नली। The duct conveying the bile from liver towards the duodenum.

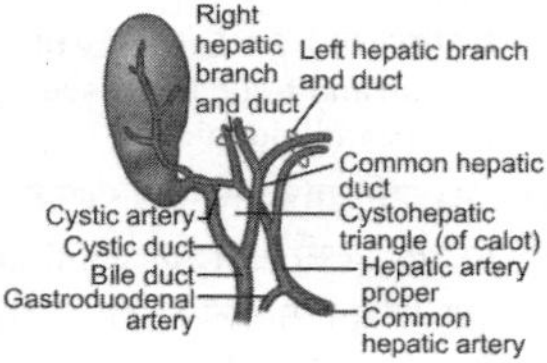

Hepatic necrosis (हिपैटिक नेक्रोसिस) यकृत का परिगलन। Necrosis of liver.

Hepaticostomy (हिपैटिकोस्टॉमी) यकृतीवाहिनी में स्थायी नाल्व्रण बनाना। To make a permanent fistula into the hepatic duct.

Hepatitis (हिपैटाइटिस) यकृती शोथ (सूजन)। Inflammation of the liver.

Hepatoblastoma (हिपैटोब्लास्टोमा) यकृतप्रस्-अबुर्द। A malignant neoplasm of the liver.

Hepatocele (हिपैटोसील) यकृत का हर्निया। Hernia of the liver.

Hepatodynia (हिपैटोडाइनिया) यकृत में दर्द होना। Pain in the liver.

Hepatogenous (हिपैटोजीनस) यकृत में उत्पन्न, यकृतजन्य। Origination in the liver.

Hepatoid (हिपैटॉयड) यकृत के आकार का। Liver-shaped.

Hepatojugular (हिपैटोजुगुलर) यकृत एवं जुगुलर शिरा सम्बन्धी। Pertaining to the liver and jugular vein.

Hepatolithiasis (हिपैटोलिथिएसिस) यकृत में अश्मिनों (पथरियों) का पाया जाना। The presence of the calculi in the liver.

Hepatology (हिपैटोलॉजी) यकृत एवं इसके रोगों का वैज्ञानिक अध्ययन। Study of the liver.

Hepatomegaly (हिपैटोमेगैली) यकृत का बढ़ जाना, यकृतवृद्धि। Enlargement of the liver.

Hepatonephritis (हिपैटोनेफ्राइटिस) यकृत एवं गुर्दे दोनों की सूजन। Inflammation of both the liver and kidneys.

Hepatopathy (हिपैटोपैथी) यकृत का कोई भी रोग। Any disease of the liver.

Hepatoptosia (हिपैटोप्टोसिया) यकृत का नीचे की ओर विस्थापित हो जाना, यकृतभ्रंश।

Downward displacement of the liver.

Hepatorrhagia (हिपैटोरेह्जिया) यकृत में या यकृत से रक्तस्राव होना। Hemorrhage into or from the liver.

Hepatorrhexis (हिपैटोरैह्क्सिस) यकृत का फट जाना। Rupture of the liver.

Hepatosplenomegaly (हिपैटोस्प्लीनोमेगैली) यकृत एवं प्लीहा वृद्धि। Enlargement of the liver and spleen.

Hepatotrophy (हिपैटोट्रॉफी) यकृत का अपक्षय या शोष होना। Atrophy of the liver.

Hepaticoenterostomy (हिपैटिकोएन्ट्रोस्टॉमी) यकृती वाहीनी एवं आँत के बीच एक छिद्र बनना। To make an opening between the hepatic duct and the intestine.

Hepatocarcinoma (हिपैटोकार्सिनोमा) यकृत का कार्सिनोमा अथवा कैंसर। Carcinoma or cancer of the liver.

Hereditary (हीयरीडीटरी) आनुवंशिक, वंशानुगत, एक पीढ़ी से दूसरी पीढ़ी में संचारित होने वाला। Transmitted from one generation to another.

Heredofamilial (हीयरीडोफेमीलियल) वंशानुगत दोष के कारण कुछ परिवारों में उत्पन्न होने वाला (रोग), अनुवंशपरिवागत। Occurring (disease) in certain families due to the inherited defect.

Hermaphrodite (हर्माफ्रोडाइट) दोनों लिंगों की जननांगी एवं लैंगिक विशिष्टताओं से युक्त प्राणी, उभयलिंगी। An individual possessing and sexual characteristics of both sexes.

Hermaphroditism (हर्माफ्रोडाइटिज्म) वह अवस्था जिसमें एक ही प्राणी में शुक्रग्रन्थि एवं डिम्बग्रन्थि दोनों के ऊतक विद्यमान रहते हैं। Existence of ovarian and testicular tissue in same individual.

Hernia (हर्निया) किसी अंग अथवा अंग के किसी भाग का अपनी गुहा जिसमें सामान्यतः वह स्थित रहता है, की दीवार से बाहर निकल आना, बहिःसरण। A condition in which part of an organ is displaced and protrudes through the wall of the cavity containing it.

(*i*) **Complete hernia** (कमप्लीट हर्निया) ऐसा हर्निया जिसमें कोश एवं उसकी अन्तर्वस्तुएँ पूर्णरूप से हर्निया-छिद्र से होकर बाहर निकल जाती है। Hernia in which the sac and its contents have

passed through the hernia opening completely.
(*ii*) **Congenital hernia** (कॉनजैनाइटल हर्निया) जन्मजात हर्निया। Hernia existing since birth.

Herniated (हर्निएटेड) हर्निया से ग्रस्त व्यक्ति अथवा हर्निया के समान बाहर को निकलने वाला। Having a hernia or protruding like a hernia.

Herniorrhaphy (हर्नियोरैह्फी) शल्य-क्रिया द्वारा हर्निया की मरम्मत करने के पश्चात् हर्निया की सिलाई करना, हर्निया सीवनी। Surgical repair of hernia with suturing.

Herniotomy (हर्नियोटॉमी) हर्निया को ठीक करने के लिए किया जाने वाला काट कर अलग करने वाला ऑपरेशन, हर्नियाछेदन। A cutting operation done for the correction of a hernia.

Herpangina (हरर्पेन्जाईना) मुख के पिछले भाग में छोटे-छोटे स्फोट तथा व्रण उत्पन्न होना, मुखीपरिसर्प। Minute vesicles and ulcers at the back of the mouth.

Herpes (हर्पीज़) त्वचा का एक शोधज रोग जिसमें त्वचा पर गुच्छों के रूप में छोटे-छोटे जलस्फोट (दाने) बन जाते हैं। An inflammatory disease of the skin marked by the formation of small recyclers in clusters.

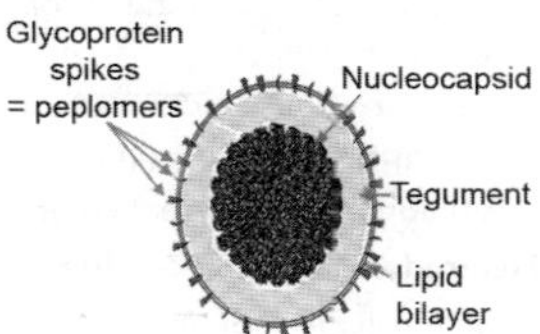

Hersage (हर्सेज) किसी परिसरीय तंत्रिका का अलग-अलग तन्तुओं में बँट जाना। Splitting of a peripheral nerve into separate fibers.

Hertz (हर्ट्ज) बारम्बारता की एक इकाई जो प्रति सैकण्ड एक-एक चक्र के बराबर है। इसका प्रतीक Hz है। A unit of frequency equal to one cycle per second; Its symbol is Hz.

Heterauxesis (हीटरौक्सेसिस) शरीर के भागों की असंग वृद्धि। Disproportionate growth to the body parts.

Heteroautoplasty (हीटरोऑटोप्लास्टी) किसी अन्य व्यक्ति से ली गई त्वचा का निरोपण करना अथवा पैबन्द करना। Grafting of the skin taken from another person.

Heterocephalus (हीटरोसिफैलस) ऐसा भ्रूण जिसके असमान परिमाण के दो सिर होते हैं। A fetus having two heads of unequal size.

Heterochromous (हीटरोक्रोमस) असामान्य भिन्न रंग वाला। Of abnormal different color.

Heterodont (हीटरोडोन्ट) विभिन्न आकृतियों के दाँतों वाला। Having teeth of different shapes.

Heterogeneous (हीटरोजीनियस) भिन्न प्रकार के पदार्थों से बना हुआ, विषमांगी, विजातीय। Composed of different kinds of substances.

Heterogenesis (हीटरोजेनेसिस) हर तीसरी पीढ़ी में भिन्न लक्षणों से युक्त सन्तान का उत्पन्न होना। Production of offspring with different characteristic in alternate generation.

Heterogeusia (हीटरोग्यूसिया) जब भोजन को मुख में रखा जाता है अथवा इसे चबाया जाता है तो एक असामान्य स्वाद का पता चलना। Perception of abnormal taste when food is placed in the mouth or when it is chewed.

Heterograft (हीटरोग्राफ्ट) उत्तक निरोप का एक ऐसा प्रकार जिसमें एक प्रजाति के जन्तु का दूसरी प्रजाति के जन्तु में स्थानान्तरित निरोप किया जाता है। A type of tissue graft in which the donor and recipient are of different species.

Heteroimmunity (हीटरोइम्यूनिटी) अन्य जाति के एण्टिजन के प्रति रोगक्षमता होना। Immunity to an antigen from another species.

Heterolalia (हीटरोलेलिया) इच्छित शब्दों के बजाय अर्थहीन शब्दों का बोलना। The use of meaningless words.

Heterologous (हीटरोलोगस) 1. उस ऊतक से बना हुआ जो सामान्यतः शरीर के उस भाग में नहीं पाया जाता, विषधर्मी। 2. भिन्न प्राणी अथवा जाति से प्राप्त कोशिकाएँ, ऊतक अथवा रक्त। 1. Made up of tissue which is not normal to that part. 2. Cells, tissue or blood obtained from a different individual or species.

Heterometropia (हीटेरोमीट्रोपिया) जिसमें दोनों आँखों में अपवर्तन भिन्न होता है। Two eyes with different refraction.

Heteromorphous (हीटरोमोर्फस) असामान्य रचना वाला, विषमरूप, विषमाकृतिक। An abnormal structure.

Heterophil (हीटरोफिल) विशिष्ट एण्टिजन के अतिरिक्त अन्य एण्टिजन से प्रतिक्रिया करने वाली एण्टीबॉडी से सम्बन्धित। An antibody reacting with other than the specific antigen.

Heterophonia (हीटरोफोनिया) आवाज का बदल जाना। Change of voice.

Heterophoria (हीटरोफोरिया) आँखों की अपनी सामान्य स्थिति से घूम जाने की प्रवृति। The tendency of the eyes to deviate from their normal position.

Heteroprosopus (हीटरोप्रोसोपस) एक सिर एवं दो चेहरों वाला भ्रूण। A fetus having one head and two faces.

Heteropsia (हीटरोप्सिया) दो आँखों में असमान दृष्टि का पाया जाना। Unequal vision in the two eyes.

Heterosexual (हीटरोसैक्सुअल) वह व्यक्ति जो लैंगिक रूप से विपरीत लिंग के व्यक्ति की ओर आकर्षित होता है। Sexually attracted to people of opposite sex.

Heterotonia (हीटरोटोनिया) तनाव अथवा तान में उतार-चढ़ाव होना। Occurrence of variations in the tension or tone.

Heterotopia (हिटरोटोपिया) किसी अंग अथवा भाग का अपने सामान्य स्थान से विस्थापित हो जाना। Displacement of an organ or part from its normal place.

Heterotrichosis (हीटरोट्राइकोसिस) शरीर पर विभिन्न रंगों के बालों का उगना। Growth of hairs of different colors on the body.

Heterotroph (हीटरोट्रॉफ) प्राणी जैसे मनुष्य जिसे अपनी वृद्धि एवं विकास के लिए जटिल कार्बनिक भोजन की आवश्यकता होती है। The organism like man requires complex organic food for growth and development.

Heterotropia (हीटरोट्रॉपिया) नेत्रविचलन। Deviation of the eyes from the normal position.

Heterozygote (हीटरोजाइगोट) किसी निर्दिष्ट लक्षण के लिए भिन्न एलीलों से युक्त प्राणी, विषमयुग्मज। An individual having different alleles for given characteristics.

Hiatus (हायटस) एक द्वार, छिद्र, रन्ध्र अथवा दरार या फटना। An opening, an aperture, a foramen or gap.

Hibernation (हाइबरनेशन) सर्दियों में काम-काज से पूर्णतया अलग रहना, शीत निष्क्रियता। A sleeping throughout the winter.

Hiccough (हिक्कफ) हिचकी, हिक्का। An involuntary spasm of the diaphragm and respiratory organ with a sudden closure of the glottis and a characteristic gulping sound.

Hidradenitis (हाइड्रेडीनाइटिस) स्वेद ग्रन्थियों की सूजन। Inflammation of the sweat gland.

Hidradenoma (हाइड्रोडीनोमा) स्वेद ग्रन्थियों का ग्रन्ध्यबुर्द। Adenoma of the sweat gland.

Hierarchy (हायरार्की) व्यक्तियों अथवा वस्तुओं के महत्त्व अथवा मूल्य के सन्दर्भ में उनका वर्गीकरण। Classification of persons or objects in order of importance.

Hierolisthesis (हाइरोलिस्थेसिस) सैक्रम का विस्थापित हो जाना। Displacement of the sacrum.

High residue diet (हाई रेजीड्य डाइट) वह आहार जिसमें उच्च मात्रा में रेशें या सेल्यूलोस उप. स्थित हो। High fiber cellulose diet beneficial for colorectal disease; diabetes and obesity.

Hillock (हिल्लोक) एक छोटा-सा उभार या उठान। A small eminence or elevation.

Hilton's line (हिल्टन लाइन) मूलाधार की त्वचा तथा गुदा की श्लेष्मिक झिल्ली के संगम पर स्थित एक सफेद रेखा। A white line at the junction of the skin of perineum and the mucous membrane of the anus.

Hilum (हाइलम) विदर, दरार, नाभि, बीज। A depression on the surface of an organ where vessels ducts.

Hindgut (हाइन्डगट) भ्रूण की वह रचना जिससे पोषण नली का शेषान्त्र से मलाशय तक का भाग विकसीत होता है, पश्चान्त्र। The embryonic structure from which the alimentary canal from ileum to the rectum develops.

Hinge joint (हिंग ज्वाइन्ट) चलसन्धि। Hinge joints are formed between two bones where the bones can only move along one axis to flex or extend.

Hip (हिप) जांघ का ऊपरी भाग, कूल्हा, नितम्ब। The upper part of the thigh.

Hip joint (हिप ज्वाइन्ट) नितम्ब-संधि। The joint of the upper part of the thigh.

Hippocrates (हिप्पोक्रेट्स) चिकित्सा शास्त्र के जनक प्रसिद्ध यूनानी कार्यचिकित्सक जिन्हें चिकित्सा के पिता के नाम से जाना जाता है। Greek physician who first established the scientific basis of medical practice, hence known as Father of Medicine.

Hirci (हिर्साइ) बगल के बाल। Axillary hair.

Hirschsprung's disease (हिरस्चसप्रंग्स डिज़ीज) अत्यधिक विस्फारित वृहदान्त्र या कोलन जो सामान्यतः जन्मजात होती है परन्तु शैशव काल या बचपन में भी हो सकती है। Extremely dilated colon which is usually congenital but may occur in infancy or childhood.

Hirsutism (हिर्स्‌टिज्म) अत्यधिक बालों का उगना अथवा असामान्य स्थानों में विषेशकर स्त्रियों में बालों का पाया जाना, अतिरोमता, पुंबतरोमता। Excessive growth of hair or the presence of hair at abnormal places especially in women.

Hissing (हिसिंग) फुफकारना जैसे साँप के द्वारा किया जाता है। Hissing noise as made by a snake.

Histamine (हिस्टामीन) शरीर के ऊतकों में स्वतः प्रकट होने वाला रासायनिक पदार्थ, जिससे रक्त चाप को कम करता है, श्वास-नलिकाओं को यह संकुचित कर देता है। A naturally occurring chemical substance in the body tissue which is a powerful stimulant of gastric secretion constrictor of bronchial smooth muscle and vasodilator.

Histiocyte (हिस्टियोसाइट) एक संयोजी उत्तक में वृहतभक्षककोशिका की उपस्थिति। A macrophage present in connective tissue.

Histiocytosis (हिस्टियोसाइटोसिस) हिस्टियोसाइटों का अधिक संख्या में रक्त में पाया जाना। Presence of histiocytes in the blood in large number.

Histochemistry (हिस्टोकैमिस्ट्री) कोशिकाओं व ऊतकों का रसायन विज्ञान। Chemistry of the cells and tissue.

Histocompatibility (हिस्टोकम्पैटीबिलिटी) रक्त आधान तथा प्रतिरोपण में दाता की कोशिकाओं का प्रापक (प्राप्तकर्ता) के रक्त द्वारा स्वीकार कर लेने का गुण अर्थात् प्राप्तकर्ता के रक्त द्वारा दाता की कोशिका नष्ट नहीं होती, वे जीवित रहती है। The quality of the cells of the donor of being accepted by the blood of the recipients in blood transfusion and transplantation, i.e. the cell of the donor remain alive and are non outrage by the blood of the recipient.

Histogenesis (हिस्टोजेनेसिस) ऊतक जनन। Origin and development of tissue.

Histogenic (हिस्टोजेनिक) ऊतकों से बना हुआ। Formed by the tissue.

Histoid (हिस्टॉयड) शरीर के किसी एक ऊतक से मिलता-जुलता। Resembling one of the tissue of the body.

Histology (हिस्टोलॉजी) ऊतक-विज्ञान। Study of microscopic structure of cell and tissue.

Histoma (हिस्टोमा) ऊतकों का एक अबुर्द। Any tumor of the tissue.

Histoplasmosis (हिस्टोप्लाज्मोसिस) हिस्टोप्लाज्मा कैप्सुलेटम नामक कवक के संक्रमण द्वारा उत्पन्न रोग जिसमें न्यूमोनिया, ज्वर हो जाता है, रक्ताल्पता हो जाती है तथा यकृत एवं प्लीहा बढ़ जाते है, हिस्टोप्लाज्मता। The disease caused by the infection of the fungus *histoplasma capsulatum* characterized by pneumonia fever anemia and enlargement of the liver and spleen.

Historrhexis (हिस्टोरैह्क्सिस) ऊतक का टूट जाना। The breaking up of the tissue.

Histotomy (हिस्टोटॉमी) हिस्टोटोम द्वारा किसी ऊतक को सूक्ष्मदर्शी-परीक्षण के लिए बहुत पतली-पतली फांकों में काटना, ऊति-उच्छेदन। To cut a tissue into very thin slices for its microscopic examination by histotome.

Histrionic (हिस्ट्रियोनिक) अचानक उत्पन्न होने वाला। Appearing suddenly.

Hives (हाइव्ज़) पित्ती उछलना। Urticaria.

Hoarseness (हौर्सनैस) आवाज में कर्कशता। A roughness or harshness of voice.

Hobnail liver (होबनेल लीवर) विशम या पर्विल सतह वाला यकृत। A liver with irregular or nodular surface.

Hodgkin's disease (हॉजकिन्स डिजीज) हॉजकिन के रोग से पीड़ितव्यक्ति जिसके ग्रैव, कक्षीय एवं वक्षंणीय लसीका पर्व बढ़े होते हैं। A protein of hodgkin's disease with enlarged cervical axillary and inguinal lymph nodes.

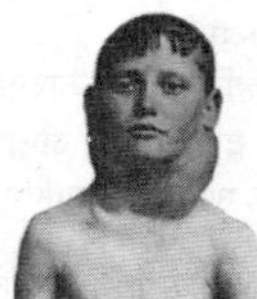

Hodophobia (होडोफोबिया) यात्रा करने का विकृत भय। Morbid fear of traveling.

Holoblastic (होबोब्लास्टिक) पूर्णतया विभाजित होने वाला। Dividing completely.

Holoendemic (होलोएण्डेमिक) किसी क्षेत्र विशेष के सभी लोगों को प्रभावित करने वाले रोग। A disease affecting all population of a particular region.

Holography (होलोग्राफी) तीनो परिमापों या आयामों में किसी वस्तु का फिल्म पर प्रतिबिम्ब प्राप्त करना। To produce a three dimensions image of an object on the film.

Holoprosencephaly (होलोप्रोसेन्सिफैली) एक अतिरिक्त गुणसूत्र द्वारा अग्रमस्तिष्क के एक खण्ड का जन्मजात अभाव। Congenital absence of one forebrain lobe caused by an extra chromosome.

Holorachischisis (होलोरेचिसकाइसिस) सम्पूर्ण कशेरूका-दण्ड की फटन होकर सुषुम्ना पूर्णतया बाहर निकल आती है। Fissure of the entire vertebral column with the protrusion of the spinal cord completely.

Holosystolic (होलोसिस्टोलिक) पूर्णप्रकुचनीय। Related to entire period of systole.

Homachronous (होमोक्रोनस) प्रत्येक पीढ़ी में एक ही समय अथवा एक ही आयु में उत्पन्न होने वाला। Occurring at the same time or at the same age in each generation.

Homan's sign (होमैन्स साइन) पैर की अंगुली का हाथ से अभिपृष्ठ-आकुंचन करने पर पिण्डली में दर्द होना जो पिण्डली में गहराई में स्थित शिराओं में धनास्त्रात होने का एक प्रारम्भिक चिन्ह है। Pain occurring in the calf on dorsiflexion of the toe passively which is an easily sign of thrombosis in deep veins of the calf.

Homaxial (होमेक्सियल) एक लम्बाई के सभी अक्षों से युक्त जैसे एक गोलाकार संरचना।
Having all axes of the same length as a sphere.

Homeopathy (होमीयोपैथी) इस सिद्धान्त पर आधारित चिकित्सा पद्धति कि कोई औषधि जो बड़ी मात्रा में स्वस्थ्य मनुष्य में किसी रोग के लक्षण उत्पन्न करती है, वही थोड़ी मात्रा में प्रयोग में लाने पर उन्ही लक्षणों को शांत करती है। A system of treatment based on the theory that large dose of a drug which produce symptoms of a disease in healthy person cures some symptoms when administered in small amounts.

Homeostasis (होमियोस्टेसिस) समास्थिति, धातु-समय।
Stability in the normal physiological state.

Homeotherm (होमियोथर्म) समतापी। Hematherm warm blended.

Homicide (होमीसाइड) हत्या, हत्यारा। Murder, murderer.

Homoblastic (होमोब्लास्टिक) एक ही प्रकार के ऊतक से उत्पन्न होने वाला। Developing from a single type of tissue.

Homodromous (होमोड्रोमस) एक ही दिशा में घूमने वाला। Moving in the same direction.

Homogeneous (होमोजीनियस) एक-सा बना हुआ, समांग। An uniform composition.

Homogenesis (होमोजेनेसिस) प्रत्येक पीढ़ी में एक ही क्रिया द्वारा उत्पत्ति। Reproduction by the same process in each generation.

Homoiotherm (होमॉयोथर्म) गर्म खून वाला जीव, उष्णरक्तक प्राणी। Warm blooded organism.

Homologue (होमोलोग) कोई भी समजात अंग अथवा शरीर का भाग। Similar in position origin and structure.

Homology (होमोलॉजी) समजात होने की अवस्था सजातीयता, समरूपता। The state of being homologous.

Homonymous (होमोनिमस) एक ही नाम वाले। Having the same name.

Homophile (होमोफिल) ऐसे एण्टीबॉडी से सम्बन्धित जो केवल एक विशिष्ट एण्टिजन के साथ ही प्रतिक्रिया करती है। Pertaining to an antibody which reacts only with a specific antigen.

Homotonic (होमोटोनिक) एक से तनाव वाला। Having a uniform tension.

Homozygous (होमोजाइगस) एक से अलीलों द्वारा उत्पन्न, समयुग्मजी। Produced by similar alleles.

Hookworm (हुकवर्म) मनुष्य की आँत में रहने वाला परजीवी एन्किलोस्टोमा ड्योडीनेल जो अंकुशकृमिरोग उत्पन्न करता है। Ancylostoma duodenale, a parasitic living in the human intestine causing ancylostomiasis.

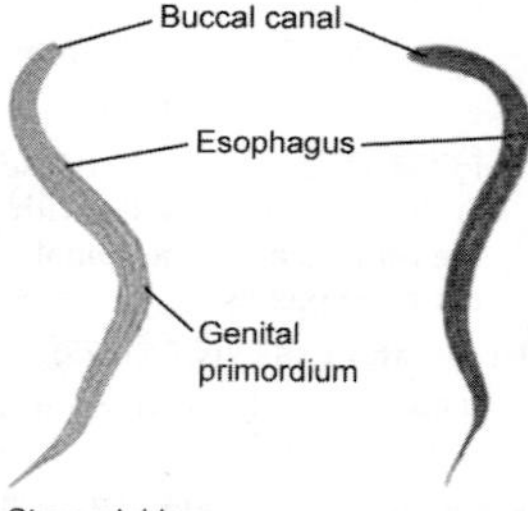

Hor decub (होर डेकूबा) सोते समय। At bed time.

Hormone (हार्मोन) किसी ग्रन्थि, अंग अथवा शरीर के भाग में उत्पन्न होने वाला एक रासायनिक पदार्थ जो रक्त के द्वारा शरीर के दूसरे भाग में लाया जाता है। A chemical substance produced

in a gland organ or part of the body which is carried through the blood to another part of the body. (*i*) **Gonadotropic hormone** (गोनाडोट्रॉपिक–हॉर्मोन) अग्र पीयूष ग्रन्थि से उत्पन्न होने वाला एक हॉर्मोन जो जननग्रन्थियों को प्रभावित करता है, जननग्रन्थिप्रेरक हॉर्मोन। A hormone produced by the anterior pituitary gland which affects the gonads.
(*ii*) **Oxytocin hormone** (ऑक्सीटोसीन–हॉर्मोन) पश्च पीयूष ग्रन्थि से उत्पन्न होने वाला एक हार्मोन जो गर्भाशय को संकुचित करता है। A hormone produced by the posterior pituitary gland which causes contraction of the uterus.
(*iii*) **Prolactin hormone** (प्रोलैक्टिन हॉर्मोन) अग्र पीयूष ग्रन्थि का एक हॉर्मोन जो दुग्ध स्राव जो उत्तेजित करता है। A hormone of the anterior pituitary gland stimulate lactation.

Hormonagogue (हार्मोनेगोग) किसी हार्मोन के उत्पादन को बढ़ाने वाला। Increasing the production of a hormone.

Hormonogenetic (हॉर्मोनोजेनटिक) हॉर्मोन को उत्पन्न करने वाला। Hormonopoitic producing hormones.

Horn (हॉर्न) त्वचा की एक कठोर, श्रंगी अतिवृद्धि जो मुख्यतया केरेटिन की बनी होती है। Cutaneous outgrowth composed chiefly of keratin.

Horner's syndrome (हॉरनर्स सिण्ड्रोम) ऐसा संलक्षण जिसमें एक ओर की पुतली संकुचित हो जाती है, पलक आंशिक रूप से नीचे को लटक जाती है, नेत्रगोलक नेत्र गुहा में धस जाता है, तथा कभी-कभी चेहरे के एक ओर पसीना नहीं आता।

A syndrome characterized by contraction of the pupil partial drooping of eyelid recession of the eyeball into the orbit of one side and sometimes loss of sweating over one side of the face.

Horsepower (हॉर्सपावर) शक्ति की एक इकाई जो 745.7 वॉट के बराबर या 550 फूट पौण्ड प्रति सेकण्ड होती है। A unit of power equal to 745.7 watt or 550 foot pounds per seconds.

Hospice (हॉसपाइस) आश्रम, शरण स्थल, ऐसा स्थान जहाँ व्यक्तियों को सेवाएं उपलब्ध करवायी जाती है। Palliative and supportive care services for terminally ill.

Hospital (हॉस्पिटल) रोगी एवं चोट खाए हुए व्यक्ति की चिकित्सा के लिए एक संस्था, चिकित्सालय, अस्पताल। An institution for the treatment of the sick and injured person.

Hospitalization (हॉस्पिटलाइजेशन) चिकित्सा के लिए किसी रोगी का अस्पताल में रखना। Placing of a patient in a hospital for the treatment.

Host (होस्ट) वह जीवधारी जिससे कोई परजीवी अपना पोषण ग्रहण करता है, परपोषी, सत्कारी। The organism from which a parasite obtains its nourishment.

Hostility (होस्टीलिटी) नाराजगी अथवा शत्रुता। Angriness or enmity.

Hottentotism (हौटेन्टोटिज्म) अजीब किस्म से हकलाकर बोलना। Abnormal form of stuttering.

Hourglass stomach (हॉवरग्लास स्टोमक) अपने केन्द्र पर पेशीय संकुचन द्वारा विभाजित आमाशय जैसा कि अक्सर आमाशय व्रण या गैस्ट्रिक अल्सर में होता है। A stomach divided by the muscular constriction at its center which often occurs in gastric ulcer.

House physician (हाउज फिजीशियन) ऐसा कार्यचिकित्सक जो किसी अस्पताल के वरिष्ठ कार्यचिकित्सक के निर्देशन में रोगियों की चिकित्सा एवं उनकी देख-भाल करता है। A physician who treats the patients and take care of them in a hospital under the direction of a senior physician.

Howell–Jolly bodies (हॉवेल-जाली बाडीज़) लाल रक्त कोशिकाओं में दिखाई देने वाले गोलाकार कण होते हैं, यह थैलेसीमिया तथा ल्यूकीमिया में पाये जाते हैं। Spherical granular in the erythrocytes thalassemia leukemia, etc.

Howk (हॉक) खखार कर गला साफ करना, खखारना। To clear the throat with a noise.

Hum (हम) एक मृदु निरन्तर होने वाली ध्वनी, क्ष्वेद। A soft continuous sound.

Human (ह्यूमन) मानव। Pertaining to man or mankind.

Human immunodeficiency virus (ह्यूमन इम्यूनोडैफीशियन्सी वायरस) ऐसा विषाणु जो इकाई एक्वार्ड इम्यूनोडैफीशियन्सी सिण्ड्रोम अर्थात् एड्स रोग उत्पन्न करता है। A virus that cause Acquired Immunodeficiency Syndrome, i.e. AIDS.

Humectants (ह्यूमैक्टेन्ट) नम बनाने वाला कारक, आर्द्रकारी। A moisturizing agent.

Humerus (ह्यूमेरस) कन्धे से कोहनी तक की हड्डी, प्रगण्डिका। The large bone of the upper arm articulating with the scapula above and the radius and ulna below.

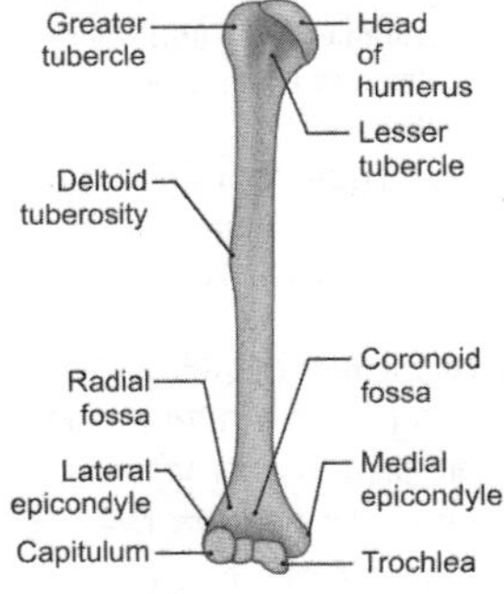

Humidity (ह्यूमिडीटी) वायुमण्डल या जलवायु में स्थित आर्द्रता या नमी। Moisture in the atmosphere.

Humor (ह्यूमर) शरीर में स्थित कोई भी तरल अथवा अर्द्ध तरल पदार्थ। A fluid or semifluid substance present in the body.

Humoral (ह्यूमोरेल) शरीर के तरलों से सम्बन्धित, देहद्रवी। Pertaining to the fluid of the body.

Humpback (हम्पबैक) कुब्ज, कुबड़ा। Kyphosis.

Hunchback (हन्चबैक) कुब्जता से ग्रस्त ऐसा व्यक्ति जिसकी कमर गोल हो जाती है। A person with the kyphosis that there is prominent rounded deformity of the back.

Hunger (हन्गर) भोजन अथवा वायु के प्राप्त करने की तीव्र इच्छा, भूख, क्षुधा। A strong desire for food or air.

Hunterian chancre (हन्टेरियन शैकर) कठिनक्षत, उपदंशक्षत। Hard syphilitic chancre.

Hutchinson's teeth (हटचिनसन्स टीथ) ऊपर वाले भेदक दांतों की दोषपूर्ण अवस्था, विषमदन्तता, ऊर्ध्व कृन्तक दाँत। Defect of the upper incisors.

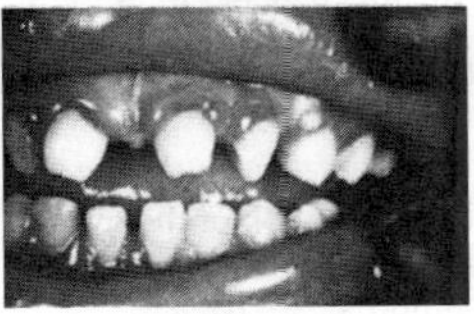

Hyaline (हायलाइन) काँच के समान एवं अर्द्ध पारदर्षक, काचाभ। Glassy and translucent.

Hyaline cartilage (हायलाइन कार्टिलेज) हड्डियों के जोड़ बनाने वाली सतहों को ढ़कने वाली काँच के समान, चिकनी एवं अर्द्धपारदर्शक एक उपास्थि जो वास्तविक उपास्थि होती है।

The glassy smooth and translucent cartilage which is true cartilage covering the articular surface or the bones.

Hyaline casts (हायलाइन कास्ट्स) मूत्र में पाये जाने वाले पीले काँच

के समान एवं पारदर्शक निर्मोच या साँचें, काचाभ निर्माक। Pale glassy and transparent casts found in the urine.

Hyalinization (हायलाइनाइजेशन) किसी ऊतक का काँच के समान पदार्थ में परिवर्तित होना, काचाभीकरण। Conversion of a tissue into a glass like substance.

Hyalinosis (हायलिनोसिस) स्फटिककलामयता। Waxy or hyaline degeneration.

Hyalitis (हायलाइट्सि) स्फटिक झिल्ली का प्रदाह, स्फटिककलाशोथ। Inflammation of the hyaloid membrane or the vitreous humors.

Hyaloditis (हायलॉयडाइटिस) विट्रियस ह्यूमर की हायलॉयड झिल्ली की सूजन। Hyalitis.

Hyaloid membrane (हॉयलोइड मेम्ब्रेन) विट्रियस ह्यूमर को ढ़कने वाली झिल्ली। The membrane enveloping the vitreous humor.

Hyalophobia (हायलोफोबिया) काँच छूने का रोगोत्पादक भय। Morbid fear of touching the glass.

Hybrid (हाइब्रिड) विभिन्न जाति के माता-पिता की संतान, संकर, दोगला। An offspring of the parents of different species.

Hybridization (हाइब्रीडाइज़ेशन) संकरों का पैदा होना। The production of hybrid.

Hybridoma (हायब्रिडोमा) संकर कोशिकाबुर्द। A tumor of hybrid cells.

Hydatid (हायडेटिड) फीताकृमियों के अण्ड़ों से निर्मित पुटी। The cyst formed by larvae of tapeworm.

Hydatid mole (हाइडेटीड मोल) जरायु अंकुरों में पुटीय ह्रास होने के कारण बहुत सी पुटियों का बनने वाला एक पिण्ड जिससे गर्भाशय में शीघ्रता से वृद्धि होती है। Degenerative process of chorionic villi with formation of multiple cysts within uterus.

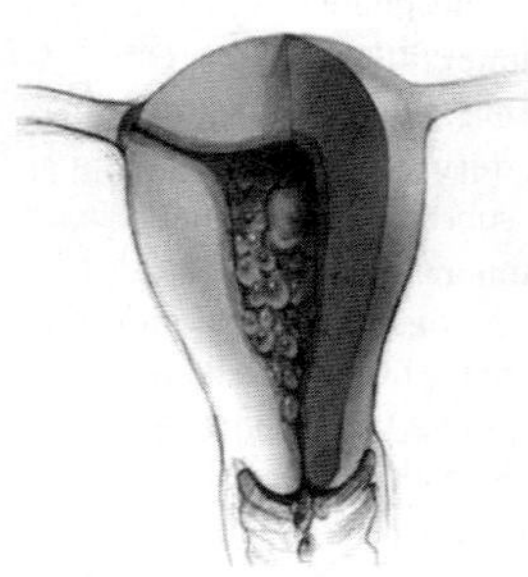

Hydatism (हाइडेटिज्म) किसी गुहा में तरल द्वारा उत्पन्न ध्वनि। The sound produced by fluid in a cavity.

Hydragogue (हाइड्रेगोग) एक विरेचक जो पतले पानी जैसे दस्त लाकर आँतों को खाली करता है जैसे मैग्नीशियम सल्फेट, जलनिस्सारक। A duragative which causes evacuation of bowels by producing watery stool, e.g. magnesium sulfate.

Hydramnios (हाइड्रेम्नियोज) उल्व-गुहा में उल्व-तरल का अधिक हो जाना जिससे गर्भाशय बहुत फैल जाता है, अति-उल्वोदकता। Excess of amniotic fluid in the amniotic cavity causing overdistention of the uterus.

Hydrarthrosis (हाइड्रारथ्रोसिस) जोड़ों में पानी भर जाना। Serous effusion into joints cavity.

Hydraulic (हाइड्रोलिक) तरल-विज्ञान। The science of fluids.

Hydrenencephaly (हाइड्रेन्सिफेली) सहज अमस्तिष्कता। Congenital absence of the cerebral hemisphere.

Hydriatric (हाइड्रियाट्रिक) पानी द्वारा रोगों का उपचार करना, जलोपचार, जलचिकित्सा। Application of water for treatment.

Hydrocarbon (हाइड्रोकार्बन) जलकार्बन, ऐसा पदार्थ जो जल व कार्बन से मिलकर बनता है। Compound made from only hydrogen and carbon.

Hydrocele (हाइड्रोसील) वृषणों में पानी भर जाना, जलवृषण। Fluid accumulation in tunica vaginalis test or sac like cavity.

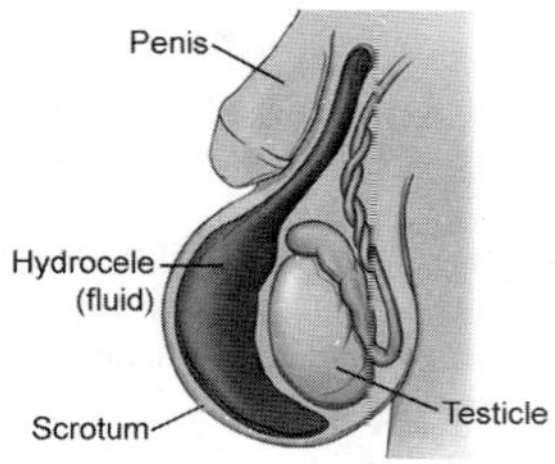

Hydrocephalus (हाइड्रोसिफैलस) सिर में पानी जमा हो जाना, जलशीर्ष। Collection of fluid in the head.

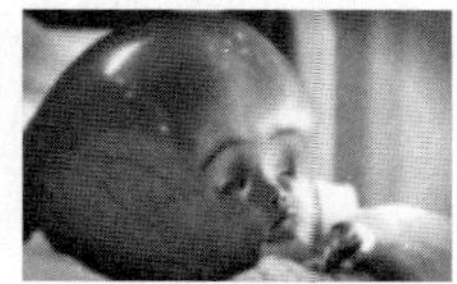

Hydrochlorate (हाइड्रोक्लोरेट) हाइड्रोक्लोरिक अम्ल का कोई भी लवण। Any salt of hydrochloric acid.

Hydrocolpos (हाइड्रोकॉल्पोस) जलयोनिपुटी। Relation cyst of vagina.

Hydrodenitis (हाइड्रोडीनाइटिस) किसी स्वेद ग्रन्थि का शोथ। Inflammation of sweet gland.

Hydrogel (हाइड्रोजेल) एक जेली जिसमें पानी होता है। A gel containing water.

Hydrogen (हाइड्रोजन) एक रंगहीन, गन्धहीन एवं स्वादहीन गैस जिसका परमाण्विक नं. 1 होता है। A colorless, odorless and tasteless gas possesing atomic no 1.

Hydrogenate (हाइड्रोजिनेट) हाइड्रोजन के साथ संयुक्त। To bring about a combination with hydrogen.

Hydrogenation (हाइड्रोजिनेशन) हाइड्रोजन मिलाकर असंतृप्त वसा को एक ठोस वसा में बदलने की क्रिया। The process of changing an unsaturated fat to a solid saturatead fat by adding hydrogen.

Hydrokinetic (हाइड्रोकाइनेटिक) तरलों में होने वाली गति एवं ऐसी गति को प्रदान करने में लगने वाले बलों से सम्बन्धित। Pertaining to the motion of fluid and the forces giving rise to such motion.

Hydrolysis (हाइड्रोलाइसिस) जलापघटन, जललयन। The splitting into more simple substance by the addition of water.

Hydromeningitis (हाइड्रोमैनिनजाइटिस) सीरमी रिसाव के साथ मस्तिष्कावरणों का शोथ। Inflammation of the meninges with serous of fusion.

Hydrometer (हाइड्रोमीटर) किसी तरल का विशिष्ट गुरूत्व या घनत्व मापने वाला एक यंत्र। An instrument for measuring the specific gravity or density of a fluid.

Hydrometra (हाइड्रोमीट्रा) गर्भाशय में जलीय तरल का इकट्ठा हो जाना। A collection of watery fluid in the uterus and vagina.

Hydromyelia (हाइड्रोमाइलिया) सुषुम्ना रज्जु की केन्द्रीय नली का चौड़ा होना, जलमेरूरज्जु। Distention of central canal of spinal cord fluid.

Hydromyelocele (हाइड्रोमाइलोसीस) एक थैली का जिससे प्रमस्तिष्क मेरू-द्रव होता, अयुक्त मेरूदण्ड से बाहर निकल आना। Protrusion of spiral CSF through spina bifida.

Hydromyoma (हाइड्रोमायोमा) जलपेश्यबुर्द। Cystic uterine fibroid

Hydronephrosis (हाइड्रोनैफ्रोसिस) मूत्रनली या गवीनी में अवरोध उत्पन्न हो जाने से मूत्र के संचित हो जाने के कारण वृक्कीय श्रेणी एवं आलवलों का फूल जाना तथा वृक्क का अपक्षय हो जाना, जलवृक्कता। Distension of the renal pelvis and calyces with the collection of urine due to obstruction in the ureter and the atrophy of the kidney results.

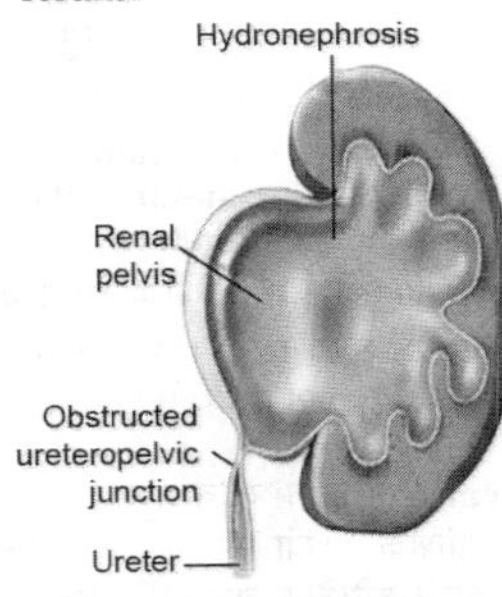

Hydropenia (हाइड्रोपीनिया) शरीर में पानी की कमी होना। Deficiency of water in body.

Hydropericarditis (हाइड्रोपैरीकार्डाइटिस) सीरमी रिसाव के साथ हृदयावरणशोथ, जलपरिहृदशोथ। Inflammation of the pericardium with serous effusion.

Hydroperitoneum (हाइड्रोपैरिटोनियम) जलपर्युदर्या, उदरावणशोफ। Ascites.

Hydrophilia (हाइड्रोफीलिया) जल का अवशोषण करने का गुण। The equality of absorbing water.

Hydrophobia (हाइड्रोफोबिया) पानी से डर लगने की बीमारी। Morbid fear of water.

Hydropneumatosis (हाइड्रोन्यूमेटोसिस) ऊतकों में तरल एवं गैस का पाया जाना जिसमें शोथ एवं वातस्फीति दोनों होते हैं। Presence of fluid and gas in the tissue producing combined edema and emphysema.

Hydropneumopericardium (हाइड्रोन्यूमोपैरीकार्डियम) हृदयावरण में तरल एवं गैस का पाया जाना। Presence of fluid and gas in the pericardium.

Hydropneumothorax (हाइड्रोन्यूमोथौरेक्स) फुस्फुसावरणी गुहा में तरल एवं गैस की विद्यमानता, जलवातवक्ष। Presence of fluid and gas in the pleural.

Hydrops (हाइड्रॉप्स) जलशोफ या शोफ, पानी वाली सूजन। Dropsy or edema.

Hydropyonephrosis (हाइड्रोपायोनेफ्रोसिस) वृक्कीय श्रोणि में पस एवं मूल का पाया जाना। Presence of pus and urine in the renal pelvis.

Hydrorrhea (हाइड्रोरिह्या) शरीर के किसी भी भाग से जैसे नाक से प्रचुर मात्रा जलीय स्राव निकलना। Copious watery discharge from any part of the body like from the nose.

Hydrosalpinx (हाइड्रोसैलिपक्स) डिम्ब वाहिनी में जलीय तरल का संचयन, जल-डिम्ब-वाहिनी। Accumulation of watery fluid in the fallopian tube.

Hydrostatics (हाइड्रोस्टोटिक्स) तरलों के साम्यावस्था में रहने पर उनके गुणों का अध्ययन। Study of the properties of fluid in equilibrium.

Hydrotaxis (हाइड्रोटैक्सिस) जल अथवा नमी की ओर अथवा उससे दूर गति करना। Motion towards or away from water or moisture.

Hydrotherapy (हाइड्रोथिरैपी) जल का प्रयोग करके रोगों की चिकित्सा करना, जल-चिकित्सा। Treatment of the disease by use of water.

Hydrothorax (हाइड्रोथोरैक्स) फुस्फुसावरणी गुहा में सीरमी तरल का इक्कठा हो जाना। The collection of serous fluid in the pleural cavity.

Hydroureter (हाइड्रोयूरेटर) मूत्रनली का असाधारण रूप से फूल जाना, जलगवीनी। Distension of ureter due to obstruction.

Hygiene (हाइजीन) स्वास्थ्य एवं इसे सुरक्षित रखने की विधियों का अध्ययन, स्वास्थ्य विज्ञान। Study of health and the methods of preserving it.

Hygroma (हाइग्रोमा) एक कोश, पुटी अथवा श्लेषपुटी जिसमें तरल भाग होती है। Arac cyst or bursa containing fluid.

Hygrometer (हाइग्रोमीटर) वायु में नमी की मात्रा मापने वाला यंत्र, आर्द्रतामापी। An instrument for measuring the amount of moisture in the air.

Hyla (हाइला) प्रमस्तिष्कीय कुल्या का एक पार्श्वीय प्रसार। A lateral extension of the cerebral aqueduct.

Hymen (हाइमन) योनि द्वार को आंशिक अथवा पूर्ण रूप से ढ़कने वाली श्लेष्मिक कला की एक परत, योनिच्छिद। A fold for mucous membrane which partially or wealthy covers the vaginal opening.

Hymenitis (हाइमेनाइटिस) योनिच्छदशोध। Inflammation of the hymen.

Hymenology (हाइमेनोलॉजी) झिल्लियों एवं उनके रोगों का विज्ञान। The science of the membranes and their disease.

Hymenorrhaphy (हाइमेनोरैह्फी) योनि को आंशिक रूप से अथवा पूर्णतया बन्द करने के लिए विदीर्ण अथवा फटे हुए योनिच्छद की सिलाई करना। The suturing of the ruptured hymen to close the vagina partially or completely.

Hymenotomy (हाइमेनोटॉमी) योनिच्छद में चीरा लगाना। To incisor the hymen.

Hyoglossal (हायोग्लोसल) कण्ठिका अस्थि एवं जिह्वा सम्बन्धी अथवा हायोग्लोसस पेशी से सम्बन्धित, कण्डिकाजिह्वा। Pertaining to the hyoid bone and tongue or to the hyoglossal muscle.

Hyoid bone (हॉयडबोन) जिह्वा के आधार पर स्थित घोड़े के नाल के आकार की हड्डी। Horse shoe-shaped bone lying at the base of the tongue.

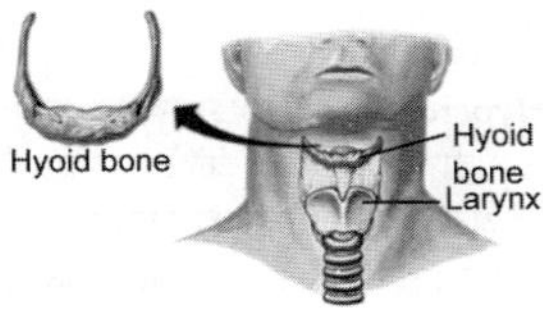

Hypaphrodisia (हाइपैफ्रोडिसीया) कामेच्छा का कम हो जाना। Decreased sexual desire.

Hyper (हाइपर) एक उपसर्ग जिसका अर्थ ऊपर अत्यधिक अथवा बढ़ा हुआ होता है। A prefix meaning above excessive or increased.

Hyperacidity (हाइपरएसिडिटी) अत्यधिक अम्लता। Excess of acid in stomach.

Hyperactivity (हाइपरएकटीविटी) अतिसक्रियता, अत्यधिक क्रियाशीलता। Increased or excessive activity.

Hyperacusis (हाइपरेकुसिस) ध्वनि के प्रति अत्यधिक संवेदनशीलता, श्रवण अतिसंवेदिता। Excessive sensitivity to sound.

Hyperadiposis (हाइपरएडिपोसिस) अत्यधिक मोटापा। Excessive fatness.

Hyperalgia (हाइपरेल्जिया) वेदना के प्रति संवेदनशीलता बढ़ जाना अर्थात् दर्द बहुत महसूस होना। Increased sensitivity to pain.

Hyperalimentation (हाइपरएलीमेन्टेशन) अतिपोषणता। Administration or consumption of nutrient beyond normal requirements.

Hyperammonemia (हाइपरअमोनीमिया) रक्त में अमोनिया का अत्यधिक पाया जाना। An excess of ammonia in the blood.

Hyperasthenia (हाइपरस्थीनिया) अत्यधिक कमजोरी। Extreme weakness.

Hyperbaric (हाइपरबेरिक) सामान्य से अधिक भार, दाब अथवा विशिष्ट गुरूत्व पर। At a greater weight pressure of specific gravity than normal.

Hyperbilirubinemia (हाइपरबिलिरूबिनीमिया) रक्त में बिलिरूबिन का अधिक पाया

जाना। Excess of bilirubin in the blood.

Hypercalcemia (हाइपरकैल्सीमिया) रक्त में कैल्सीयम का अधिक पाया जाना। Excess of calcium in the blood.

Hypercalciuria (हाइपरकैल्सीयूरीया) मूत्र में कैल्सीयम का अधिक पाया जाना। An excess of calcium in the urine.

Hypercapnia (हाइपरकैप्निया) रक्त में कार्बन डाइऑक्साइड का अधिक पाया जाना। An excess of carbon dioxide in the blood.

Hypercementosis (हाइपरसिमेन्टोसिस) दन्त मूलों के सिमेन्ट की अतिवृद्धि। Overgrowth of the cement of the roots.

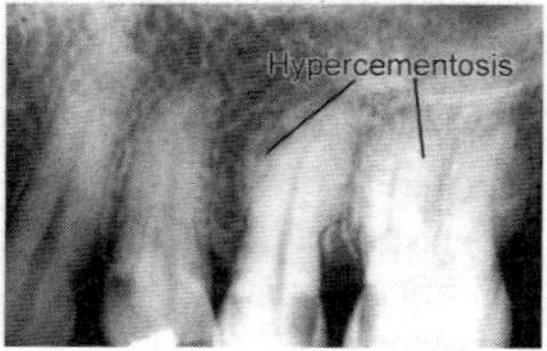

Hyperchloremia (हाइपरक्लोरीमिया) रक्त में अत्यधिक मात्रा में क्लोराइडों का पाया जाना। Excessive amount of chlorides in the blood.

Hypercholesterolemia (हाइपरकोलेस्ट्रोलीमिया) रक्त में अधिक कोलेस्ट्रॉल की विद्यमानता। Excessive of cholesterol in the blood.

Hypercholia (हाइपरकोलिया) अत्यधिक पित्त या बाइल का बनना। Excessive secretion of bile.

Hyperchromatic (हाइपरक्रोमेटिक) अत्यधिक वर्णकता से युक्त। Marked with excessive pigmentation.

Hypercoagulability (हाइपरकौगुलेबिलिटी) रक्त के जमने की क्षमता का बढ़ जाना, अतिस्कन्दनता। Increased ability of the blood to coagulate.

Hypercorticism (हाइपरकॉटिसिज्म) एड्रीनल ग्रन्थि के कॉर्टेक्स से अत्यधिक हार्मोनों का उत्पन्न होना। Excessive production of adrenal cortical hormones.

Hypercryalgesia (हाइपरक्रोयेल्जेसिया) ठण्ड के प्रति अत्यधिक संवेदनशीलता। Excessive sensitivity to cold.

Hypercyesis (हाइपरसाइसिस) एक से अधिक भ्रूण का गर्भाशय में स्थित होना। Presence of more than one fetus in uterus.

Hyperdicrotic (हाइपरडाइक्रोटिक) असामान्य रूप से द्विस्पन्दी। Abnormally dicrotic.

Hyperdipsia (हाइपरडिप्सिया) प्यास अधिक लगना। Intense thirst.

Hyperdontial (हाइपरडोन्टियल) सामान्य संख्या से अधिक संख्या में दाँतों का पाया जाना। Presence of more than normal number of teeth.

Hyperemesis (हाइपरेमेसिस) अत्यधिक उल्टियाँ होना, अतिवमन। Excessive vomiting

Hyperemesis gravidarum (हाइपरेमेसिस ग्रेविडेरम) गर्भावस्था में होने वाली अत्यधिक उल्टियाँ, ग्रभिणी अतिवमन। Excessive vomiting during pregnancy.

Hyperemia (हाइप्रीमिया) रक्ताधिक्य अथवा शरीर के किसी भाग में रक्त का अधिक हो जाना, त्वचा की लाली से जिसका पता चलता है। Congestion or an excess of blood in a part of the body shown by redness of the skin.

Hypererethism (हाइपरेरेथिज्म) अत्यधिक क्षोभ्यता तथा चिड़चिड़ापन। Excessive irritability.

Hyperergy (हाइपेरेर्गी) अत्यन्त तीव्र एलर्जी। Extreme allergy.

Hyperesthesia (हाइपरेस्थीसिया) उद्दीपद जैसे वेदना अथवा स्पर्श के प्रति बढ़ी हुई संवदेनशीलता, अतिसंवेदिता। Increased sensitivity to stimulation such as pain or touch.

Hyperextension (हाइपरैक्सटेन्सन) अत्यधिक प्रसार। Excessive extension.

Hyperfibrinogenemia (हाइपरफाइब्रिनो जीनीमिया) रक्त में अधिक फाइब्रिनोजन का पाया जाना। An excessive of fibrinogen in the blood.

Hypergalactia (हाइपरगैलेक्टिया) अत्यधिक दूध का बनना। Excessive secretion of milk.

Hypergia (हाइपर्जिया) एलर्जनों के प्रति संवेदनशीलता का कम हो जाना। Diminished sensitivity of allergens.

Hyperglycemia (हाइपरग्लाइसीमिया) रक्त में शुगर का बढ़ जाना। Increase of sugar in the blood as in diabetes.

Hypergonadism (हाइपरगोनाडिज्म) लिंग ग्रन्थियों की बढ़ी हुई क्रियात्मक सक्रियता जिससे कालपूर्व लैंगिक विकास होता है। Increase functional activity of the sex gland with precocious sexual development.

Hyperhidrosis (हाइपरहाइड्रोसिस) अत्यधिक पसीना आना। Excessive sweating.

Hyperhydration (हाइपरहाइड्रेशन) शरीर में पानी का बढ़ जाना। Excess of water in the body.

Hyperinflation (हाइपरन्फ्लेशन) किसी भी अंग विशेषकर फेफड़ों में वायु का बहुत भर जाना। Excessive of air in any organ especially the lungs.

Hyperinsulinism (हाइपरइन्सुलिनिज्म) इन्सुलिन की अधिकता के कारण होने वाली दुरावस्था, अतिइन्सुलिनता। Morbid condition through excess of insulin.

Hyperkalemia (हाइपरकेलीमिया) रक्त में पोटेशियम का अधिक पाया जाना। An excess of potassium in the blood.

Hyperkeratosis (हाइपरकेरेटोसिस) बाह्यत्वचा की श्रृंगी परत अथवा आँख के कॉर्निया की अतिवृद्धि। Overgrowth of the horny layer of the epidermis or of the cornea of the eye.

Hyperkinesia (हाइपरकाइनीसिया) अत्यधिक बढ़ी हुई शारीरिक क्रियाशीलता। Highly increased physical activity.

Hyperlipemia (हाइपरलाइपीमिया) रक्त में अत्यधिक मात्रा में वसा या चर्बी का होना। Excessive quantity of fat in the blood.

Hyperlipoproteinemia (हाइपरलाइपोप्रोटीनिमीया) रक्त में अधिक लाइपोप्रोटीन का पाया जाना। Excess of lipoprotein in the blood.

Hyperlogia (हाइपरलोगिया) अत्यधिक बातें बनाना। Excessive talkativeness.

Hyperlucent (हाइपरल्यूसैन्ट) अतिअर्द्धपारदर्शक।

Hypermelanosis (हाइपरमेलेनोसिस) त्वचा में अत्यधिक मेलेनिन वर्णक का जमा हो जाना जो सामान्यतः गर्भावस्था में, जीर्ण वृक्कीय पात में, जीर्ण कण्ड़ में तथा ACTH उत्पादक अबुर्दों आदि के द्वारा होता है। Excessive deposition of melanin pigment in the skin which is generally caused in pregnancy, chronic renal failure, chronic pruritus and by ACTH producing tumors.

Hypermenorrhea (हाइपरमेनोरिह्या) अत्यधिक आर्तव-स्राव होना। Excessive menstrual bleeding.

Hypermetabolism (हाइपरमेटाबोलिज्म) बढ़ा हुआ चयापचय। Increased metabolism.

Hypermetria (हाइपरमीट्रिया) अत्यधिक पेशीय सक्रियता। Excessive muscular activity.

Hypermetropia (हाइपरमीट्रोपिया) दूरदृष्टिता। Hyperopia.

Hypermimia (हाइपरमीमिया) बोलते समय बहुत अधिक हाव-भाव दिखाना। Speaking accompanied by a great number of gestures.

Hypermnesia (हाइपरम्नेसिया) अति-स्मृति। Exaggeration of memory.

Hypermobility (हाइपरमोबिलिटी) बढ़ी हुई गतिशीलता। Increased mobility.

Hypermyesthesia (हाइपरमायेस्थीसीया) पेशी अतिसंवेदिता। Muscular hyperesthesia.

Hypernatremia (हाइपरनेट्रीमिया) रक्त में सोडियम का अधिक पाया जाना। Excessive of sodium in the blood.

Hyperonychia (हाइपरोनीकिया) नाखूनों की अतिवृद्धि, अतिनखता। Hypertrophy of the nails.

Hyperorchidism (हाइपरऑर्काइडिज्म) शुक्र–ग्रन्थियों की अत्यधिक क्रियात्मक सक्रियता। Excessive functional activity of the testis.

Hyperosinophilia (हाइपरओसिनोफिलिया) रक्त में इओसिनोफिलों की संख्या में अत्यधिक वृद्धि हो जाना। Marked increase in the number of esosinophils in the blood.

Hyperosmia (हाइपरोस्मिया) दुर्गन्ध के प्रति अत्यधिक संवेदनशीलता। Excessive sensitivity to the foul smell.

Hyperosmolarity (हाइपरऑस्मोलेरिटी) किसी घोल जैसे रक्त में परासरणीय सक्रिय कणों की असामान्य रूप से बढ़ी हुई सान्द्रता। Abnormally increased concentration of the osmotically active particles in solution, e.g. in blood.

Hyperostosis (हाइपराॅस्टोसिस) अस्थि ऊतक का अत्यधिक बढ़ना, अस्थ्यर्बुद। A hypertrophy of bone tissue, exotasis.

Hyperparasite (हाइपरपैरासाइट) एक परजीवी जो दूसरे परजीवी पर रहता है। A parasite living upon another parasite.

Hyperparathyroidism (हाइपरपैराथाइरॉयडिज्म) पैराथाइरॉयड ग्रन्थियों की अत्यधिक सक्रियता के कारण होने वाला रोग, अतिपरावटुता। The condition due to excessive activity of the parathyroid glands.

Hyperpathia (हाइपरपैथिया) संवेदी उद्दीपनों के प्रति बढ़ी हुई संवेदनशीलता। Increased sensitivity to sensory stimuli.

Hyperperistalsis (हाइपरपैरिस्टैल्सिस) आँतों का अत्यधिक क्रमांनुकुचन गतियाँ होना। Excessive peristaltic movement of the intestine.

Hyperphasia (हाइपरफेजिया) बात-चीत करने की तीव्र इच्छा। Intense desire for talking.

Hyperphosphaturia (हाइपरफॉस्फेचूरिया) मूत्र में फास्फेटों का अधिक पाया जाना।

Presence of phosphates in the urine in excess.

Hyperphonia (हाइपरफोनिया) स्वर रज्जुओं के क्षोभण से हकलाना। Stuttering or stammering due to irritability of the vocal cords.

Hyperphoria (हाइपरफोरिया) नेत्र ऊर्ध्वाविचलन प्रवृत्ति। Anopsia anophoria.

Hyperphosphatasemia (हाइपरफॉस्फेटेसीमिया) रक्त में एल्कैलाइन फॉस्फेट का बढ़ जाना। Increased alkaline phosphatase in the blood.

Hyperphosphatemia (हाइपरफॉस्फेटीमिया) रक्त में फॉस्फोरस का बढ़ जाना।

An excess of phosphorus in the blood.

Hyperphrenia (हाइपरफ्रेनिया) मानसिक सक्रियता का बढ़ जाना। Accelerated mental activity.

Hyperpigmentation (हाइपरपिग्मन्टेशन) अति-वर्णकयुक्तता, अतिवर्णकता। Increased pigmentation.

Hyperpituitarim (हाइपरपिट्यूटेरिज्म) पीयूष ग्रन्थि के अग्र खण्ड की अति सक्रियता के फलस्वरूप उत्पन्न दशा, अतिपीयूषिकता। The condition resulting from increased activity of the anterior lobe of the pituitary gland.

Hyperplasia (हाइपरप्लेसिया) शरीर के किसी अंग अथवा भाग की उसकी कोशिकाओं की संख्या में वृद्धि होने के कारण होने वाली अतिवृद्धि। Overgrowth of an organ or a part of the body due to marked increase in the number of its cells.

Hyperplastic (हाइपरप्लेस्टिक) अतिविकसन से सम्बन्धित। Pertaining to hyperplasia.

Hyperploidy (हाइपरप्लॉयडी) एक गुणसूत्र से युक्त होने और इस प्रकार गुणसूत्रों के संतुलित सैटों से रहित रहने की अवस्था।

The condition of having one extra chromosome and thus not balanced sets of chromosome.

Hyperpnea (हाइपर्निया) जल्दी-जल्दी एवं गहरे सांस लेने में असामान्य वृद्धि, अतिश्वसन। Abnormal increase in rate and depth of respiration.

Hyperpraxia (हाइपरप्रैक्सिया) अत्यधिक मानसिक सक्रियता एवं बेचैनी। Excessive mental activity and restlessness.

Hyperprolactinemia (हाइपरप्रोलैक्टीनीमिया) रक्त में प्रोलेक्टिन हॉर्मोन का बढ़ जाना।

An increase of prolactin hormone in the blood.

Hyperproteinemia
(हाइपरप्रोटीनिमिया) रक्त में प्रोटीन का बढ़ जाना। An excess of protein in the blood.

Hyperproteinuria
(हाइपरप्रोटीनूरिया) मूत्र में अधिक प्रोटीन का होना। Excess of protein in the urine.

Hyperptyalism (हाइपरटायालिज्म) थूक बहुत आना। Excessive secretion of saliva.

Hyperpyrexia (हाइपरपाइरेक्सिया) शरीर का उच्च तापमान अतिज्वर, तेज बुखार। Very high temperature of the body.

Hyperreflexia (हाइपररिफ्लैक्सिया) प्रतिवर्त क्रियाओं का बढ़ जाना। Exaggerated reflex action.

Hyperresonance (हाइपररेजोनैन्स) शरीर के किसी क्षेत्र का परिताड़न करने पर उत्पन्न बढ़ा हुआ अनुनाद। An increased resonance produced on precussion of an area of the body.

Hyper-resonant (हाइपर-रेजोनैन्ट) परिताड़न करने पर अतिअनुनादी। Over resonant on precussion.

Hypersecretion (हाइपरसिक्रिशन) अत्यधिक स्राव, अतिस्राव। Excessive secretion.

Hypersensibility
(हाइपरसैन्सीबिलिटी) अति संवेदी। Hypersensitivity to a foreign protein or drug.

Hypersexuality
(हाइपरसैक्सुआलिटी) काम वासना का बढ़ जाना। Excessive sexual desire.

Hypersomania (हाइपरसोमानिया) अत्यधिक सोना तथा आलस में पड़े रहना, अतिनिद्रा। Excessive sleeping or drowsiness.

Hypersplenism (हाइपरस्प्लीनिज्म) प्लीहा की अति सक्रियता। Increased activity of the spleen.

Hypersthenic (हाइपर्स्थीनिक) अतिबल वाला। Having great strength or tonicity.

Hypersthenuria (हाइपर्सथेनूरिया) बढ़ी हुई सान्द्रता का अर्थात् गाढ़े मूत्र का विसर्जन होना जो अधिकतर निर्जलीकरण अथवा पसीने में अत्यधिक तरल के निकल जाने के कारण होता है। Excretion of the urine of high concentration usually due to dehydration or excess loss of fluids in the sweat.

Hypersusceptibility
(हाइपरससेप्टीबिलिटी) आसानी से अधिक प्रभावित होने की अवस्था। The state of being affected greatly.

Hypertension (हाइपरटैन्शन) उच्च रक्त-चाप जिसमें सिस्टोलिक पारे के 140 मि.मि. से ऊपर तथा डायस्टोलिक पारे के 90 मि.मि. से ऊपर होता है। Increased blood pressure in which systolic is above 140 mm and diastolic is above 90 mm of mercury.

Hypertensor (हाइपरटैन्सर) रक्तचाप बढ़ाने वाला एक कारक। An agent raising the blood pressure.

Hyperthecosis (हाइपरथीकोसिस) डिम्बग्रन्थि में ग्राफी पुटकों की थीका या पिधान कोशिकाओं का अतिविकसन होना।

Hyperplasia of the theca cell of the Graafian follicles in the ovary.

Hyperthelia (हाइपरथीलिया) दो से अधिक चूचुकों का होना। Presence of more than two nipples.

Hyperthermia (हाइपरथर्मिया) तीव्र ज्वर या अतिज्वर, अतिताप। Hyperpyrexia or very high fever.

Hyperthrombinemia (हाइपरथ्रॉम्बिनीमिया) रक्त में थ्रोम्बिन का बढ़ जाना।

An excess of thrombin in the blood.

Hyperthymia (हाइपरथाइमिया) बहुत भावुक हो जाना। To become very emotional.

Hyperthyroidism (हाइपरथाइरॉयडिज्म) थॉयरॉइड ग्रन्थि की अत्यधिक बढ़ी हुई क्रियाशीलता जिसमें नेत्रोत्सेधी गलगण्ड हो जाता है जिसमें नेत्र गोलक बाहर को निकल जाते हैं। अणुट-अतिक्रियता। Hyperactivity of the thyroid gland marked by exophthalmic goiter in which the eyeballs are protrudeal the enlargement of thyroid gland.

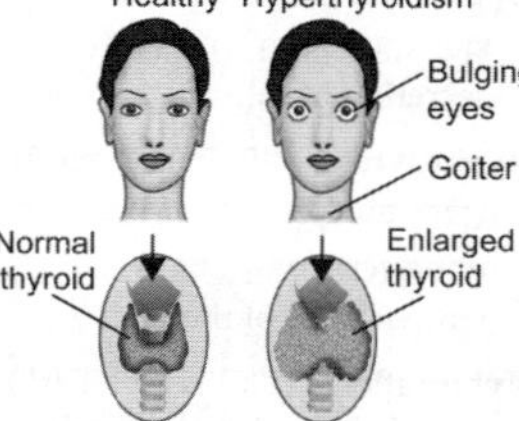

Hypertonia (हाइपरटोनिया) धमनियों अथवा पेशियों की तान बढ़ जाना, अतितानता। Increased tone of the arteries or muscle.

Hypertonic (हाइपरटोनिक) वह जिसकी तान बढ़ी होती है, अतितनावी। Having increased tone.

Hypertrichosis (हाइपरट्राइकोसिस) बालों का अधिक उगना, रोमातिवृद्धि, अतिरोमता।

Growth of hair in excess.

Hypertrophy (हाइपरट्रॉफी) शरीर का अस्वाभाविक रूप से

बढ़ना, अतिवृद्धि। Unnatural enlargement of a part or organ of the body.

Hyperuricemia (हाइपरयूरिसीमिया) रक्त में यूरिक अम्ल की अधिकता। Excess of uric acid in the blood.

Hypervascular (हाइपरवेस्कुलर) अतिवाहिकामय, अतिरक्तधर। Excess vascularity.

Hyperventilation (हाइपरवैन्टीलेशन) असामान्य रूप से बढ़ा हुआ फुफ्फुसीय संवातन, अतिसंवातन। Abnormally increased pulmonary ventilation.

Hyperviscosity (हाइपरविस्कोसिटी) अत्यधिक श्यानता अथवा चिपचिपाहट जैसे रक्त की। Excessive viscosity or adhering property as of the blood.

Hypervitaminosis (हाइपरविटामिनोसिस) किसी एक अथवा अधिक विटामिनों के अधिक खाने से उत्पन्न दशा, अतिविटामिनता। The condition caused by ingestion of one or more vitamins in excess.

Hypervolemia (हाइपरवोलेमिया) रक्तायतनवृद्धि, रक्तबहुलता। Increase in the circulating blood volume

Hipsisteno Cephalus (हिप्सीस्टेनो सिफैलस) एक ऊँचे और तंग सिर वाला। Having a high narrow head.

Hypesthesia (हाइपिसथिसिया) अल्पसमवेदित। Diminished sensitivity to stimulation.

Hypha (हाइफा) किसी कवक का कवकजाल बनाने वाले सूत्रों में से एक कवक तन्तु। One of the ligaments compassing the mycelium of a fungus.

Hyphema (हाइफीमा) नेत्र के अग्र कोष्ठ में रक्तस्राव होना, अग्रकक्षरक्तता। Hemorrhage in the anterior chamber of the eye.

Hypnagogic (हिप्नेगोगिक) निद्राकारी अथवा नींद लाने वाला। Hypnotic producing sleep.

Hypnagogic state (हिप्नेगोगिक स्टेट) सोने एवं जागने के बीच की अवस्था। A state between sleeping and awakening.

Hypnodontics (हिप्नोडोन्टिक्स) कृत्रिम निद्रा द्वारा किसी दन्त-रोग की चिकित्सा करना। The treatment of a dental disease by hypnosis.

Hypnology (हिप्नोलॉजी) निद्रा का वैज्ञानिक अध्ययन। Scientific study of sleep.

Hypnosis (हिप्नोसिस) कृत्रिम निद्रा, सम्मोहन। Artificial sleep.

Hypnotic (हिप्नोटिक) निद्राकर अथवा निद्रा लानेवाला। Inducing sleep.

Hypnotism (हिप्नोटिज्म) सम्मोहित करने की क्रिया। The act of induring hypnosis.

Hypoacidity (हाइपोएसिडिटी) आमाशय में हाइड्रोक्लोरिक अम्ल की कमी हो जाना। Deficiency of hydrochloric acid in the stomach.

Hypoacusis (हाइपोएकुसिस) ध्वनि उद्दीपनों के प्रति कुछ घटी हुई संवेदनशीलता। Slightly diminished sensitivity to sound stimuli.

Hypoalbuminemia (हाइपोएल्बुमिनिमिया) रक्त में एलब्यूमिन की कमी हो जाना, अल्पएल्ब्यूमिनरता। Decreased albumin in the blood.

Hypoaldosteronism (हाइपोएल्डोस्टेरोनिज्म) शरीर में एल्डोस्टेरोन की कमी हो जाना। Deficiency of aldosterone in the body.

Hypoalimentation (हाइपोएलीमेन्टेशन) अपर्याप्त पोषण। Insufficient nourishment.

Hypocalcemia (हाइपोकैल्सीमीया) रक्त में कैल्सियम घटकर सामान्य से नीचे हो जाना। Decrease of calcium in the blood below normal.

Hypocalciuria (हाइपोकैल्सियूरिया) मूत्र में कैल्सियम का घट जाना। Diminished calcium in the urine.

Hypocapnia (हाइपोकैप्निया) अल्पकैप्नियता। Decreased CO_2 in blood.

Hypochloremia (हाइपोक्लोरिमिया) अल्पक्लोरीनता। Decreased chloride content in blood.

Hypochlorhydria (हाइपोक्लोरहाइड्रिया) जठर-रस में हाइड्रोक्लोरिक एसिड की कमी होना। Deficiency of hydrochloric acid in the stomach.

Hypochlouria (हाइपोक्लोयूरिया) मूत्र में क्लोराइडों की कमी। Diminished chlorides in the urine.

Hypochondriac (हाइपोकॉण्ड्रियक) रोगभ्रम से ग्रस्त व्यक्ति। Person affected with hypochondriasis.

Hypochondrium (हाइपोकॉण्ड्रियम) अधः पर्शुकप्रदेश, कोख। Two superior regions of the abdomen just below the short ribs.

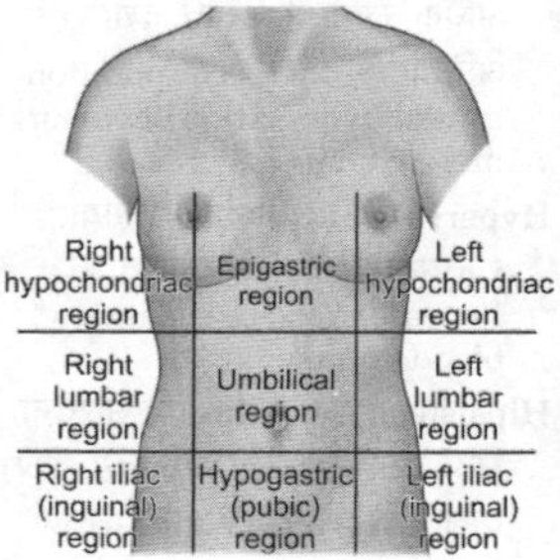

Hypochromasia (हाइपोक्रोमेसिया) लाल रक्त कोशिकाओं में हीमोग्लोबिन की कमी हो जाना। Deficiency of hemoglobin in the red blood cells.

Hypocinesia (हाइपोसाइनीसिया) चलने-फिरने की शक्ति कम हो जाना। Diminished power of movement.

Hypocorbia (हाइपोकार्बिया) रक्त में कार्बन डाइऑक्साइड की कमी हो जाना। Decreased CO_2 in blood.

Hypocythemia (हाइपोसाइथीमिया) रक्त में लाल रक्त कोशिकाओं की संख्या घट जाना। Deficiency in the number of red blood cells in the blood.

Hypodermic (हाइपोडर्मिक) त्वचा के नीचे प्रविष्ट जैसे कोई अधस्त्वक् या हाइपोडर्मिक इन्जैक्शन। Inserted under the skin as a hypodermic injection.

Hypodontia (हाइपोडॉन्शिया) दाँतों का विकास कम होना अथवा उनका पूर्ण अभाव। Diminished development or absence of teeth.

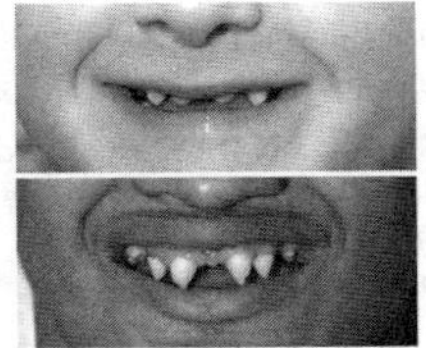

Hypodynamia (हाइपोडाइनेमिया) असामान्य रूप से घटी पेशीय शक्ति। Abnormally diminished muscular power.

Hypoergia (हाइपोएर्जिया) किसी भी उद्दीपन के प्रति संवेदनशीलता का कम हो जाना। Diminished sensitivity to any stimulus.

Hypoexophoria (हाइपोएक्सफोरिया) आँखो का नीचे एवं साइड की ओर घूम जाना। Deviation of the visual axes downward and laterally.

Hypofunction (हाइपोफंक्शन) अल्पक्रिया, कार्याल्पता। Decreased function

Hypogammaglobulinemia (हाइपोगामाग्लोबुलिनीमिया) रक्त में गामाग्लोबुलियों की कमी जो अर्जित अथवा जन्मजात हो सकती है। Deficiency of gammaglobulins in the blood which may be acquired or congenital.

Hypogastrium (हाइपोगैस्ट्रियम) उदर का निचला अन्दरूनी भाग। The lower interior part of the abdomen.

Hypogenetics (हाइपोजेनेटिक्स) शरीर की दोषपूर्ण रचना होने से सम्बन्धित। Pertaining to hypogonesis.

Hypoglossal (हाइपोग्लोसल) जीभ के नीचे स्थित। Situated below the tongue.

Hypoglottis (हाइपोग्लॉटिस) जीभ की निचली सतह। Under surface of the tongue.

Hypoglycemia (हाइपोग्लाइसीमिया) रक्त में ग्लूकॉज की कमी होना। Deficiency of glucose in the blood.

Hypohepatica (हाइपोहिपैटिका) यकृत के कार्य में कमी हो जाना। Deficient liver function.

Hypokalemia (हाइपोकेलीमिया) रक्त में पोटेशियम की कमी होना। Deficiency of potassium in the blood.

Hypokinesia (हाइपोकाइनीसिया) किसी उद्दीपन के प्रति प्रेरक प्रतिक्रिया या असामान्य रूप से कम हो जाना, अल्पगतिकता। Abnormally diminished motor reaction to a stimulus.

Hypolemmal (हाइपोलेमल) किसी झिल्ली के नीचे स्थित। Situated below a membrane.

Hypolipidemic (हाइपोलाइपीडेमिक) रक्त की लाइपिड सान्द्रता को कम करने वाला। Decrease the lipid concentration of the blood.

Hypoliposis (हाइपोलाइपोसिस) ऊतकों में वसा की कमी होना। Deficiency of fat in the tissue.

Hypomagnesemia (हाइपोमैग्नीसीमिया) रक्त में मैग्नीसियम की कमी होना। Deficiency of magnesium in the blood.

Hypomenorrhea (हाइपोमैनोरिह्या) ऋतुस्राव में कमी होना। Aligomenorrhea.

Hypomorph (हाइपोमॉर्फ) ऐसा व्यक्ति जिसकी धड़ की लम्बाई के अनुपात में टाँगे छोटी होती है। The person possessing short legs in proportion to the length of trunk.

Hyponatremia (हाइपोनेट्रीमिया) रक्त में सोडियम की कमी। Deficiency of sodium in the blood.

Hyponoia (हाइपोनोइया) मानसिक क्रिया का मन्द पड़ जाना। Sluggish mental activity.

Hypoparathyroidism (हाइपोपैराथायरॉयडिज्म) अल्पपरावटुता। A pathological state due to partial loss or insufficient parathyroid tissue.

Hypopharynx (हाइपोफेरिक्स) अधोग्रसनी, अधोकण्ड। Laryngopharynx.

Hypophoria (हाइपोफोरिया) एक आँख के दृष्टि अक्ष का नीचे की ओर झुक जाना। Downward deviation of the visual axis of one eye.

Hypophosphatemia (हाइपोफॉस्फेटीमिया) रक्त में

फॉस्फेटों की कमी। Deficiency of phosphates in the blood.

Hypophyseal (हाइपोफाइजीयल) पीयूष ग्रन्थि से सम्बन्धित। Pertaining to the pituitary gland.

Hypophysectomy (हाइपोफाइसैक्टमी) पीयूषिक उच्छेद। Excision of the pituitary gland.

Hypophysis (हाइपोफाइसिस) जतूक या स्फैनॉयड अस्थि के पर्याणिका या टर्शिका में स्थित एक अन्तःस्रावी ग्रन्थि जो अग्र एवं पश्च दो खण्ड़ों से बनी होती है जो पीयूषिका-वृन्त द्वारा मस्तिष्क के अधश्चेतक से जुड़े होते हैं, पीयूष ग्रन्थि। Hypophysis cerebri of of the pituitary gland on endocrine gland situated in the sella turcica of the sphenoid bone consisting of two portion anterior and posterior lake attached to hypothalamus of the brain by hypophyseal stalk.

Hypophysitis (हाइपोफाइजाइटिस) पीयूष ग्रन्थि की सूजन। Inflammation of the pituitary gland.

Hypopigmentation (हाइपोपिगमैन्टेशन) वर्णकता कम हो जाती है। Diminished pigmentation.

Hypopituitarism (हाइपोपिट्यूटेरिज्म) पीयूष ग्रन्थि से विशेषकर अग्र खण्ड से हॉर्मोनों के स्राव में कमी हो जाने से उत्पन्न दशा, पीयूषिका अल्पक्रियता। The condition resulting from diminition in the secretion of hormones from the pituitary gland especially from the anterior lobe.

Hypoposia (हाइपोपोसिया) तरलों का सेवन कम करना। Diminished intake of fluids.

Hypoproteinemia (हाइपोप्रोटीनिमिया) रक्त में प्रोटीन की कमी, अल्पप्रोटीनरक्तता। Deficiency of protein in the blood.

Hypopyon (हाइपोपायोन) नेत्र के अग्र कोष्ठ में पस इकट्ठा हो जाना। Accumulation of pus in the anterior chamber of the eye.

Hyposialadenitis (हाइपोसियालेडीनाइटिस) अवअधोहनुज लार-ग्रन्थि का शोथ। Inflammation of the submandibular salivary gland.

Hyposmia (हाइपोस्मिया) गन्ध संवेदनशीलता का कम हो जाना, अल्प-घ्राणता। Diminished sensitivity of smell.

Hypospodia (हाइपोस्पोडिया) मूत्र-मार्ग का जन्मजात पुरुष में शिश्न की निचली सतह पर तथा स्त्री में योनि में खुलना, अधोमूत्रमार्गता।

Opening of the urethra into the under surface of the penis in male and into the vagina in female congenitally.

Hyposthenia (हाइपोस्थीनिया) दुर्बलता कमजोरी। Weakness.

Hypostasis (हाइपोस्टेसिस) शरीर के किसी आश्रित भाग अथवा निचले अंगों में तरल पदार्थ या रक्त परिसंचरण का घट जाना, अधःस्थिति।
The accumulation of blood or its solid components in parts of an organ or body due to poor circulation.

Hyposynergia (हाइपोसिनर्जिया) शक्तिहीन सामंजस्य। Poor coordination.

Hypotension (हाइपोटेन्शन) प्रकुंचनीय तथा अनुशिथिलनीय रक्तदाब का सामान्य से कम हो जाना, अल्प-रक्तदाब। Abnormally low blood pressure.

Hypotensor (हाइपोटैन्सर) दाबह्रासी साधन। A hypotensive agent.

Hypothalamus (हाइपोथैलेमस) अधःश्चेतक। A part of the diencephalon below the thalamus.

Hypothenor (हाइपोथीनर) हथेली पर अल्जा हड्डी की ओर लघु अँगुली के नीचे स्थित एक मांसल उभार, कनिष्ठामूल। A fleshy eminence on the palm on the side of ulna bone below the little finger.

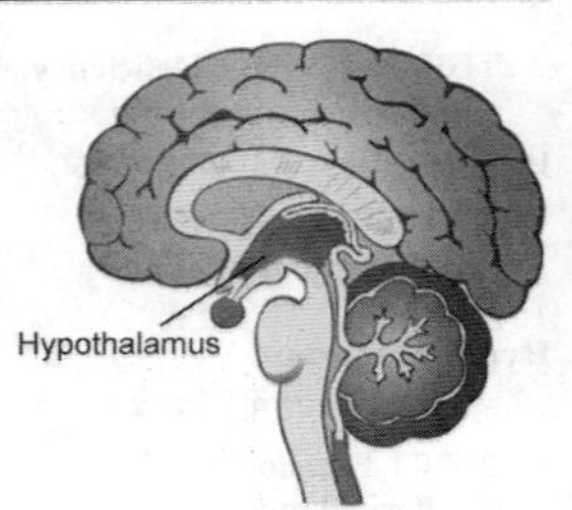

Hypothalamus

Hypothermia (हाइपोथर्मिया) अल्पोष्णता, उल्पताप, अल्पतप्तता। A state of lowered temperature of the body.

Hypothesis (हाइपोथीसिस) अनुमान या परिकल्पना। Supposition or assumption.

Hypothrombinemia (हाइपोथ्रॉम्बिनीमिया) रक्त में थ्रॉम्बिन की कमी होना। Deficiency of thrombin in the blood.

Hypothymism (हाइपोथाइमिज्म) थायमस ग्रन्थि की क्रियाशीलता में कमी हो जाना। Diminished activity of the thymus gland.

Hypothyroidism (हाइपोथाइरॉयडिज्म) अवटु ग्रन्थि की अपूर्ण क्रिया अथवा पूर्ण निष्क्रियता। Imperfect or complete loss of the function of the thyroid gland.

Hypotonia (हाइपोटोनिया) पेशियों की तान घट जाना, अल्पतनाव। Diminished tone of the muscles.

Hypotrichosis (हाइपोट्राइकोसिस) बालों की कमी होना, अल्परोमता। Deficiency of hair.

Hypotrophy (हाइपोट्रॉफी) शरीर के ऊतकों की वृद्धि अस्वाभाविक रूप से कम होना। Degeneration and atrophy of tissue.

Hypotympanum (हाइपोटिम्पैनम) मध्यकर्ण-गुहा का मध्य कर्ण-कला के स्तर से नीचे का भाग। The post of the cavity of the middle ear beneath the level of the tympanic membrane.

Hypouricuria (हाइपोयूरिकूरिया) मूत्र में यूरिक एसिड की कमी होना। Deficiency of uric acid in the urine.

Hypoventilation (हाइपोवैन्टीलेशन) फुफ्फुसीय वायुकोशों में प्रवेश करने वाली वायु की मात्रा कम हो जाना। Reduction in the amount of air entering to the pulmonary alveoli.

Hypovitaminosis (हाइपोविटामिनोसिस) भोजन में किसी विटामिन की कमी से उत्पन्न होने वाली दशा। The condition developed by the deficiency of a vitamin in the diet.

Hypovolemia (हाइपोवोलीमिया) शरीर मे खून की मात्रा कम होना, अल्पायतनरक्तता। Hypovolemia is a state of decreased blood volume.

Hypovolia (हाइपोवोलिया) जलांश का घट जाना। Diminished water content.

Hypoxemia (हाइपोक्सीमिया) रक्त का अपर्याप्त ऑक्सीकरण होना। Insufficient oxygenation of the blood.

Hypoxia (हाइपोक्सिया) शरीर के ऊतकों में ऑक्सीजन की कमी होना, अल्प-ऑक्सीजनता। Deficiency of oxygen in the body tissue.

Hypsokinesis (हिप्सोकाइनेसिस) खड़े होने पर पीछे को गिर जाना जैसा कि सकम्प पक्षाघात में देखा जाता है। To fall backward when standing. Seen in paralysis agitans.

Hypsophobia (हिप्सोफोबिया) ऊँचाई से डर। Fear of being at great heights.

Hystereurysis (हिस्टीरेयूरिसिस) गर्भाशय के मुँह का चौड़ा करना। Dilation of the mouth of the uterus.

Hysterography (हिस्टीरोग्रांफी) प्रसव काल में गर्भाशय के संकोचों की तीव्रता एवं उनकी बारम्बारता

का लेखा-चित्र अभिलेखन करना। Graphic recording of the frequency and intensity of the uterine contraction during labor.

Hysteria (हिस्टीरीया) स्नायु तन्त्र के आंगिक अथवा जैव रोग से रहित मानसिक वियोजन के फलस्वरूप उत्पन्न दशा जिसमें शारीरिक लक्षण एवं चिन्ह प्रकट होते हैं। A condition resulting from mental dissociation without organic disease of the nervous system presenting physical symptoms and sign.

Hysteroid (हिस्टीरॉयड) हिस्टीरिया के समान। Resembling tending towards hysteria.

Hysteric (हिस्टीरिक) हिस्टीरिया से ग्रस्त व्यक्ति। The person affected hysteria.

Hystero-oophorectomy (हिस्टीरो-ओफोरिक्टामी) एक या दोनों डिम्बग्रन्थियों के साथ गर्भाशय को काट कर अलग कर देना। Removal of the uterus with the one or both ovaries.

Hysterocele (हिस्टीरोसील) गर्भाशय का बहिःसरण या हर्निया। Hernia of the uterus.

Hysterectomy (हिस्टीरेक्टॉमी) गर्भाशय को शल्यक्रिया द्वारा काटकर अलग कर देना, गर्भाशयोच्छेदन। Surgical removal of the uterus.

Hysterogram (हिस्टोरोग्राम) गर्भाशय का एक्स-रे चित्र। X-ray film of the uterus.

Hysteromania (हिस्टीरॉमेनिया) स्त्रियों में सम्भोग की इच्छा का बढना, स्त्रीकामोन्माद। Lascivious, increased sexual desire in a woman.

Hysterometry (हिस्टीरोमीट्री) गर्भाशय के परिमाण को मापना। To measure the size of the uterus.

Hysteromyoma (हिस्टीरोमायोमा) गर्भाशय का पेश्याबुर्द अथवा तन्तुपेशीअबुर्द। Myoma or fibromyoma tumor of the uterus.

Hysteromyomectomy (हिस्टीरोमायोमेक्टॉमी) गर्भाशय के तान्तव अबुर्द को काटकर अलग करना। Excision of a fibroid tumor of the uterus.

Hysteropathy (हिस्टीरोपैथी) गर्भाशय का कोई भी रोग। Any disease of the uterus.

Hysterorrhaphy (हिस्टीरोरैह्फी) गर्भाशय की सिलाई करना। Suturing of the uterus.

Hysterorrhexis (हिस्टीरोरैह्क्सि) गर्भाशय का विशेषकर गर्भावस्था में फट जाना। Rupture of the uterus especially in pregnancy.

Hysterosalpingectomy (हिस्टीरोसेल्पिन्जेक्टॉमी) गर्भाशय–डिम्बवाहिनी उच्छेदन। To remove the uterus with the fallopian tube by surgery.

Hysterosalpingography (हिस्ट्रोसेल्पिन्जोग्राफी) गर्भाशय डिम्बवाहिनी चित्रण। Radiography of the uterus and fallopian tubes after introducing a radiopaque substance into these organs.

Hysterosalpingostomy (हिस्टीरोसेल्पिन्जोस्टॉमी) किसी डिम्ब वाहिनी का गर्भाशय के साथ सम्मिलन। Anastomosis of a fallopian tube with the uterus.

Hysteroscope (हिस्टीरोस्कॉप) जरायुदर्शी, गर्भाशयदर्शी। An instrument for visual examination of the uterine cavity.

Hysterospasm (हिस्टीरोस्पाज्म) गर्भाशय में ऐंठन आ जाना। Spasm of the uterus.

Hysterotomy (हिस्टीरोटॉमी) गर्भाशय में चीरा लगाना। To make an incision into the uterus.

Hysterotrachelectomy (हिस्टीरोटेकीलेक्टॉमी) गर्भाशयग्रीवा को काट कर अलग कर देना। Excision of the cervix of the uterus.

Hysterotrachelorrhaphy (हिस्ट्रोट्रेकीलोरैह्फी) गर्भाशयग्रीवा की सिलाई करना। Suturing of the uterine cervix.

Hysterotrachelotomy (हिस्टीरोट्रेकीलोटॉमी) गर्भाशयग्रीवा में चीरा लगाना। To make an incision into the uterine cervix.

Hysterovaginectomy (हिस्टीरोवेजाइनेक्टॉमी) गर्भाशययोनि-उच्छेदन। Excision of both uterus and vagina.

Hystriciasis (हिस्ट्रीसियसिस) बालों का एक रोग जिसमें वे सीधे खड़े रहते है, केशोनुत्तानता। A hair disease in which they stand in erect stage.

I

Iamatology (ऐमेटोलॉजी) औषधि-विज्ञान। Science of medicines.

Iateria (ऐटीरिया) चिकित्सा विधान। Therapeutics.

Iatraliptics (ऐट्रेलिप्टिक्स) मालिश द्वारा रोगों की चिकित्सा करना। Treatment of the disease by massage. (*i*) **Iatrogenic** (ऐट्रोजेनिक) औषधीय एंवम शल्य चिकित्सा क्रिया करते समय रोगी में कोई भी मानसिक रोग एंव शारीरिक रोग उत्पन्न हो जाना। Adverse body effect induced drug procedure of the doctor.

Ice-bag (आईस-बैग) बर्फ से भरी जलरूद्ध रबर की थैली जो किसी स्थान को ठण्डा करने के लिए प्रयोग में लायी जाती है। A water tight rubber bag containing ice used for applying cold locally.

Ichnogram (इक्नोग्राम) खड़े रहने की स्थिति में पाँव का लिया गया निशान। A footprint taken while standing.

Ichor (आइकोर) किसी जख्म से निकलने वाला पतला पानी जैसा बदबूदार स्राव। Thin fetid watery discharge from a wound.

Ichoremia (आइकोरीमिया) पूतिजीवरक्तता या रक्त विशाक्तता। Septicemia or blood poisoning.

Ichthyophobia (इक्थायोफोबिया) मछली का विकृत भय। Morbid fear of fish.

Ichthyosis (इक्थायोसिस) मछली के समान सूखी, खुरदरी। Fish like dry, rough.

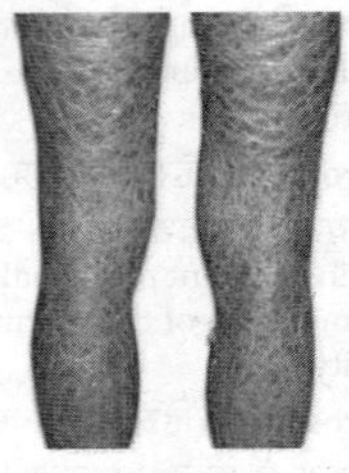

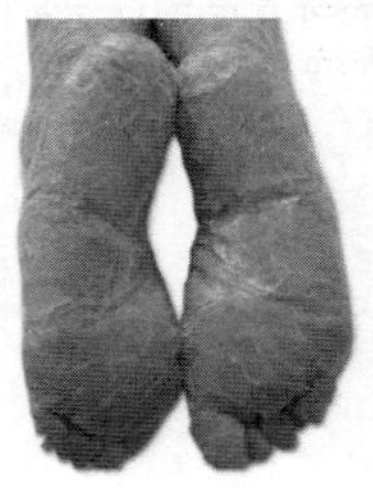

Ictal (इक्टल) आघात सम्बन्धी, आघातजनित । Relating to or caused by a stroke or seizure.

Icteric (इक्टेरिक) कामला से सम्बन्धित । Pertaining to jaundice.

Icterohepatitis (इक्टीरोहिपैटाइटिस) यकृत शोथ जिसके साथ कामला हो जाती है । Inflammation of the liver with jaundice.

Icteroid (इक्ट्रॉयड) कामला या पीलिया के समान । Resembling jaundice.

Icterus (इक्ट्रस) कामला या पीलिया । Jaundice.

Ictus (इक्टस) अचानक आक्रमण, मुक्का, धक्का या आघात । Sudden attack, stroke, blow or stroke.

Id (इड) रोग की मुख्य विक्षति से दूर प्रकट होने वाले त्वचा विस्फोट का संकेत देने वाला प्रत्यय । Suffix indicating a skin rash appearing remote from the main lesion of the disease.

Idea (आइडिया) भावना या विचार । A mental image or conception.

Ideal (आइडीयल) आदर्श रूप । Perfect type.

Ideation (आइडीएशन) सोचने अथवा विचार बनाने की क्रिया, चिन्तन । The process of thinking or formation of ideas.

Ideology (आइडीयोलॉजी) विचारों का विज्ञान । The science of ideas.

Idiocy (इडियोसी) जड़बुद्धिता, मूर्खता या मूढ़ता । A condition of severe mental deficiency.

Idioglossia (इडियोग्लोसिया) दोषयुक्त उच्चारण जिसमें अर्थहीन स्वर ध्वनियाँ निकलती हैं । Defective articulation with the emittance of meaningless vocal sound.

Idiopathic (इडियोपैथिक) बिना किसी ज्ञात कारण के उत्पन्न होने वाला, अज्ञात हेतुक । Occurring without any known cause.

Idiophrenic (इडियोफ्रेनिक) स्वमनोजात । Relating to or originating in the mind or brain alone.

Idiosyncrasy (इडियोसिन्क्रेसी) एक आदत अथवा शारीरिक या मानसिक गुण जिसके द्वारा कोई व्यक्ति दूसरों से भिन्न होता है । A habit or physical or mental peculiarity by which a person differs from others.

Idiot (इडियट) निर्बुद्धि अथवा पूर्ण मूर्ख, बेवकूफ, मूढ़ । A person with severe mental deficiency.

Idiotrophic (इडियोट्रॉफिक) अपना पोषण स्वयं प्राप्त करने की क्षमता रखने वाला । Capable of securing its own nourishment.

Idioventricular (इडियोवेन्ट्रिकुलर) हृदनिलयी, हृद्नियल सम्बन्धी । Pertaining to the cardiac ventricles.

Iduria (आयोडूरिया) आयोडीन का मूत्र में उत्सर्जित होना। Excretion of iodine in the urine.

Igneous (इग्नियस) अग्नि सम्बन्धी। Pertaining to or containing fire.

Ilectomy (इलियक्टॉमी) शेशान्त्रोच्छेदन। Excision of the ileum.

Ileitis (इलियाइटिस) इलियम का शोथ। Inflammation of the ileum.

Ileocecostomy (इलियोसीकास्टॉमी) इलियम एवं सेकम के बीच शल्य-क्रिया द्वारा एक छिद्र बनाना। Surgical formation of an opening between the ileum and the cecum.

Ileocolitis (इलियोकोलाइटिस) इलियम एवं कोलन की सूजन। Inflammation of the ileum and colon.

Ileocolostomy (इलियोकोलोस्टॉमी) शल्य-क्रिया द्वारा इलियम एवं कोलन के बीच सम्मिलन। Surgical anastomosis between the ileum and the colon.

Ileoileostomy (इलियोइलियोस्टॉमी) इलियम के एक भाग एवं दूसरे भाग के बीच सम्मिलन। Anastomosis between one

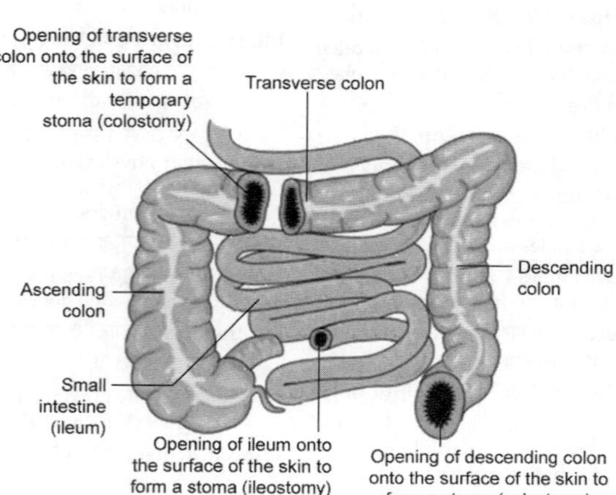

Ileocolostomy

part and the other part of the ileum.

Ileorrhaphy (इलियोरैह्फी) इलियम की सिलाई करना। Suture of the ileum.

Ileostomy (इलियोस्टॉमी) शल्य-क्रिया द्वारा उदर-भित्ति से होकर इलियन में से एक मार्ग बनाना, शेषान्त्रछिद्रीकरण। Surgical formation of a passage through the abdominal wall into ileum.

Ileotomy (इलियोटॉमी) इलियम में एक चीरा लगाना। To make an incision into the ileum.

Ileus (इलियस) आन्त्रवरोध, आँत में रूकावट पैदा हो जाना। Intestinal obstruction.

Iliac (इलियक) इलियम या श्रोणिफलक सम्बन्धी। Pertaining to the ileum.

Iliac crest (इलियक क्रेस्ट) कूल्हा, इलियम हड्डी का ऊपरी स्वतन्त्र किनारा। Hip, upper free margin of the iliac bone.

Iliac fossa (इलियक फोसा) श्रोणि की इलियक या श्रोणिफलक के गड्ढों में से एक। One of the depression of the iliac bone of the pubis.

Iliac region (इलियक रीजन) अधोजठर प्रदेश अथवा हाइपोगैस्ट्रियम के किसी भी ओर का वंक्षण क्षेत्र। Inguinal region on either side of the hypogastrium.

Iliac spine (इलियक स्पाइन) इलियम के चार कंटकों में से कोई सा एक जिनके नाम अग्रज एवं पश्चज अधोवर्ती कंटक तथा अग्रज एवं पश्चज अर्ध्ववर्ती कंटक है। Anyone of the four spines of the ileum, normally the anterior and posterior inferior spines; and the anterior and posterior superior spines.

Iliofemoral (इलियोफीमोरल) इलियक एवं फीमर हड्डी से सम्बन्धी। Pertaining to the iliac and the femur bone.

Iliosciatic (इलियोसियाटिक) इलियम एवं इस्कियम सम्बन्धी। Pertaining to the ileum and ischium.

Illness (इलनैस) बीमारी या रोग, अस्वस्थता। Sickness, unhealthiness.

Illumination (इल्युमिनेशन) शरीर के किसी भाग अथवा अंग का या किसी वस्तु का निरीक्षण करने हेतु उसे प्रदीप्त करना, प्रदीप्ति। The lighting up of a part or an organ of the body or an object for inspection.

Illusion (इल्यूज़न) भ्रम, भ्रांति। False perception.

Ima (इमा) सबसे नीचे। Lowest.

Image (इमेज) किसी वस्तु की तस्वीर जैसे कि किसी लैन्स अथवा शीशे में दिखाई देती है, प्रतिबिम्ब। The picture of an object such as that produced by a lense or mirror.

Imagination (इमेजिनेशन) उन वस्तुओं, व्यक्तियों अथवा स्थानों के विषय में विचार बनाना जिनका पहले से कोई पता नहीं होता, मन की कल्पना। The formation of ideas about the things, person or places which are not known previously.

Imaging (इमेजिंग) नेदानिक उद्देश्यों से किसी तस्वीर अथवा प्रतिबिम्ब का बनाना। The production of a picture or an image for diagnostic purpose.

Imbalance (इम्बैलेन्स) असंतुलन। Out of balance.

Imbecile (इम्बेसाइली) जड़बुद्धि, अल्पबुद्धि, अल्पमति। Feeble in mind.

Imbibition (इम्बीबिशन) किसी ठोस के द्वारा द्रव का अवशोषण होना, अन्तः शोषण। Absorption of fluid by a solid.

Imbricated (इम्ब्रीकेटेड) एक दूसरे के ऊपर चढ़े हुए। Overlapping like.

Immature (इम्मेच्योर) अपरिपक्व। Not fully developed.

Immedicable (इमेडिकेबिल) असाध्य, जख्म जो भरा ना जा सकता है। The wound which cannot be healed.

Immersion (इमर्सन) शरीर को पानी या अन्य तरल में डुबो देना। The dipping of the body under water or the fluid.

Immiscible (इम्मिससाइबल) मिश्रण के अयोग्य। Not capable of being mixed.

Immobility (इम्मोबीलीटी) अकड़न, जकड़न, ऐंठन। Incapable of motion.

Immobilization (इम्मोबिलाइजेशन) शरीर के किसी भाग को गति करने के अयोग्य बनाने की क्रिया। The process of making a part unable to move.

Immune (इम्यून) शारीरिक द्रवों में उत्पन्न एण्टीबॉडियों अथवा कोशिकीय रोगक्षमता का उत्पन्न होना, रोगक्षम। Protected from or resistant to a disease due to the formation of humoral antibodies.

Immunifacient (इम्यूनिफेसिएन्ट) रोगक्षमकारी, प्रतिरक्षाकारी। Producing immunity.

Immunity (इम्यूनिटी) रोगक्षमता। The capacity of the body to resist infection.

(*i*) **Cellular immunity** (सेलुलर-इम्यूनिटी) उपार्जित रोगक्षमता

जिसमें लिम्फोसाइट के कार्य की प्रधानता होती है, कोशिकीय रोगक्षमता। Acquired immunity in which the rate of the lymphocytes predominates.

(*ii*) **Congenital immunity** (कॉनजेनाइटल इम्यूनिटी) जन्मजात रोगक्षमता। Immunity present since birth.

Immunization (इम्यूनाइजेशन) किसी रोग की रोगक्षमता बनाने अथवा किसी व्यक्ति के रोगक्षमता बनने की क्रिया, रोगक्षमीकरण। The process of rendering a patient immune or of becoming immune.

Immuno (इम्यूनो) रोगक्षम, रोगक्षमता का संकेत देने वाला एक उपसर्ग। A prefix indicating immune, immunity.

Immunoassay (इम्यूनोएसे) शरीर के तरलों में प्रोटीनों की मात्रा को मापना जिनका सम्बन्ध किसी एण्टिजन के अपनी विशिष्ट एण्टीबॉडी के साथ प्रतिक्रिया करने से होता है। Measure the amount of proteins in the body fluid concerned with the reaction of an antigen with its specific antibody.

Immunobiology (इम्यूनोबायोलॉजी) जीव-विज्ञान की वह शाखा जिसमें संक्रामक रोगों, अंगों के प्रतिरोपण, एलर्जी, स्वरोगक्षमता तथा कैन्सर आदि के प्रति रोगक्षम अनुक्रिया का अध्ययन किया जाता है। The branch of biology dealing with the study of immune response to the infections disease, transplantation of organs, allergy, autoimmunity and cancer, etc.

Immunochemistry (इम्यूनोकैमिस्ट्री) रोगक्षमीकरण का रसायनशास्त्र। Chemistry of immunization.

Immunocompetence (इम्यूनोकॉम्पीटैन्स) किसी एण्टिजन के उद्दीपन के प्रति किसी रोगक्षम अनुक्रिया को उत्पन्न करने की क्षमता। Capability of developing an immune response to stimulation by an antigen.

Immunocyte (इम्यूनोसाइट) कोई भी लिम्फॉयड कोषिका जो एण्टिजन से प्रतिक्रिया करके एण्टीबॉडी उत्पन्न करती है। Any lymphoid cell reacting with the antigen to produce antibody.

Immunodiagnosis (इम्यूनोडायग्नोसिस) विशिष्ट रोगक्षम अनुक्रियाओं का प्रयोग करके रोगों का निदान करना। To make diagnosis of the disease by using specific immune response.

Immunoelectrophoresis (इम्यूनोइलैक्ट्रोफोरेसिस) विधुतकण-

संचालन द्वारा शरीर के तरलों में प्रोटीन एवं एण्टीबॉडियों की मात्रा एवं उनकी विशिष्टता की जाँच करने की एक विधि। A method of investigating the amount and character of protein and antibodies in the body fluid by electrophoresis.

Immunofluorescence (इम्यूनोफ्लूओरेसैन्स) प्रतिदिप्ति या फ्लुओरेसैन्स द्वारा ऊतकों में एण्टिजन के स्थान का पता लगाने वाली एक विधि। A method of determining the location of antigen in the tissue by fluorescence.

Immunogen (इम्यूनोजन) कोई भी पदार्थ जो किसी एण्टीबॉडी के बनने को प्रोत्साहित करता है। Any substance which stimulates the formation of an antibody.

Immunogenetics (इम्यूनोजेनेटिक्स) किसी व्यक्ति की रोक्षम अनुक्रिया को नियन्त्रित करने वाले जीनी या आनुवंशिक कारकों का तथा इन कारकों के पीढ़ी दर पीढ़ी संचरण अध्ययन। The study of the genetic factor controlling the immune response of a person and the transmission of these factors from generation.

Immunogenic (इम्यूनोजेनिक) रोगक्षमता उत्पन्न करने वाला, रोगक्षमताजनक। Producing immunity.

Immunogenicity (इम्यूनोजेनीसिटी) रोगक्षमता उत्पन्न करने का किसी पदार्थ का गुण, रोगक्षमताजनकता। The property of a substance to produce immunity.

Immunoglobulin (इम्यूनोग्लोबुलिन) लिम्फोसाइटों तथा प्लाज्मा कोशिकाओं से बनने वाली एक प्रकार की प्रोटीन जो एण्टीबॉडी के रूप में कार्य करती है एवं सीरम तथा शरीर के अन्य तरलों एवं ऊतकों में पायी जाती है। A type of the protein acting as an antibody formed by the lymphocytes and plasma cells found in the serum and in another body fluid and tissue.

Immunohematolgy (इम्यूनोहीमैटोलोजी) स्वरोगक्षम एवं रक्त रोगों का अध्ययन। The study of the autoimmune and blood disease.

Immunology (इम्यूनोलॉजी) रोगक्षमता के सभी पहलुओं का अध्ययन रोगक्षमताविज्ञान। The study of all the aspects of immunity.

Immunopathology (इम्यूनोपैथोलॉजी) रोगों के प्रति रोगक्षम अनुक्रिया के फलस्वरूप ऊतकों में होने वाले परिवर्तनों का अध्ययन। The study of the changes in the tissue resulting from immune response to disease or allergic reactions.

Immunopathy (इम्यूनोपैथी) रोगक्षमता विकृति। An immunity disorder.

Immunostimulant (इम्यूनोस्टिमुलैन्ट) एण्टीबॉडी के बनने को उत्तेजित करने वाला पदार्थ। A substance stimulating the formation of antibody.

Immunostimulation (इम्यूनोस्टिमुलेशन) किसी रोगक्षम अनुक्रिया का उत्तेजित होना। Stimulation of an immune response.

Immunosuppresant (इम्यूनोसप्रेसैन्ट) रोगक्षम अनुक्रिया को कम करने वाला। Suppressing immune response.

Immunotherapy (इम्यूनोथिरेपी) पहले से निर्मित एण्टीबॉडी के प्रयोग से किसी व्यक्ति का रोगक्षमीकरण करना। Immunization of a person by the administration of the performed antibodies.

Immunotoxin (इम्यूनोटॉक्सिन) एक प्रतिजीवविष। An antitoxin.

Immunotropic (इम्यूनोट्रॉपिक) रोगक्षम अनुक्रिया को बढ़ाने वाला। Enhancing the immune response.

Impaction (इम्पैक्शन) कसकर फँसे रहने की अवस्था, अंतर्घट्टन। The condition of being tightly wedged.

Impalpable (इम्पैल्पेबिल) स्पर्श करने से जिसका पता न चलता हो। Not detectable by touch.

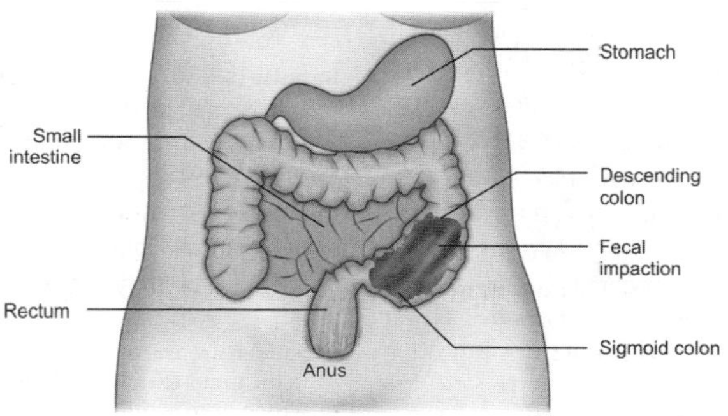

Impaction

Imperative (इम्प्रेटिव) अनैच्छिक, जो अपनी इच्छा से नियन्त्रित न किया जा सके। Involuntary, not controlled by the will.

Imperception (इम्परसेप्सशन) कोई विचार बनाने में असमर्थता। Inability to form an idea.

Imperforate (इम्पर्फोरेट) अछिद्री, छिद्रहीन। Without an opening.

Imperforation (इम्पर्फोरेशन) छिद्रहीन होने अथवा बन्द रहने की अवस्था। The state of being without opening or being blood.

Impervious (इम्पर्वियस) अप्रवेश्य, अगम्य। Impenetrable.

Impetigo (इम्पेटिगो) पीब वाली फुंसियों से युक्त चर्म रोग, सपूयचर्मस्फोट। A superficial highly contagious skin infection.

Implant (इमप्लान्ट) निरोपित अथवा निवेशित। To graft or insert.

Implosion (इमप्लोजन) आकस्मिक निपात। A sudden collapse.

Imponderable (इम्पौण्डेरेबिल) जिसे तौला अथवा नापा न जा सकता हो जैसे गर्मी। Unable to be weighed or measured as heat.

Impotent (इम्पोटैन्ट) नपुंसक, नामर्द। Sexual weak man to active penile erection.

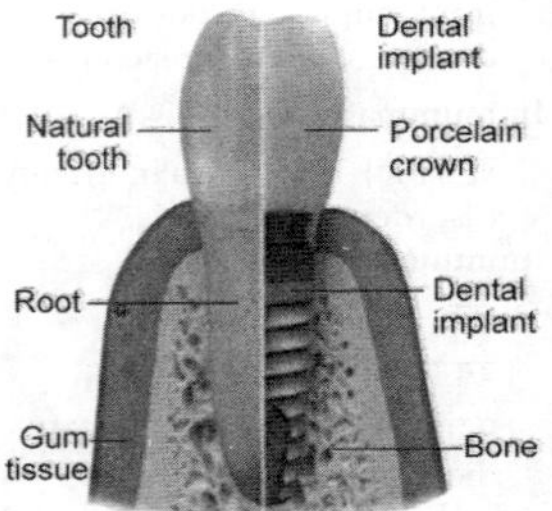

Implant (tooth implant)

Impregnate (इम्प्रीग्नेट) गर्भाधान करना, संसेचन करना। To render pregnant, cause to conceive.

Impression (इम्प्रेशन) एक अंग की सतह पर दूसरे अंग के पकड़ने वाले दबाव से हल्का-सा गड्ढा। A slight depression made on the surface of an organ by pressure exerted by another.

Impulse (इम्पल्स) अचानक बलपूर्वक आगे को ढकेलने की क्रिया। The act of driving forward with sudden force.

Impulsion (इमपल्सन) कुछ गलत कार्य एंवम अपराध करने के लिए विचार उत्पन्न होना। Sudden arousal of an idea in the mind to do something wrong or to commit crime.

In dies (इन डाइज) प्रतिदिन। Daily.

In extremis (इन एक्ट्रीमिस) मृत्यु के क्षण, मरणासन्न। At the point of death.

In situ (इन सिटू) अपने सामान्य स्थान में, उद्‌गम स्थान में सीमित। In its normal place, confined to the site of origin.

In utero (इन यूटिरो) गर्भाशय के अन्दर। Inside the uterus.

In vitro (इन वाइटरो) अन्तःकाचपत्री, कांच के अन्दर, कृत्रिम वातावरण में। In the glass, in an artificial environment.

In vivo (इन वाइवो) जीवित ऊतक के अन्दर अन्तर्जीवी। In the living body or tissue.

Inaction (इनेक्शन) किसी उद्‌दीपन के प्रति अनुक्रिया बिल्कुल न होना अथवा कम होना। Total absence of or decreased response to any stimulus.

Inactivate (इनएक्टिवेट) निष्क्रिय कर देना, विनाश, नष्ट । Destruction, destroy.

Inanimate (इनैनिमेट) निर्जीव, मृत। Lifeless, dead.

Inanition (इनैनीशन) लम्बे समय तक उपवास करने अथवा अल्प पोषण द्वारा उत्पन्न क्षीणता की अवस्था। A debilitated condition due to prolonged starvation or under nutrition.

Inappetence (इनैप्पीटैन्स) खाना खाने की इच्छा न होना या भूख न लगना। Lack of desire for food or loss of appetite.

Inarticulate (इनार्टिकुलेट) सन्धियों से रहित। Having no joints.

Inassimilable (इनएसिमिलेबल) स्वांगीकरण योग्य न हो अथवा शरीर के द्वारा जिसका उपयोग न हो सकता हो। Not assimible or which is unable to be utilized by the body.

Incarcerated (इन्कार्सिरेटेड), बाधित। Confined, constricted, strangulated.

Incarceration (इन्कार्सिरेशन) सीमित करना, संकुचन। Confinement constriction or imprisonment.

Incest (इनसेस्ट) खूनी रिश्तों से लैंगिक सम्भोग करना। Sexual intercourse between blood relations.

Inchondritis (इनकॉण्ड्राइटिस) किसी तन्तूपास्थि का शोथ। Inflammation of a fibrocartilage.

Incidence (इनसिडेन्स) आघटन, आंकड़ा। The number of new cases of a disease in a population over period of time.

Incineration (इन्साइनेरेशन) अग्नि द्वारा नष्ट होना। Destruction by fire.

Incinerator (इन्साइनेरेटर) अग्नि द्वारा नष्ट करने वाला, भस्मक। Destroying by fire.

Incipient (इनसिपियेन्ट) आरंभमाण, प्रारम्भिक। Commencing, beginning.

Incise (इन्साइज) तेज औजार से काटना। To cut with a sharp instrument.

Incisor (इन्सीजर) युवा व्यक्ति के प्रत्येक जबड़े के अगले चार काटने वाले दांतों में से एक, कृतन्क। One of the four front cutting teeth in each jaw of an adult.

Incisura (इन्सीजूरा) भंगिका। An incision, a slit or notch.

Inclination (इनक्लीनेशन) सामान्य से झुकाव अथवा लम्बरूप से झुकाव। Leaning from the normal or from the vertical.

Inclusion (इन्क्लूजन) अन्तर्वेशन, अन्तर्विष्ट। The state of being enclosed or included.

Inclusion bodies (इन्क्लूजन बॉडीज) निस्पन्दी अथवा छनने योग्य विषाणुओं के संक्रमण में कुछ कोशिकाओं के कोशिका द्रव्य के केन्द्रक में स्थित पिण्ड, अन्तःस्थ पिण्ड। The bodies present in the nuclear of cytoplasm of certain cells in the infection of filterable viruses.

Incoagulability (इनकौगुलेबिलिटी) जमने में असमर्थता। Inability to be coagulated.

Incoherence (इनकोहीरैन्स) असंगति, असम्बद्धता। The condition of being not connected.

Incoherent (इनकोहीरैन्ट) जो चिपका हुआ न हो, असंलग्न। Not adherent, disjointed.

Incombustible (इनकोम्ब्यूस्टीबल) अदह्य, अदहनीय, दुर्दह्य। Incapable of being burnt.

Incompatible (इनकॉम्पैटिबल) विरोधी कार्य करने वाला। Not being in harmony.

Incompetence (इनकॉम्पीटैन्स) शरीर के किसी अंग अथवा भाग की सामान्य कार्य ठीक प्रकार से करने में अक्षमता। Inability of an or part of the body to perform normal function properly.

Incompetent (इनकॉम्पीटैन्ट) वैधानिक रूप से अपने कार्य करने में अक्षम व्यक्ति जो मन्द बुद्धि अथवा पागल हो सकता है, अक्षम। Legally unable person to perform his/her duties who may be mentally retarded or insane.

Incontinence (इनकॉन्टीनैन्स) मस्तिष्क अथवा सुषुम्ना रज्जु में हुई क्षति के कारण या अवरोधिनी अथवा संकोचिनी पर नियन्त्रण न रहने के कारण उत्सर्गी पदार्थों। Inability to retain the excretory products such as urine, feces, semen or milk, etc. due to loss of sphincter control. (*i*) **Fecal incontinence** (फीकल इनकॉन्टीनैन्स) मल एवं वायु का अनियन्त्रित रूप से निकलना। Involuntary passage of feces and flatus.

Incontinence of milk (इनकॉन्टीनैन्स ऑफ मिल्क) अत्यधिक दुग्ध स्राव होना। Excessive milk flow.

Incoordination (इनकोआर्डिनेशन) शरीर के परस्पर सम्बन्धित अंगों एवं भागों का एक दूसरे के साथ मिलकर कार्य न करना, असमंजन। Nonfunctioning harmoniously of the interrelated organs and parts of the body.

Incorporation (इनकॉर्पोरेशन) दो या अधिक पदार्थो का संयुक्त होकर एक समांग पिण्ड बनाना, संयोजन। Combination of two or more substances to form homogeneous most.

Increment (इनक्रिमेन्ट) वृद्धि। A change in the value of a variable.

Incrustation (इनक्रस्टेशन) पपड़ियों, खुरन्ट अथवा परतों का बनना, पर्पटीभवन। Formation of trusts, scabs or scales.

Incubation (इनक्यूबेशन) संक्रमण से लेकर रोगलक्षण प्रकट होने तक की अवधि। The period that elapses between the introduction of morbid principle into the system and the development of disease.

Incubator (इनकयूबेटर) ऊष्मायन। A device for rearing prematurely born children or for the cultivation of bacteria.

Incudiform (इनक्यूडीफोर्म) इनकस हड्डी की आकृति वाला। Incus shaped.

Incurable (इनक्योरेबल) असाध्य, ठीक न होने वाला। The disease which cannot be cured.

Incus (इनकस) मध्यकर्ण की तीन में से एक कोमल हड्डी, स्थूणक। The name of one of the three ossicles of the middle ear.

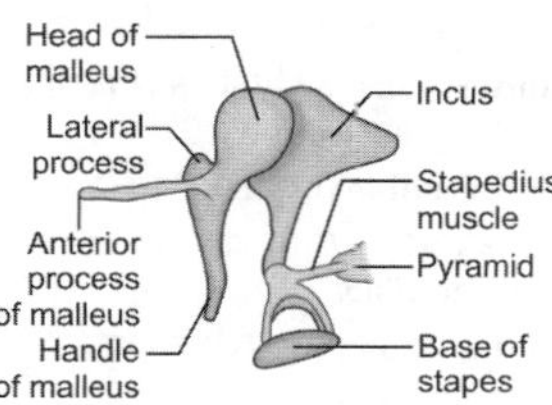

Indentation (इन्डैन्टेशन) एक खाँचा, दाँत अथवा गड्डा। A notch or depression.

Index (इण्डैक्स) हाथ की प्रथम अथवा तर्जनी अँगुली। The first or forefinger.

Indian hemp (इण्डियन हैम्प) भाँग। Cannabis indica.

Indicator (इण्डीकेटर) रासायनिक विश्लेषण में कोई पदार्थ जो कर्ण

परिवर्तन द्वारा तथा किसी pH की उपलब्धि पर किसी रसायन के प्रकट होने अथवा उसके लुप्त होने का संकेत देता है, संकेतक। In chemical analysis, a substance which indicate the appearance or disappearance of a chemical by color change or attainment of a certain pH.

Indifferent (इनडिफ्रैन्ट) सामान्य उद्दीपनों के प्रति अनुक्रिया न करने वाला, अविभेदी। Not responsive to normal stimuli.

Indiffusible (इन्डिफ्यूजिबल) अविसरणीय। Unable to be diffused.

Indigenous (इण्डीजीनस) स्वदेशीय। Native to country.

Indigestible (इन्डाइजेस्टिबल) अपाच्य, न पचने योग्य। Not digestible.

Indigestion (इन्डाइजेशन) भोजन का पाचन न होना। Failure of digestion.

Indium (इण्डियम) एक धातु तत्व। A metallic element.

Indole (इण्डोल) मल में पाया जाने वाला एक ठोस, स्फटिकाम पदार्थ जो आँत में ट्रिन्प्टोफेन के जीवाणुज विघटन का उत्पाद होता है और जिससे मल से एक विशेष प्रकार की गंध आती है। A solid crystalline substance, the product of bacterial decomposition of tryptophan in odor in the intestine found in the feces by a peculiar odor arise from the feces.

Indolent (इण्डोलैन्ट) आलसी या सुस्त, अकर्मण्य। Lazy inactive.

Indolent ulcer (इन्डोलैन्ट अल्सर) वह जख्म जो धीरे-धीरे भरता है परन्तु उसमें दर्द नहीं होता। The ulcer that heals slowly but it is not painful.

Induction (इन्डक्शन) कुछ कराने की क्रिया, प्रेरण जैसे गर्भाशय संकोचक औषधियों का प्रयोग करके प्रसव कराना। The process of using something as induction of labor by the use of oxytocic drugs.

Inductor (इन्डक्टर) प्रेरक, संचालक। An agent bringing about induction, an organism.

Inductotherm (इन्डक्टोथर्म) विद्युत धारा ज्वर उत्पन्न करने वाला एक उपकरण, ज्वर प्रेरक उपकरण। An apparatus for producing fever by electricity.

Indurated (इन्ड्यूरेटेड) सख्त किया गया। Hardened.

Induration (इन्ड्यूरेशन) कठोर या सख्त बनाने की क्रिया। Process of hardening.

Indwelling (इण्ड्वैलिंग) लम्बे समय तक शरीर के भीतर रहने वाला,

जैसे निकास नली। Remaining inside the body as a catheter.

Inebriant (इनेब्रिएन्ट) कोई भी मादक वस्तु। An intoxicant.

Inebriation (इनेब्रिएशन) शराब पीने की आदत। Drunkness, habit of drinking liquor.

Inelastic (इनैलास्टिक) जो लचीला न हो। Not elastic.

Inert (इनर्ट) निष्क्रिय, रसायन विज्ञान में, दूसरे रसायनों से प्रतिक्रिया न करने वाला। Inactive in chemistry not reacting with other chemical.

Inertia (इनर्शिया) निष्क्रियता, जड़त्व अथवा स्वतः गतिशीलता में असमर्थता। Inactivity or inability to move spontaneously.

Infancy (इन्फैन्सी) जीवन के प्रारम्भ के एक वर्ष का काल, शैशव। The period of first one year of life.

Infant (इन्फैन्ट) जन्म से लेकर एक वर्ष तक की आयु का बच्चा, शिशु। The child from the time of birth to one year of age. (*i*) **Newborn infant** (न्यूबौर्न इन्फैन्ट) जन्म के पश्चात् प्रथम दो से चार सप्ताह की अवधि का शिशु। The infant during the first two to four weeks after birth. (*ii*) **Preterm infant** (प्रीटर्म इन्फैन्ट) गर्भावस्था के 37वें सप्ताह की पूर्ण होने से पूर्व पैदा होने वाला शिशु। The infant born before the completion of 37th weeks of pregnancy.

Infanticide (इन्फैन्टीसाइड) किसी शिशु को मारने वाला। The killer of an infant.

Infantile (इन्फैन्टाइल) शैशव अथवा किसी शिशु से सम्बन्ध। Pertaining to infancy or an infant.

Infantilism (इन्फैन्टीलिज्म) शिशुता, शैशव। The persistence of infantile characteristics into the adult life.

Infarct (इन्फार्क्ट) शरीर के किसी ऊतक का वह स्थान जिसकी धमनीय रक्त आपूर्ति रूक जाने से उसका परिगलन हो जाता है। Area of necrosis consequent to cessation of blood supply.

Infarctectomy (इन्फार्कटेक्टॉमी) शल्य-क्रिया द्वारा किसी रोधगतिलांश को निकाल देना। Surgical removal of an infarct.

Infarction (इन्फार्कशन) किसी रोधगतिलांश का बनना या रोधगलन। The formation of an infarct.

Infect (इन्फैक्ट) संक्रमण होना या करना। The communication of a disease.

Infected (इनफैक्टेड) संक्रमण से ग्रसित, संक्रमित। Affected with infection.

Infection (इनफैक्शन) संक्रमण, संसर्ग, उपसर्ग, छूत की बीमारी।

Invasion of the body by the germs, viruses or parasites. (*i*) **Acute infection** (एक्यूट इनफैक्शन) कुछ देर के लिए अचानक होने वाला संक्रमण। The infection occurring suddenly for short duration. (*ii*) **Chronic infection** (क्रोनिक-इनफैक्शन) जीर्ण संक्रमण। Infection of long duration. (*iii*) **Fungus infection** (फन्गास-इनफैक्शन) किसी कवक द्वारा उत्पन्न संक्रमण। Infection caused by a fungus.

Infectious (इन्फैक्शियस) संक्रमण उत्पन्न करने वाला संक्रमक। Causing infection.

Infective (इन्फैक्टिव) संक्रमण उत्पन्न करने में सक्षम, संक्रमी। Capable of producing infection.

Infecundity (इन्फैकण्डिटी) स्त्री में बांझपन, बध्यता। Barrenness sterility in woman.

Inferiority complex (इन्फीरियरिटी कॉम्पलैक्स) हीन भावना। Feeling on oneself inferior to others.

Infestation (इन्फैस्टेशन) कष्ट, दुःख। Trouble.

Infiltration (इन्फिल्ट्रेशन) किसी पदार्थ की किसी ऊतक अथवा पदार्थ से होकर गुजरने एवं किसी कोशिका, ऊतक अथवा अंग में जमा होने कि क्रिया। इस प्रकार जमा हुआ पदार्थ भी, अन्तःसंचरण। The process of passing of a substance through a tissue or a substance and being deposited in a cell tissue or an organ also the material so deposited. (*i*) **Adipose infiltration** (एडीपोस इन्फिल्ट्रेशन) वसीय अतःसंचरण, ऊतकों में वसा या चर्बी का जमा होना। Falty infiltration deposition of fat in the tissue.

Infirmary (इन्फर्मरी) जीर्णरोगीशाला। A place in a large institution for the care of those who are ill.

Inflammation (इन्फ्लेमेशन) शरीर के किसी भाग की लाली या सूजन, जिसके साथ प्रायः उत्राप, दर्द और ज्वर विद्यमान रहता है, शोथ प्रदाह। A redness or swelling of any part of the body usually attended with heat pain and fever. (*i*) **Acute inflammation** (एक्यूट इन्फ्लेमेशन) अचानक उत्पन्न होने एवं कुछ ही काल के लिए रहने वाला शोथ, तीव्र शोथ। Inflammation of sudden onset and of short duration. (*ii*) **Fibrinous inflammation** (फाइब्रिनस इन्फ्लेमेशन) शोथ जिसके निःस्राव में अत्यधिक मात्रा में फाइब्रिन होता है, फाइब्रिनी

शोथ। Inflammation marked by exudates containing a great amount of fibrin.

Inflation (इन्फ्लेशन) फुलाव अथवा शरीर के किसी अंग अथवा भाग को वायु, गैस अथवा तरल से फुलाने की क्रिया, वातस्फीति। Distention or the act of distending an organ or part of the body with air gas or fluid.

Inflator (इन्फ्लेटर) वायु से किसी अंग को फुलाने वाला एक उपकरण। An apparatus for distending an organ with air.

Inflection (इन्फ्लेक्शन) अन्दर की ओर मुड़ा हुआ, अन्तर्गति। A binding inward, inflexon.

Influenza (इन्फ्ल्यूएंजा) श्वसन पथ का एक तीव्र सांसर्गिक विषाणुजनक संक्रमण। An acute contagious viral infection of the respiratory tract.

Influenzal (इन्फ्ल्यूएंजल) इन्फ्यूएंजा से सम्बन्धित। Pertaining to influenza.

Infra (इन्फ्रा) एक उपसर्ग जिसका अर्थ नीचे से नीचे या कम अथवा बाद होता है, अव-निचला। A prefix meaning below, under, beneath or inferior to or after.

Infraglotic (इन्फ्राग्लोटिक) कण्ठद्वार या घंटी के नीचे। Below the glottis.

Inframammary (इन्फ्रानैमेरी) स्तन ग्रन्थि के नीचे। Below the mammary gland.

Infrapubic (इन्फ्राप्यूबिक) जघनास्थि से नीचे। Below the pubis.

Infrared (इन्फ्रारेड) अदृष्टिगोचर ऊष्मा किरणें जिनकी तरंग दैर्ध्य स्पेक्ट्रम के अन्त में लाल रंग की तरंग-दैर्ध्य से बड़ी होती है, इनकी तरंग दैर्ध्य 75–1000 म्यू। Invisible heat rays of wavelength greater than that of the red end of the spectrum having leave length of 75–1000 μ.

Infraversion (इन्फ्रावर्जन) आँख का नीचे की ओर घूम जाना। Downward deviation of the eye.

Infundibular (इन्फण्डीबुलर) कीप सम्बन्धी। Pertaining to the infundibulum.

Infusion (इन्फ्यूजन) किसी पदार्थ के घुलनशील सक्रिय तत्वों को प्राप्त करने के लिए उसे गर्म अथवा ठण्ड़े पानी में भिगोना। The steeping of a substance into hot or cold water to obtain its soluble active elements.

Ingestion (इन्जैशन) अशन, अन्तर्ग्रहण। The act of taking food or medicine into the stomach, the taking of particles by phagocytic cells.

Ingredient (इन्ग्रेडिएन्ट) किसी यौगिक अथवा मिश्रण का कोई

भाग, अवयव। Any part of a compound or a mixture.

Ingrowing (इन्ग्रोइंग) भीतर की ओर वृद्धि करने वाला। Growing inwards.

Ingrown nail (इन्ग्रोन नेल) ऐसा नाखून जिसका किनारा कोमल ऊतक में वृद्धि कर जाता है, जिससे दर्द होता है। The nail with the edge grown into the soft tissue causing inflammation and pain.

Inguen (इन्गुइन) वंक्षण प्रदेश। The groin.

Inguinal (इन्गुवाइनल) वंक्षण प्रदेश सम्बन्धी। Pertaining to groin.

Inguinal gland (इन्गुवाइनल-ग्लैण्ड) वंक्षण प्रदेश में स्थित लसीका पर्व। Lymph nodes in the groin region.

Inguinal ring (इन्गुवाइनल रिंग) वंक्षण वलय। गहन वंक्षण वलय जो वंक्षण-नाल का उदर के भीतर खुलने वाला मुख होता है। Deep inguinal ring, the opening of the inguinal canal in the interior of the abdomen.

Inguinolabial (इन्गुवाइनोलेबियल) वंक्षण एवं भगोष्ठ सम्बन्धी। Pertaining to the groin and the labium.

Inguinoscrotal (इन्गुवाइनोस्क्रोटल) वंक्षण एवं वृषण सम्बन्धी। Pertaining to the groin and the scrotum.

Inhalation (इनहैलेशन) वायु, वाष्प अथवा किसी गैस को फेफड़ों में खींचना। Draw in of air, vapor or gas into the lungs.

Inhaler (इनहेलर) औषधियों को सांस के साथ खींच कर अन्दर फेफड़ों में पहुँचाने के लिए एक उपकरण, श्वसित्र। An apparatus for administering the medicines by inhalation into the lungs.

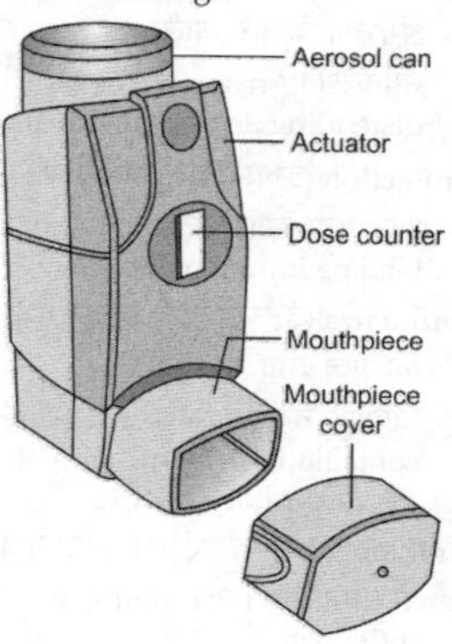

Inherent (इनहीयरैन्ट) प्राकृतिक, परिस्थितियों के परिणाम स्वरूप नहीं, वंशानुगत। Intrinsic, not neutral as a result of circumstances.

Inheritance (इनहेरीटैन्स) वंशागति। Something hereditary acquired through eggs and sperms.

Inhibin (इन्हीबिन) शुक्रग्रन्थि में सीरोटोलाइ कोशिकाओं द्वारा तथा डिम्बग्रन्थि में ग्रेन्यूलोसा कोशिकाओं द्वारा स्रावित एक हार्मोन जो अग्रज पीयूश ग्रन्थि द्वारा पुटक-उद्दीपक हॉर्मोन के स्रावण को कम कर देता है। A testicular hormone that inhibits its secretion by pituitary.

Inion (इनियन) बाह्य पश्चकपालिक प्रोद्वर्ध (उभार), पश्चकपाल बिन्दू। External occipital protuberance.

Iniopagus (इनियोपेगस) दो भ्रूण जो पश्चकपाल पर जुड़े होते है। Two fetuses fused at the occiput.

Initial (इनिसियल) प्रारम्भिक, आरम्भिक। Beginning.

Initis (इनाइटिस) किसी पेशी के पदार्थ का शोथ। Inflammation of the substance of muscle.

Inject (इन्जैक्ट) शरीर अथवा शरीर के किसी भाग में इन्जैक्शन द्वारा तरल पहुँचाना। Introducing fluid into the body or a part of the body by injection.

Injection (इन्जैक्शन) अतःपेशी, अवत्वक् अथवा अंतःशिरा मार्ग द्वारा बलपूर्वक किसी तरल को किसी अंग में अथवा शरीर के किसी भाग में प्रविष्ट करना। The forcing of a fluid into an organ or a part of the body by intramuscular, subcutaneous or intravenous route.

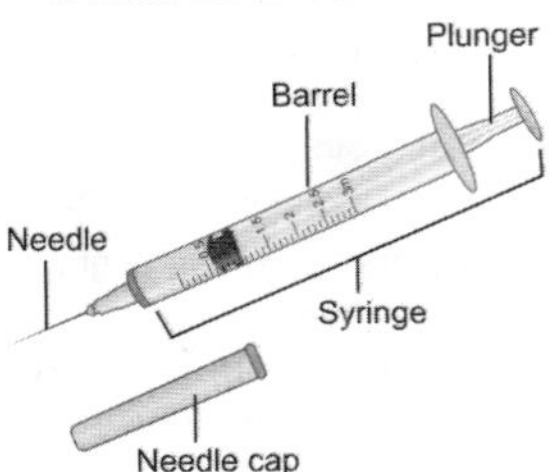

Injector (इन्जैक्टर) इन्जैक्शन लगाने के लिए एक यंत्र। An instrument for making injection.

Injury (इन्जरी) क्षति, क्षतिग्रस्तता, चोट, घाव। A wound or hurt or any damage to body.

Inlay (इनले) किसी ऊतक दोष में भरा जाने वाला ठोस पदार्थ अथवा किसी दन्त गुहा की आकृति के अनुरूप दाँत से बाहर बना भरावन जिसे दाँत में भर कर चिपका दिया जाता है। A solid material filled into a tissue defector, a filling corresponding the shape of a tooth cavity mode outside the tooth and then cemented it into the tooth.

Inosemia (इनोसेमिया) रक्त में फ्राइब्रिन का अधिक पाया जाना। An excess of fibrin in the blood.

Innate (इन्नेट) प्राकृतिक, स्वाभाविक। Inherent.

Innervate (इनर्वेट) किसी अंग की नाड़ी आपूर्ति को उत्तेजित करना। To stimulate the nerve supply of an organ.

Innervation (इनर्वेशन) शरीर के किसी भाग की तंत्रिका आपूर्ति अथवा तंत्रिका उद्‌दीपन। The nerve supply or the nerve stimulation of a part of the body.

Innocent (इन्नोसैन्ट) हानिरहित या सुदम। Harmless or benign.

Innocuous (इन्नोकुअस) अहानिकर। Innocent.

Innominate (इन्नोमिनेट) नाम रहित, बेनामी। Nameless.
(*i*) **Innominate Bone** (इन्नोमिनेट बोन) नितामबास्थि, श्रोणिफलक। The hip bone including the pubis ilium and ischium.

Inoculate (इनक्यूलेट) रोपण करना, संरोपण करना। To inject microorganism serum or toxic materials into body.

Inoculation (इनोकुलेशन) टीका, टीकाकरण, संरोपण, टीका लगाना। The introduction of specific virus into the systems.

Inoculum (इनॉकूलम) टीके के द्वारा प्रविष्ट किया जाने वाला पदार्थ, संरोप। The substance introduced by inoculation.

Inocyst (इनोसिस्ट) एक तन्तुमय सम्पूट। A fibrous capsule.

Inodorous (इनॉडोरस) गन्धहीन। Having no smell.

Inogenesis (इनोजेनेसिस) तन्तुमय ऊतक का बनना। Formation of fibrous tissue.

Inoperable (इनऑपरेबल) जिसका ऑपरेशन नहीं किया जा सकता है। That which is not suitable to be operated.

Inositis (इनोसाइटिस) तन्तुमय ऊतक का शोध। Inflammation of librous tissue.

Inotropic (इनोट्रॉपिक) पेशीय संकुचनशीलता के बल को प्रभावित करने वाला, पेशीप्रेरक, पेश्याकुंचप्रभावी। Affecting the force of muscular contractility.

Inquest (इनकुएस्ट) किसी अचानक एवं अप्रत्याशित होने वाली मृत्यु के ढंग की किसी चिकित्सा परीक्षक के सामने की जाने वाली कानूनी जाँच-पड़ताल, अपमृत्यु-समीक्षा। A legal inquiry made before a medical examiner into the manner of sudden and unexpected death.

Insane (इनसेन) विक्षिप्त, पागल। Mentally deranged.

Insanitary (इनसेनीटरी) अस्वास्थ्यकर। Unhealthful.

Insanity (इनसेनिटी) उन्माद, पागलपन, विक्षिप्त। A legal term for any mental illness characterized by inability to distinguish between right and wrong.

Insatiable (इनसेटिएबिल) सन्तुष्ट न हो सकने वाला। Unable to be satisfied.

Inscription (इन्सक्रिप्शन) किसी नुस्खे का मुख्य भाग जिसमें औषधियों के नाम एवं उनकी मात्राएँ लिखी होती है, औषधि निर्देश। The main part of a prescription containing the name and dose of the medicine.

Insect (इन्सैक्ट) फाइलम आर्थ्रोपोडा का एक वर्ग जिसके जीवों के शरीर के तीन स्पष्ट विभाजन-सिर, वक्ष एवं उदर होते हैं, तीन जोड़े संयुक्त पैर होते हैं तथा साधारणतया दो जोड़े पंख होते हैं। A class of the phylum arthropoda whose organism are characterized by three distinct body divisions as head, thorax and abdomen, three pairs of jointed legs and usually two pairs of wings.

Insecticide (इन्सैक्टीसाइड) वह औषधि या पदार्थ जो कीटों को मारता है, कीटनाशक। An agent which kills the insects.

Insectivorous (इन्सैक्टीवोरस) कीट-भक्षी। Insect eating.

Insecurity (इसिक्यूरिटी) असुरक्षा। Feeling of helplessness apprehension.

Insemination (इन्सेमीनेशन) सम्भोग के दौरान वीर्य का शिश्न से निकल कर योनि या ग्रर्भाशयग्रीवा में जमा होना। Deposition of semen from the penis into vagina or the cervix during intercourse.

Insenescence (इनसेनेसेन्स) वृद्ध होने की क्रिया। The process of growing old.

Insensible (इनसेन्सीबिल) अचेत, विवेकहीन अथवा वह व्यक्ति जिसमें संवेदनशीलता का अभाव होता है, संज्ञाहीन। Unconscious or the person with loss of sensibility.

Insertion (इनसर्शन) अंदर रखने अथवा निरोपण की क्रिया। The act of putting in or implantation.

Insidious (इन्सीडियस) धीरे-धीरे बढ़ने वाला। Developing slowly.

Insight (इनसाइट) स्वयं सोचना समझना। Self-understanding.

Insolation (इनसोलेशन) ऊश्माघात अथवा सूर्याघात, लू लगना। Heat stroke or sunstroke.

Insoluble (इन्सोलयूबिल) अघुलनशील। Unable to dissolved.

Insomnia (इनसोम्नियां) अनिद्रा, नींद न आना। Sleeplessness.

Insomniac (इन्सोम्निएक) अनिद्रा से पीड़ित व्यक्ति। The person suffering from insomnia.

Inspirator (इन्सपिरेटर) एक प्रकार का श्वसित्र। A type of respirator or inhaler.

Instep (इनस्टेप) पांव का मेहराब के समान अभिमध्य भाग। Archlike medial portion of the foot.

Instillation (इन्सटीलेशन) बूँद-बूँद करके किसी तरल को डालना, बिन्दु पातन। Pouring a liquid drop by drop.

Instillator (इन्सटीलेटर) तरल को बूँद-बूँद करके डालने वाला उपकरण। An apparatus for introducing liquid drop by drop.

Instinct (इन्सटिंक्ट) कुछ वातावरणीय दशाओं एवं उद्दीपनों के प्रति किसी विशेष प्रकार से प्रतिक्रिया करने की वंशानुगत प्रवृति, सहत-वृत्ति। The inherited tendency to react to certain environmental condition and stimuli particular way.

Instinctive (इन्सटिंक्टिव) सहजवृत्ति द्वारा ज्ञात, सहज-ज्ञान मूलक। Determind by instinct.

Instrumentation (इन्सट्रूमैन्टेशन) यंत्रों द्वारा किसी कार्य को सम्पन्न करना। Performance of a work with instruments.

Instussusceptum (इन्टुसस्सेप्टम) आन्तान्त्र प्रवेश में भ्रंश हुआ आँत का भाग, आन्त्रविष्टांश। The portion of the intestine prolapsed in intussusception.

Insufficiency (इनसफीसियन्सि) अपर्याप्तता, कमी। Inadequacy of function.

Insufflate (इन्सूफ्लेट) हवा, गैस पाउडर को फूंक मारकर या श्वांस खींच कर शरीर गुहा मे भरना। The air, gas blow into some opening upon some part of the body.

Insula (इन्सुला) द्विपिका। The oval-shaped region of the cerebral cortex.

Insulator (इन्सुलेटर) अपरिचालक पदार्थ, रोधी। The material method restricts the transfer of heat and electricity resistance.

Insulin (इन्सुलिन) अग्नाश्य का एक द्रव्य जिसकी कमी से मधुमेह रोग हो जाता है। The internal secretion of the islets of Langerhans situated within the pancreas.

Insulinase (इन्सुलिनेस) इन्सुलिन को निष्क्रिय बनाने वाला एक एन्जाइम। An enzyme that inactivates insulin.

Insulinemia (इन्सुलिनीमिया) रक्त में इन्सुलिन का अधिक पाया जाना। Excess of insulin in the blood.

Insulinogenesis (इन्सुलिनोजेनेसिस) अग्नाशय के लैगरहैन्स के द्वीप समूहों से इन्सुलिन की उत्पत्ति एवं उसकी मुक्ति होना। The production and release of insulin by the islets of Langerhans of the pancreas.

Insulinogenic (इन्सुलिनोजेनिक) इन्सुलिन द्वारा उत्पन्न। Caused by insulin.

Insulinoid (इन्सुलिनॉयड) इन्सुलिन के समान अथवा इन्सुलिन के गुणों से युक्त। Resembling insulin or having the properties of insulin.

Insulitis (इन्सुलाइटिस) अग्नाशय के लैंगरहैन्स के द्वीप समूहों का शोथ। Inflammation of the islets of langerhans of the pancreas.

Integration (इन्टिग्रेशन) जोड़ना या मिलाना, युग्मन। The joining or bringing together.

Integument (इन्टेगुमेन्ट) त्वचा, आच्छद, अध्यावरण। A covering or skin.

Integumentory (इन्टेगुमेन्टरी) त्वचीय। अच्छद या त्वचा सम्बन्धी, अध्यावरणी। Cutaneous or dermal pertaining to the integument.

Intellect (इनटैलेक्ट) बुद्धि, ज्ञान, प्रज्ञा। The faculty of thinking, understanding.

Intellectual (इन्टैलैक्चुअल) मस्तिष्क सम्बन्धी। Pertaining to the mind.

Intelligence (इन्टैलीजेन्स) समझने एवं समस्याओं को सुलझाने की योग्यता, बुद्धि। Ability to understand and to solve the problems.

Intelligence quotient (इन्टैलीजेन्स क्योशिएन्ट) किसी व्यक्ति से पूछे गये चुने हुए प्रश्नों के प्रति उसके उत्तरों द्वारा उस व्यक्ति का पता लगाया गया बुद्धि का सूचक। The index of intelligence of a person determined by his/her answers to the selected questions.

Intensity (इन्टेंसिटी) उच्च तनाव, ऊर्जा अथवा कार्य, विस्तार, प्रसार। A high tension energy or activity extension.

Intention (इन्टैन्शन) विहोरण अथवा भरने का ढंग। Manner of healing. (e.g. the healing process on the wound.

Interatrial (इन्टरेट्रियल) हृदय के अलिन्दों के बीच, अतंराअलिन्दी। Between the atria of the heart.

Interbrain (इन्टरब्रेन) अंतर्मस्तिष्क, थैलेमेन्सीफेलोन। Thalamencephalon.

Intercalated (इन्टरकैलेटेड) बीच में प्रविष्ट किया गया। Inserted between.

Intercapillary (इन्टरकैपिलरी) केशिकाओं के बीच में। Between the capillaries.

Intercerebral (इन्टरसेरीब्रल) दो प्रमस्तिष्क गोलार्द्धों के बीच। Between the two cerebral hemispheres.

Interchange (इन्टरचेंज) विनिमय, परस्पर बदलना। To exchange with each other; to alternate.

Intercodence (इन्टरकौडेन्स) दो बड़ी नियमित नाड़ी स्पन्दों के बीच एक अतिरिक्त स्पन्दन का उत्पन्न होना। Occurrence of an extra beat between the two regular pulse beats.

Intercourse (इन्टरकोर्स) परस्पर विनिमय, सम्पर्क या संचरण। Mutual exchange, communication.

Intercrural (इन्टरक्रूरल) दो टाँगों के बीच। Between two legs.

Intercurrent (इन्टरकरन्ट) किसी अन्य रोग की अवधि के दौरान उत्पन्न होने एवं अवधि को रूपांतरित करने वाला, मध्यवर्ती। Accruing during and modifying the course of another disease.

Interdentium (इन्टरडैन्टियम) दो आस-पास के दाँतों के बीच का जगह। The space between two adjacent teeth.

Interface (इन्टर्फेस) दो कायों की एक उभयनिष्ठ सीमा बनाने वाली सतह, अंतरापृष्ठ। A surface forming a common boundary of two bodies.

Intergluteal (इन्टरग्लूटियल) नितम्बों के बीच। Between two buttocks.

Interictal (इन्टरिक्टल) रोगाक्रमणों अथवा ग्रहों के बीच उत्पन्न होने वाला। Accruing between the attacks or the seizures.

Interlabial (इन्टरलेबियल) होठों अथवा किन्हीं भी दो भगोष्ठों के बीच। Between the lips or any two labia.

Interlobitis (इन्टरलोबाइटिस) फुफ्फुसीय खण्ड़ों के पृथक करने वाले वाले फुफ्फुसावरणों का शोथ। The inflammation of the pleura reporting the pulmonary lobes.

Intermammary (इन्टरमैमरी) स्तनों के बीच। Between the breasts.

Intermediary (इन्टरमीडियरी) दो कायों के बीच स्थित। Situated between the two bodies.

Intermenstrual (इन्टरमैन्सट्रुअल) मासिक धर्मों के बीच। Between the menstrual periods.

Intermission (इन्टरमीशन) मध्यान्तर, सविरामता। An interval, intermittency.

Intermittent (इन्टरमिटैन्ट) समय-समय पर निश्क्रिय हो जाना, सविरामी। Becoming inective periodically. (*i*) **Intermittent fever** (इन्टरमिटैन्ट फिवर) सविराम ज्वर, विरामी ज्वर। A fever with periods of apyrexia.

Intermural (इन्टरम्यूरल) किसी अंग के दीवारों के बीच। Between the walls of an organ.

Intermuscular (इन्टरमस्कुलर) पेशीयों के बीच, अंतरापेशी। Between the muscles.

Internalization (इन्टरनलाइजेशन) एक मानसिक प्रक्रिया जिसमें अन्य लोगों का महत्त्व, उनके दृष्टिकोण एवं स्टैण्डर्ड अज्ञानतावश अपने जैसे समझ लिए जाते हैं। A mental process in which the values, attitudes and standards of others are unconsciously taken as one's own.

Internatal (इन्टरनेटल) नितम्बों के बीच। Between the buttocks.

Interneurons (इन्टरन्यूरोन्स) अन्तमरातंत्रिकाणु। A neurons situated in between neuron.

Internist (इन्टरनिस्ट) आन्तरिक चिकित्सा में विशेषज्ञ। Specialist in internal medicine.

Interoceptive (इन्ट्रोसेप्टिव) शरीर में उत्पन्न होने वाली संवेदनाओं से सम्बन्धित। Pertaining to the sensation arising within the body.

Interomittent (इन्टरोंमिटेन्ट) रुक-रुक कर किसी गुहा अथवा शरीर में पहुँचाने अथवा इन्जैक्शन लगाने वाला। Conveying or injecting into a cavity or body.

Interosseous (इन्टरोंसियस) अस्थियों के बीच, अन्तरास्थिक। Between the bones

Interpalpebral (इन्टरपैल्पीब्रल) आँख की पलकों के बीच। Between the eyelids.

Interparietal (इन्टरपैर इटल) पार्श्विका या पैराइटल अस्थियों के बीच। Between the parietal bones.

Interphase (इन्टरफेज़) दो क्रमबद्ध कोशिका विभाजनों के बीच का समय। The interval between two successive cell division.

Interposition (इन्टरपोजिशन) शरीर के भागों के बीच में निवेशन। Insertion between the parts of the body.

Interpretation (इन्टरप्रिटेशन) व्याख्या, विवरण। Analysis, description.

Intersection (इन्टरसैक्शन) वह स्थान जहाँ पर एक रचना दूसरी

को पार करती है। A site where one structure crosses another.

Interseptal (इन्टरसैप्टल) दो पटों के बीच। Between two septa.

Intersex (इन्टरसैक्स) वह व्यक्ति जिसमें पुरूष एवं स्त्री दोनों की द्वितीयक लैंगिक विशिष्टताएँ होती है, उभयलिंगी। An individual having both male and female secondary sexual characteristics.

Interspinal (इन्टरस्पाइनल) कंटक अथवा मेरूदण्ड के दो कंटक-प्रवर्धों के बीच। Between two spinous processes of the spine.

Interstice (इन्टरस्टिस) किसी ऊतक अथवा रचना में एक छोटा स्थान या दरार, अन्तराल। A small space or gap in a tissue or structure.

Interstitium (इन्टरस्टीटियम) शरीर के भागों, ऊतकों अथवा कोशिकाओं के बीच बहुत छोटा स्थान। Very small place between the body parts, tissue or cells.

Intertriginous (इन्टरट्राइजीनस) त्वग्वलिशोथ से ग्रस्त। Affected by intertrigo.

Intertrigo (इन्टरट्राइगो) रगड़ खाने से त्वचा की विपरीत सतहों पर उत्पन्न होने वाला एक त्वकरक्तिम विस्फोट, त्वग्वलिशोथ। Any erythematous eruption accruing on the opposite surfaces of the skin from friction or rubbing.

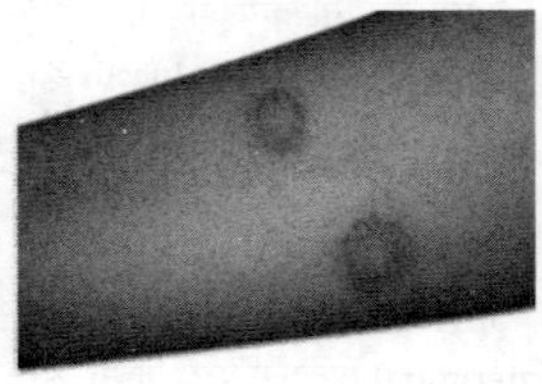

Intertrochanteric (इन्टरट्रोकेन्ट्रिक) उरू अस्थि या फीमर हड्डी के बड़े एवं छोटे ट्रोट्रन्टरों के बीच स्थित, अन्तरागण्डकी। Situated between the greater and lesser trochanters of the femur.

Interureteral (इन्टरयूरेट्रल) गवीनियों अथवा सूत्रनलियों के बीच। Between the ureters.

Interval (इन्टरवल) दो वस्तुओं अथवा शरीर के दो भागों के बीच का स्थान। The space between two objects or parts of the body.

Intervention (इन्टरवेन्शन) व्यवधान, मध्यस्थता। An interposition medication.

Interventricular (इन्टरवेन्ट्रीकुलर) हृदय के निलयों के बीच, अन्तरानिलयी। Between the ventricles of the heart.

Intestinal flora (इन्टेस्टाइनल फ्लोरा) आँत में सामान्य रूप से पाये जाने वाले अविकारी जीवाणु जो उपकारक होते हैं। Bacteria present in intestine that synthesize vitamins.

Intestinal obstruction (इन्टेस्टाइनल ऑब्सट्रक्शन) आँत की अवकाशिका का अवरोध। Blockage of the lumen of the intestine.

Intestinal perforation (इन्टेस्टाइनल पर्फोरेशन) आँत में छेद का बनना। Formation of a hole in the intestine.

Intestine (इन्टेस्टाइन) पोषण नली अथवा भोजन नली का वह भाग जो आमाशय के जठरनिर्गम द्वारा गुदा तक फैला होता है, आन्त्र। The part of the alimentary canal extruding

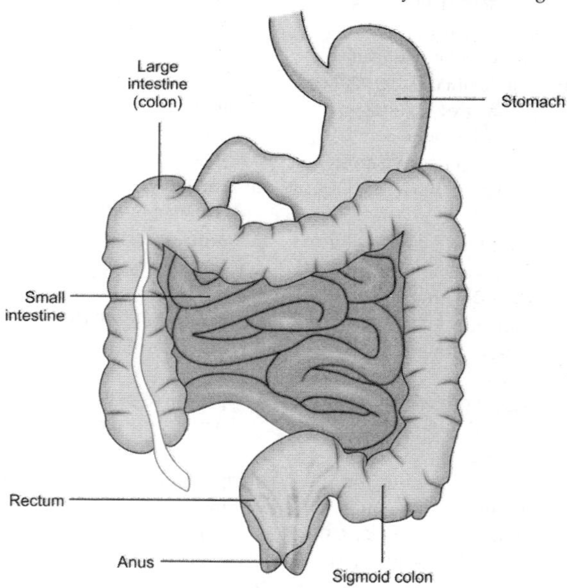

Intestine

from the pyloric opening of the stomach to the anus and divided into two parts.

Intima (इन्टिमा) किसी रचना की सबसे भीतरी परत जैसे किसी रक्त वाहिनी की सबसे भीतरी परत, अन्तःअस्तर। Tunica intima, innermost coat of a structure as of a blood vessel.

Intoxication (इन्टॉक्सीकेशन) मादक अथवा विषाक्त होने की अवस्था, मादकता। The state of being intoxicated or poisoned.

Intra-abdominal (इन्ट्राएब्डोमिनल) उदर के अन्दर, अन्तरूदरीय। Within the abdomen.

Intra-alveolar (इन्ट्रा-एल्वियोलर) वायुकोष्ठों के भीतर। Inside the alveoli.

Intra-atrial (इन्ट्रा-एट्रियल) हृदय के अलिन्द अथवा आलिन्दों के भीतर। Within the atrium or atria.

Intracardiac (इन्ट्राकार्डियक) हृदय के अन्दर, अन्तःहृदी। Within the heart.

Intracarpal (इन्ट्राकार्पल) मणिबन्ध का कलाई के अन्दर। Within the wrist.

Intrad (इन्ट्राड) अन्दर की ओर। Inwardly.

Intradural (इन्ट्राडयूरल) दृढ़तानिका या ड्यूरा मेटर के भीतर अथवा उसमें बन्द। Within or enclosed by the dura mater.

Intragastric (इन्ट्रागैस्ट्रिक) आमाशय के भीतर। Within the stomach.

Intralesional (इन्ट्रालीजनल) किसी विक्षति के भीतर। Within a lesion.

Intralocular (इन्ट्रालोकुलर) किसी संरचना की गुहा के भीतर। Within the cavity of any structure.

Intramedullary (इन्ट्रामेडयूलरी) मस्तिष्क के मेडुला ऑब्लांगेटा में स्थित। Within the medulla oblongata of the brain.

Intramural (इन्ट्राम्यूरल) किसी अंग की दिवारों के भीतर, अन्तर्भितिक। Within the walls of an organ.

Intranatal (इन्ट्रानेटल) प्रसवकालीन। At the time of birth.

Intraocular (इन्ट्राऑकुलर) नेत्रगोलक के भीतर। Within the eye ball.

Intraovarian (इन्ट्राओवेरियन) डिम्बग्रन्थि के भीतर। Within the ovary.

Intrapartum (इन्ट्रापार्टम) प्रसव के समय उत्पन्न होने वाला। Accruing during delivery.

Intraperitoneal (इन्ट्रापैरीटोनियल) पर्युदर्या-गुहा या पैरीटोनियम-गुहा के अन्दर। Within the peritoneal cavity.

Intrapsychic (इन्ट्रासाइकिक) मस्तिष्क में उत्पन्न होने वाला

जैसे कलहों या झगड़ों का उद्‌गम मस्तिष्क से होता है। Oridinating in the mind such as conflicts.

Intra-rectal (इन्ट्रारैक्टल) मलाशय के भीतर। Within the rectum.

Intrathecal (इन्ट्राथीकल) किसी आवरण के अन्दर, मेरूदण्ड-नाल के भीतर। Within a sheath, within the spinal.

Intratympanic (इन्ट्राटिम्पैनिक) मध्यकर्ण-गुहा के अन्दर। Within the tympanic cavity.

Intrauterine-contraceptive device (इन्ट्रायूटेराइन-कॉन्ट्रासेप्टिव डिवाइस) प्लास्टिक तथा ताँबे आदि का बना एक उपकरण जो गर्भधारण को रोकने के लिए लम्बे समय तक गर्भाशय में रखा जाता है। An apparatus made up of plastic and copper, etc. placed in the uterus for a long time to prevent conception.

Intravasation (इन्ट्रावेज़ेशन) रक्त वाहिनियों में बाह्य पदार्थो का प्रवेश करना। The entrance of foreign substance into the blood vessels.

Intravenous (इन्ट्रावेनस) शिरा के भीतर, अन्तःशिराभ। Within a vein.

Intravenous infusion (इन्ट्रावेनस इन्फ्यूजन) तुरन्त असर लाने के लिए किसी विलयन का किसी शिरा में इन्जैक्शन लगाना जैसे रक्तस्राव। Injection of a solution into a vein to gain the immediate affect as in hemorrhage.

Intravital (इन्ट्रावाइटल) जीवन में उत्पन्न होने वाला अनतजीर्वित। Accruing during life.

Intravitam (इन्ट्रावाइटम) जीवन में। During life.

Intrinsic (इन्ट्रिन्जिक) किसी भाग में पूर्णरूप से स्थित अथवा केवल उसी भाग से सम्बन्धित जो आवश्यक एवं प्राकृतिक होता है, अन्तःस्थ। Belonging to or embedded in essential nature of a thing.

Intrinsic factor (इन्ट्रिन्जिक फैक्टर) एक पदार्थ जो पेट से स्रावित होता है जो शरीर में Vit B_{12} को अवशोषित करने में मदद करता है। Substance present in the gastric juice that facilitates absorption of vit B_{12}.

Introceptor (इन्ट्रोसेप्टर) एक संवेदी तंत्रिका अन्त जो शरीर के भीतर स्थित रहता है और आन्तरिक अंगों से आवेगों को संचरित करता है, अंतःसंवेदी A sensory nerve ending located within the body and transmits impulses from the internal organ.

Introducer (इन्ट्रोडयूज़र) किसी नालशलाका या कैथीटर आदि किसी यन्त्र को प्रविष्ट करने वाला एक उपकरण। An apparatus which introduces some instrument as catheter.

Introflexion (इन्ट्रोफ्लैक्शन) अन्दर की ओर एक झुकाव। A bending inwards.

Introitus (इन्ट्रॉयटस) किसी नली अथवा गुहा में कोई द्वार या प्रवेश मार्ग। An opening or enhance into a canal or cavity.

Introjection (इन्ट्रोजैक्शन) एक मानसिक प्रक्रिया जिसमें अज्ञानतावश प्रिय एवं अप्रिय बाह्य वस्तुएँ किसी व्यक्ति के मस्तिष्क में समा जाती है। A mental process in which favorable and unfavorable external things are unconsciously taken within oneself.

Intromission (इन्ट्रोमिशन) शरीर के एक भाग का दूसरे में निवेशन अथवा रखना। The insertion or placing of one part of the body into another part.

Introspection (इन्ट्रोस्पैक्शन) अपने अन्दर झांक कर देखना। Looking within oneself.

Introversion (इन्ट्रोवर्जन) किसी अंग का बाहर से अन्दर की ओर घूम जाना। The turning of an organ from outside inward.

Introvert (इन्ट्रोवर्ट) बाहर से भीतर की ओर घूमा हुआ अंग। The organ turned from outside inward.

Intrusion (इन्ट्रूशन) आँख का अन्दर की ओर नाक की ओर घूम जाना। Rotation of the eye inward towards the nose.

Intubation (इन्टूयूबेशन) शरीर के किसी भाग विशेष कर वायु प्रवेश करने के लिए स्वरयंत्र में किसी नली या ट्यूब का निवेशन करने की क्रिया, नलिका प्रवेश। Insertion of a tube into a body part especially into the larynx for entrance of air.

Intuition (इन्ट्यूशन) अन्तर्ज्ञान, सहजज्ञान। Instinct.

Intumesence (इन्ट्मिसेन्स) बढ़ने या फूलने की। Swelling up or enlarging.

Intussusception (इन्टुसस्सेप्शन) आँत के किसी भाग का आँत के ठीक नीचे स्थित अन्य किसी भाग की अवकाशिका में भ्रंश, आन्त्रान्त्र प्रवेश। Intussception invagination the prolapse of one part of the intestine into the lumen of another part situated just below the intestine.

Intussuscipiens (इन्टुसस्सीपिएन्स) आन्तान्त्र प्रवेश में आँत का

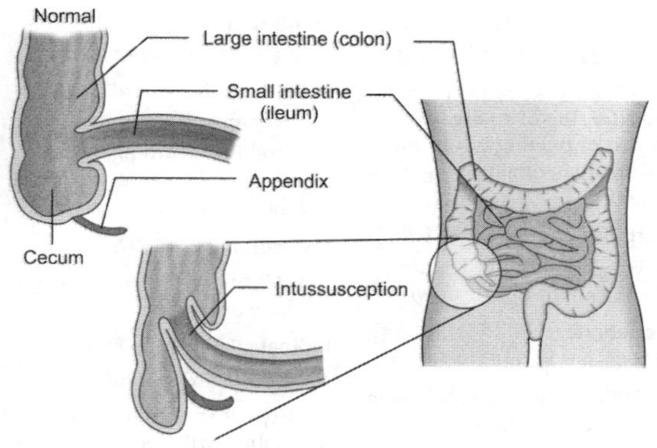

Intussusception

वह भाग जो दूसरे भाग को ग्रहण करता है। The portion of the intestine in the intussusceptions which receives the other portion.

Inunction (इननक्शन) इस प्रकार त्वचा में रगड़ा गया मरहम अथवा कोई औषधियुक्त पदार्थ। The ointment or a medicated substance so rubbed into the skin.

Invaginate (इन्वेजिनेट) आच्छदित करना अथवा आवरण से ढकना। To ensheath.

Invalid (इनवेलिड) अपंग, अशक्त, दुर्बल, कमजोर। A sick person confined to bed or wheelchair.

Invasion (इन्वैसन) संक्रामी जीवों का शरीर में प्रवेश करना एवं ऊतकों में उनका फैल जाना, रोगाक्रमण। The entrance of infectant organism into the body and their distribution into the tissue.

Invasive (इन्वैसिव) शरीर में प्रवेश करने एवं ऊतकों में फैलने के गुण से युक्त जैसे कि कुछ सूक्ष्मजीव होते हैं। Having the property to enter the body and to spread in the tissue as are some microorganisms.

Invermination (इनवर्मिनेशन) आन्त्र-कृमियों द्वारा कष्ट होना, कृमि-रूग्णता। Infestation by intestinal worms.

Inversion (इन्वर्जन) किसी अंग अथवा भाग के सामान्य सम्बन्ध का उल्टा हो जाना या किसी

अंग अथवा भाग का जैसे गर्भाशय का अन्दर से बाहर को निकल आना। Reversal of the normal relationship of an organ or a part or twining inside out of an organ or a part, e.g. the uterus.

Invert (इनवर्ट) भीतर से बाहर की ओर घुमाना, अंतर्वर्त। To turn inside out or upside down.

Invertebrate (इनवर्टिब्रेट) ऐसे जन्तु जिनके कशेरूकादण्ड नहीं होता, अपृष्ठवंशी। The animals having no vertebral column.

Inverted image (इनवर्टेड इमेज) उल्टा प्रतिबिम्ब। Image which is turned upside down.

Investing (इन्वैस्टिंग) किसी चादर अथवा आवरण जैसे ऊतक के द्वारा चारों ओर से ढकने वाला। Encircling with a sheath or covering as tissue.

Investment (इन्वैस्टमेन्ट) एक आवरण अथवा चादर। A covering or sheath.

Inveterate (इनविट्रेट) दुःसाध्य, असाध्य, चिरस्थाई, लाइलाज। Chronic firmly seated habit.

Involucrum (इनवोल्यूक्रम) विविक्तच्छद, आवरण। An enveloping membranes, an envelope.

Involuntary (इन्वॉलन्ट्री) अनैच्छिक। Independent of the will.

Involution (इन्वोल्यूशन) अन्दर की ओर चक्कर खा जाना या घूम जाना। प्रसव के पश्चात् गर्भाशय का परिमाण में घट जाना। A rolling or turning inwards, reduction in size of the uterus following delivery.

Involutional (इन्वोल्यूशनल) प्रत्यावर्तन सम्बन्धी। Pertaining to the involution.

Iodinate (आयोडिनेट) आयोडीन से चिकित्सा करना अथवा उससे संयुक्त करना। To treat or combine with iodine.

Iodism (आयोडिज्म) आयोडीन अथवा इसके यौगिकों के अधिक समय तक एवं अधिक मात्रा में प्रयोग करते रहने से उत्पन्न दशा, आयोडात्यय। The condition produced by prolonged and excessive use of iodine or its compounds.

Iododerma (आयोडोडर्मा) आयोडीन के द्वारा उत्पन्न कोई भी त्वचा रोग। Any skin disease due to iodine.

Iodophilia (आयोडोफीलिया) वह दशा जिसमें कुछ कोशिकाएँ जैसे बहुरूपी केन्द्रीकीय श्वेत रक्त कोशिकाएँ, कुछ विकृतिजन्य अवस्थाओं जैसे जीव विषरक्तता और गम्भीर रक्ताल्पता में आयोडीन या

आयोडाइडों से अभिरंजित होने पर भूरे–से लाल रंग से रंगे जाने को प्रदर्शित करती है। The condition in which certain cells as polymorphonuclear white blood cells in certain pathological conditions as toxemia and severe anemia show diffuse brownish red coloration or staining with iodine or iodides.

Ion (आयन) विद्युत-चार्ज का वहन करने वाला कण। The particle carrying an electric charge.

Ionization (आयोनाइजेशन) किसी पदार्थ का घोल में आयनों में विघटित हो जाना। Dissociation of a substance in solution into ions.

Ionogen (आयोनोजन) कोई भी वस्तु जो आयनो में पृथक हो सकती है। Anything that dissociates into ions.

Ionophoresis (आयनोफोरेसिस) आयनसंचलन। Electrophoresis.

Iophobia (आयोफोबिया) विषयुक्त होने का विकृत भय। Morbid fear of being poisonous.

Ipsilateral (इप्सीलेट्रल) समपार्श्वी, समपार्श्विक। On the same side.

Iralgia (आइरैल्जिया) उपतारा या परितारिका में दर्द होना। Iridalgia, pain in the iris.

Iridalgia (आइरिडैल्जिया) परितारिकार्ति। Iralgia.

Iridauxesis (आइरिड्योक्सेसिस) परितारिकावमोटन। Thickening of the iris following plastic iritis.

Iridectome (आइरिडैक्टोम) उपतारा या परितारिका उच्छेदन में उपतारा को काटने वाला एक यंत्र। An instrument for cutting the iris in iridectomy.

Iridectomy (आईरिडेक्टॉमी) परितारिका के किसी भाग को शल्यक्रिया द्वारा काटकर अलग कर देना, परितारिका उच्छेदन, उपतारा-उच्छेदन। Surgical removal of a portion of the iris.

Iridemia (आईरिडीमिया) परितारिका से रक्तस्राव होना। Hemorrhage term of the iris.

Irideremia (आईरिडेरीमिया) आँख की पुतली अथवा उपतारा का अभाव, अपरितारकता। An iris so rudimentary that it seems to be absent, aniridia.

Irides (आईराइड्स) आइरिस का बहुवचन। Plural of iris.

Iridium (आइरिडियम) धनातु। A white silvery metallic element.

Iridocapsulitis (आईरिडे कैप्सूलाइटिस) परितारिका एवं लैन्स के कैप्सूल का शोथ। Inflammation of the iris and the capsule of the lens.

Iridocele (आईरिडोसील) स्वच्छमण डल या कॉर्निया से होकर परितारिका के कुछ भाग का

बाहर निकल आना। Protrusion of a portion of the iris through the cornea.

Iridocoloboma (आईरिडोकोलोबोमा) परितारिका की जन्मजात फटन या दरार। Congenital fissure of the iris.

Iridocorneal (आइरिडोकॉर्नियल) परितारिका एवं स्वच्छमण्डल सम्बन्धी। Pertaining to the iris and cornea.

Iridocyclectomy (आइरिडोसाइक्लेटोमी) परितारिका एवं रोमपिण्ड या सिलयरी बॉडी के कुछ भाग को शिल्यक्रिया द्वारा काट कर अलग कर देना। Surgical removal of a part of the iris and the ciliary body.

Iridocyclitis (आइरिडोसाइक्लाइटिस) परितारीक एवं सिलयारी बॉडी की सूजन, परितारिका-रोमक पिण्डशोथ। Inflammation of the iris and the ciliary body.

Iridodialysis (आइरिडोडायलायसिस) पारितारिक का अपने चिपकावों अथवा संलग्नताओं से पृथक्करण, परितारिका विग्लन। The separation of the iris from its attachments.

Iridodonesis (आईरिडोडोनेसिस) आँख की पुतली की कम्पन। Agitated motion or trembling of the iris.

Iridokeratitis (आइरिडोकेराटाइटिस) परितारिका एवं स्वच्छमण्डल का शोथ। Inflammation of iris and the cornea.

Iridokinesis (आइरिडोकाइनेसिस) पारितारिका का संकुचन एवं प्रसारण। Contraction and expansion of the iris.

Iridomalacia (आईरिडोमैलेशिया) परितारिका का मुलायम होना। Softening of the iris.

Iridopathy (आईरिडोपैथी) आँख की परितारिका का कोई भी रोग। Any disease of the iris of the eye.

Iridorhexis (आईरिडोरैह्क्सिस) परितारिका का फट जाना अथवा अपने लगाव के स्थान से चिर जाना। Rupture or the tearing away of the iris from its attachment.

Iridotasis (आईरिडोटेसिस) ग्लोकोमा की चिकित्सा में शल्यक्रिया द्वारा परितारिका को फैलाना। To stretch the iris by surgery in the treatment off glaucoma.

(*i*) **Iridotomy** (आइरिडोटॉमी) परितारिका में चीरा लगाना, परितारिकाच्छेद। To make an incision into the iris. The surgical processes

Iridovulsion (आईरिडोएवल्जन) परितारिका का फट जाना। A tearing away of the iris.

Iris (आईरिस) आँख की पुतली, उपतारा। The colored layer of the eye surrounding the pupil.

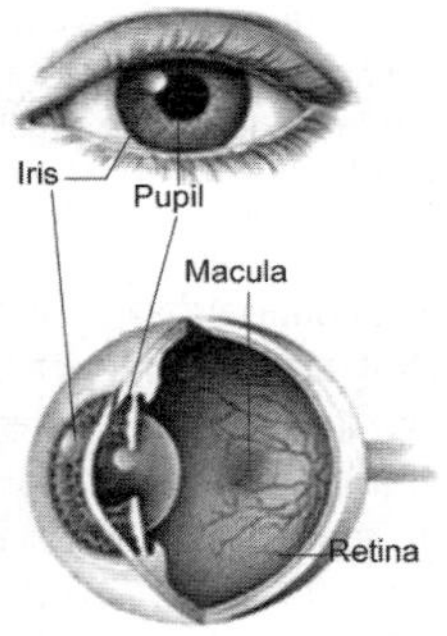

Iritis (आईराइटिस) परितारिकाशोथ। Inflammation of the iris.

Iron (आयरन) अयस, लोहा, लौह। Ferrum, a metallic element of grey color.

Irradiation (इरैडिएशन) रोगों की चिकित्सा एवं उनके निदान के लिए विकिरण ऊर्जा, किरणन। Exposure to radiant energy as X-ray ultraviolet rays light and heat.

Irrational (इरैशनल) अपरिमेय, अयुक्त। Unreasonable or unreasoning, not rational.

Irreducible (इरैड्यूसिबल) अखण्डनीय, अलघुकरणीय, अलघुकारी। Not reducible incapable of being made smaller or simpler.

Irrigation (इर्रीगेशन) जल अथवा अन्य किसी तरल की धार से धुलाई करना, धावन। The washing by a stream of water or other fluid.

Irrigator (इर्रीगेटर) जल अथवा अन्य किसी तरल से शरीर के किसी भाग अथवा गुहा के धोने के काम आने वाला एक उपकरण। An apparatus used in washing a part or cavity of the body with water or some other fluid.

Irritability (इर्रीटेबिलिटी) उद्दीपनों के प्रति असामान्य सम्वेदनशीलता, क्षोभशीलता या चिड़चिड़ापन। Abnormal sensitiveness to stimuli.

Irritable (इर्रीटेबल) किसी उद्दीपन के प्रति प्रतिक्रिया करने में सक्षम। Capable of reacting to a stimulus.

Irritation (इर्रीटेशन) उत्तेजित करने का कार्य, क्षोभण। The act of stimulating.

Ischemia (इस्कीमिया) किसी रक्त वाहिनों में संकुचन हो जाने अथवा उसमें अवरोध उत्पन्न हो जाने से किसी भाग की रक्त आपूर्ति में स्थायी न्यूनता हो जाना। Temporary deficiency of blood supply in a part due to constriction or obstruction of a blood vessels.

Ischemic (इस्कीमिक) स्थानिक अरक्तता सम्बन्धी, अरक्तताजन्य। Pertaining to ischemia.

Ischialgia (इस्कियेल्जिया) आसनास्थि में दर्द होना। Pain in the ischium.

Ischiatitis (इस्कियाटाइटिस) इस्कियम हड्डी या आसनास्थि की सूजन। Inflammation of the ischium.

Ischiodynia (इस्कियोडाइनिया) इस्कियम में दर्द होना। Pain in the ischium.

Ischiofibular (इस्कियोफिबुलर) इस्कियम एवं फिबुला हड्डी से सम्बन्धित। Pertaining to the ischium and the fibula bone.

Ischionitis (इस्कियोनाइटिस) इस्कियम हड्डी के गण्डक का शोथ। Inflammation of the tuberosity of the ischium bone.

Ischiosacral (इस्कियोसैक्रल) इस्कियम एवं सैक्रम सम्बन्धी। Pertaining to the ischium and the sacrum.

Ischuretic (इस्कूरेटिक) मूत्र-त्याग के बन्द हो जाने अथवा मूत्र को ठहर जाने को दूर करने वाला। Relieving the suppression or retention of urine.

Island (आईलैण्ड) कोशिकाओं का एक गुच्छ अथवा ऊतक का एक पृथक टुकड़ा। A cluster of cells or an isolated piece of tissue.

Isoagglutination (आईसोएग्लुटिनेशन) उसी जाति के अन्य सदस्य के रक्त की एग्लुटिनिनों द्वारा लाल रक्त कोषिकाओं का समूहन। Agglutination of the red blood cells by agglutinins from the blood of another member of the same species.

Isoagglutinin (आईसोएग्लुटिनिन) किसी सीरम में विद्यमान कोई एण्टीबॉडी जो किसी जाति के प्राणि की लाल रक्त कोशिकाओं का समूहन करती है जिससे वह उत्पन्न होती है। An antibody in a serum which agglutinates the red blood cells of the individual of the same species from which it is derived.

Isoantigen (आइसोएन्टिजन) समप्रतिजन। An antigenic substance that occurs only in some individual of a species.

Isobaric (आईसोबेरिक) उसी विशिष्ट गुरूत्व वाला जिससे इसकी तुलना की जाती है। Of the same specific gravity with which it is compared.

Isochromatic (आइसोक्रोमेटिक) एक रंग से युक्त। Having the same color.

Isochronal (आइसोक्रोनल) नियमित समयान्तरों में कार्य करने अथवा उत्पन्न होने वाला। Acting or accruing at regular intervals.

Isochronia (आइसोक्रोनिया) घटनाओं की समय, गति या बारम्बारता के दृष्टिकोण से उनकी वार्तालाप का आदान-प्रदान। The correspondency of events with respect to time, rate or frequency.

Isocoria (आइसोकोरिया) दोनों आँखों की पुतलियों के परिमाण में बराबर होने की अवस्था। The condition of the pupils of the eyes of being equal in size.

Isocytosis (आइसोइटोसिस) कोशिकाओं के विशेषकर लाल रक्त कोशिकाओं के परिमाण में बराबर होने की दशा। The condition of the cells of being equal in size especially of red blood cells.

Isodactylism (आइसोडैक्टाइलिज्म) हाथ अथवा पैर की बराबर लम्बाई की अंगुलियों से युक्त होने की दशा। The condition of having fingers or toes of equal length.

Isodiametric (आइसोडायामीट्रिक) बराबर व्यास वाला, समव्यासमापी। With equal diameters.

Isodontic (आइसोडोन्टिक) बराबर परिमाण के दाँतों वाला। Having teeth of equal size.

Isodynamic (आइसोडाइनामिक) बराबर की शक्ति वाला, समबल। With equal strength.

Isoelectric (आइसोइलैक्ट्रिक) समविभावी, समविद्युतविभव, समविभव। Equally electric throughout.

Isogamete (आइसोगैमेट) एक कोशिका जो उसी प्रकार की कोशिका में संयोजन करके जनन करती है। A cell that through fusion with a similar cell reproduction.

Isogamy (आइसोगैमी) समयुग्मकों अथवा समान कोशिकाओं के संयोजन के फलस्वरूप जनन होना। Reproduction resulting from union of isogamete or identical cells.

Isogeneric (आइसोजेनेरिक) एक ही प्रकार का अथवा एक ही जाति का। Of the same kind or belonging to the same species.

Isogenesis (आइसोजेनेसिस) विकास, प्रक्रियाओं में समानता। Similarity in the developmental process.

Isoiconia (आइसोइकोनिया) किसी वस्तु के प्रतिबिम्ब क दोनों आँखों में बराबर होना। Equality of the image of an object in both eyes.

Isoimmunization (आइसोइम्यूनाइज़ेशन) आइसोएण्टिजनो की अनुक्रिया में किसी व्यक्ति में एण्टीबॉडियों का उत्पन्न होना। Development of antibodies in an individual in response to isoantigens.

Isolation (आइसोलेशन) पृथक करने की क्रिया अथवा पृथक हो जाने की अवस्था। The act of isolating or state of being isolated.

Isologous (आइसोलोगस) उत्पत्ति सम्बन्धी दृष्टिकोण से एक समान। Isogenic genetically identical.

Isolophobia (आइसोलोफोबिया) अकेले रहने का भय। Fear of being alone.

Isomer (आइसोमर) समावयवी पदार्थ। The isomeric substance.

Isomerism (आइसोमरिज्म) समावयविता, समावयवता। Having an identical chemical composition.

Isomerization (आइसोमेरीज़ेशन) समवयवीमय, समावयवीकरण। A process in which one isomer is formed from another.

Isometric (आइसोमीट्रिक) बराबर की लम्बाई-चौड़ाई वाला, सममितीय। Of equal dimensions.

Isometropia (आइसोमीट्रोपिया) दोनो आँखों का एक ही अपवर्तन। Same refraction of the two eyes.

Isomorphous (आइसोमोर्फस) एक-सी शक्ल वाला, समाकार। Having the same shape.

Isophoria (आइसोफोरिया) नेत्रअविचलन प्रवृत्ति। A state in which the tension of the vertical muscle of each eye is equal and the visual lines lie in the horizontal plane.

Isopia (आइसोपिया) दोनों नेत्रों में समदृष्टि अर्थात् दोनों आँखों से बराबर दिखाई देना। Equal vision in both the eyes.

Isosexual (आइसोसैक्सुअल) एक ही लिंग से सम्बन्धित अथवा एक ही लिंग की विशिष्टता। Pertaining to characteristic of the same sex.

Isosmotic (आइसोस्मोटिक) एक से परासरणी दाब वाला। Having the same omotic pressure.

Isotonic (आइसोटोनिक) समरासारी, समतानी, समतानिक। Having equal tension.

Isotope (आइसोटोप) रासायनिक तत्वों की किसी श्रृंखला में से एक जिनके रासायनिक गुण एक समान होते हैं परन्तु अपने परमाणु भार एवं विद्युत-आवेश में वे भिन्न होते हैं। One of a series of chemical elements which have the same chemical properties but differ in their atomic weight and electric charge.

Isotropic (आइसोट्रोपिक) समदिक्, समवृत्तिक। Single refractive, isotropus.

Issue (इशू) सन्तान, पस या मवाद रक्त अथवा अन्य पदार्थ का स्राव। Offspring, a discharge of pus blood or other matter.

Isthmitis (इस्थमाइटिस) संकीर्ण संयोजक अथवा संकीर्ण पथ की सूजन। Inflammation of the isthmus.

Isthmus (इस्थमस) दो बड़े पिण्डों अथवा भागों को जोड़ने वाला एक तंग मार्ग, संकीर्णपथ, संकीर्ण संयोजक। A narrow passage connectivity of the two larger bodies or parts.

Itch (इच) कण्ड्, खुजली, खारिश, खाज। Irritation of skin inducing desire to scratch.

IV (आई. वी.) अन्तःशिराभ। Intravenous.

J

Jab (जैब) किसी नुकीली सामग्री से भोंकना (चुभोना)। Stabbing with something pointed material.

Jaborandi (जैबोरेंडी) स्वेदन-पत्र। The leaves of various species of pilocarpus trees of Brazil.

Jacket (जैकेट) मेरूदण्ड को अचल बनाने अथवा विकृतियों को सही करने के लिए धड़ पर कसी जाने वाली प्लास्टर ऑफ पेरिस की एक पट्टी, बाह्यवरण। A bandage of Plaster of Paris applied to trunk to immobilize the spinal column or to correct deformities.

Jackscrew (जैकस्क्रव) एक पेंच के द्वारा कार्य करने वाला उपकरण जो दन्त-चाप को फैलाने अथवा अस्थिभंग के पश्चात् अस्थि के टुकड़ों की स्थिति सही करने के काम आती है। A device operated by means of a screw used to expand the dental arch or for correcting the position of the bone fragments after fracture.

Jacksonian epilepsy (जैक्सोनियन इपिलैप्सी) एक स्थानिक प्रकार का अपस्मार जिसमें ग्रह (झटके) शरीर के केवल किसी सीमित भाग में ही उत्पन्न होते है। A localized form of epilepsy in which the seizures accrue only in a limited portion of the body.

Jacquemier's sign (जैकोमीयर्स साइन) गर्भावस्था में योनि की श्लेष्मिक काला या नीले या हल्के बैंगनी रंग का हो जाना। Blue or black coloration of the vaginal mucous membrane in pregnancy.

Jactitation (जेक्टीटेशन) तीव्र रोग में शरीर का इधर-उधर को भागना, तड़पन। Restless, to and fro movement of the body in acute illness.

Jaeger's test types (जेगर्स टेस्ट टाइप्स) निकट दृष्टि की जाँच के लिए किसी कार्ड पर छपी हुई विभिन्न परिमाणों के टाइपों की लाइनें। Lines of types of various sizes printed on card for testing the near vision.

Jagged (जैग्ड) दाँतेदार या खाँचेदार। Notched.

Jargon (जारगोन) अपरिचित शब्दों का जो विज्ञान के किसी विशेष क्षेत्र के व्यक्तियों के लिए विशेष तौर से होता है, बोलना।

Speech or writing of unfamiliar word which are particular to a person in a special field of science.

Jarvis's snore (जारविस स्नोर) नासा-गुहाओं में स्थित वृद्धियों को अलग करने वाला एक यंत्र। An instrument for removing the growth in the nasal cavities.

Jaundice (जॉण्डिस) कामला, पीलिया, पाण्डुरोग, कॅवल, कमल। Bile pigment in the blood and tissue giving them a yellow appearance icterus.
(*i*) **Congenital jaundice** (कॉनजेनाइटल जॉण्डिस) जन्मजात कामला। Jaundice accruing since birth.
(*ii*) **Hepatocellular jaundice** (हिपैटोसेलुलर जॉण्डिस) यकृत कोशिकाओं पर आघात पहुँचने अथवा उनके रोग के कारण होने वाली कामला। Jaundice due to injury to or disease of the liver.
(*iii*) **Infectious jaundice** (इन्फैक्शियस जॉण्डिस) संक्रामक यकृतशोध में होने वाली कामला। Jaundice accruing in infectious hepatitis.
(*iv*) **Obstructive jaundice** (ऑब्सट्रक्टिव जॉण्डिस) पित्त के यकृत से ड्योडिनम में होने वाले बहाव में होने वाले किसी यांत्रिक अवरोध के परिणामस्वरूप उत्पन्न कामला, रूद्वपति कामला। Jaundice resulting from some mechanical obstruction in the flow of bile from liver to the duodenum.

Jaw (जा) हनु, जबड़ा। The maxilla.
(*i*) **Cracking jaw** (क्रैकिंग जा) ऐसा जबड़ा जिसके गति करने के दौरान सामान्य या रोगग्रस्त शंख-अधोहनुक सन्धि में एक ध्वनि सुनाई देती है। A jaw in which a sound is heard in the normal or diseased temporomandibular joint during movement of the jaw. (*ii*) **Lock jaw** (लॉक जा) जबड़े की पेशियों की तनाव युक्त ऐंठन जैसाकि धनुस्तम्भ या टेटनस में देखी जाती है, हनुस्तम्भ। Tonic spasm of the jaw muscles as seen in tetanus.

Jejunal (जेजुनल) जेजुनम सम्बन्धी। Pertaining to the jejunum.

Jejunitis (जेजुनाइटिस) जेजुनम का शोध, मध्यान्त्र शोध। Inflammation of the jejunum.

Jejunocolostomy (जेजुनोकोलोस्टॉमी) जेजुनम एवं कोलन के बीच शल्यक्रिया द्वारा एक मार्ग बनाना। Formation of a passage by surgery between the jejunum and the colon.

Jejunoileitis (जेजुनोइलियाइटिस) जेजुनम एवं इलियन का शोध, मध्यशेषान्त्रशोध। Inflammation of the jejunum and ileum.

Jejunoileostomy (जेजुनोइलियोस्टॉमी) जेजुनम एवं इलियन के बीच एक मार्ग बनाना। Formation of a passage between the jejunum and ileum.

Jejunoplasty (जेजुनोप्लास्टी) प्लास्टीक सर्जरी द्वारा जेजुनम की मरम्मत करना। Repairing of the jejunum by plastic surgery.

Jejunorrhaphy (जेजुनोरैह्फी) जेजुनम की शल्यक्रिया द्वारा मरम्मत करना। Surgical repair of the jejunum.

Jejunotomy (जेजुनोटॉमी) जेजुनम में एक चीरा लगाना। To make an incision into the jejunum.

Jejunum (जेजुनम) बीच की छोटी आँत, मध्यान्त्र। A protein of small intestine between duodenum and ileum.

Jelly (जेली) एक कोमल, गाढ़ा, चिपचिपा अर्द्धठोस पिण्ड। A soft, thick, sticky semisolid mass.

Jerk (जर्क) पेशी में अचानक होने वाली गति, प्रतिक्षेप, झटका। A sudden muscular movement. (*i*) **Achilles jerk, Ankle jerk** (एलिकस जर्क, एन्क्लि जर्क) एलिकस टैण्डन को ठोंकने पर पिण्डली की पेशियों का संकुचित होना। Contraction of the calf muscles accruing on striking achilles tendon. (*ii*) **Knee jerk** (नी जर्क) जब घुटना समकोण पर आंकुचित हुआ होता है तो पटेलर टैण्डन पर ठोंकने पर पैर की निचले भाग में आगे की ओर प्रतिक्षेप या झटके आना, जाना प्रतिक्षेप। The forward jerking of the lower leg upon striking the patellar tendon when the knee is floral right angle.

Jerking (जर्किंग) जिसमें प्रतिक्षेप या झटके आते हो, प्रतिक्षेपक। Making sudden movements.

Joint (ज्वाइंट) संधि या जोड़। An articulation the site of junction or union between two or more bones. (*i*) **Arthrodial joint** (आर्थोडियल ज्वाइंट) संसर्पी सन्धी। Gliding joint (*ii*) **Ball and socket joint** (बाल एण्ड साकेट ज्वाइंट) ऐसा जोड़ जिसमें एक हड्डी का गोल सिरा दूसरी हड्डी की गुहा में फिट हो जाता है

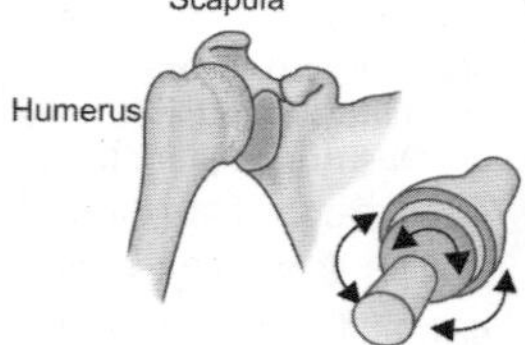

Ball and socket

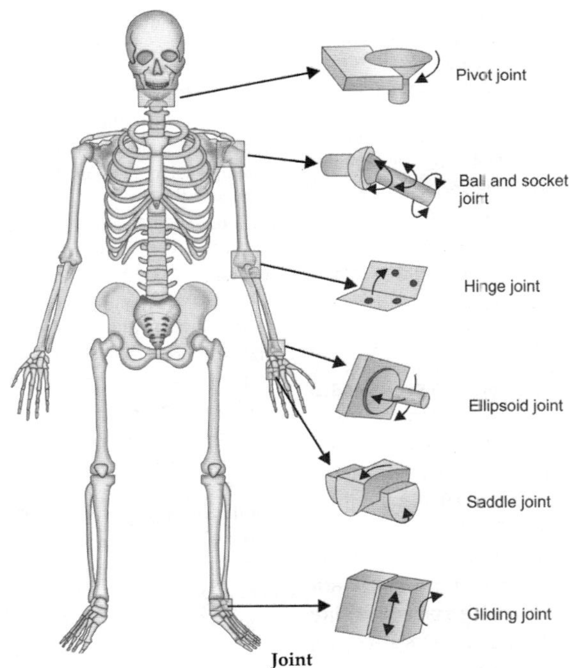

Joint

जैसे कूल्हे का जोड़, उलूखन संखि। Enathrosis multiaxial the joint in which the round and of a bone fits into the cavity of another bone, e.g. hip joint. (*iii*) **Charcot's joint** (चार्कोट्'स ज्वाइन्ट) हड्डी का अवशोषण। The refers to progressive degeneration of a weight bearing joint, a process marked by bony destruction, bone resorption, and eventual deformity.

(*iv*) **False joint** (फाल्स ज्वाइंट) किसी अस्थि भंग के पश्चात् बनने वाला जोड़। The joint formed after a fracture. (*v*) **Hinge joint** (हिंग ज्वाइन्ट) ऐसा जोड़ जो केवल आगे और पीछे को घूमता है जैसे कोहनी संध्ि, कोर संधि।

Ginglymoid joint, a joint which moves forward and backward only as elbow joint. (*vi*) **Pivot joint** (पाइवट ज्वाइन्ट) धुराग्र संधि। A joint that permits rotation of a bone rotator joint. (*vii*) **Saddle joint** (सैडल ज्वाइन्ट) ऐसा जोड़ जिसमें एक हड्डी के सिरे की सतह उन्नतोदार होती है जबकि इसके विपरीत ओर की नातेदार होती है। Receptive joints the joint in which the surface of one boney end in convex which that of its opposite side is concavey. (*viii*) **Synarthrodial joint** (साइनार्थ्रोडियल ज्वाइंट) अचल संधि। Immovable joint.

Joint capsule (ज्वाइंट केप्सूल) किसी चल संधि में हड्डियों के सिरों को बन्द करने वाली थैलीनुमा एक संरचना जिसमें एक बाह्य तन्तुमय परत होती है तथा एक भीतरी श्लेषक-कला की परत होती है। इसमें श्लेषक तरल भरा होता है। A saclike structure enclosing the bony ends in a movable joint consisting of an outer fibrous layer and an inner layer of the synovial membrane it contains synovial fluid.

Joule (जूल) एक एम्पियर विद्युत धारा द्वारा एक ओहम के प्रतिरोध के विरूद्ध एक सेकण्ड में किया गया कार्य। Work done in one second by an electric current of 1 amp against a resistance of one ohm.

Jugal (जुगल) जुड़ा हुआ या गण्डास्थि अथवा गाल से सम्बन्धित। United or pertaining to the malar or zygomatic bone or the check.

Jugal bone (जुगल बोन) गण्डास्थि। Malar or zygomatic bone.

Jugular (जुगुलर) गर्दन सम्बन्धी, ग्रीवाशिरा। Pertaining to the neck, jugular vein.

Jugular process (जुगुलर प्रोसेस) पश्चकपालिक अस्थि से शंखास्थि की ओर निकलने वाला एक उभार। A projection from the occipital bone towards the temporal bone.

Jugular veins (जुगुलर वेन्स) ग्रीवा क्षेत्र की शिराएं। Veins of the neck region.

Jugulation (जुगुलेशन) चिकित्सा द्वारा किसी रोग का एकदम रूक जाना। Sudden arrest of a disease by the treatment.

Jugulum (जुगुलम) गर्दन अथवा गला। Neck or throat.

Jugum (जुगुम) दो संरचनाओं को जोड़ने वाला एक कटक या खातिका। A ridge or furrow connecting the two structures.

Juice (जूस) किसी जन्तु, मनुष्य अथवा पौधे के किसी भी भाग

से निकाला गया सत्व, स्रावित अथवा उत्सर्जित कोई भी तरल जैसे—जठर रस। Any fluid extracted, secreted or excreted from any part of an animal, a man or a plant, e.g. gastric juice.

Junction (जन्कशन) दो भागों की संयोग का अथवा उनके एक दूसरे के पास आने का स्थान जैसे म्यूकोक्यूटेनियस जन्कशन जो त्वचा एवं श्लेष्मिक कला के बीच का संगम होता है। The place of union or coming together of two parts, e.g. mucocutaneous junction, a junction between the skin and the mucous membrane.

Jurisprudence medical (जुरिसप्रुडैन्स, मेडिकल) विधि-शास्त्र जिसका चिकित्सीय प्रैक्टिस में उपयोग होता है, चिकित्सीय विधि-शास्त्र। The science of law as applied to the practice of medicine.

Justomajor (जस्टोमेजर) सामान्य से बड़ा। Bigger than normal.

Juvenile (ज्वेनाइल) बचपन अथवा युवास्था से सम्बन्धित। Pertaining to the childhood or youth.

Juvenile delinquent (ज्वैनाइल डेलिन्कुएन्ट) ऐसा किशोर जो असामाजिक अथवा अपराधिक कार्य करता है और जिस पर माँ-बाप का कोई नियंत्रण नहीं होता। An adolescent who commits antisocial or criminal acts and cannot be controlled by his parents.

Juxta (जक्सटा) एक उपसर्ग जिसका अर्थ 'पास में स्थित' होता है। A prefix meaning situated near.

Juxta-articular (जक्सटा-आर्टिकुलर) किसी जोड़ के पास स्थित। Situated near a joint.

Juxtaposition (जक्सटापोजिशन) समीपवर्ती स्थिति, सान्निध्य। Adjacent position.

Juxtapyloric (जक्सटापाइलोरीक) जठरनिर्गम के पास। Near the pylorus.

Juxtavesical (जक्सटावैसाइकल) मूत्राशय के पास स्थित। Situated near the urinary bladder.

K

K (के) पोटेशियम का रासायनिक प्रतीक। Chemical symbol for Potassium.

Kakosmia (केकोस्मिया) दुर्गन्ध की अनुभूति होना जो वास्तव में विद्यमान नहीं होती। Cacosmia perception of foul smell which actually does not exist.

Kakotrophy (कैकोट्रॉफी) कुपोषण। Malnutrition.

Kala-azar (कालाजार) एक कशाभयुक्त एककोशिकीय जन्तु लीशमैनिया डोनोवैनाई जो संक्रमित बालु मक्षिका या सैण्डफ्लाई के काटने से संचारित होता है, के द्वारा उत्पन्न संसार के उष्णकटिबन्धी एवं अवऊष्ण-कटिबन्धी प्रदेशों में फैलने वाला एक प्राणघातक संक्रामक रोग जिसमें ज्वर होता है रक्ताल्पता एवं क्षीणता हो जाती है तथा प्लीहा एवं यकृत बढ़ जाते हैं। Protozoal tropical disease caused by leishmania donovani manifesting with lever lymphadenopathy and hepatosplenomegaly with darkening of skin.

Kalimeter (कैलीमीटर) किसी पदार्थ की क्षारीयता को मापने वाला उपकरण। A device for determining alkalinity of a substance.

Kaliopenic (कैलियोपैनिक) रक्त में पोटेशियम की कमी हो जाने से सम्बन्धित। Pertaining to kaliopenia.

Kalium (कैलियम) पोटेशियम। Potassium.

Kaliuresis (कैलियूरेसिस) पोटेशियम का मूत्र में उत्सर्जित होना। Excretion of potassium in the urine.

Kanner syndrome (केनर सिण्ड्रोम) आन्मकेन्द्रित शिशु। Autism infantile.

Kaolin (केओलिन) जलयोजित एल्युमीनियम सिलीकेट जिसका अवशोषक के रूप में शामक एवं नमी का अवशोषण करके अतिसार के रक्षक के रूप में प्रयोग होता है। Clay powder containing hydrated aluminum silicate used as absorbent and used as protector in diarrhea.

Karyo (कैरियो) एक उपसर्ग जिसका अर्थ किसी कोशिका का केन्द्रक होता है। A prefix meaning nucleus of a cell.

Karyocyte (कैरियोसाइट) एक केन्द्रक युक्त लाल रक्त कोशिका, मूललोहित कोशिका। A nucleated red blood cells.

Karyogenic (कैरियोजेनिक) केन्द्रक को बनाने वाला। Forming the nucleus.

Karyoklasis (कैरियोक्लेसिस) कोशिका केन्द्रक का अवखण्डन। Disintegration of the cell.

Karyolysis (कैरियोलाइसिस) केन्द्रकसंलयन। Chromatolysis.

Karyon (कैरियोन) किसी कोशिका का केन्द्रक। The nucleus of a cell.

Karyopyknosis (कैरियोपिकनोसिस) किसी कोशिका केन्द्रक का सिकुड़ जाना तथा क्रोमैटिन का संघनित होना। Shrinkage of a cell nucleus with condensation of the chromatin.

Karyorrhexis (कैरियोरैह्क्सिस) कोशिका केन्द्रक के फट जाने पर क्रोमेटिन का छोटे-छोटे कणों में अवखण्डित हो जाना, केन्द्रकभंग। Karyoclasis the disintegration of the chromatin into small granules on rupture of the cell nucleus.

Karyosome (कैरियोसोम) एक कोशिका जो केन्द्रकों में विभाजित नहीं होती। Irregular clump of nondividing chromatin in cell nucleus.

Kata (कैटा) एक उपसर्ग जिसका अर्थ नीचे, पीछे, विपरीत अथवा उल्टी क्रिया होता है। A prefix meaning down, back, against or reversing process.

Kathisophobia (कैथिसोफोबिया) नीचे बैठने का भय। Fearing of sitting down.

Kegel exercise (केगल एक्सरसाइज) स्त्रियों के मूलाधार की पेशियों को शक्तिशाली बनाने के लिए किये जाने वाले व्यायाम जो शिशु जन्म की प्रक्रियाओं एवं लैंगिक आनन्द में सहायता करते हैं। An exercise for strengthening the pubococcygeal levator ani muscles in control of urinary and fecal incontinence.

Kelectome (कैलेक्टोम) परीक्षण के लिए किसी अबुर्द पदार्थ को निकालने वाला एक यंत्र। An instrument for removing a piece of a tumor substance for examination.

Keloid (कीलॉयड) किसी चोट लगने अथवा ऑपरेशन के पश्चात् या मुहासा निकलने के बाद त्वचा में उठा हुआ, लाल, मोटा एवं कठोर व्रणचिन्ह। Hypertrophic, raised firm thick scar following trauma or surgical incision

Kelvin scale (कैल्विन स्केल) एक तापमान मापनी जिसमें जीरो सैल्सियस पैमाने के ऋणात्मक 273° के बराबर होता है।

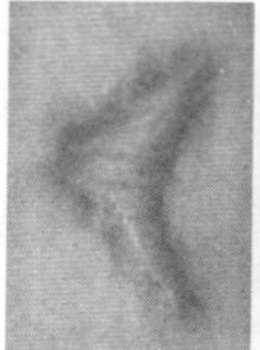
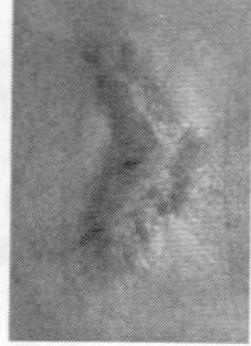

Keloid

Temperature scale in which absolute zero is equal to minus 273° on Celsius scale.

Kenophobia (कीनोफोबिया) खाली स्थानों का विकृत भय। Morbid fear of empty.

Keratalgia (कैराटेल्जिया) स्वच्छमण्डल में दर्द होना। Pain in the cornea.

Keratectomy (केराटेक्टॉमी) स्वच्छमण्डल के किसी भाग को शल्यक्रिया द्वारा काटकर अलग कर देना। Excision of a portion of the cornea.

Keratiasis (केराटिएसिस) त्वचा पर श्रृंगी अधिमांसों का बनना। Formation of the horny warts on the skin.

Keratin (केराटिन) बाह्यत्वचा, बाल एवं नाखूनों में पाया जाने वाला एक कठोर प्रोटीन पदार्थ। A hard protein substance found in the epidermis hair and nails.

Keratinase (केराटिनेज़) केराटिन का जलअपघटन करने वाला एक एन्जाइम। A enzyme which hydrolyzes the keratin.

Keratinization (केराटिनाइज़ेशन) कठोर अथवा श्रृंगी बनने की क्रिया, केराटिनीकरण। The process of becoming hard or horny.

Keratinocyte (केराटिनोसाइट) त्वचा की कोई भी कोशिका जो केराटिन का निर्माण करती है। Any cell of the skin which synthesize the keratin.

Keratinous (केराटिनस) केराटिन से बना हुआ अथवा उसकी प्रकृति का केराटिनी। Composed of or of the nature of keratin.

Keratitis (केराटाइटिस) स्वच्छमण्डलशोथ, कॉर्निया की सूजन। Inflammation of the cornea. (*i*) **Actinic keratitis** (एक्टिनिक केराटाइटिस) स्वच्छमण्डल या कॉर्निया की अल्ट्रावॉयलेट प्रकाश से होने वाली प्रतिक्रिया के रूप में उत्पन्न होने वाला स्वच्छमण्डलशोथ। Keratitis accruing as a reaction of the cornea to ultraviolet light.

Keratitis bullosa (केराटाइटिस बुलोसा) स्वच्छमण्डल पर छालों का बन जाना, स्फोटी स्वच्छमण्डलशोथ। The formation of bleds upon the cornea. (*i*) **Mycotic keratitis** (माइकोटिक केराटाइटिस) कवक संक्रमण द्वारा उत्पन्न स्वच्छमण्डलशोथ। Inflammation of the cornea caused by fungus infection.

(*ii*) **Trachomatous keratitis** (ट्रेकोमेटस केराटाइटिस) रोहों में होने वाला स्वच्छमण्डलशोथ। Keratitis accruing in trachoma.

Keratocele (केराटोसील) किसी आघात अथवा व्रण के फलस्वरूप कार्निया से होकर डेस्मेट की झिल्ली का बाहर निकल आना। Protusion of Descemet's membrane through the cornea as a result of injury or ulcer.

Keratocentesis (केराटोसेन्टेसिस) कॉर्निया का छिद्रीकरण। Puncture of the cornea.

Keratoconjunctivitis (केराटोकन्जन्क्टीवाइटिस) स्वच्छमण्डल या कॉर्निया एवं नेत्रश्लेष्मा का शोथ। Inflammation of cornea and conjunctiva.

Keratoconus (केराटोकोनस) कॉर्निया के केन्द्रीय भाग का शंक्वाकार रूप से बाहर निकलना, शंकुक-स्वच्छमण्डल। Conical protrusion of the central portion of the cornea.

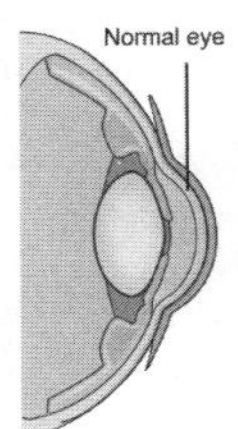

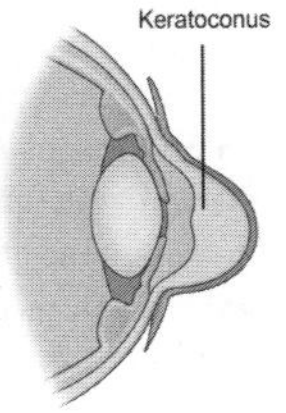

Keratodermatitis (केराटोडर्मेटाइटिस) त्वचा की श्रृंगी परत का शोथ। Inflammation of horny layer of the skin.

Keratodermia (केराटोडर्मिया) हथेली व पैरों की तल्वे की स्ट्रेटम कॉर्नियम की अतिवृद्धि। Hypertrophy of stratum corneum of palms and soles of feet.

Keratohelcosis (केराटोहेल्कोसिस) कॉर्निया में जख्म बन जाना। Ulceration of the cornea.

Keratohemia (केराटोहीमिया) कॉर्निया में रक्त का पाया जाना। Presence of blood in the cornea.

Keratoid (कैराटॉयड) श्रृंगी अथवा स्वच्छमण्डल ऊतक से मिलता-जुलता। Horny or resembling corneal tissue.

Keratolysis (केराटोलाइसिस) त्वचा की श्रृंगी परत का उखड़ जाना अथवा झड़ जाना। Loosening or shedding of the horny layer of the skin.

Keratoma (केराटोमा) किण या कील, श्रृंगी वृद्धि। A callosity horny growth.

Keratomalecia (केरेटोनैलेशिया) विटामिन 'ए' की कमी में कॉर्निया का मुलायम हो जान। Softening of the cornea in vitamin A deficiency.

Keratometer (केराटोमीटर) कॉर्निया की वक्रताओं को मापने वाला यंत्र। An instrument for measuring the curves of the cornea.

Keratometry (केराटोमीट्री) कॉर्निया वक्रताओं को मापना, स्वच्छमण्डलमिति। Measurement of the corneal curves.

Keratomycosis (केराटोमाइकोसिस) कॉर्निया का कवक संक्रमण स्वच्छमण्डलकवकता। Fungal infection of the cornea.

Keratopathy (केराटोपैथी) कॉर्निया का कोई भी अशोथज रोग। Any noninflammatory disease of the cornea.

Keratoplasty (केराटोप्लास्टी) स्वच्छमण्डल या कॉर्निया की प्लास्टिक सर्जरी अथवा कॉर्निया-निरोपण। Plastic surgery on the cornea or cornea grafting.

Keratoplastyoptic (केराटोप्लास्टीऑप्टिक) कॉर्निया-व्रणाचिन्ह को अलग करके उसे कॉर्निया ऊतक से पुनः स्थापित करना। To remove the corneal scar and replace it with corneal tissue. (*i*) **Refractive keratoplasty** (रिफ्रेक्टिव-केराटोप्लास्टी) ऐसी कॉर्निया की प्लास्टिक सर्जरी जिसमें नेत्र को अपवर्तन दोष को दूर करने के लिए कॉर्निया की आकृति रूपान्तरित कर दिया जाता है। Treatment of myopia or hypermetropia by reshaping corneal curvature either by multiple incision or as in keratomileusis.

Keratorrhexis (केराटोरैह्क्सिस) कॉर्निया का फट जाना। Rupture of cornea.

Keratoscope (केराटोस्कोप) कॉर्निया का दृष्टि-परीक्षण करने वाला एक यंत्र। An instrument for examination of cornea.

Keratose (केराटोस) श्रृंगी। Horny.

Keratosis (केराटोसिस) कोई भी श्रृंगीय वृद्धि। Any horny growth. (*i*) **Actinic keratosis** (एक्टीनिक-केराटोसिस) सूर्य प्रकाश के प्रति अत्यधिक अनावृत होने से उत्पन्न त्वचा की श्रृंगीय वृद्धि जो दुर्दम भी हो सकती है, विकीरणशील केरेटिनता। The horny growth of the skin caused by excessive exposure to sunlight which may also become malignant.

Keratosis lingue (केराटेसिस लिंग्यू) जिह्वा की श्वेतशल्कता। Leukoplakia of the tongue.

Keratosis pilaris (केराटोसिस-पाइलेरिस) लोम-केरेटिनता। A horny formation around the hair follicle. (*i*) **Senile K.** (सेनाइल–केराटोसिस) वृद्ध व्यक्तियों की शुष्क एवं रूक्ष त्वचा। Dry harsh skin of the old people.

Keratotome (केराटोटोम) कॉर्निया में चीरा लगाने वाला चाकू, स्वच्छमण्डल छुरिका। A knife for corneal incision.

Keratotomy (केराटोटॉमी) कॉर्निया में चीरा लगाना। To make an incision into the cornea.

Kerion (केरियॉन) टिनीय केपिटीस द्वारा उत्पन्न कपाल का कवक संक्रमण जिसमें शोथयुक्त दलदला पिण्ड बन जाता है। A lesion secondary to tinea capitis.

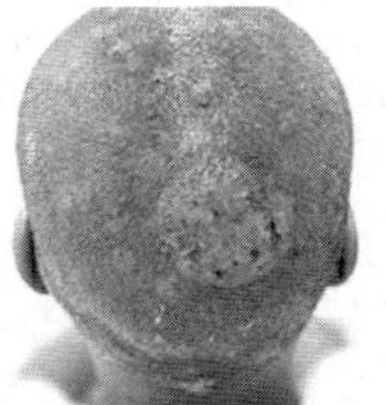

Kernig's sign (कर्निग्स साइन) नितम्बसन्धि तथा कोहनी की सिकुड़न, जानु, मैनिनजाइटिस का एक चिन्ह है।
Reflex spasm and pain in hamstrings when attempting to extend the knee after flexion of hip a sign of meningitis.

Ketoacidosis (कीटोएसिडोसिस) कीटोन कणों की अधिकता से होने वाली अम्लरक्तता। Acidosis due to excess of ketone bodies.

Ketoaciduria (कीटोएसिडूरिया) मूत्र में कीटों अम्लों की विद्यमानता। Presence of ketoacidosis in the urine.

Ketogenesis (कीटोजेनेसिस) कीटोन कणों का बनना, कीटोनजनन। Production of ketone bodies.

Ketolysis (कीटोलाइसिस) कीटोन कणों का विघटित हो जाना, कीटोनलयन। The dissolution of ketone bodies.

Ketone (कीटोन) कार्बोनील ग्रुप (c = o) से युक्त एक पदार्थ जो मधुमेह एवं भूखे रहने की स्थिति में यकृत में ग्लाइकोजन की कमी के कारण वसा चयापचय के अन्तिम उत्पादों वसीय अम्लों के आंशिक ऑक्सीकरण से यकृत में बनता है। A substance containing carbonyl group (c = o) attached to two carbon atoms, e.g. acetone, the ketones are end products of fat metabolism.

Ketone bodies (कीटोन बॉडीज) वसीय अम्लों के ऑक्सीकरण से बना यौगिकों का एक वर्ग जिसमें एसिटोएसिटिक एसिड, बीटा-हाइड्रॉक्सीब्यूट्रिक एसिड

एवं एसिटोन होते है। A group of compounds produced during oxidation of fatty acid and include acetones, β-hydroxybutyric acid and acetoacetic acid.

Ketonemia (कीटोनीमिया) रक्त में कीटोन कणों का अधिक पाया जाना। Presence of ketone bodies in the blood in excess quantity.

Ketonuria (कीटोन्यूरिया) मूत्र में कीटोन कणों का पाया जाना, कीटोनमेह। Presence of ketone bodies in the urine.

Ketoplasia (कीटोप्लासिया) कीटोनों का बनना। Formation of ketones.

Ketose (कीटोस) कीटोनों से युक्त कोई भी कार्बोहाइड्रेट। A carbohydrate containing the ketones.

Ketosis (कीटोसिस) शरीर में कीटोन कणों का जमा हो जाना, कीटोनमयता। Accumulation of ketone bodies in the body.

Ketotic (कीटोटिक) कीटोनमयता से सम्बन्धित। Pertaining to the ketosis.

Kidney (किडनी) वृक्क, गुर्दा। Urine secreting organ.

(*i*) **Atrophic kidney** (एट्रॉफिक किडनी) ऐसा वृक्क जो अपर्याप्त रक्त परिसंचरण और या वृक्काणुओं के अभाव में परिमाण में छोटा हो जाता है। A kidney that is reduced in size because of inadequate blood circulation and or loss of nephrons. (*ii*) **Contracted kidney** (कॉन्ट्रेक्टेड किडनी) जीर्ण अन्तरालीय वृक्कशोथ में छोटा हुआ वृक्क। Small kidney in chronic interstitial nephritis. (*iii*) **Ectopic kidney** (एकटोपिक किडनी) अस्थानिक वृक्क। Kidney at abnormal site. (*iv*) **Fatty kidney** (फैटी किडनी) वसीय ह्रास से युक्त वृक्क। Kidney with fatty degeneration. (*v*) **Horseshoe kidney** (हार्सशू किडनी) अश्वनाल वृक्क। A congenital union of the kidneys. (*vi*) **Floating kidney** (फ्लोटिंग किडनी) चल वृक्क। Movable kidney.

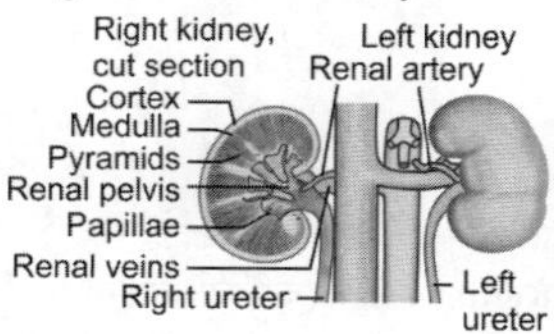

Kidney failure (किडनी फैल्योर) वृक्कपात। Diminished function of the kidney.

Kidney stone (किडनी स्टोन) वृक्काश्म, गुर्दे की पथरी, वृक्काश्मरी। Presence of calculus in the pelvis of kidney.

Kilo (किलो) एक हजार का संकेत देने वाला उपसर्ग। A prefix indicating one thousand.

Kilocycle (किलोसाइकिल) एक हजार चक्कर प्रति सेकण्ड। One thousand cycles per second.

Kilogram (किलोग्राम) 1000 ग्राम का भार। A weight of 1000 gms.

Kilogram-meter (किलोग्राम-मीटर) एक किलोग्राम भार को एक मीटर उठाने के लिए किया जाने वाला कार्य। The work done to raise one kilogram weight to one meter.

Kilohertz (किलोहर्टज) विद्युत में एक हजार चक्रों की एक इकाई। In electricity, a unit of one thousand cycles.

Kilojoule (किलोजूल) एक हजार जूल। One thousand joule.

Kiloliter (किलोलीटर) एक हजार लीटर। One thousand liter.

Kilometer (किलोमीटर) 1000 मीटर अथवा 3280.83 फीट या 0.62 मील। 1000 meters or 3280.83 feet or 0.62 of a mile.

Kilowatt (किलोवाट) एक हजार वाट के बराबर विद्युत-शक्ति की एक इकाई। A unit of electrical energy equal to one thousand watts.

Kimmelstiel Wilson syndrome (काइमेलस्टाइल विल्सन सिण्ड्रोम) एक ऐसा संलक्षण जो मधुमेह के रोगी में उत्पन्न हो सकता है जिसमें उच्च रक्तचाप, सार्वदैहिक शोफ एवं मूत्र में प्रोटीन की मात्रा कम हो जाती है। Nodular glomerulosclerosis in long standing diabetes mellitus with hypertension, edema, retinal lesions and proteinuria.

Kinanesthesia (काइनेनेस्थीसिया) गति की अनुभूति होने में असमर्थता। Inability to perceive the sensation of movement.

Kinematics (काइनेमेटिक्स) गति-विज्ञान। Science of motion.

Kinematograph (काइनेमेटोग्राफ) गतिमान वस्तुओं का चित्रण करने के लिए एक उपकरण जिसका रोग निदान में प्रयोग किया जाता है। A device for viewing photographs of objects in motion used in diagnosis.

Kinesalgia (काइनेसेल्जिया) पेशीय गति होने पर दर्द होना। Pain accruing on muscular movement.

Kinescope (काइनेस्कोप) आँख के अपवर्तन की जाँच करने वाला एक उपकरण। An apparatus for testing the refraction of the eye.

Kinesiatrics (काइनेसियाट्रिक्स) गतिरोग-विशेषज्ञ, गतिरोग-चिकित्सा। Treatment involving active and passive movement.

Kinesics (काइनेसिक्स) शरीर की गतियों का अध्ययन। The study of the body movements.

Kinesiology (काइनेसियोलॉजी) शरीर की पेशीय गतियों का वैज्ञानिक अध्ययन। Scientific study of the muscular movements of the body.

Kinesiotherapy (काइनेसियोथिरैपी) व्यायाम द्वारा रोगों की चिकित्सा करना। Treatment of disease by exercise.

Kinesophobia (काइनेसोफोबिया) गति होने का विकृत भय। Morbid fear of movements.

Kinesthesia (काइनेस्थीसिया) वह संवेद जिसके द्वारा स्थिति, भार एवं गति का ज्ञान होता है, गतिसंवेदना। Ability to perceive extent direction and weight of movement.

Kinetic (काइनेटिक) गति सम्बन्धी उसे उत्पन्न करने वाला गतियुक्त, गतिज। Pertaining to or consisting of motion.

Kinetochore (काइनेटोकोर) गुणसूत्र बिन्दु। Centromere.

Kinetocyte (काइनेटोसाइट) परिभ्रमण करने वाली कोशिका। A wondering cell.

Kink (किंक) किसी नली जैसे आँत अथवा मूत्रनली आदि में एक अप्राकृतिक मोड़। An unnatural bend in a tube as in the intestine or ureter, etc.

Kinking (किकिंग) ऐठंन। Twisting.

Klieg eye (क्लाइग आई) वह नेत्र जिसमें चलचित्र अथवा टेलीविजन फिल्म बनाने में प्रयुक्त तीव्र प्रकाश के प्रति अनावृत होने से नेत्रश्लेष्म-कलाशोथ, अश्रु स्रावण एवं प्रकाशासह्यता हो जाती है। Conjunctivitis lacrimation and photophobia from exposure to intense lights as used in making of television and film shooting.

Klumpke's paralysis (क्लम्पकीज पैरालाइसिस) अग्रबाहु के पक्षाघात के साथ अपक्षय। Paralysis with atrophy of the forearm.

Kneading (नीडिंग) गूँथने का कार्य। Act of working for dough.

Knee (नी) फीमर की टीबिया के साथ बनी संधि जो आगे की ओर पटेला, हड्डी या नी कैप से ढकी होती है, जानु, घुटना। Femorotibial articulation covered anteriorly with patella. (*i*) **Housemaid's knee** (हाउज़मेड्'स नी) पटेला हड्डी के आगे श्लेषपुटी या वसा का शोथ जिसके भीतर तरल संचित हो जाता है। Bursitis of bursa anterior to patella due to prolonged kneeling.

Knee cap (नी कैप) पटेला हड्डी, जानुका। Patella bone.

Knee joint (नी ज्वाइंट) फीमर एवं टिबिया हड्डियों का जोड़, जानु सन्धि, घुटने का जोड़। The articulation of the femur and the tibia bone.

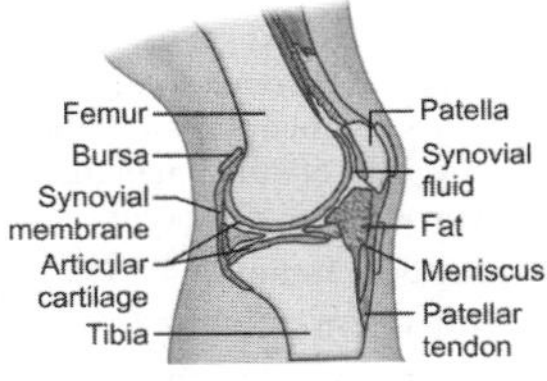

Kneipp cure (नीप क्योर) जल चिकित्सा। Hydrotherapy.

Knob (नौब) उभार अथवा पर्विका। A protuberance or nodule.

Knock knee (नौक नी) बहिर्नत जानु, संघट्ट जानु। A crooked knee, genu valgum.

(*i*) **Locked knee** (लॉक्ड नी) ऐसी दशा जिसमें टाँग को प्रसारित नहीं किया जा सकता। ऐसा अक्सर अर्द्धचन्द्राकार उपास्थि के विस्थापित के कारण होता है। Inability to extend the leg due to torn semilunar cartilage.

Knot (नॉट) शरीर रचना विज्ञान में, किसी संरचना की वृद्धि जिससे उभार या पर्व के समान रचना निकल आती है। In anatomy, enlargement of a structure forming a knob like structure.

(*i*) **False knot** (फाल्स नॉट) नाभि की रक्त वाहिनियों के चक्करदार होने के फलस्वरूप उत्पन्न नाभि-रज्जु का एक बाह्य फुलाव। An external bulging of the umbilical cord resulting from coiling of the umbilical blood vessels. (*ii*) **True knot** (ट्रु नॉट) भ्रूण के नाभि-रज्जु के किसी फंदे से होकर रपट जाने से बन जाने वाली गांठ, वास्तविक गांठ। A knot formed by the fetus slipping through a loop of the umbilical cord.

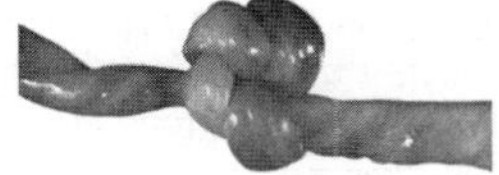

Knotting (नॉटिंग) गाँठों का बनना। Formation of knots.

Knuckle (नकल) किसी भी अंगुल्यस्थि-संधि के पृष्ठ तल का उठान, अँगुली की गांठ। Prominence of the dorsal aspect of any phalangeal joint.

Koilonychia (कोइलोनीकिया) हाथ की अँगुलियों के नाखूनों का दुष्पोषण या अपविकास जिसमें नाखून पतले एवं नतोदार हो जाते हैं। किनारे उठे हुए होते हैं, दर्बी नख। Dystrophy of the finger nails in which they become thin and concave with raised margins.

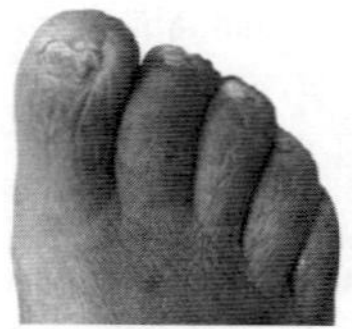

Koilosternia (कोइलोस्टर्नियां) कीपाकार वक्ष से युक्त होना। The condition of having funnel-shaped chest.

Kolp (कोल्प) योनि को संकेतिक करने वाला एक उपसर्ग। A prefix indicating vagina.

Koplik's spots (कोपलिक्स स्पॉट्स) मीजिल्स या खसरा के प्रकट होने से पूर्व मुख की श्लेष्मिक कला पर नीलापन किए हुए सफेद केन्द्रो से युक्त छोटे-छोटे लाल धब्बे। Small red spots with bluish white centers on the mucous membrane of the mouth before the rash appears in measles.

Kopophobia (कोपोफोबिया) थकान का असामान्य भय। Abnormal fear of tiredness.

Kraurosis vulvae (क्रौरोसिस वल्वी) अधिकतर वृद्ध स्त्रियों के बाह्य जननांगों का शुष्क होना व सिकुड़ जाना। A condition in which the atrophy and shrinkage of the cutaneous layer of the skin of the vagina and vulva. Mostly occured in old age women's.

Krourasis (क्रोरोसिस) त्वचा एवं श्लेष्मिक कला का अपक्षय होने के परिणामस्वरूप उनके शुष्क होने एवं उनमें झुर्री पड़ने अथवा उनके सिकुड़ जाने की दशा विशेषकर भग की। Atrophy and dryness of skin and mucous membrane especially of vulva malignant degeneration may occur.

Krukenberg tumor (क्रूकेनबर्ज ट्यूमर) दुर्दमडिम्बग्रन्थ्यबुर्द, डिम्बाशय का एक दुर्दम अर्बुद। Secondary malignant tumor of the ovary.

Kussmaul's breathing (कुस्मौल्य ब्रीदिंग) तीव्र मधुमेही अम्लरक्तता तथा सन्यास या गहन मूर्च्छा में हाँफते हुए बहुत गहरे-गहरे सांस लेना। Very deep gasping respiration in severe diabetic acidosis and coma.

Kwashiorkor (क्वाशियोरकोर) बच्चों में तीव्र प्रोटीन अल्पता के कारण उत्पन्न एक रोग जिसमें आलस, वृद्धि के रूक जाने, मानसिक दुर्बलता, संक्रमणों के प्रति बढ़ी हुई सुग्राहता, शोफ, त्वकशोथ जिसके साथ त्वचा एवं बालों के वर्णक में परिवर्तन हो जाते है तथा यकृत में वृद्धि। A condition due to severe protein deficiency in children characterized by the symptoms of lethargy, retarted growth, mental deficiency, increased within the skin and hair pigment and enlargement of the liver.

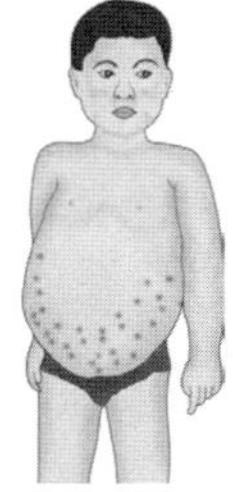

Kymograph (काइमोग्राफ) हृदय या मध्यपट अथवा डायफ्राम की गतियों के प्रसार का अभिलेख करने वाला एक एक्स-रे उपकरण। गतिलेखी।
A radiographic apparatus for recording the range of movement of the heart or diaphragm.

Kymoscope (काइमोस्कॉप) रूधिरधारादर्शीयंत्र। An instrument for studying the blood current.

Kyphorachitis (काइफोरेकाइटिस) बालास्थिविकार में वक्ष एवं मेरूदण्ड की विकृति जिसमें पीठ में कूबड़ निकल आता है। Deformity of the thorax and spinal column in rickets resulting in the development of a hump at the back.

Kyphoscoliosis (काइफोस्कोलियोसिस) पृष्ठपार्श्वकुब्जता।
Combined kyphosis and scoliosis.

Kyphosis (काइफोसिस) मेरूदण्ड की वक्षीय क्षेत्र में अत्यधिक वक्रता जिसमें पीछे की ओर उन्नोतोदरता हो जाती है। अर्थात् उभार निकल आता है, कुब्जता, कुबड़ापन।
Humpback increased curvature of the spinal column in the thoracic region with convexity backwards.

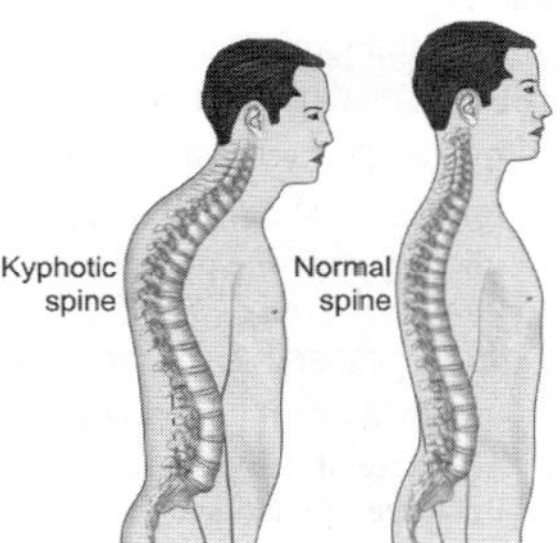

Kyphosis

Kyphotic (काइफोटिक) कुब्जता या कुबड़ेपन से ग्रस्त अथवा कुब्जता सम्बन्धी। Affected by or pertaining to kyphosis.

L

L and A (एल एण्ड ए) नेत्रों की पुतलियों की प्रकाश एवं समंजन के प्रति प्रतिक्रिया। The reaction of the pupils of the eyes to light and accommodation.

Lamina cribrosa (लामिना क्रीब्रोसा) चालनीवत् फलक, चालनीरूप फलक। A cribriform plate of ethmoid bone.

LA (Left atrium) (ला) बॉया आलिन्द। Left atrium.

Labial (लेबियल) होठों से सम्बन्धित। Pertaining to the lips.

Labile (लेबाइल) अस्थिर, चलायमान, एक से दूसरे स्थान को खसक जाने वाला। Not fixed, unstable, gliding from one place to another.

Lability (लेबीलिटी) अस्थिरता अथवा परिवर्तनशील होने की अवस्था। The state of being not fixed or unstable or changeable.

Labioalveolar (लेबियोएल्वियोलर) होठों एवं दन्त गर्तिकाओं से सम्बन्धित। Pertaining to the lips and sockets of the tooth.

Labioglossolaryngeal (लेबियोग्लोसोलेरिन्जीयल) होंठ, जिह्वा एवं ग्रसनी या गले से सम्बन्धित। Pertaining to the lips, tongue and pharynx.

Labiomental (लेबियोमेंटल) निचले होंठ एवं हड्डी से सम्बन्धित। Pertaining to the lower lip and the chin.

Labiomycosis (लेबियोमाइकोसिस) होंठों का कवक रोग। Fungus disease of the lip.

Labioplasty (लेबियोप्लास्टी) ओष्ठसंधान। Plastic surgery on a lip.

Labium (लेबियम) मांसल किनारा अथवा होंठ, ओष्ठ, भगोष्ठ। A fleshy border or a lip.

Labium oris (लेबियम ओरिस) मुख के होंठ। Lips of the mouth.

Labor (लेबर) स्त्री में वह क्रिया जिसके द्वारा भ्रूण गर्भाशय से योनि से होते हुए शरीर के बाहर निकल जाता है। प्रसव। Function in female by which the fetus is expelled from the uterus through vagina on the outside of the body.

(*i*) **Arrested labor** (एरेस्टेड-लेबर) गर्भाशय जड़त्व अथवा गर्भाशय की निश्क्रियता, श्रोणि में अवरोध उत्पन्न हो जाने

अथवा सार्वदैहिक रोग में निष्फल सामान्य प्रसव। Failure of the normal labor due to uterine inertia obstruction of the pelvis or systemic disease.

(*ii*) **Dry labor** (ड्राइ लेबर) शुष्क प्रसव, जिसमें गर्भाशय की सिकुड़न आरम्भ होने से पहले ही उत्वकोष फट जाता है तथा उल्व-द्रव शिशु के साथ ही बाहर निकल आता है। Labor after spontaneous loss of practically all of the amniotic fluid.

(*iii*) **False labor** (फाल्स लेबर) ऐसे संकुचन होना जिनसे गर्भाशयग्रीवा विस्फारित नहीं होती तथा भ्रूण का प्रस्तुत होने वाला भाग नीचे नहीं उतरता। Contraction which do not produces dilation of the cervix of the uterus and descension of the presenting part of the fetus. (*iv*) **Induced labor** (इनड्यूसड लेबर) जिसमें प्रसव यंत्रों की सहायता के अतिरिक्त अन्य साधन भी अपनायें जाते है। प्रेरित प्रसव। That brought on by artificial means.
(*v*) **Postmature labor** (पोस्टमेच्योर लेबर) सम्भावित तिथि से दो या अधिक सप्ताह पश्चात् होने वाला प्रसव, दीर्घ प्रसव। Occurring two weeks or more after expected date of delivery.
(*vi*) **Precipitate labor** (प्रेसीपिटेट लेबर) शीघ्रता से अर्थात दो-तीन घण्टे के भीतर हो जाने वाला प्रसव, सहसा प्रसव, आकस्मिक प्रसव। Labor accruing very rapidly, i.e. within two to three hours
(*vii*) **Spontaneous labor** (स्पौन्टेनियस लेबर) स्वाभाविक प्रसव, स्वतः प्रसव, स्वतः प्रवर्तित प्रसव। That requiring no artificial aid.

Labrum (लेब्रम) होंठ अथवा होंठ के समान संरचना। Lip or liplike structure.

Labyrinth (लैबीरिन्थ) अन्तःकर्ण जो अस्थिल एवं कला-गहनों से मिलकर बनता है, गहन। The internal ear consisting of osseous or bony and membranous labyrinths.
(*i*) **Membranous labyrinth** (मेम्ब्रेनस लेबीरिन्थ) कला-गहन। The membranous cavity within the osseous labyrinth.

(*ii*) **Osseous labyrinth** (ऑसियस लेबीरिन्थ) अस्थि-गहन। The bony portion of the internal ear, bony labyrinth.

Labyrinthectomy (लैबिरिन्थैक्टॉमी) गहन-उच्छेदन। Excision of the labyrinth.

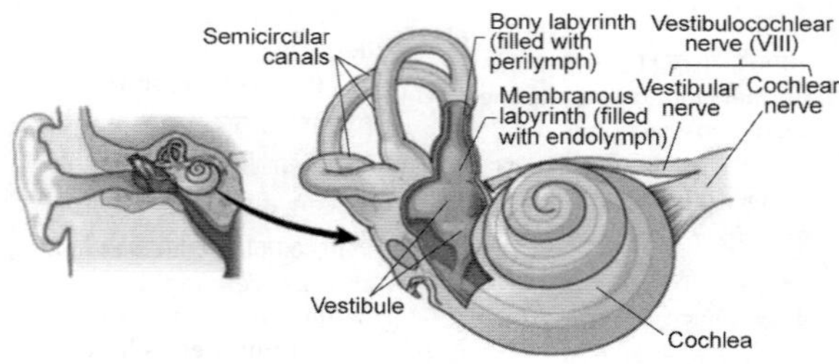

Labyrinth

Labyrinthitis (लैबिरिन्थाइटिस) गहन का शोथ। Inflammation of the labyrinth.

Labyrinthotomy (लैबिरिन्थोटॉमी) गहन में चीरा लगाना। To make incision into the labyrinth.

Lacerable (लैसीरेबल) विदीर्ण (कटे-फटे) हो जाने के सक्षम। Capable of being lacerated.

Laceration (लैसीरेशन) फाड़ना, व्रव अथवा माँस की अव्यवस्थित फटन, विदार। The act of tearing wound or irregular tear of the flesh.

Lacrimal (लैक्रीमल) आँसुओं से सम्बन्धित। Pertaining of the tears.

Lacrimation (लैक्रीमेशन) आँसुओं का बनना एवं बाहर निकलना, आश्रुस्रवण। Secretion and discharge to the tears.

Lacrimonasal (लैक्रीमोनेजल) अश्रुप्रवाही ग्रंथी एवं नासिका सम्बन्धी। Pertaining to the lacrimal gland and the nose.

Lacrimotomy (लैक्रीमोटॉमी) अश्रु-कोश अथवा अश्रुवाहिनी में चीरा लगाना। To make an incision into the lacrimal sac or duct.

Lactacidemia (लैक्टासिडीमिया) रक्त में लैक्टिक एसिड का अधिक पाया जाना। Excess of lactic acid in the blood.

Lactalbumin (लैक्टेल्ब्युमिन) एल्ब्यूमिन दूध की एक घुलनशील प्रोटीन है जो दूध को गर्म करने पर दूध की सतह के ऊपर एक झिल्ली की भाँति जम जाता है। Albumin, a soluble protein of milk which coagulate and appears as a film on the surface of milk, when milk is heated.

Lactic acid (लेक्टिक एसिड) दुग्धाम्ल, दुग्धक्षार। Acid that causes the souring of the milk.

Lactiferous (लैक्टीफेरस) दुग्ध का स्त्रवण एवं वाहन करने वाला, दुग्धजन। Secreting and carrying milk.

Lactifuge (लैक्टीफ्यूज) दुग्ध स्रवण को रोकने वाला, दुग्धशोषक। Stopping milk secretion.

Lactinated (लैक्टीनेटेड) दुग्ध शर्करा से युक्त अथवा उससे तैयार किया गया। Containing of or prepared with milk sugar.

Lactivorous (लैक्टीवोरस) दूध पर जीवित रहने वाला। Living upon milk.

Lactogen (लैक्टोजन) कोई भी पदार्थ जो दूध के उत्पादन को बढ़ाता है। An agent that stimulate milk production or secretion.

Lactogenic (लैक्टोजेनिक) दुध की मात्रा बढ़ाने वाला, दुग्धजनक, दुग्धवर्धक। Stimulating milk production.

Lactoglobulin (लैक्टोग्लोबुलिन) दुग्ध में पाई जाने वाली ग्लोबिन (प्रोटीन)। A globulin (protein) found in the milk.

Lactoscope (लैक्टोस्कोप) दुध की गुणवत्ता एवं शुद्धता की जाँच करने वाला एक यंत्र। An instrument for examining the quality and purity of milk.

Lactose (लैक्टोज़) दुग्ध शर्करा जिसके जल अपघटन से ग्लूकोज एवं गैलेक्टोज बनते हैं। Sugar of milk which on hydrolysis yields glucose and galactose.

Lactosuria (लैक्टोसूरिया) मूत्र में लैक्टोस का पाया जाना, लैक्टोज़मेह। Presence of lactose in urine.

Lacuna (लैक्यूना) उपास्थि अस्थि अथवा शरीर के अन्य किसी अंग में दोष अथवा दरार। Defects or gap in the cartilage bone or any other organ of the body.

Laennec's cirrhosis (लोनेकस सिरहोसिस) बहुत दिनों से शराब अधिक पीने से सम्बद्ध यकृत सिरहोसिस। Cirrhosis of the liver associated with chronic excessive intake of alcohol.

Lag (लैग) किसी उद्दीपन के प्रयोग करने एवं इसके फलस्वरूप उत्पन्न प्रतिक्रिया के बीच बीता समय। The time elapsed between application of a stimulus and the resulting reaction.

Lageniform (लैग्नीफोर्म) कुप्पी के आकार का। Flask shaped.

Lagophthalmos (लैगॅप्थाल्मोस) आँखों को पूर्णतया बन्द करने में अक्षम, अलप–निमेर्शी। Unable to close the eyes.

Laliatry (लैलियाट्री) वाक विकारों का अध्ययन एवं उनकी चिकित्सा करना। Study and treatment of the speech disorders.

Lallation (लैलेशन) बड़बड़ाना, शिशुओं की भाँति बोलना, हकलाना। The babbling, infantile form of speech.

Lalophobia (लैलोफोबिया) हकलाने के डर से बोलने का विकृत भय। Morbid fear to speak due to fear of stammering.

Lalorrhea (लैलोरिह्या) वाणी का अति प्रवाह। Excessive flow of speech.

Lame (लेम) पंगु, लॅंगड़ा। Cripple by leg.

Lamella (लैमीला) एक पतली प्लेट अथवा परत जैसी हड्डी की। पटलिका, पत्तक, पक्षक। Thin plate layer or sheet as of compact bone.

Lamellar (लैमीलर) पत्तकी, पटलित। Disposed in lamellas scaly.

Lamina (लैमीना) एक पतली, चपटी परत या झिल्ली, पटल, पत्तदल, आवरण, अस्तर, फलिका। A plate or thin sheet of material.

Lamina spiralis (लैमीना स्पाइरैलिस) सर्पिल फलक। The spiral partition dividing the cochlear cavity.

Lamina terminalis (लैमीना टर्मिनेलिस) अन्त्य फलक। The thin sheet of tissue forming the anterior border of the third ventricle, median portion the wall of the fore-brain vesicle consists a thin lamina.

Laminated (लैमीनेटेड) परतों में व्यवस्थित। Arrange in layers.

Laminitis (लैमीनाइटिस) किसी पटल अथवा फलक का शोथ। Inflammation of a lamina.

Laminotomy (लैमीनोटॉमी) किसी कशेरूका के किसी फलक को विभाजित करना। Division or partial removal of vertebral lamina.

Lamp (लैम्प) कृत्रिम दिपक, कृत्रिम रूप से रोशनी उत्पन्न करने वाला यंत्र। A device producing light artificially.

Lancet (लेन्सेट) कुन्तिका, छोटा, दो धार वाला शल्यक्रिया सम्बन्धी चाकू। A small surgical blade used for making small drainage incisions.

Lancinating (लेन्सीनेटिंग) तेज अथवा काटने वाला जैसे कोई दर्द होता है, विदीर्णकारी। Sudden sharp transient pain as if tearing into pieces.

Laniary (लैनियरी) फाड़ने के योग्य जैसे रदनक दाँत। Capable for tearing as the canine teeth.

Lanolin (लैनोलिन) भेड़ की ऊन से प्राप्त एक शुद्ध, वसा के समान

पदार्थ जिसका मरहम के आधार के रूप में प्रयोग किया जाता है, ऊर्ण वसा। A purified fatlike substance obtained from the wool of sheep used as an ointment base.

Lanugo (लैनुगो) भ्रूण के शरीर पर स्थित रोआदार बाल, गर्भरोम। Fine hair on the body of the fetus.

Laparocele (लैपरोसील) एक उदरीय बहिःसरण। An abdominal hernia.

Laparocystectomy (लैपरोसिस्टेक्टॉमी) गर्भाशय से बाहर स्थित भ्रूण की अथवा किसी पुटी को उदर में चीरा लगाकर अलग करना। Removal of extra-uterine fetus or cyst through an abdominal incision.

Laparocystodotomy (लैपरोसिस्टोडोटॉमी) उदरीय भित्ती से होकर मूत्राशय में चीरा लगाना। To make an incision into the urinary bladder through the abdominal wall.

Laparohepatotomy (लैपरोहिपैटोटॉमी) उदरीय भित्ति से होकर यकृत में चीरा लगाना। To make an incision into the liver through the abdominal wall.

Laparohysteropexy (लैपरोहिस्टीरोपैक्सी) गर्भाशय का उदरीय भित्ति के साथ स्थिरीकरण। Fixation of the uterus with the abdominal wall.

Laparomyomectomy (लैपरोमायोमेक्टॉमी) पेट में चीरा लगाकर पेशीय ऊतक को काटना। To cut the muscular tissue through an abdominal incision.

Laparoscope (लैपरोस्कोप) उदर-जाँच के लिए प्रयुक्त किया जाने वाला यंत्र। An instrument for examining the abdomen.

Laparotomy (लैपरोटॉमी) पेट का ऑपरेशन उदर-छेदन। An abdominal incision.

Lapatoscope (लैपटोस्कोप) कोशिका कलाओं की मोटाई के मापने वाला एक उपकरण। An apparatus for measuring the thickness of cell membranes.

Larva (लार्वा) अण्डे से निकलने के पश्चात् तथा प्यूपा में रूपान्तरित होने से पूर्व जिससे वह युवा रूप में बाहर निकलता है, किसी कीट का विकासशील रूप। A developing form of an insect after it has emerged from an egg and before it transforms into a pupa from which it emerges as an adult.

Larvicide (लार्वीसाइड) कीट लार्वो को मारने वाला एक कारक, लार्वानाशी। An agent that kills the insect larva.

Laryngalgia (लैरिन्जैलजिया) स्वरयंत्र में दर्द होना। Pain in the larynx.

Laryngectomy (लैरिन्जेक्टॉमी) शल्यक्रिया द्वारा स्वरयंत्र को अलग करके निकाल देना, स्वरयन्त्र उच्छेदन। Surgical removal of the larynx.

Laryngismus (लैरिन्जिस्मस) स्वरयंत्र की ऐंठन। Spasm of the larynx.

Laryngitis (लैरिन्जाइटिस) स्वरयंत्र का शोथ। Inflammation of the larynx.

Laryngocele (लैरिन्गोसील) एक जन्मजात वायु कोश जो स्वरयंत्र की गुहा से सम्बन्धित होता है और गर्दन के ऊपर बाहर को फूला हुआ दिखाई देता है, स्वरयंत्र विपुटी। A congenital air sac connection with the cavity of the larynx which may bulge outward on the neck.

Laryngoedema (लैरिन्गोइडीमा) एलर्जीजन्य प्रतिक्रिया द्वारा उत्पन्न स्वर-यंत्र की सूजन। Swelling of the larynx caused by an allergic reaction.

Laryngogram (लैरिन्गोग्राम) स्वरयंत्र का एक्स-रे चित्र। X-ray film of the larynx.

Laryngomalacia (लैरिन्गोमेलेसिया) स्वरयंत्र-मृदुता, स्वरयंत्र की कोमलता। The science of the larynx.

Laryngoparalysis (लैरिन्गोपैरालाइसिस) स्वरयंत्र का पक्षाघात। Paralysis of the larynx.

Laryngophony (लैरिन्गोफोनी) ग्रसनी का परिश्रवण करने पर सुनाई देने वाली स्वर ध्वनियाँ। Vocal sounds heard on auscultation to the pharynx.

Laryngoplasty (लैरिन्गोप्लास्टी) स्वरयंत्र की प्लास्टिक सर्जरी द्वारा मरम्मत करना। Repair of the larynx by plastic surgery.

Laryngorrhagia (लैरिन्गोरैह्जिया) स्वरयंत्र से रक्तस्राव होना। Hemorrhage from the larynx.

Laryngoscopy (लैरिन्गोस्कोपी) स्वरयंत्र के भीतर का नेत्र परिक्षण, स्वरयंत्रदर्शन। Visual examination of the interior of the larynx.

Laryngospasm (लैरिन्गोस्पाज्म) स्वरयंत्र की पेशियों की ऐंठन स्वरयंत्राकर्श। Spasm of the muscle of the larynx.

Laryngostomy (लैरिन्गोस्टॉमी) स्वरयंत्र छिद्रीकरण। To establish a permanent opening into the larynx through the neck.

Laryngotracheitis (लैरिन्गोट्रेकाइटिस) स्वरयंत्र एवं श्वास प्रणाली का शोथ। Inflammation of the larynx and trachea.

Laryngotracheobronchitis (लैरिन्गोट्रेकियोब्रोन्काइटिस) स्वरयंत्र, श्वासप्रणाल एवं श्वासनिकाओं का प्रदाह, स्वरयंत्र श्वासप्रणाल श्वसनीशोथ। Inflammation of the larynx, trachea and bronchi.

Larynx (लैरिक्स) स्वरअंग, स्वरयंत्र। The organ of voice.

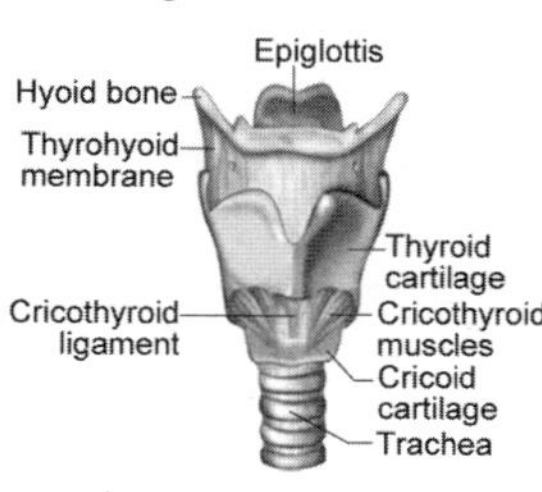

Laser (लेज़र) ऐसा उपकरण जिसमें लेजर किरण निकलती है तथा जिसका उपयोग सूक्ष्म शल्यकर्म, नेत्र रोगविज्ञान, चर्मरोगविज्ञान तथा अनेको नैदानिक कार्य-विधियों आदि में किया जाता है। An apparatus that emits laser beam used in microsurgery, ophthalmology, dermatology and various diagnostic procedures, etc.

Lassitude (लेसीट्यूड) थकान। Weariness, exhaustion.

Latency (लेटेन्सी) गुप्त रहने की अवस्था। The state of being latent.

Latent (लेटेन्ट) सुशुप्तावस्था में पड़ा हुआ अथवा गुप्त। Dormant or concealed.

Lateral (लेट्रल) किसी पार्श्व से सम्बन्धित, पाशर्विक, पार्श्वीय। On the side of the body.

Lateroabdominal (लेटेरोएब्डोमिनल) शरीर के पार्श्व एवं उदर से सम्बन्धित। Pertaining to the side of the body and the abdomen.

Lateropulsion (लेटेरोपल्शन) एक ओर नीचे गिरने की अनियंत्रित प्रवृत्ति। Involuntary tendency to fall down to one side.

Laterotrusion (लेटेरोटॉर्जन) एक ओर को ऐंठ जाना। A twisting to one side.

Lavage (लैवाज) धावन, प्रक्षालन, पानी से धोना। Washing out of body cavity irrigation.

Law (लॉ) किसी घटना के एक वैज्ञानिक कथन जो सभी स्थानों पर सत्य होता है, सिद्धान्त, नियम, विधान, कानून, संहिता। A scientific statement for an occurrence which is found to be true uniformly, principle.

Lax (लैक्स) तनाव रहित, शिथिल, यह आंत्र गतियों के लिए प्रयोग किया जाता है। Without tension, loose, side of intestinal movements.

Laxation (लैक्सेशन) आंत्र गतियाँ। Intestinal movements.

Laxative (लैक्सेटिव) जुलाब लाने वाली दवा, दस्तावर दवा, मृदुविरेचक। Agent promoting or stimulating bowel movement.

Lean body mass (लीन बॉडी माँस) शरीर के भार में से उसमें स्थित वसा के भार को घटाने से प्राप्त भार। Body weight without fat content.

Leap (लीप) कूदना, उछलना, कुदाना। To jump, to spring, to cause jump.

Lecithin (लैसीथिन) शरीर तथा पौधों में पाया जाने वाला पदार्थ, योक। A phosphorized substance occurring widely in the body and in plant tissues.

Lectulus (लैक्टुलस) बिस्तर। Bed.

Leg (लैग) टांग, जंघा, अधःशाखा, अधःभुजा। The lower extremity especially from the knee down.

Legitimacy (लेजिटिमेसी) वैधानिक होने की दशा। The condition of being legal.

Leiomyoma (लीयोमायोमा) आरेखीपेशी अबुर्द। A tumor of unstrapped muscular fibers.

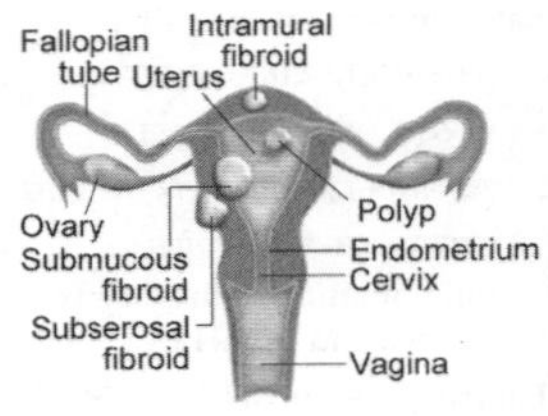

Leiomyomatosis (लीयोमायोमेटोसिस) शरीर में बहुत से आरेखी पेशीअबुदों के होने की अवस्था। The state of being many leiomyomas in the body.

Leiomyosarcoma (लीयोमायोसार्कोमा) आरेख पेशी अबुर्द एवं सार्कोमा दोनों संयुक्त। Combined leiomyoma and sarcoma.

Leiotrichous (लीयोट्राइकस) चिकने अथवा सीधे बालों वाला। Having smooth or straight hairs.

Leishmaniasis (लीशमैनिएसिस) लीशमैनिया की किसी जाति के संक्रमण जैसे लीशमैनिया ट्रॉपिका के संक्रमण से उत्पन्न त्वचीय सीश्मैनियता। Infection with a species of leishmania as cutaneous leishmaniasis caused by infection with Leishmania tropica.

Length (लैंथ) दो बिन्दुओं के बीच की दूरी की माप, लम्बाई, आयाम। The measurement of distance between two point.

(*i*) **Crown heel length** (क्राउन–हील लैंथ) भ्रूण अथवा नवजात शिशु में सिर के शीर्ष से एड़ी तक की दूरी। Fetal or infant length from crown to heel.

Length of stay (लैंथ ऑफ स्टे) किसी अस्पताल में भर्ती होने तथा वहाँ से छुट्टी होने के बीच के दिनों की संख्या। The number of days between admission and discharge from a hospital.

Lens (लेंस) ताल, वीक्ष, आँख का पर्दा। A transparent convex and concave disk shaped substance usually glass.

(*i*) **Biconcave lens** (बाइकोनकेव लैन्स) उभयावत्तल लैंस। One concave on both surface.

(*ii*) **Contact lens** (कॉन्टैक्ट लैन्स) कॉच अथवा कृत्रिम रूप से तैयार सामग्री का एक वक्र लैन्स जिसे दृष्टि दोषों को दूर करने के लिए आँख पर लगाया जाता है। सम्पर्क लैन्स। Resin lens lifting directly on cornea. (*iii*) **Photochromatic lens** (फोटोक्रोमेटिक लैन्स) प्रकाशवर्णी लैंस। Lens that darkens on exposure to ultraviolet light used in sunglasses. (*iv*) **Trial lens** (ट्रॉयल लैन्स) दृष्टि परिक्षण के लिए प्रयोग में लाया जाने वाला कोई भी लैन्स। Any lens used in testing the vision.

Lentectomize (लैन्टेक्टोमाइज) ऑपरेशन के द्वारा आँख के लैन्स को निकाल देना। To remove the lens of the eye by surgery.

Lenticonus (लैन्टीकोनस) लैन्स की अग्र अथवा पश्च सतह का जन्मजात शंक्वाकार उभार, शंकुक लैन्स। Congenital conical bulging of the anterior or posterior surface of the lens.

Lentiform (लैन्टीफॉर्म) लैन्स की आकृति वाला। Shaped like a lentil or lens of eye.

Lentigo (लैन्टिगों) मेचक, वर्णक, धब्बा, दाग। A brown macule resembling a freckle.

Leontiasis (लियोनटिएसिस) लैप्रोमायुक्त कुष्ठ में चेहरे का शेर के चेहरे की भांति दिखाई देना। Lion like appearance of the face in lepromatous leprosy.

Lepothrix (लैपोथ्रिक्स) एक रोग जिसमें बाल का काण्ड एक कड़े, शल्कीय त्वग्वसीय पदार्थ में बन्द हो जाता है। A disease in which the shaft of the hair is enclosed in hard scaly sebaceous matter.

Leprid (लैप्रिड) गुलिकाभ कुष्ठ की त्वचा विक्षति। Skin lesion of tuberculoid leprosy.

Lepromatous (लैप्रोमेटस) कुष्ठिक सम्बन्धी, कुष्ठाबुर्दवत्। Pertaining to lepromas.

Lepromatous leprosy (लैप्रोमेटस लैप्रोसी) कुष्ठिका-कुष्ठ। Leprosy in which natural cutaneous lesions are infiltrate. (*i*) **Tuberculoid leprosy** (ट्यूबरकुलॉयड लैप्रोसी) यक्ष्मिकाभ कुष्ठ, गुलिकाभ कुष्ठ। A benign stable and resistant form of leprosy.

Leprostatic (लैप्रोस्टेटिक) कुष्ठाणुरोधक। Inhibiting the growth of mycobacterium leprae.

Leprosy (लैप्रोसी) कुष्ठ, कोढ़, कुष्ठाणुओं द्वारा फैलने वाला रोग। A chronic transmissible disease caused by the mycobacterium leprae.

Leptocephalia (लैप्टोसिफैलिया) वह व्यक्ति जिसकी खोपड़ी असामान्य रूप से लम्बरूप में लम्बी एवं तंग होती है। The person having an abnormally vertically elongated narrow skull.

Leptocyte (लैप्टोसाइट) टार्गेट कोशिका, कृशलोहितकोशिका। Target cell.

Leptodactyle (लैप्टोडैक्टाइली) हाथ अथवा पैर की अँगुलियों का असामान्य रूप से पतला हो जाना। Unusual slenderness of fingers.

Leptomeninges (लैप्टोमैनिन्जीज) पाया-एराक्नॉयड मेटर का एक साथ बोला जाना। Pia-arachnoid membranes together.

Leptophonia (लप्टोफोनिया) आवाज की कमजोरी। A weak thin quality of voice.

Leptoprosopia (लैप्टोप्रोसोपिया) चेहरे का तंग होना। Narrowness of the face.

Leptorhine (लैप्टोराइ्इन) पतली नाक वाला। Having a slender nose.

Leptosome (लैप्टोसोम) पतला एवं हल्का-फुल्का व्यक्ति। A person with a slender, thin or frail body.

Leresis (लेरेसिस) बुढ़ापे में बात अधिक करना। Talkativeness in old age.

Lesbian (लैसबियन) स्त्री समलिंगकामुक। A homosexual women.

Lesion (लीज़न) शरीर के किसी भाग का कार्य न करना। A pathological alteration in structure or function of an organ. (*i*) **Focal lesion** (फोकल लीज़न) स्थानिक विक्षति। Lesion of a small definite area. (*ii*) **Peripheral lesion** (पैरीफेरल लीजन) परिसरीय तंत्रिकाओं की विक्षती। Lesion of peripheral nerves. (*iii*) **Vascular lesion** (वैस्कुलर-लीजन) किसी रक्तवाहिनी की विक्षती। Lesion of a blood vessels.

Lethal (लीथल) घातक, मारक, प्राणघातक। Deadly capable of causing death.

Lethargy (लिथार्जी) सुस्ती या आलस्य। Sluggishness or drowsiness.

Leukapheresis (ल्यूकेफेरेसिस) रोगी से प्राप्त रक्त से श्वेत रक्त कोशिकाओं को पृथक करना तथा फिर शेष रक्त को वापिस रोगी में चढ़ा देना। To separate the white blood cells from the withdrawn blood and then remainder of the blood transfused back into the patient.

Leukemia (ल्यूकीमिया) रक्तोत्पादक अंगों का प्रगतिशील दुर्दम रोग जिसमें रक्त में श्वेत रक्त कोशिकाएं एवं उनकी पूर्वगामी कोशिकाएँ संख्या में बहुत बढ़ जाती है, रक्त कैन्सर, अधि श्वेतकोशिकारक्तता, श्वेतरक्तता। Progressive malignant disease of the blood forming organs marked by the increase in the number of white blood cells and their precursor in the blood; blood cancer.

Leukemid (ल्यूकेमिड) ल्यूकीमिया से सम्बद्ध त्वचा का कोई भी अविशिष्ट विस्फोट जिसमें ल्यूकिमिया कोशिकाएं हो सकती है अथवा नहीं भी हो सकती। A nonspecific cutaneous lesion containing infiltration of leukemic cells.

Leukemogen (ल्यूकीमोजन) ल्यूकीमिया उत्पन्न करने वाला कोई भी पदार्थ। Any substance producing leukemia.

Leukemoid (ल्यूकीमॉयड) श्वेतरक्ताभ। Of the nature of leukemia.

Leukoblast (ल्यूकोब्लास्ट) श्वेतकोषिकाणुप्रसू। The germ of leukocyte.

Leukoblastosis (ल्यूकोब्लास्टोसिस) रक्त में अत्यधिक संख्या में अपरिपक्व श्वेत कोशिकाओं का पाया जाना। Abnormal proliferation of leukocytes in blood.

Leukocyte (ल्यूकोसाइट) श्वेतकोशिका, श्वेताणु। A white blood corpuscle or white blood cells.

Leukocytes

Lymphocytes

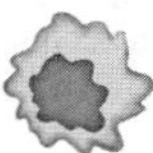
Macrophage

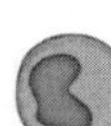
Neutrophil

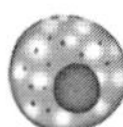
Eosinophil

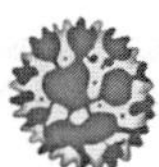
Basophil

Leukocytoblast (ल्यूकोसाइटोब्लास्ट) वह कोशिका जिसमें कोई श्वेत रक्त कोशिका उत्पन्न होती है। The earliest recognizable leukocyte precursor.

Leukocytoid (ल्यूकोसाइटॉयड) श्वेत रक्त कोशिका से मिलता-जुलता। Resembling a leukocyte.

Leukocytolysis (ल्यूकोसाइटोलाइसिस) श्वेत रक्त कोशिकाओं का नष्ट होना। Destruction of the white blood cells.

Leukocytosis (ल्यूकोसाइटोसिस) कुछ समय के लिए रक्त में श्वेत रक्त कोशिकाओं का बढ़ जाना जो अधिकतर किसी संक्रमण में होता है। श्वेतकोशिका बहुलता। A transient increase in number of white blood cells in the blood which occurs generally in some infection.

Leukocytotoxin (ल्यूकोसाइटोटॉक्सिन) श्वेत कोशिका जीवविष, श्वेत रक्त कोशिकाओं को नष्ट करने वाला जीवविष। Any substance that selectively damages leukocytes.

Leukocytotoxis (ल्यूकोसाइटोटोक्सिस) श्वेत रक्त कोशिकाओं का संक्रमण के स्थान या चोट की ओर अथवा उनसे दूर को गति करना। Migration of leukocytes to the site of inflammation and injury.

Leukocyturia (ल्यूकोसॉइटयूरिया) श्वेत कोशिका जीवविष, मूत्र में श्वेत रक्त कोशिकाओं को नष्ट करने वाला जीवविष का पाया जाना। Presence of WBC in the urine.

Leukoderma (ल्यूकोडर्मा) त्वचा की वर्णकयुक्तता का स्थानीय अभाव, श्वेत कुष्ठ। Lack of normal skin pigmentation.

Leukodystrophy (ल्युकोडिस्ट्रॉफी) मस्तिष्क के श्वेत द्रव्य का काठिन्य, श्वेत मस्तिष्क दुष्पोषण। Sclerosis of the white matter of brain.

Leukoencephalitis (ल्यूकोएन्सीफैलाइटिस) मस्तिष्क के श्वेत द्रव्य का शोथ। Inflammation of the white matter of brain.

Leukoencephalopathy (ल्यूकोएन्सीफैलोपेथी) मस्तिष्क के श्वेत द्रव्य का कोई भी रोग। Any disease of the white matter of brain.

Leukoma (ल्यूकोमा) घनी, श्वेत स्वच्छमण्डलीय अपारदर्शिता, श्वेत फुल्ली। Dense white scar of cornea.

Leukomyelitis (ल्यूकोमायलाइटिस) सुशुम्ना रज्जु के श्वेत द्रव्य का शोथ। Inflammation of the white matter of the spinal cord.

Leukonecrosis (ल्यूकोनेक्रोसिस) श्वेत कोथ। White gangrene.

Leukopedesis (ल्यूकोपेडेसिस) श्वेत रक्त कोशिकाओं का रक्त वाहिनियों की दीवारों से होकर गुजरना। Migration of lymphocytes through wall of blood vessels.

Leukopenia (ल्यूकोपीनिया) श्वेत कोशिकाल्पता, रक्त में श्वेत रक्त कोशिकाओं का कम हो जाना। Abnormal decrease in number of leukocytes in blood.

Leukoplakia (ल्यूकोप्लेकिया) मुँह के अन्दर सफेद चकते बन जाना। श्वेतशल्कता। The formation of white spots or plates on the epidermis of epithelium also called Smoker's patches.

Leukopoiesis (ल्यूकोपॉयसिस) श्वेत कोशिकाजनन। Formation growth and maturation of leukocytes.

Leukorrhea (ल्यूकोरिह्या) गर्भाशयग्रीवा नलिका अथवा योनि से सफेद या पीलापन लिए हुए चिपचिपे स्राव का निकलना, श्वेतप्रदर। Abnormal white non bloody discharge from vagina.

Leukotaxis (ल्यूकोटेक्सिस) कृत्रिम रूप से श्वेताणुओं की वृद्धि होना, श्वेतकोशिकाकर्शण। Artificially produced leukocytosis.

Leukotomy (ल्यूकोटॉमी, खण्डछेदन, मस्तिष्क खण्डछेदन। Transorbital frontal labotomy.

Leukotoxic (ल्यूकोटॉक्सिक) श्वेत रक्तकोशिकाओं के लिए विनाशकारी। Destructive to the leukocytes.

Leukous (ल्यूकस) सफेद, विशेषकर त्वचा से सम्बन्धित। White, especially relating to the skin.

Levator (लीवेटर) शरीर के किसी अंग अथवा भाग को उठाने वाला पेशी। A muscle that raises up the part into which it is inserted.

Levocardia (लीवोकार्डिया) हृदय की सामान्य स्थिति के लिए प्रयोग में लाया जाने वाला शब्द जब अन्य अन्तरांग उलट जाते है। The term used for the normal position of the heart when other viscera are inverted.

Levoduction (लीवोडक्शन) किसी आँख का बाई ओर को घूम जाना। Movement of an eye to the left side.

Levophobia (लीवोफोबिया) शरीर के बाई ओर स्थित वस्तुओं का विकृत भय। Morbid fear of the things on the left side of the body.

Levorotatory (लीवोरोटेटरी) बाई ओर को घुमाने वाला, वामावर्ती।

Causing to turn towards the left.

Levulosemia (लीव्यूलोसीमिया) रक्त में फ्रक्टोज का पाया जाना। Presence of fructose in the blood.

LGA (एल जी ए) गर्भायु से बड़ा। Large for gestational age.

Liability (लियाबिलिटी) कानूनी उत्तरदायित्व। Legal responsibility.

Libido (लिबिडो) कामलिप्सा, कामोत्तेजना, वासना। Sexual desire or appetite.

Lichen (लाइकेन) शैवाक, पिटकमय, त्वकशोथ। A popular inflammation of the skin; aggravated or obstinate eczema.

Lid (लिड) आँख की पलक, वर्त्म। The eyelid.

Lie (लाइ) माता के लम्ब अक्ष की अपेक्षा गर्भाशय में स्थित भ्रूण के लम्ब अक्ष की स्थिति। The position of the long axis of fetus in the uterus with respect to mother.

Lien (लाइन) प्लीहा या तिल्ली। Spleen.

Lienculus (लाइनकुलस) अतिरिक्त प्लीहा।Accessory spleen.

Lienitis (लाइनाइटिस) प्लीहाशोध, तिल्ली का प्रदाह। Inflammation of spleen.

Lienomyelogenous (लाइनोमाइलोजीनस) प्लीहा एवं अस्थि मज्जा दोनों से उत्पन्न होने वाला। Produced from both the spleen and bone marrow.

Lienorenal (लाइनोरीनल) प्लीहा एवं वृक्क संबंधी। Pertaining to spleen and kidney.

Liensure (लाइसैनस्योर) चिकित्सा में प्रैक्टिस करने के लिए किसी को लाइसैन्स प्रदान करना। To grant a licence to perform medical practice.

Lientery (लाइनटेरी) दस्त आना जिसमें मल में अपचित भोजन होता है। Diarrhea in which the stool contains undigested food.

Life (लाइफ) जन्म एवं मृत्यु के बीच का समय। The time span between birth and death.

Ligament (लिगामैंट) तन्तुमय संयोजी ऊतक की एक बन्धनी जो अस्थियों, उपास्थियों तथा अन्य संरचनाओं को जोड़ती है तथा प्रावरणी अथवा पेशियों को सहारा देने या उन्हें संलग्न करने का कार्य करती है। स्नायु, बन्ध। A band of fibrous connective tissue which connect the bones cartilages and other structure and serves for support or for attachment of fascia or muscles.

(*i*) **Broad ligament** (ब्रॉड लिगामेन्ट) गर्भाशय के पार्श्वीय

किनारों से संलग्न पैरीटोनियम की तहें, पृथु स्थयु। Folds of peritoneum attached to the lateral borders of the uterus. (*ii*) **Inguinal ligament** (इन्गवाइनल लिगामैन्ट) इलियम के अग्र ऊर्ध्व कंटक से जघनास्थि के कंटक तक जाने वाला स्नायु, वंक्षणीय स्नायु। The ligament running from the anterior superior spine of the ilium to the spine of the pubis. (*iii*) **Round ligament** (राउण्ड लिगामैन्ट) गोल स्नायु। The hip of liver, forearm and uterus consist of round ligament. (*iv*) **Suspensory ligament** (सस्पेन्सरी लिगामेन्ट) निलम्बी स्नायु। The suspensory ligament of the crystalline lens. (*v*) **Triangular ligament** (ट्राइएंगुलर लिगामेन्ट) त्रिकोण स्नायु। The triangular ligament of the urethra.

Ligamentopexis (लिगामैंटोपैक्सिस) गर्भाशय का गोल स्नायु निलम्बन। Suspension of the uterus on the round ligament.

Ligate (लाइगेट) बन्ध लगाना, बाँधना। To apply a ligature.

Ligation (लाइगेशन) बंधन, आवेष्ठन। Application of a ligature.

Ligator (लाइगेटर) गहन भागों में विद्यमान वाहिनियों का बंधन करने के लिए प्रयोग में लाया जाने वाला एक यंत्र। A surgical instrument facilitating ligation superficial or deep.

Ligature (लाइगेचर) बाँधने अथवा कसने की क्रिया। Process of binding or tying.

Light (लाइट) प्रकाश, रोशनी, बत्ती। The agent which produces vision.

Lightening (लाइटनिंग) भ्रूण के प्रस्तुत होने वाले भाग का नीचे उतर कर श्रोणि में आ जाना। हल्कापन, अपरोहण। The descent of fetus deeper into pelvis.

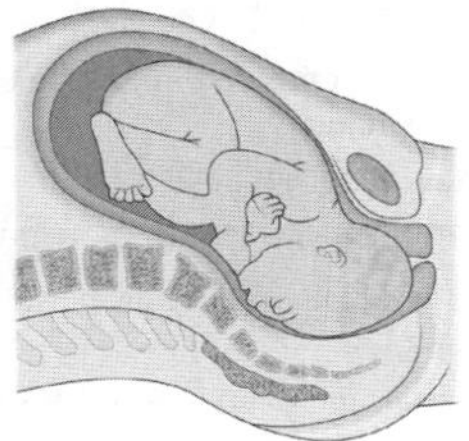

Limb (लिम्ब) बाहु या टांग अथवा कोई शाखा। An arm or leg or an extremity.

Liminal (लिमीनल) जिसे मुश्किल से ही जाना जा सकता है। Hardly perceptible.

Limp (लिम्प) लंगड़ा कर चलना। To walk lamely.

Linea (लीनिया) रेखा, किसी रचना की सतह पर एक संकरा खुरदरा किनारा अथवा धारी या लकीर। A line, a long thin mark, ridge, crease.

Linea alba (लीनिया एल्बा) उदर के मध्य में उरोस्थि से जघनास्थि तक संयोजी ऊतक की एक श्वेत रेखा, उदरमध्य रेखा। A white line of the connective tissue in the middle of the abdomen from sternum to the pubis.

Linea nigra (लीनिया नाइग्रा) गर्भावस्था के बाद के भाग के दौरान उदर पर दिखाई देने वाली नाभि के ऊपर से जघनास्थियों तक जाने वाली एक काली रेखा। Pigmented linea alba of pregnancy.

Linear (लीनियर) किसी रेखा से सम्बन्धित अथवा रेखा के समान, रेखित। Having the properties of a line.

Lingual (लिंग्वुअल) जिह्वा सम्बन्धी, जीभ की शक्ल वाला। Pertaining to the tongue, tongue-shaped.

Lingulectomy (लिंग्वुलेक्टॉमी) जिह्वा खण्ड़क उच्छेदन। Surgical resection of lingual of left upper lobe.

Linguopapillitis (लिंग्वोपैपीलाइटिस) जीभ के किनारों का सूज जाना अथवा उनमें जख्म बन जाना। Inflammation of the tongue and the gingival.

linguopulpal (लिंग्वोपल्पल) बनायी गई किसी गुहा की जिह्वापरक एवं मज्जा की सतहों से सम्बन्धित। Pertaining to the lingual and pupal surface of a formed cavity.

Liniment (लिनीमैंट) औषधिय तरल जो दर्द को दूर करने अथवा क्षोभण का प्रतिकार करने हेतु त्वचा पर मालिश करने के काम आता है, विलैपन, मलहम, मर्ध। An only medicinal liquid applied on skin by friction as an counter irritant.

Lining (लाइनिंग) किसी भी वस्तु का भीतरी आवरण, अस्तर। Inner covering of anything.

Linitis (लाइनाइटिस) आमाशय का शोथ। Inflammation of the lining of the stomach.

Linkage (लिंकेज) किसी रासायनिक यौगिक में विभिन्न परमाणुओं के बीच सम्बन्ध। The connection between the different atoms in chemical compounds.

Linseed (लिंसीड) अलसी, तीसी। Flax seed, linum.

Lint (लिंट) नरम रेशमी पट्टी, जो घावों की मरहम पट्टी करने के काम आती है।

Line well-scraped for dressing sores and wounds.

Lip (लिप) मुख व ऊपरी अथवा निचला मांसल किनारा, होंठ। Upper or lower fleshy margin of mouth.

Lipacidemia (लाइपेसिडीमिया) रक्त में वसीय अम्लों का अधिक पाया जाना। Excess of fatty acids in blood.

Liparocele (लाइपेरोसील) अण्डकोशीय बहिःसरण जिसमें वसा होती है, वसार्बुद। Scrotal hernia containing fat, fatty tumor.

Lipase (लाइपेस) वसा को खण्डित करने वाला एक एन्जाइम। Enzyme that catalyzes hydrolysis of fat.

Lipectomy (लाइपेक्टॉमी) वसीय ऊतकों को शल्यक्रिया द्वारा काट कर निकाल देना। Excision of fatty tissue.

Lipemia (लाइपीमिया) वसारक्तता, रक्त में वसा की बढ़ी हुई मात्रा। Presence of fat in the blood.

Lipid (लाइपिड) वसाभ, चर्बी जैसा, वसासम। Fat like lipid.

Lipidolytic (लाइपिडोलाइटिक) लाइपिड का विघटन या संलयन करने वाला। Causing lysis of lipid.

Lipidosis (लाइपिडोसिस) लाइपिड चयापचय का कोई भी विकार। Any disorder of lipid metabolism.

Lipiduria (लाइपिडूरिया) मूत्र में लाइपिडों का पाया जाना। Presence of lipids in the urine.

Lipoarthritis (लाइपोआर्थराइटिस) किसी सन्धि के वसीय ऊतक का शोथ। Inflammation of fatty tissue of a joints.

Lipoatrophy (लाइपोएट्रोफी) शरीर के अवखक् वसीय ऊतकों का अपक्षय जैसे कि इन्सुलिन का इन्जैक्शन लगाने के स्थान पर हो जाता है। Atrophy of subcutaneous tissue at sites of insulin injection.

Lipochondroma (लाइपोकॉण्ड्रोमा) वसीय एवं उपास्थि तत्वों, दोनों से बना अबुर्द। A tumor composed of both fatty and cartilaginous elements.

Lipodystrophy (लाइपोडिस्ट्रॉफी) वसा चयापचय का कोई भी दोष, वसादुष्पुष्टि। Any defect of fat metabolism.

Lipoferous (लाइपोफेरस) वसा को उत्पन्न अथवा वाहन करने वाला। Producing or carrying fat.

Lipogenesis (लाइपोजेनेसिस) वसा या चर्बी का बनना। Formation of fat.

Lipoid (लाइपॉयड) वसा के समान, लाइपिड। Fat like lipid.

Lipoidosis (लाइपॉयडोसिस) शरीर के ऊतकों में अत्यधिक मात्रा में लाइपॉयडों के जमा हो जाने से उत्पन्न दशा। Condition caused by the accumulation of excessive amount of lipoids in the body tissue.

Lipolysis (लाइपोलाइसिस) वसा का विघटन होना, वसा-अपघटन। Chemical breaking down of fat.

Lipoma (लाइपोमा) सुदम वसीय अबुर्द, वसाबुर्द। Adipoma, benign fatty tumor.

Lipomatasis (लाइपोमेटोसिस) ऐसा रोग जिसमें ऊतकों में अबुर्द के समान वसा जमा हो जाती है, वसाबुर्दता। Liposis obesity to the condition in which there is tumor like deposition of fat in the tissue.

Lipomeningocele (लाइपोमैनिन्जोसील) एक मस्तिष्कावरण-हर्निया, जिसके ऊपर स्थित एक वसाबुर्द होता है। A meningocele associated with an overlying lipoma.

Lipomeria (लाइपोमेरिया) किसी भुजा का जन्मजात अभाव। Congenital absence of a limb.

Lipopenia (लाइपोपीनिया) शरीर में लाइपिडों की कमी होना। Deficiency of lipids in the body.

Lipophage (लाइपोफेज) ऐसी कोशिका जो वसा को निगल जाती है अथवा उसका अवशोषण करती है। A cell which ingests or absorbs fat.

Lipophilic (लाइपोफिलिक) वसारागी। Fat soluble.

Lipoproteinemia (लाइपोप्रोटीनीमिया) रक्त में लाइपोप्रोटीनो का अधिक पाया जाना। Presence of an excess of lipoprotein in the blood.

Lipoproteins (लाइपोप्रोटीन) लाइपिड रक्त में परिसंचरण नहीं कर सकते, ये साधारण प्रोटीन के साथ संयुक्त हो जाते है। यह संयोजन लाइपोप्रोटीन कहलाता है। लाइपोप्रोटीनों के रूप में लाइपिड रक्त में परिसंचरण करते है। Lipids are unable to circulate in the blood they combine with the simple proteins, this combination is called lipoprotein. In the form of lipoprotein, lipids are transported in the blood.

Liposis (लाइपोसिस) वसामयता, मेदुरता, वसीय अनतःस्यन्दन। Adiposis fatty infiltration.

Lipostomy (लाइपोस्टॉमी) मुख का जन्मजात अभाव तथा बहुत छोटा होना। Congenital absence or very smallness of the mouth.

Lipotropic (लाइपोट्रॉपिक) वसाप्रेरक। Having an affinity for lipids.

Lipotropin (लाइपोट्रॉपिन) वसीय ऊतक से वसा को संचारित करने वाला पीयूष ग्रन्थि का एक हार्मोन। A hormone secrete from pituitary gland that cause release of fatty acids from fat.

Lippes loop (लिपेज़ लूप) एक प्रकार का अन्त-गर्भाशयी गर्भनिरोधक साधन। A type of intrauterine contraceptive device.

Lipping (लिपिंग) सन्धि के हासीय रोग में किसी अस्थिल अतिवृद्धि का विकसीत होना। The development of a bony overgrowth in osteoarthritis.

Lipuria (लाइपूरिया) मूत्र में वसा का पाया जाना, वसामेह। Presence of fat in the urine.

Liqorrhea (लिक्वोरिह्या) द्रव का प्रवाह। The flow of liquid.

Liquefaction (लिक्वीफैक्शन) किसी ठोस का द्रव में परिवर्तन, द्रवण, तरलीकरण। Conversion of a solid into a liquid.

Liquer (लिक्वर) शरीर के कुछ तरलों के लिए प्रयोग में लाया जाने वाला एक शब्द जैसे लिक्वर एम्नाई। लिक्विड, तरल, शराब। A term applied to certain body fluid, e.g. liquor amnii, liquid, wine.

Liquescent (लिक्वीसेन्ट) द्रव बनने वाला। Becoming liquid.

Lisping (लिस्पिंग) अस्पष्ट बोलना, तुतलाना। To speak imperfectly, to speak with lips.

Lissotrichy (लिसोट्राइकी) सीधे बालों का होना। The condition of having straight hair.

Lithectomy (लिथेक्टॉमी) शल्यक्रिया द्वारा किसी पथरी को निकालना। Surgical removal of a calculus.

Lithiasis (लिथिएसिस) पथरियों का बनना, अश्मरीयता। Formation of stones.

Lithocenosis (लिथोसीनोसिस) पथरियों के कुचले हुए छोटे-छोटे टुकड़ों की मूत्राशय से बाहर निकालना। Removal of the crushed small pieces of calculi from the urinary bladder.

Lithodialysis (लिथोडायालाइसिस) किसी घोलक का इन्जैक्शन लगाकर पथरियों को मूत्राशय में घोल देना। Dissolution of calculi in the urinary bladder by injection of a solvent.

Lithogenesis (लिथोजेनेसिस) पथरियों का बनना। Formation of calculi.

Lithokonion (लिथोकोनियन) मूत्राशय में स्थित पथरियों का चूरा कर देने वाला एक यंत्र।

An instrument for powdering the vesical calculi.

Litholysis (लिथोलाइसिस) अश्मलयन, अश्मविघटन। Lithodialysis.

Lithometra (लिथोमेट्रा) गर्भाशयी ऊतक का अस्थिभवन होना। Ossification of the uterine tissue.

Lithonephritis (लिथोनैफ्राइटिस) पथरियों के क्षोभण से उत्पन्न वृककशोथ। Inflammation of the kidney due to irritation of the calculi.

Lithopedion (लिथोपीडियन) गर्भाशय में स्थित भ्रूण का कैल्सीकृत होना। A retained calcified fetus.

Lithotomy (लिथोटॉमी) पथरियों को बाहर निकालने के लिए किसी वाहिनी अथवा अंग में चीरा लगाना। An incision into duct or organ for removing stone.

Lithotripsy (लिथोट्रिप्सी) मूत्राशय अथवा मूत्रमार्ग में किसी पथरी को कुचलना।
The crushing of a calculus in the bladder or urethra.

Lithotrite (लिथोट्राइट) मूत्राशय में स्थित पथरी को कुचलने वाला एक यंत्र।
An instrument for crushing a stone in the urinary bladder.

Lithuria (लिथूरिया) मूत्र में यूरिक एसिड या यूरेट का अधिक पाया जाना। Excess of uric acid and urates in the urine.

Litmus (लिटमस) अम्लता या क्षारता का सूचक वनस्पति वर्णक, नीलवर्ण काई, शैवाल। A vegetable pigment used as an indicator of acidity or alkanity.

Litter (लिटर) रोगी अथवा जख्मी व्यक्ति को ले जाने वाला स्ट्रेचर। A stretcher for transporting the invalid.

Littritis (लिटराइटिस) मूत्रमार्गीय ग्रन्थियों की सूजन। Inflammation of the urethral glands.

Livedo (लिवीडो) नीललांछन, विशेष रूप से किसी ऊतक पर। A small bluish spot in a tissue.

Liver (लीवर) उदर के ऊपरी भाग में दाई ओर मध्यपक्ष या डायाफ्राम के ठीक नीचे स्थित एक बड़ी, चार खण्डो वाली गहरे लाल रंग की ग्रन्थि जिसका वजन लगभग 1200 से 1600 ग्राम होता है जिसका मुख्य कार्य पित्त या बाइल बनाना है। Large four lobes

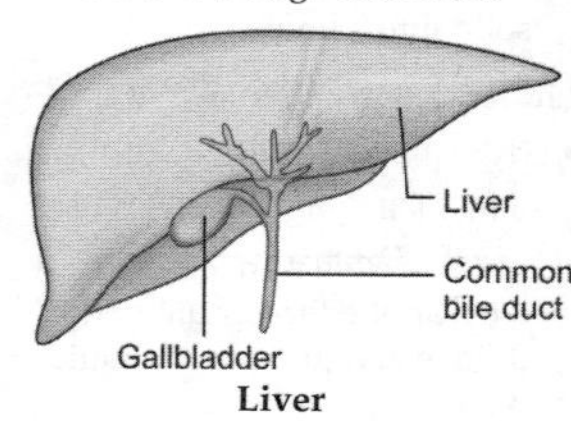

Liver

dark red gland weighing about 1200 to 1600 gms, situated in the upper part of the abdomen on the right side just beneath the diaphragm of which the main function is to secrete bile. (*i*) **Amyloid liver** (एमाइलॉड लीवर) श्वेतसारिक यकृत, मण्डाभ यकृत। Enlargement of the liver due to the deposition of an albuminous substance.

(*ii*) **Cirrhosis liver** (सिरहोसिस लीवर) तन्तुमय ऊतक एवं पर्विकाओं के बनने से कठोर बना हुआ यकृत। Hardened liver due to the formation of fibrous tissue and nodules.

(*iii*) **Fatty liver** (फैटी लीवर) यकृत की कोशिकाओं में वसा के जमा हो जाने से बढ़ा हुआ यकृत। Enlarged liver due to deposit of fat in its cells.

(*iv*) **Floating liver** (फ्लोएटिंग लीवर) चल यकृत, आसानी से विस्थापित हो जाने वाला यकृत। An easily displaced liver.

(*v*) **Nutmeg liver** (नटमैग लीवर) यकृत का जीर्ण निष्क्रिय रक्तधिक्य जिससे केन्द्रीय प्रतिहारी क्षेत्र लाल हो जाता है तथा एक पीला-सा परिसरीय मण्डल होता है। Liver affected by chronic vascular congestion as in CHF.

(*vi*) **Polycystic liver** (पोलिसिस्टिक लीवर) बहुत से पुटीयों से युक्त यकृत। Liver containing many cysts.

Lividity (लिविडिटी) त्वचा विवर्णता, नीलापन। Skin discoloration as a bruise.

Livor mortis (लिवोर मॉर्टिस) मृत्यु के पश्चात् शरीर के आश्रित भागों की विवर्णता। Discoloration of the dependent parts of the body after death.

Loa Loa (लोआ-लोआ) फाइलेरिया का विशिष्ट रूप। A specific form of filariasis.

Lobe (लोब) किसी अंग अथवा ग्रन्थि का बहुत कुछ स्पष्ट सीमा वाला भाग जो सीमाओं द्वारा पृथक रहता है। खण्ड या पाली। A more or less well-defined portion of an organ or a glands separated by boundaries. (*i*) **Caudate lobe** (कोडेट लोब) पुच्छक-केन्द्रक खण्ड। The caudate lobe is an independent part of the liver, situated upon the posterior-superior surface of the liver on the right lobe of liver.

(*ii*) **Frontal lobe** (फ्रॉन्टल लोब) ललाट–खण्ड। That part of the cerebral hemisphere is in form of the central and above of the brain fissures called sylvian fissure.

(*iii*) **Hepatic lobe** (हैपैटिक लोब) यकृत खण्ड। The lobe of the liver. (*iv*) **Occipital lobe** (ऑक्सीपीटल लोब) पश्चकपाल। Caudal region of either hemicerebrum. (*v*) **Olfactory lobe** (ऑलफेक्ट्री लोब) घ्राण-खण्ड। The rhinencephalon. (*v*) **Optic lobe** (ऑप्टिक लॉब) अक्षि-खण्ड। The optic lobes of the brain. (*vi*) **Parietal lobe** (पैराइटल लोब) पार्श्विका खण्ड। That part of the cerebral hemisphere back of the central and above the sylvian fissures. (*vii*) **Quadrate lobe** (क्वॉड्रेट लोब) चतुस्त्र खण्ड। A small lobe on inferior surface of liver between gallbladder and ligamentum teres. (*viii*) **Temporal lobe** (टैम्पोरल लोब) शंख खण्ड। The part of the cerebral hemisphere lying below the sylvian fissure.

Lobes of the cerebrum

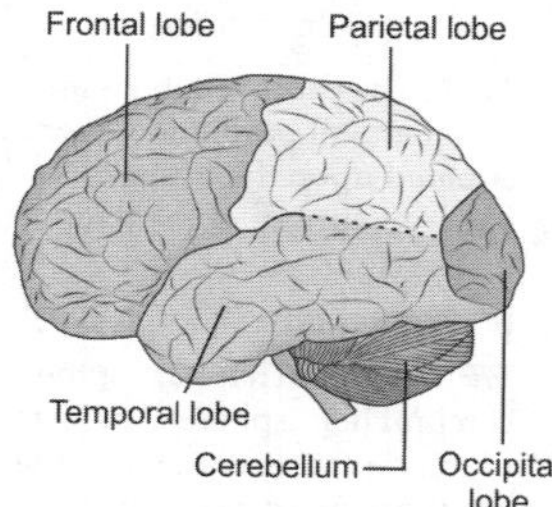

Lobectomy (लोबेक्टॉमी) किसी अंग अथवा ग्रन्थि के किसी खण्ड को शल्यक्रिया द्वारा काट कर अलग कर देना। Excision of a lobe of organ or a gland.

Lobitis (लोबाइटिस) किसी खण्ड का शोथ। Inflammation of a lobe.

Lobulated (लोब्युलेटेड) खण्ड़ों अथवा खण्डकों से बना हुआ। Consisting of or divided into lobes and lobules.

Lobule (लोब्यूल) एक छोटा खण्ड अथवा किसी खण्ड को बनाने वाले छोटे-छोटे विभाजनों में से एक खण्डक। A small lobe or one of the smaller divisions making up a lobe.

Lochia (लोकिया) योनि से निकलने वाला स्राव। The vaginal discharge.

Lochia alba (लोकिया अल्बा) योनि द्वारा श्वेत सूतिस्राव। The whitish flow from vagina that takes place from about the seventh day after delivery.

Lochia rubra (लोकिया रूब्रा) योनि द्वारा स्राव जो कि प्रसवोत्तर के पहले तीन से पाँच दिन तक होता है। जो कि गहरे लाल रंग का होता है जिसमे मुख्यतः लाल रक्त काणिकाँए होती है। The first three to five days of postpartum vaginal bloody discharge with very bright red color and it contains a huge amount of red blood cells.

Lochia serosa (लोकिया सिरोसा) योनि द्वारा सीरमी सूतिस्राव। The pink or brown tinged color uterine discharge accruing about the fifth day after delivery.

Lochiorrhea (लोकियोरैह्या) सूतिस्राव का अत्यधिक बहना, विपुल सूतिस्राव। Excessive flow of lochia.

Lockjaw (लॉकजा) जबड़े की पेशियों की तनाव के साथ ऐंठन जैसे कि धनुस्तम्भ या टेटनस में देखी जाती है। Tonic spasm of the jaw muscles as seen in tetanus.

Locomotor (लोकोमोटर) चलन सम्बन्धी, गतिज। Pertaining to locomotion.

Loculation (लोक्युलेशन) छोटी-छोटी गुहाओं का बनना। Formation of small cavity.

Loculus (लोकुलस) एक छोटा-गुहाओं का बनना। A small space or cavity.

Locus (लोकस) एक बिन्दु अथवा स्थान किसी गुणसूत्र पर किसी जीन का स्थान, स्थली। A place or spot as the specific site occupied by gene in the chromosome.

Logadectomy (लोगेडेक्टॉमी) नेत्रश्लेष्मा के किसी भाग को शल्यक्रिया द्वारा काट कर अलग कर देना। Excision of a portion of the conjunctiva.

Logamnesia (लोगेम्नेसिया) लिखे हुए या बोले गए शब्दों को समझने में असमर्थता। Inability to understand written or spoken words.

Logoclony (लोगोक्लोनी) किसी शब्द के अन्तिम अक्षर को बार-बार दुहराना। Intermittent repetition of the last syllable of a word.

Logoneurosis (लोगोन्यूरोसिस) कोई भी विक्षिप्ति जिसमें वाक् विकार होना विशेषता होती है, वाक-तंत्रिका विक्षिप्ति। Any neurosis marked by speech disorders.

Logorrhea (लोगोरिह्या) अधिक बात करना। Logomania.

Loin (लॉयन) पसलियों एवं श्रोणि के बीच पीठ का निचला एवं पार्श्वों का भाग, कटि-प्रदेश। The lower part of the back and sides between ribs and the pelvis.

Lophotrichous (लोफोट्राइकस) एक सिरे पर कषाभों के गुच्छों से युक्त। Having bunches of flagella at one end.

Lordasis (लॉर्डोसिस) रीढ़ की हड्डी का आगे की ओर झुकना, अग्रकुब्जता। Anterior convex curvature of the spine, lordona.

Lotion (लोशन) शरीर पर बाह्य प्रयोग के लिए तरल औषधीय योग। Liquid medicinal preparation for external use to the body.

Loupe (लोउप) बढ़ाकर दिखाने वाला लैन्स, आवर्धक लैन्स। A magnifying lens.

Louse (लाऊस) यूका, जूँ। Pediculus.

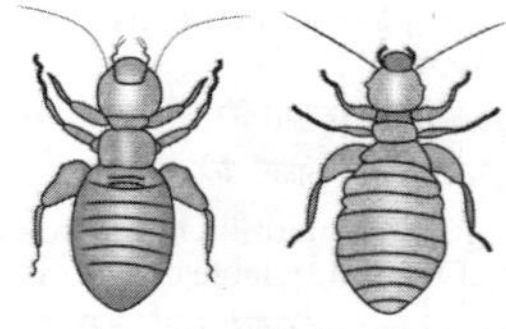

Lox (लौक्स) द्रव ऑक्सीजन। Liquid oxygen.

Lozenge (लोजेन्ज) औषधियुक्त चूसने की गोली, चूष। Troche, medicinal sucking tablet.

Lubb-dupp (लब–डप) परिश्रवण करने पर हृदय की सुनाई देने वाली दो ध्वनियाँ। The two heart sound heard on auscultation.

Lubricant (लुब्रीकेन्ट) रगड़ को कम करने के लिए चिकना बनाने वाला जैसे कोई तेल या ग्रीस, स्नेहक। Making smooth as an oil or grease to lessen the friction.

Lucent (ल्यूसैन्ट) चमकदार साफ, अर्द्ध-पारदर्शक। Shining, clear, translucent.

Lucid (ल्यूसिड) स्वच्छ मस्तिष्क। Clear mind.

Lucifugal (ल्यूसिफ्यूगल) तेज रोशनी से दूर भागने वाला। Repelled by bright light.

Lucipetal (ल्यूसिपीटल) तेज रोशनी की ओर आकर्षिक होने वाला। Attracted to bright light.

Luetic (लुईटिक) उपदंशग्रस्त, आतशकग्रस्त। Syphilitic.

Lumbago (लम्बेगो) कटि-प्रदेश में शूल, कटि-वेदना, कमरदर्द। Pain in the lumbar region.

Lumbar (लम्बर) कटि-सम्बन्धी। Pertaining to the loins.

Lumbocostal (लम्बोकॉस्टल) कमर एवं पसलियों से सम्बन्धित, कटिपर्शुकी। Pertaining to the loins and ribs.

Lumboiliac (लम्बोइलियक) कटि एवं वक्षण-क्षेत्र से सम्बन्धित। Pertaining to the lumbar and inguinal regions.

Lumbosacral (लम्बोसैक्रल) कटि एवं त्रिकास्थि प्रदेश सम्बन्धी। Pertaining to the lumb and sacral regions.

Lumbrical (लम्ब्रीकल) वर्मी-कृमि। Vermiform.

Lumbricoid (लम्ब्रीकॉयड) गोलकृमि से मिलता-जुलता। Resembling a roundworm.

Lumbricosis (लम्ब्रीकोसिस) आन्त्र-कृमियों का संक्रमण। Infection with ascarides.

Lumen (ल्यूमैन) अवकाशिका, कुहर, कोटर। The space inside a tubular structure.

Luminal (ल्यूमिनाल) किसी अवकाशिका जैसे रक्त वाहिनी की अवकाशिका से संबंधित। Pertaining to a lumen as that of a blood vessels.

Luminescence (ल्यूमिनेसैन्स) ऊष्मा की उत्पत्ति हुए बिना प्रकाश की

उत्पत्ति। Production of light without production of heat.

Luminiferous (ल्यूमिनीफेरस) प्रकाश को उत्पन्न करने अथवा उसका वाहन करने वाला। Producing or carrying light.

Luminous (ल्यूमिनस) प्रकाशमान, चमकीला। Giving of light.

Lumpectomy (लम्पेक्टॉमी) स्तन के किसी अर्बुद को शल्यक्रिया द्वारा काट कर कर निकाल देना। Excision of a tumor from the breast.

Lunar (ल्यूनर) चन्द्रमा सबंधी, एक माह से सम्बन्धित, द्वारा निर्धारित। Pertaining to the moon, a month, determined by.

Lunate (ल्यूनेट) चन्द्राकार अथवा अर्द्ध-चन्द्राकार। Moon-shaped or crescentic.

Lung (लंग) फुफ्फुस, फेफड़ा। One of the two organs of respiration.

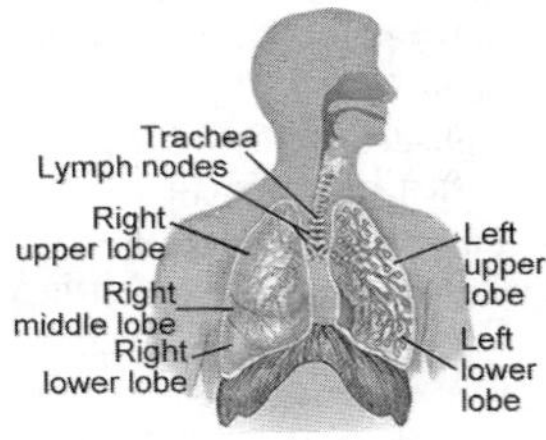

Lunula (ल्यूनुला) चन्द्रक, नरवगर्त, नरवचन्द्रिका। The semicircular white area at the root of the nails.

Lupiform (ल्यूपीफोर्म) ल्यूपस के समान। Resembling lupus.

Lupus (ल्यूपस) कोई भी जीर्ण, प्रगतिशील त्वचा रोग जिसमें जख्म बनने लगते है। Any chronic progressive ulcerative skin disease.

Lupus erythematosus (ल्यूपस इरीदेमेटोसस) रक्तिम त्वग्यक्ष्मा, रक्तिम-लूपस। An autoimmune disease in which the human immune system becomes hyperactive and attacks healthy tissues in many parts of the body.

Lupus vulgaris (ल्यूपस वल्गेरिस) चर्मक्षय, त्वग्यक्ष्मा। Typical lupus. A chronic and progressive form of skin tuberculosis that affects the head and neck area, lower extremities and gluteal area.

Luteal (ल्यूटीयल) पीत-पिण्ड से सम्बन्धित अथवा इसके या इसके हॉर्मोन के गुणों वाला। Pertaining to or having the property of the corpus luteum or its hormone.

Luteinic (ल्यूटिनिक) डिम्बग्रन्थि के पीत-पिंड से सम्बन्धित। Pertaining to the corpus luteum of the ovary.

Luteinization (ल्यूटिनाइजेशन) वह क्रिया जिसके द्वारा डिम्बोत्सर्जन

के पश्चात् डिम्बग्रन्थि-पुटक पीत- पिण्ड में बदल जाता है। The process by which after ovulation an ovarian follicle is converted into the corpus luteum.

Luteogenic (ल्यूटियोजेनिक) पीत-पिण्डों को उत्पन्न करने वाला। Producing corpora lutas.

Luteolysis (ल्यूटियोलाइसिस) पीत-पिण्ड का विनाश। Destruction of corpus luteum.

Luteoma (ल्यूटियोमा) ल्यूटिन कोशिकाओं से युक्त डिम्बग्रन्थि का एक अबुर्द, पीतपिंडबुर्द। An ovarian tumor containing lutein cells.

Luteotropic (ल्यूटियोट्रॉपिक) पीत-पिंड के बनने को उत्तेजित करने वाला। Stimulating formation of the corpus luteum.

Lux (लक्स) पीत, पीला। Yellow.

Luxation (लक्सेशन) किसी सन्धि की सन्धिच्युति। Dislocation of a joint.

Lycopene (लाइकोपेन) टमाटरों एवं अन्य लाल फलों का कैरोटीन के समान लाल वर्णक। The red carotenoid pigment of tomatoes and other fruits.

Lymph (लिम्फ) लसीका। A gland of the body separated by the blood and carried by the lymphatic vessels.

Lymph node (लिम्फ नोड) लसीका-वाहिनियों के पथ के बीच-बीच में लसीका-ऊतक के एकत्रित होने से बना एक गोलपिण्ड। A rounded body consisting of accumulation of lymphatic tissue found in the course of lymphatic vessels.

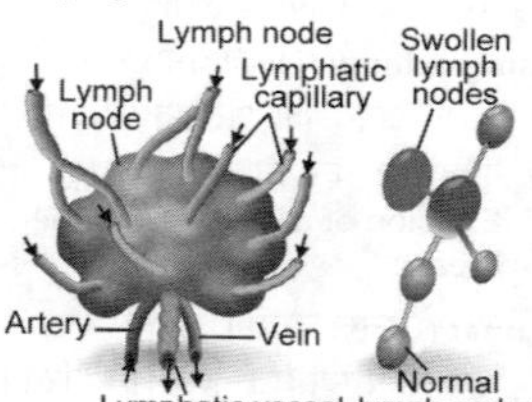

Lymphaden (लिम्फैडेन) लसीका पर्व। Lymph node.

Lymphadenectasis (लिम्फेडीनेक्टेसिस) किसी लसीका पर्व का बढ़ना। Enlargement of lymph node.

Lymphadenectomy (लिम्फेडीनेक्टॉमी) लसीका पर्वोच्छेदन। Excision of lymph node.

Lymphadenitis (लिम्फेडीनाइटिस) लसीका पर्वो की सूजन। Inflammation of lymph node.

Lymphadenocele (लिम्फेडीनोसील) किसी लसीका पर्व की पुटी। Cyst of a lymph node.

Lymphadenoma (लिम्फाडीनोमा) गण्डमाला, कण्ठमाला। A tumor node of lymphoid tissue.

Lymphadenopathy (लिम्फेडीनोपैथी) लसीकापर्व विकृति। A disease stage of lymph node.

Lymphadenosis (लिम्फेडीनोसिस) लसीका ग्रन्थिलता। Overgrowth of lymphatic glands.

Lymphadenotomy (लिम्फेडीनोटॉमी) किसी लसीका पर्व में चीरा लगाना। To make an incision into a lymph node.

Lymphagogue (लिम्फेगोग) लसीकावर्धक। Stimulating the production of flow of lymph.

Lymphangiectasis (लिम्फेन्जिएक्टेसिस) लसीका वाहिनीयों का विस्फारण, लसीका-वाहिकास्फीति। Dilatation of the lymphatic vessels.

Lymphangiography (लिम्फेन्जियोग्राफी) लसीकावाहिनीचित्रण। A description of the lymphatic vessels.

Lymphangioma (लिम्फेन्जियोमा) लसीका वाहिकाबुर्द। Tumor composed of lymphatic vessels.

Lymphangiophlebitis (लिम्फेन्जियोफ्लेबाइटिस) लसीकावाहिनियों एवं शिराओं का शोथ। Inflammation of the lymphatic vessels and veins.

Lymphangitis (लिम्फेन्जाइटिस) लसीका वाहिनियों की सतह का शोथ। Inflammation of the walls of the lymphatic vessels.

Lymphaticostomy (लिम्फोटिकोस्टॉमी) किसी लसीका वाहिनी में छिद्र बनाना। To make an opening into a lymphatic duct.

Lymphatolytic (लिम्फेटोलाइटिक) लसीका वाहिनियों का विनाशकारी। Destructive to lymphatic ducts.

Lymphization (लिम्फाइज़ेशन) लसीका का उत्पन्न होना। Production of lymph

Lymphoblast (लिम्फोब्लास्ट) वह कोशिका जिससे कोई लसीकाकोशिका या लिम्फोसाइट बनती है, लसीका कोशिकाप्रसू। The cell which gives rise to a lymphocyte.

Lymphoblastoma (लिम्फोब्लास्टोमा) लसोका कोशिकाप्रसूअबुर्द। A young immature cell that matures into a lymphocyte.

Lymphocyte (लिम्फोसाइट) लसीकाकोशिका, लसकोशिका। A white cell found in the lymph nodes, a lymph cell.

Lymphocytoma (लिम्फोसाइटोमा) लसीका कोशिकाबुर्द। A circumscribed nodule or mass of mature lymphocytes.

Lymphocytopenia (लिम्फोसाइटोपीनिया) रक्त में लसीकाकोशिकाओं की संख्या घट जाना। Reduction of the number of lymphocytes in the blood.

Lymphocytopiesis (लिम्फोसाइटोपॉयसिस) लसीकाकोशिकाओं का उत्पन्न होना। Production of lymphocytes.

Lymphocytosis (लिम्फोसाइटोसिस) लसीका कोशिकाबहुलता। Lymphocytomia.

Lymphocytotoxin (लिम्फोसाइटोटॉक्सिन) लिम्फोसाइटों को नष्ट करने वाला एक जीवविष। A toxin, destructive to lymphocytes.

Lymphodenography (लिम्फोडीनोग्राफी) लसिकापर्वचित्रण। X-ray examination of lymph nodes.

Lymphoepithelioma (लिम्फोइपिथिलियोमा) लसीकाउपकलाबुर्द। Rapidly growing malignant pharyngeal tumor.

Lymphogenesis (लिम्फोजेनेसिस) लसीका की उत्पत्ति। Production of lymph.

Lymphogranuloma venereum (लिम्फोग्रेनुलोमा वेनेरियम) एक रजित संक्रामक रोग जिसमें जननांगों पर एक जख्म बन जाता है। A tropical venereal disease caused by the formation of an ulcer on the genital organ.

Lymphoid (लिम्फॉयड) लसीका तथा लसीका ऊतक के समान, लसीकाभ। Resembling lymph or lymph tissue.

Lymphokinesis (लिम्फोकाइनेसिस) लसीका का शरीर में परिसंचरण। Circulation of lymph in the body.

Lymphoma (लिम्फोमा) लसीकाबुर्द। A tumor arising from the lymphoid tissue in the body.

Lymphomatosis (लिम्फोमेटोसिस) शरीर में बहुत सा लसीकाबुर्दों का बनना। Formation of multiple lymphomas in the body.

Lymphopoietic (लिम्फोपॉयटिक) लिम्फोसाइटों को बनाने वाला। Forming lymphocytes.

Lymphorrhea (लिम्फोरिह्या) लसीकास्राव। Secretion of lymph, lymphorrhagia.

Lymphosarcomatosis (लिम्फोसार्कोमेटोसिस) ऐसी दशा जिसमें बहुत से लसीका-सार्कोमा विद्यमान होते है। The condition characterized by the presence of multiple lymphosarcomas.

Lymphostasis (लिम्फोस्टेसिस) लसीका प्रवाह का रूक जाना। Stoppage of lymph flow.

Lymphotoxis (लिम्फोटैक्सिस) लिम्फोसाइटों को आकर्षित करने अथवा दूर हटा देने का गुण। The induction of lymphocyte movement.

Lymphotropic (लिम्फोट्रॉपिक) लसीका कोशिकाओं के प्रति आकर्षित। Attracted to lymph cells.

Lymphuria (लिम्फूरिया) मूत्र में लसीका का पाया जाना। Presence of lymph in the urine.

Lyogel (लायोजैल) ऐसी जेली जिसमें पानी बहुत होता है। A gel containing much water.

Lyse (लाइस) अपघटन करना। To cause lyses.

Lysine (लाइसिन) एक प्रकार का एमिनो अम्ल जो कि कुछ खाद्य पदार्थो मे पाया जाता है जैसे कि, फंलियां, पनीर, माँस, दूध इत्यादि An amino acid found in the protein of foods like beans, cheese, meat, milk, etc.

Lysine (लाइसीन) प्राकृतिक रूप में पाया जाने वाला एक अमीनो एसिड जो वृद्धि एवं ऊतकों की मरम्मत के लिए आवश्यक होता है। A natural amino acid which is essential for growth and repair of tissue.

Lysis (लाइसिस) किसी कोशिका का नष्ट होना अथवा उसका अपघटन होना। Destruction or decomposition of a cell or other substance.

Lysogen (लाइसोजन) वह जो किसी लाइसिन को उत्पन्न करता है। That produces lysine.

Lysozyme (लाइसोजाइम) आँसुओं, लार एवं पसीने तथा शरीर के अन्य स्रावों में पाया जाने वाला एक एन्जाइम है। An antibacterial enzyme present in tears saliva, sweat and other body secretion.

Lyssa (लाइस्सा) अलर्क, जलातंक। Rabies, hydrophobia.

M

M (एम) 1. मीटर 2. बूंद। 1. Meter 2. Minim.

Ma (एमए) मेन्टल एज का संक्षिप्त रूप। Mental age.

Macerate (मैसीरेट) भिगोकर मुलायम करना। To soften by soaking.

Macies (मेसीज़) शेष, अनुपयोगी। Atrophy, wasting.

Macrencephalia, Macrencephaly (मैक्रेनसीफेलिया, मैक्रेनसीफेली) मस्तिष्क का असमान्य रूप से बड़ा हो जाना। Abnormal enlargement of the brain.

Macrobiosis (मैक्रोबायोसिस) दीर्घायु। Long life.

Macroblast (मैक्रोब्लास्ट) एक असामान्य रूप से बड़ी एवं केन्द्रक युक्त लाल रक्त कोशिका। An abnormally large, nucleated red blood cell.

Macroblepharia (मैक्रोब्लेफेरिया) बड़ी-बड़ी पलकें। Abnormal enlargement of the eyelid.

Macrocheilia (मैक्रोचीलिया) होंठो का अत्यधिक विकास होना। Extremely large lips.

Macrocheiria (मैक्रोकाइरिया) हाथों का अत्यधिक बड़ा होना। Extremely large hands.

Macrocyst (मैक्रोसिस्ट) एक बड़ी पुटी। A large cyst.

Macrocythemia (मैक्रोसाइथीमिया) खून में अधिक संख्या में वृहतलों का पाया जाना। Presence of large number of macrocytes.

Macrocytosis (मैक्रोसाइटोसिस) हित कोशिकाओं का पाया जाना। Presence of macrocytes in the blood.

Macrodactyly (मैक्रोडैक्टिली) हाथ व पैरो की अंगुलियों का असामान्य रूप से बढ़ जाना। An uncommon condition in which fingers and toes are abnormally large due to over growth of the underlying bone and soft tissue. Mostly occured in infants.

Macrogamete (मैक्रोगैमेट) दो संयुग्मियों में से बड़ा संयुग्मी। The mature female cell in propagation reproduction in sporozoa.

Macrogametocyte (मैक्रोगैमेटोसाइट) वृहतयुग्मकों को उत्पन्न करने वाली कोशिका। A cell producing macrogametes.

Macroglobulin (मैक्रोग्लोबुलिन) उच्च अणु-भार। A globulin of high molecular weight, about 10,00,000.

Macroglobulinemia (मैक्रोग्लोबुलिनीमिया) खून में मैक्रोग्लोबुलिन का ज्यादा

पाया जाना। Excess of macroglobulins in the blood.

Macroglossia (मैक्रोग्लोसिया) जीभ का ज्यादा बढना। Excessive development of the tongue.

Macrography (मैक्रोग्राफी) बड़े-बड़े अक्षरों में लिखना। Writing in large letters.

Macromelia (मैक्रोमीलिया) एक या अधिक भुजाओं का बड़ा हो जाना। Enlarged limbs.

Macromelus (मैक्रोमीलस) लम्बी भुजाओं वाला व्यक्ति। The person having large limbs.

Macronychia (मैक्रोनीकिया) हाथ की अंगुलियों के नाखूनों का बहुत अधिक लम्बा हो जाना। Excessive length of the fingernails.

Macrophage (मैक्रोफेज) अमीबाभ भक्षक-कोशिकाएं, बृहत्भक्षक-कोशिका। A large nucleated leukocyte.

Macropsia (मैक्रोप्सिया) आँखों की ऐसी बीमारी जिसमें हर वस्तु बड़ी नजर आती है। Any disease of the eye in which objects appear enlarged.

Macroscopic (मैक्रोस्कोपिक) महावीक्षिणीय। Relating to macroscopy.

Macrostomia (मैक्रोस्टोमिया) अत्यधिक चौड़ा मुँह। Excessively wide mouth.

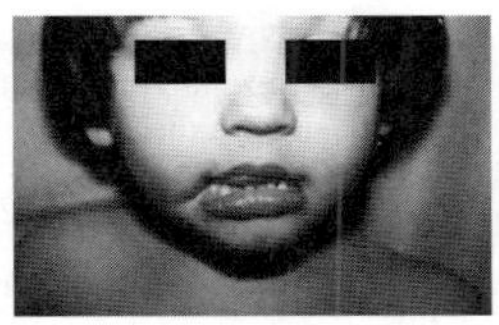

Macrotia (मैक्रोटिया) कानों का असामान्य रूप से बढ़ जाना। Abnormal enlargement of the ears.

Macula (मैकुला) चकता, धब्बा। A spot.

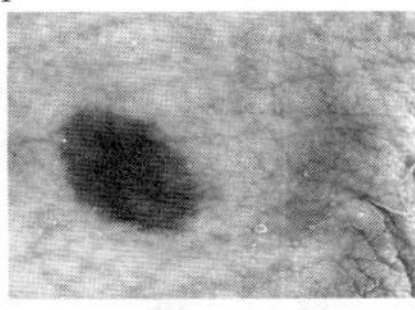

Macule (मैकुल) बिन्दु या धब्बा। Macula.

Maculopapular (मैकुलोपेपुलर) चिनी-पटकीय। The presence of macule and raised palpable papules of the skin.

Maculopathy (मैकुलोपेथी) पीतबिन्दु विकृति। Any pathological condition of the yellow spot.

Mad (मैड) पागल। Insane, rabid.

Madarosis (मैडेरोसिस) पलकों का अभाव। Loss of the eyelashes.

Maduromycosis (मडुरोमाइकोसिस) शरीर के अन्य भागों में जीर्ण कवक संक्रमण के कारण सूजन

तथा फोड़े, नासूर बन जाते है। A chronic disease, affecting feet draining sinuses discharging yellow to black granules.

Maggot (मैगट) किसी मक्खी का लार्वा-रूप। The larva-form of fly.

Magnesia (मैगनेशिया) एक प्रकार का सफेद चूर्ण। An oxide of magnesium.

Magnesium (मैगनेशियम) एक रासायनिक तत्व। An element in chemistry, magnesium.

Magnetism (मैग्नेटिज्म) चुम्बकीय आकर्षण शक्ति। The property of magnet.

Magnification (मैग्नीफिकेशन) सूक्ष्मदर्शी के द्वारा देखते समय बड़ा करने की क्रिया। The enlarging power of a microscope.

Magnitude (मैग्नीट्यूड) परिमाण या प्रसार। Size or extent.

Maim (मेम) 1. घायल कर देना। 2. हाथ अथवा पैर का प्रयोग करने से वंचित कर देना। 1. To injure seriously. 2. To deprive of the use of a part, such as arm or leg.

Mal (माल) बीमारी। Illness.

Mala (माला) गाल, जबड़ा। The cheek, The cheekbone.

Malabsorption (मालाएब्जाप्शन) अपावशोषण। Poor or disordered absorption.

Malacia (मैलेशिया) किसी भाग की कोमलता। Softening of a part.

Maladjustment (मालएडजस्टमैट) कुसमायोजन। Bad or poor adaption to any environment.

Malady (मैलेडी) बीमारी। A disease.

Malaise (मैलेस) व्याकुलता, घबराहट। Feeling of bodily discomfort or uneasiness.

Malar (मेलर) गण्ड संबंधी अथवा हनु। Pertaining to, or belonging to the cheeks.

Malaria (मलेरिया) विषमज्वर। A febrile disease caused by a blood parasite.

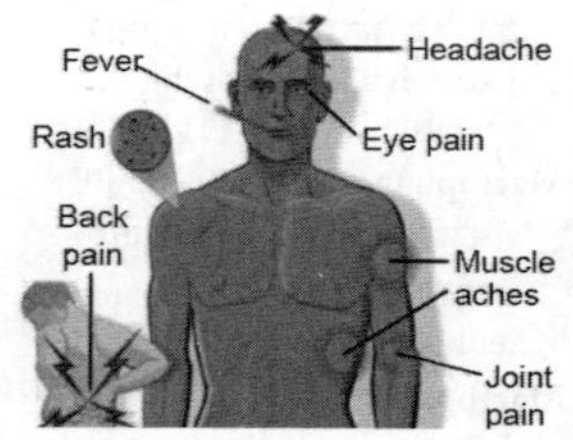

Maldigestion (मालडाइजेशन) पाचन की गड़बड़ी। Incomplete or impaired digestion.

Male (मेल) पुरूष। Denoting the sex that produces gametes, especially spermatozoa, with which a female may be fertilized or inseminated to produce offspring.

Malformation (मालफोर्मेशन) विकृति, कुरचना। Deformity.

Malfunction (मालफंक्शन) अनुचित, अस्वाभाविक क्रिया, दुष्क्रिया। Disordered, inadequate or abnormal function.

Malic-acid (मैलिक एसिड) सेवों, नासपतियों आदि का अम्ल। The acid of apples, pears, etc.

Malignant (मैलिग्नैन्ट) घातक, दुर्दम। Dangerous, virulent.

Malinger (मैलिंगर) छलरूग्णता, हरजाना प्राप्त करने के लिए बीमार बनने का बहाना करना। To pretend to be sick to gain sympathy, to get free from the work or to receive compensation.

Malingerer (मैलिंग्रर) छलरोगी। One feigning injury or illness.

Malleable (मैलिएबिल) दबाव से आकृति में बदल जाने वाला, आघातवर्ध्य। Capable of being changed in shape by pressure.

Malleation (मैलिएषन) नर्तन रोग। Chorea, hammering of the hands.

Malleolar (मैलियोलर) गुल्फ-संबंधी। Pertaining to the malleollus.

Malleolus (मैलियोलस) टखने का जोड़। A hammer, head-shaped process of bones.

Mallet (मैलेट) हथौड़ी। Hammer.

Malleus (मैलियस) हथौड़े के आकार जैसी कान की छोटी हड्डी। A small hammer-shaped bone of the internal-ear.

Malnutrition (मालन्यूट्रीशन) कुपोषण, असंतुलित भोजन लेना। The poor assimilation of nutrition.

Malocclusion (मालोक्लुजन) कुधारणा, ऊपरी एवं निचले जबड़े के दाँतों की कुस्थिति एवं उनका आपस में ठीक से न मिलना। Malposition and imperfect contact of the teeth of the upper and lower jaw.

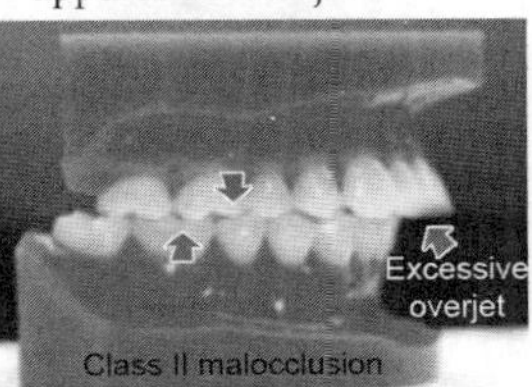

Class II malocclusion

Malpighian body (मैल्पीघियन बॉडी) गुर्दे में पाये जाने वाले क्षुद्र कण। Small corpuscles found in the kidney.

Malpractice (मालप्रैक्टीस) दुष्टाचार, हानिप्रद एवं अनुचित चिकित्सा। Injurious and improper practices.

Malrotation (मालरोटेशन) कुघूर्णन। Development failure of rotation in the normal direction and to normal degree, most common to digestive tract.

Malt (माल्ट) अनाज का सीरा। Partially fermented

barley-seed, the starch being converted into grape-sugar.

Maltose (माल्टोस) माल्ट शर्करा। A sugar derived from the action of diastase on barley.

Malunion (मालयूनियन) किसी टूटी हुई हड्डी के टुकड़ों का गलत जुड़ जाना। Faulty union of the fragments of a fractured bone.

Mamma (मैमा) स्तन। The breast, the milk secreting organ.

Mammal (मैमल) स्तनपायी, मैमालिया वर्ग का जन्तु जिसके स्तन होते है। Animal of the class mammalia having breasts.

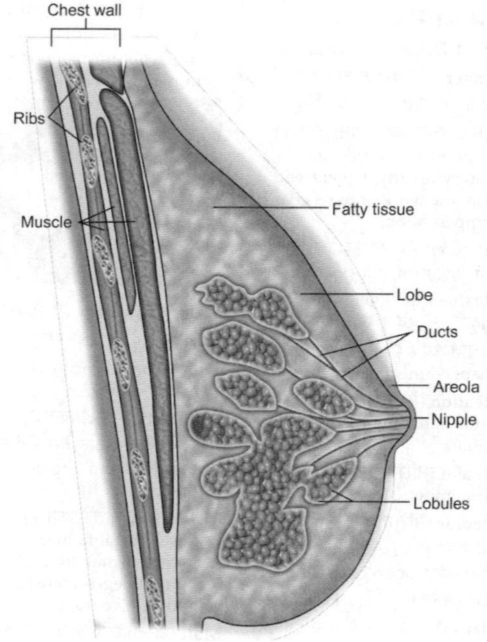

Mamma

Mammillated (मैमीलेटेड) चूचुक के समान उभारों से युक्त। Having nipple like prominences.

Mammilliplasty (मैमीलीप्लास्टी) किसी चूचुक पर प्लास्टिक सर्जरी करना। Plastic surgery on a nipple.

Mammillitis (मेम्मीलिटिस) चूचुकशोथ। Inflammation of nipple.

Mammitis (मैमाइटिस) स्तनों का प्रदाह। Inflammation of the breasts.

Mammogram (मैमोग्राम) स्तन का एक्स-रे चित्र। X-ray of the breast.

Mammography (मैमोग्राफी) स्तन का एक्स-रे परीक्षण। X-ray examination of the breast.

Mandible (मैण्डीबल) निचला जबड़ा। The lower jaw.

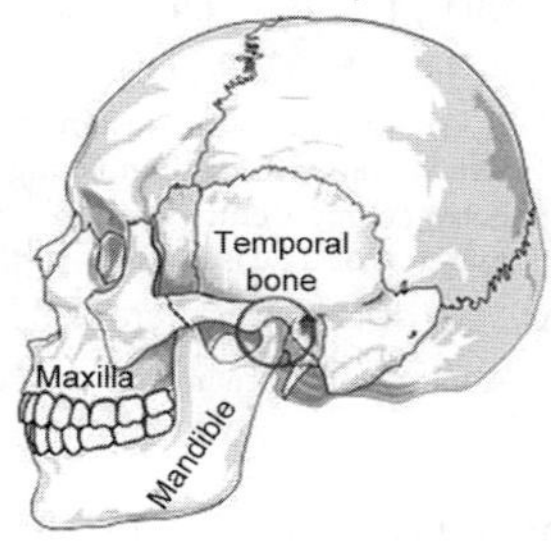

Mane (मैन) सुबह, प्रातःकाल। Morning.

Maneuver (मैन्युवर) कोई भी बुद्धि का कार्य। A skillful or dextrous procedure.

Mange (मैन्ज) पशुओं को होने वाली चमड़ी की एक बीमारी। A skin disease of animals.

Mania (मैनिया) पागलपन। Raving or furious madness.

Maniac (मैनियक) सनकी, पागल। Affected Mania.

Manifestation (मैनीफेस्टेशन) अभिव्यक्ति, प्रकाशन। Revelation, disclosure of characteristic signs or symptoms of a disease.

Manikin (मैनीकिन) शरीर रचना विज्ञान की पढ़ाई में प्रयोग में आने वाला मानव शरीर। A model of the human body or its parts used in teaching anatomy.

Manipulation (मैनीपुलेशन) हाथों से किया जाने वाला उपचार। Skillful or dextrose treatment by using the hands.

Manometer (मैनोमीटर) दाबमापी, तरल पदार्थो तथा गैसों के दबाव को मापने वाला यंत्र। An instrument for measuring the pressure of liquids or gases.

Mantoux-test (मेन्टॉक्स टेस्ट) माण्टू परीक्षण। A form of tuberculin test that injects the test material between the layers of the skin.

Manubrium (मैनुब्रियम) वक्ष के ऊपर की हड्डी। The upper bone or portion of the sternum.

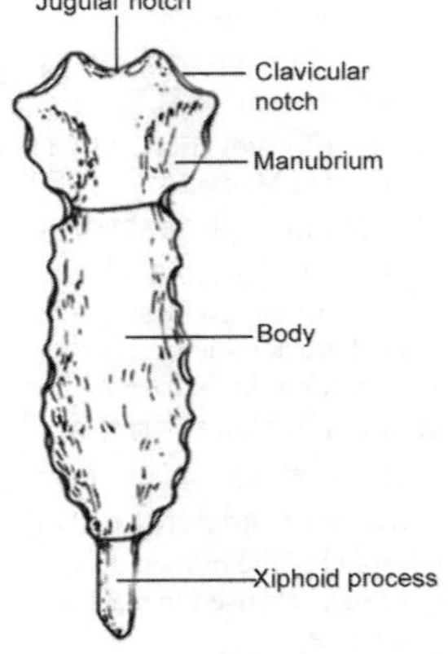

Manus (मैनस) हाथ। Hand.

Marasmus (मैरस्मस) सूखा रोग। Atrophy, undernourishment causing a child's weight to be significantly low for their age.

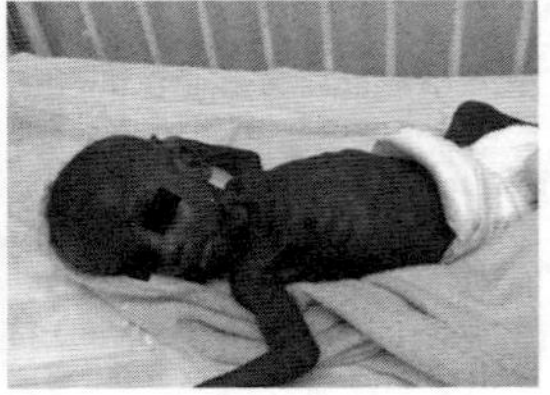

Margin (मार्जिन) परिसीमा, सीमा। A border or edge of any surface.

Margination (मार्जिनेशन) क्षतिग्रस्त स्थान पर शोथ की प्रथम अवस्था में श्वेत रक्त कोशिकाओं का एकत्रित होना तथा उनका रक्त वाहिनियों की दीवारों पर चिपक जाना। Adhesion of leukocytes to the walls of the blood vessels in the first stage of inflammation.

Margosa (मार्जोसा) नीम। The Indian neem tree.

Marihuana (मैरीहुआना) भाँग। Canna.

Marijuana (मैरीजुआना) गाजाँ। Cannabis sativa.

Mark (मार्क) चिन्ह, धब्बा, तिल। Sign, a spot, mole.

Marker (मार्कर) 1. चिन्ह करने वाला उपकरण 2. प्रत्यक्ष रूप से एक से दिखाई देने वाले पदार्थ।

1. An apparatus or substance which marks. 2. Distinguishing between apparently similar material or diseases.

Marrow (मैरो) लम्बी हड्डियोंकी चर्बी। A fatty substance in the cavities of long cylindrical bones.

Masculine (मैस्कुलाइन) पुरूष संबंधी। Relating to or marked by the characteristics of male sex.

Mask (मास्क) नाक और मुंह को ढकने का नकाब। A bandage covering the face.

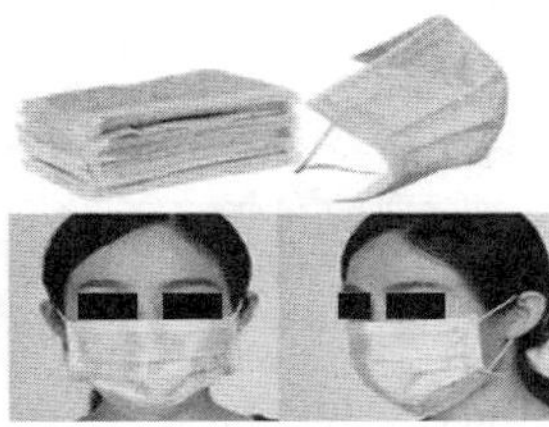

Masochism (मेसोचिस्म) परपीड़ितकामुकता। A form of sexual perversion with delights in cruel treatment.

Masochist (मेसोचिस्ट) परपीड़नकामुक। The passive person in the practice of masochism.

Mass (मास) बहुत से, समूह। A lump of matter.

Massage (मसाज) मालिश। Stroking, kneading, for the relief of pain or muscular stiffness.

Masseter (मैसेटर) मुख को बंद करने वाली एवं चबाने की मुख्य पेशी। The muscle that closes the mouth and is principal muscle for mastication.

Masseur (मैसियर) 1. मालिश करने वाला आदमी 2. मालिश करने का यंत्र। 1. The man who performs massage. 2. An instrument for massage.

Mastectomy (मास्टेक्टॉमी) स्तन को शल्यक्रिया द्वारा काट कर अलग कर देना। Excision of the breast.

Masticate (मैस्टीकेट) चबाना। To chew.

Mastication (मैस्टीकेशन) चबाना। The act of chewing.

Mastigophora (मैस्टीगोफोरा) प्रारंभिक जीव। One of the classes of protozoa.

Mastitis (मैस्टाइटिस) स्तनों का प्रदाह स्तनशोथ। Inflammation of the mammary gland in the breast or udder.

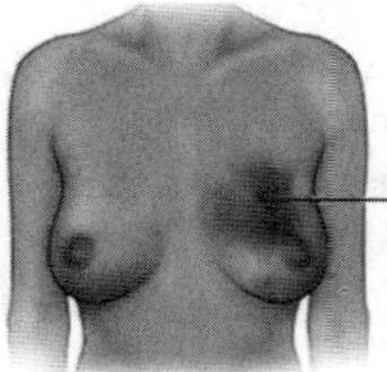

Mastocytogenesis (मास्टोसाइटोजेनेसिस) मास्ट कोशिकाओं का बनना एवं उनका विकास होना। Formation and development of mast cells.

Mastocytoma (मैस्टोसाइटोमा) मास्ट कोशिकाओं का इकट्ठा हो जाना जो एक अबुर्द के समान प्रतीत होता है। Accumulation of mast cells resembling a tumor.

Mastocytosis (मैस्टोसाइटोसिस) मास्ट कोशिकाओं का स्थानीय संचय। Local or systemic accumulation of mast cells.

Mastodynia (मैस्टोडाइनिया) स्तन में दर्द होना। Pain in the breast.

Mastoidectomy (मैस्टॉयडेक्टॉमी) कर्णमूल प्रवर्ध को शल्यक्रिया द्वारा काट कर अलग कर देना। Excision of the mastoid cells or of the mastoid process.

Mastoiditis (मैस्टॉयडाइटिस) कोशिकाओं का शोथ। Inflammation of the mastoid antrum and the cells.

Mastomenia (मैस्टोमीनिया) मासिक धर्म के समय स्तनों से रक्त बहना। Vicarious menstruation from the breast.

Mastoptosis (मैस्टोप्टोसिस) स्तनों का लटक। Sagging of the breasts.

Masturbation (मास्टरबेशन) हाथों से जननांगों को रगड़कर या मलकर लैंगिक उत्तेजना के चरमोत्कर्ष पर पहुँचना। To achieve the climax of the sexual excitement by friction of the genital organs by hands.

Materia (मैटीरिया) पदार्थ या वस्तु। Substance or matter.

Maternal (मैटर्नल) 1. माता से संबंधित 2. माता से उत्पन्न। 1. Pertaining to the mother. 2. Generate/inherit from a mother.

Maternity (मैटरनिटी) प्रसूति, मातृत्व। According to the rules of the motherhood.

Mating (मैटिंग) विपरीत लिंग के व्यक्तियों का विशेषकर जनन के लिए मिलन। Pairing of the individuals of the opposite sex, especially for reproduction.

Matrix (मैट्रिक्स) आधात्री, आधारक, गर्भाशय। A mold, the cavity in which anything is formed, the uterus.

Matron (मैट्रन) किसी अस्पताल की अध्यक्षा। The woman superintendent of a hospital.

Matter (मैटर) स्राव, पीब। Pus collected in or emitted from an abscess, pustule, etc.

Maturation (मैचुरेशन) परिपक्वता। Ripening.

Mature (मैच्योर) 1. परिपक्व 2. पूर्ण विकसित। 1. Fully developed or ripened. 2. To become fully developed.

Maxilla (मैक्जिला) ऊपर वाला जबड़ा। The bone of the upper jaw.

Maximum (मैक्सिमम) उच्चतम, अधिकतम। The highest or the largest quantity.

Meal (मिल) भोजन। Food consumed at regular intervals or at a specific time.

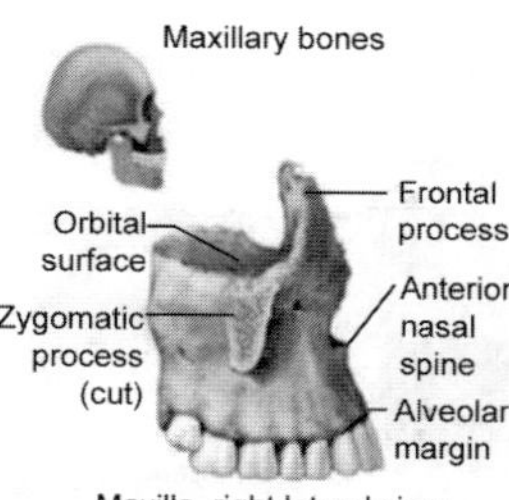

Maxilla, right lateral view

Maxilla

Mean (मिन) माध्यम। The average or general tendency of a set of values.

Measles (मिजल्स) खसरा। Rubeola morbilli.

Meatoplasty (मिटोप्लास्टी) कर्णकुहरसंधान। A plastic surgery on a meatus.

Meatorrhaphy (मिटोर्हफी) मूत्रमार्गमुखसीवन। Closing by suture of the wound made by performing a meatotomy.

Meatotomy (मिटोटॉमी) मूत्रमार्गमुखछेदन। Cutting of the urinary meatus.

Meatus (मिटस) छेद, मुख। A passage, an opening.

Mechanics (मेकेनिक्स) यान्त्रिकी। The science of the action of the forces in promoting motion or equilibrium.

Mechanism (मेकेनिज्म) क्रियाविधि। A natural or established process by which something takes place or is brought about.

Mecometer (मीकोमीटर) नवजात शिशुओं की माप लेने वाला एक यंत्र। An instrument for measuring the length of newborn infants.

Meconium (मीकोनियम) नवजात शिशु का प्रथम मल। The first feces of a newborn infant.

Medial (मीडियल) मध्यवर्ती। Pertaining to or near the middle.

Median (मीडियन) मध्यम। The middle or mesial.

Mediastinitis (मीडियास्टाइनाइटिस) मध्य स्थानिका प्रदाह। Inflammation of the mediastinum.

Mediastinum (मीडियास्टाइनम) किसी अंग के दो मुख्य भागों के बीच स्थित एक पुट। The central space in chest bounded anteriorly by sternum, posteriorly by vertebral column and laterally by pleural sacs.

Medicament (मीडिकामेन्ट) औषधि, औषधद्रव्य। A remedy or medicine.

Medicate (मेडिकेट) 1. औषधियों द्वारा किसी रोग की चिकित्सा करना। 2. औषधि से पूर्ति करना। 1. To treat a disease with the drugs. 2. To impregnate with the medicine.

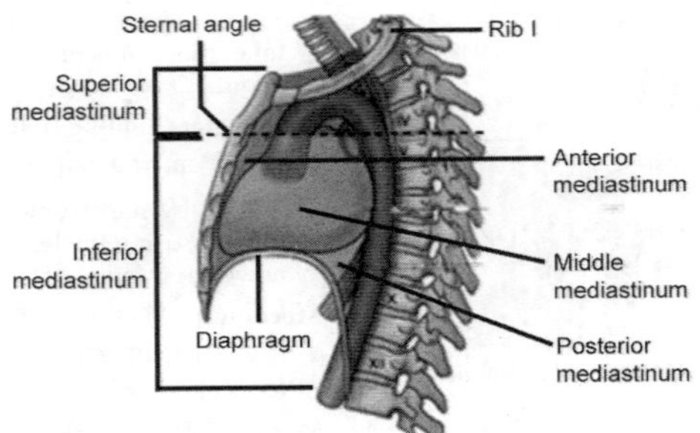

Mediastinum

Medicated (मेडिकेटेड) औषधियुक्त। Impregnated with a medicine.

Medicine (मेडीसिन) चिकित्सा-शास्त्र। The science and art of healing and preventing disease.

Medicolegal (मेडिकोलीगल) व्यवहार आयुर्विज्ञान संबंधी। Pertaining to a matter that involves both medicine and low.

Medium (मीडियम) माध्यम। A substance used in bacteriology for the growth of organisms.

Medulla (मेडुला) मडजा, अस्थि-गह्वरों के अंदर रहने वाला कोमल पदार्थ। The marrow in various cavities.

Medullated (मेडुलेटेड) मेडुला से युक्त। Containing marrow or medulla.

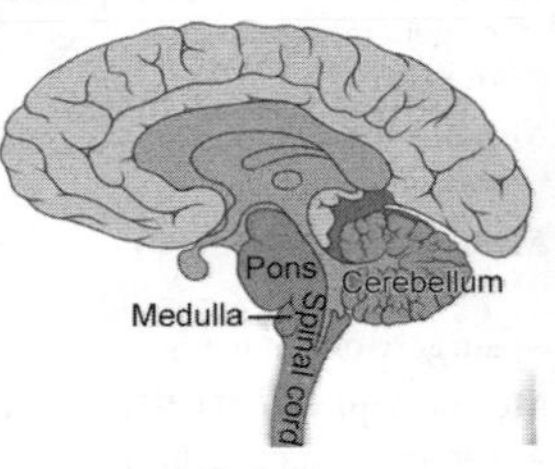

Medulla

Medulloepithelioma (मेडुलोइपिथीलियोमा) ग्लोमा। Glioma, neuroepithelioma.

Megacolon (मेगाकोलन) बड़ी आंत की फैली हुई अवस्था। Condition of dilated and elongated colon.

Megakaryocyte (मेगाकेरियोसाइट) महामूललोहित कोशिका। A cell having a large nucleus.

Megalgia (मेगल्जिया) बहुत तेज दर्द उठना। Severe pain.

Megaloblast (मेगालोब्लास्ट) एक बड़ी, केन्द्रक युक्त असामान्य लाल रक्त कोशिका। A large sized blood-corpuscle.

Megalomania (मेगालोमैनिया) मनोविक्षिप्त जिसमें कोई व्यक्ति अपने को बड़ा आदमी समझने लगता है। A psychosis characterized by thinking for one self as the greatman.

Megaloureter (मेगालोयूरेटर) मूत्रनली का विस्फारित हो जाना। Dilatation of the ureter.

Megavitamin (मेगाविटामिन) सामान्य दैनिक आवश्यकता से अधिक कोई विटामिन। A vitamin in excess of the normal daily requirement.

Megavolt (मेगावोल्ट) 10 लाख वोल्ट। One million volts.

Megrim (मेग्रीम) आधे सिर का दर्द। One-sided headache.

Meiosis (मीयोसिस) अर्धसूत्रीविभाजन। The cell division during maturation of sex cells in which two nuclear cell divisions occur in quick succession, thus forming four gemetes each containing half the number of chromosomes.

Melalgia (मेलेल्जिया) भुजाओं में तंत्रिकाशूल होना। Neuralgia in the limbs.

Melancholia (मेलन्कोलिया) व्यक्ति किसी चिंता में डूबा रहता है तथा असामान्य रूप से मानसिक एवं शारीरिक सक्रियता रूक जाती है। A condition characterized by severe depression as manifested by loss of pleasure in all activities early morning awakening, anorexia and feeling of guilt.

Melanic (मेलेनी) मेलेनिन-अबुर्द संबंधी। Relating to melanoma.

Melanin (मेलेनिन) आँखों, बालों आदि में प्रकट होने वाला एक काला वर्णक। A dark pigment occurring naturally, though in varying amounts, in skin or in body parts, such as eyes, hair, etc.

Melanoblast (मेलेनोब्लास्ट) तंत्रिका-शिखा से उत्पन्न होने वाली एक कोशिका जो मेलेनिन कोशिका में विकसित होती है। A cell originating from the neural crest, which develops into a melanocyte.

Melanocyte (मेलेनोसाइट) मेलेनिन बनाने वाली कोशिका। Melanin-forming cell.

Melanogen (मेलेनोजन) एक रंगहीन पदार्थ जिसको मेलेनिन में बदला जा सकता हैं। A colorless substance that can be converted into melanin.

Melanoma (मेलेनोमा) मेलेनिन-कोशिकार्बुद, एक वर्णकयुक्त तिल अथवा मेलेनिन उत्पन्न करने वाली कोशिकाओं से उत्पन्न होने वाला सुदम या दुर्दम-अबुर्द। A pigmented mole benign or malignant tumor arising from cell forming melanin.

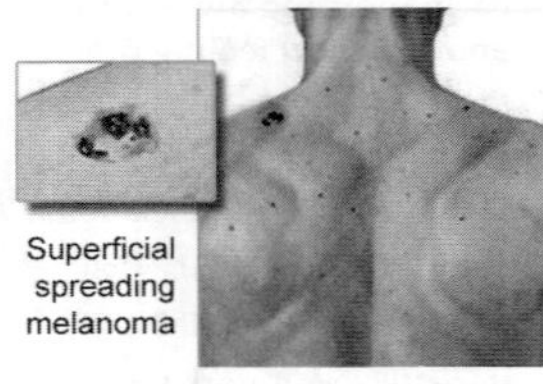
Superficial spreading melanoma

Melanonychia (मेलेनोनीकिया) नाखूनों का काला पड़ जाना। Black pigmentation of the nails.

Melanoplakia (मेलेनोप्लेकिया) जिह्वा एवं मुख की श्लेष्तिक कला पर वर्णक चकतो का बन जाना। Formation of pigmented patches on the tongue and mucous membrane the mouth.

Melanosis (मेलेनोसिस) काले-काले घाव। An abnormal deposit of black matter in the various parts of the body.

Melasma (मेलाज्मा) त्वचा की किसी भी प्रकार की विवर्णता। Any type of the discoloration of the skin.

Melitis (मेलीइटिस) गालों का प्रदाह। Inflammation of the cheeks.

Mellitus (मेलाइटस) शहद। Applied to sweet taste of urine in diabetes.

Melomelia (मीलोमेलिया) ऐसी कुरचना जिसमें भ्रूण की सामान्य भुजाओं से एक या अधिक अल्पवर्धित भुजाएँ संलग्न रहती है। A malformation in which the fetus has one or more rudimentary limbs attached to the normal limbs.

Meloschisis (मीलोस्काइसिस) एक जन्मजात कटा हुआ गाल। A congenitally cleft cheek.

Melotia (मीलोटिया) कान का गाल पर जन्मजात विस्थापन। Congenital displacement of the ear on the cheek.

Membrane (मेम्ब्रेन) झिल्ली, पर्दा। A thin flexible substance investing many internal and some external parts of the body.

Memory (मेमोरी) स्मृति, यादाश्त। Remembrance, recollection the mental registration, retention and recall of the past experience, knowledge and ideas.

Menacme (मीनेक्मी) किसी स्त्री के जीवन का वह काल जिसमें मासिक धर्म होता है। The period of a woman's life during which menstruation occur.

Menarche (मीनार्क) मासिक धर्मों के शुरू होने का समय जो साधारणतया 11 वर्ष से 18 वर्ष तक होता है। When the menstrual periods commence and other bodily changes occur.

Meninges (मैनिन्जीज) मस्तिष्कावरक झिल्लियाँ। The surrounding membranes of the brain and the spinal cord.

Meningism (मैनिन्जिज्म) मस्तिष्क एवं सुषुम्ना रज्जु के क्षोभण से मस्तिष्कावरणों के वास्तविक शोथ के अभाव में मस्तिष्कावरणशोथ के चिन्ह एवं लक्षणों का प्रकट होना। Appearance of the signs and symptoms of meningitis without actual inflammation of the meninges due to irritation of the brain and spinal cord.

Meningitis (मैनिन्जाइटिस) मस्तिष्कावरक झिल्ली का प्रदाह। Inflammation of the covering membrane of the brain and the spinal cord.

Meningocele (मैनिन्जोसील) मस्तिष्कावरण हर्निया। A protrusion of meninges.

Meningocele Meningomyelocele

Skin
Meninges
Spinal cord
Cerebro-spinal fluid
A
Skin
Spinal cord
Cerebro-spinal fluid
Spinal nerves
B

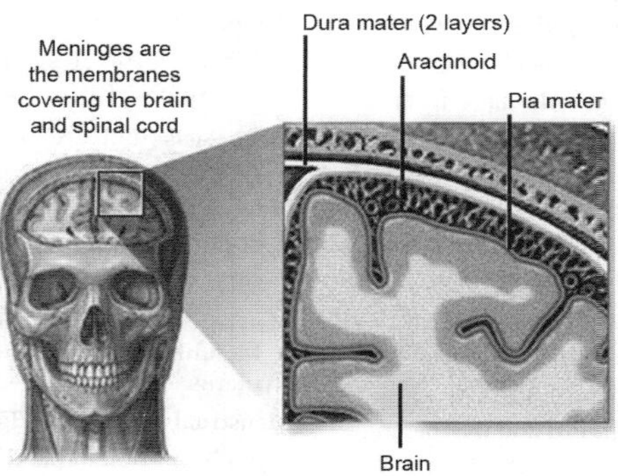

Meninges

Meningococcemia (मैनिन्जोकॉक्सीमिया) रक्त में मैनिन्जोकॉक्सों का पाया जाना। Presence of meningococci in the blood.

Meningoencephalitis (मैनिन्जोएनसिफेलाइटिस) मस्तिष्क तथा उसकी झिल्लियों का प्रदाह। Inflammation of the brain and its membranes.

Meningoencephalomyelitis (मैनिन्जोएनसिफेलोमायलाइटिस) मस्तिष्क सुषुम्ना रज्जु एवं उनके आवरणों का शोथ। Inflammation of the brain spinal cord and meninges.

Meningoencephalopathy (मैनिन्जोएनसिफेलोपैथी) मस्तिष्कावरणों एवं मस्तिष्क का कोई भी रोग। Any disease of the meninges and the brain.

Meningomyelitis (मैनिन्जोमायलाइटिस) सुषुम्ना रज्जु एवं मस्तिष्कावरणों का शोथ। Inflammation of the spinal cord and the meninges.

Meningomyelocele (मैनिन्जोमायलोसील) कशेरूका-दण्ड में स्थित किसी छिद्र से होकर सुषुम्ना रज्जु एवं मस्तिष्कावरणों का बाहर निकल आना। Protrusion of the spinal cord and the meninges through an opening in the vertebral column.

Meniscectomy (मैनिस्केक्टॉमी) घुटने की नवचन्द्रक उपास्थि को शल्यक्रिया द्वारा काटकर अलग कर देना। Excision of the meniscus cartilage of the knee.

Meniscus (मैनिस्कस) जानु-सन्धि की अर्ध चन्द्राकार उपास्थि। A semilunar cartilage particularly in the knee-joint.

Menopause (मीनोपॉज) रजोनिवृत्ति, मासिक धर्म या ऋतुस्राव का रूक जाना। Cessation of menstruation.

Menophania (मीनोफेनिया) प्रथम रजोदर्शन। The very first menses.

Menorrhagia (मैनोरेह्जिया) अतिरिक्त स्राव मासिक धर्म के समय अत्यधिक रक्तास्राव होना। Excessive menstruation.

Menorrhalgia (मैनोरेह्ल्जिया) ऋतुस्राव के दौरान पेट में बहुत तेज दर्द होना। Dysmenorrhea.

Menostasis (मीनोस्टेसिस) रजोरोध। Amenorrhea.

Menoxenia (मीनोक्सीनिया) असामान्य ऋतुस्राव या मासिक धर्म। Abnormal menstruation.

Menses (मैन्सेस) मासिक धर्म। Monthly blood flow from the uterus.

Menstrual (मेंस्ट्रुअल) मासिक धर्म संबंधी। Pertaining to the menstruation.

Menstruation (मेंसट्रुएशन) मासिक धर्म। Menses.

Mensual (मैन्सुअल) मासिक। Monthly.

Mensuration (मैन्सुरेशन) मापन-क्रिया। The process of measuring.

Mental (मैन्टल) मानसिक। Pertaining to the mind.

Mentation (मैन्टेशन) मानसिक-सक्रियता। Mental activity.

Mentum (मैन्टम) ठुड्ढी। The chin, union.

Mephitic (मेफाइटिक) दुर्गन्ध छोड़ने वाला। Emitting foul smell.

Meralgia (मेराल्जिया) जांघ में दर्द होना। Pain in the thigh.

Mercury (मरक्यूरी) पारा। A white heavy liquid metal.

Meridrosis (मेरीड्रोसिस) किसी स्थान-विशेष पर पसीना आना। Local perspiration.

Merocoxalgia (मीरोकॉक्सैल्जिया) जाँघ एवं कूल्हे में दर्द होना। Pain in the thigh and the hip.

Meromelia (मीरोमेलिया) किसी भुजा के किसी भाग का जन्मजात अभाव। Congenital absence of a part of a limb.

Meropia (मीरोपिया) आंशिक अंधता। Partial blindness.

Merosmia (मीरोस्मीया) गंध का बोध होने में असमर्थता। Inability to perceive certain odors.

Merotomy (मीरोटॉमी) खण्डों में विभाजित करना। Divide into the segments.

Merozoite (मीरोजाइट) अंशाणु। Any segment resulting from splitting up of the schizont in the asexual form of protozoa reproduction.

Mesaortitis (मीसएओर्टाइटिस) महाधमनी के मध्य अस्तर का शोथ। Inflammation of the middle coat of the aorta.

Mesentery (मीजेन्ट्री) आंतों को बांधने वाली एक झिल्ली। A membrane in the cavity of the abdomen which sustains and encompasses the intestines.

Mesoappendix (मीजोएपेण्डिक्स) उण्डुकपुच्छ की छोटी आंत्र-योजनी। The short mesentery of the vermiform appendix.

Mesocardium (मीजोकार्डियम) हृद्योजनी। The layers of splanchnic mesoderm which support the heart of the embryo.

Mesocephalic (मीजोसिफेलिक)
1. मध्यमस्तिष्क संबंधी।
2. मध्यम-परिमाण के सिर वाला।
1. Pertaining to the midbrain.
2. Having a medium sized head.

Mesocolon (मीजोकोलन) कोलन को पष्च उदरीय भित्ति से जोड़ने वाली आंत्रयोजनी। Mesentary connecting the colon with the posterior abdominal wall.

Mesocolopexy (मीजोकोलोपैक्सी) स्थिरीकरण अथवा अनावश्यक गतिशीलता एवं वृहदान्त्रयोजनी के नीचे गिरने को ठीक करने के लिए वृहदान्त्रयोजनी का निलंबन। Suspension of fixation of the mesocolon to correct the unnecessary mobility and ptosis.

Mesocord (मीजोकॉर्ड) अपरा से संलग्न नाभि-रज्जु का भाग। The portion of the umbilical cord attached to the placenta.

Mesoderm (मीजोडर्म) मध्यजनस्तर, अंतर्जन तथा बहिर्जन अस्तरों के बीच का भाग। The middle layer of the blastoderm.

Mesoduodenum (मीजोड्योडिनम) ड्योडिनम को उदरीय भित्ति से जोड़ने वाली आंत्र योजनी। The mesentery of the primitive duodenum.

Mesoepididymis (मीजोइपिडीडिमिस) अण्डधर कंचुक की एक तह जो कभी-कभी अधिवृषण को शुक्रग्रंथि से जोड़ती है। A fold of tunica vaginalis which sometimes connects the epididymis to the testis.

Mesogastrium (मीजोगेस्ट्रीयम) जहर योजनी। In embryo, the mesentery in relation to be dilated portion of the enteric canal which is the future stomach.

Mesognathous (मीजोग्नेथस) ऐसा चेहरा जिसमें जबड़ा बाहर निकला रहता है। Having a face slightly projecting jaw.

Mesometrium (मीजोमीट्रियम) गर्भाशय पेशी। The broad ligament.

Mesophilic (मीजोफिलिक) मध्यम तापमान (15°से. से 42°से. तक) पर सबसे अधिक वृद्धि करने वाला जैसे कुछ जीवाणु करते है। Growing best at moderate temperature (15 °C to 42 °C) as do some bacteria.

Mesorectum (मीजोरैक्टम) मलाशय-योजनी। Mesentery of the rectum.

Mesorrhine (मीजोराइन) मामूली-सी चौड़ी नाक वाला। Having a nose of moderate width.

Mesosalpinx (मीजोसैल्पिंक्स) डिम्ब वाहिनी-योजनी। The upper part of the broad ligament.

Mesotendon (मीजोटैण्डन) किसी कण्डरा को इसके तन्तुमय ऊतक आवरण से जोड़ने वाला संयोजी-ऊतक आवरण। Mesotendineum, a fold of synovial membrane connecting a tendon to its synovial sheath.

Mesothelioma (मीजोथिलियोमा) मध्यकला से विकसित होने वाली कोई भी रसौली। Any tumor developed from the mesothelium.

Mesovarium (मीजोवेरियम) डिम्बग्रंथि योजनी, पैरीटोनियम तह का वह भाग जो डिम्बग्रंथि की अग्र सीमा को प्रथस्नायु की पश्च परत से जोड़ता है। Peritoneal fold joining the ovary with the broad ligament.

Meta (मेटा) परिवर्तन अथवा रूपान्तरण को निर्दिष्ट करने वाला एक उपसर्ग। A prefix denoting a change or transformation.

Metabolism (मेटाबोलिज्म) चयापचय, शरीर की वह क्रिया जिसमें भोजन ऊतक-तत्वों में परीणित होता है। The process of transferring food-stuff into tissue elements and energy for use in the body growth, repair and general function.

Metabolite (मेटाबोलाइट) चयापचयक। A substance formed in metabolism.

Metacarpus (मेटाकार्पस) कलाई और उंगलियों के मध्य स्थित हड्डियाँ। The five bones which forms the palm of hand between the wrist and fingers.

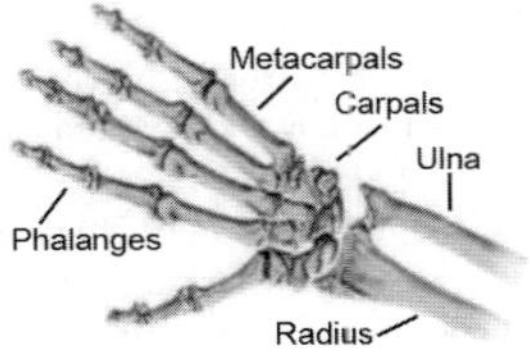

Metachromatic (मेटाक्रोमेटिक) विविधरंजकता संबंधी। Relating to metachromatism.

Metachysis (मेटाकायसिस) शरीर में रक्त डालना। The transfusion of blood.

Metacyesis (मेटासियेसिस) परागर्भाशय-सगर्भता। Extrauterine gestation.

Metal (मेटल) धातु, सोना, चांदी लोहा, आदि। A substance as gold, sliver, iron, etc.

Metamorphopsia (मेटामोर्फोप्सिया) दृष्टिदोष दोष जिसमें हर वस्तु टेढ़ी नजर आती है। A visual defect with an apparent distortion of objects.

Metamorphosis (मेटामॉरफोसिस) भौतिक रूप, संरचना या विशेष रूप से विकासीय अवस्थाओं में होने वाले रूपान्तरण और रचनात्मक परिवर्तन। Developmental change of physical form, structures, or substance.

Metamyelocyte (मेटामायलोसाइट) मध्यमज्जा कोशिका। A myelocyte that look like a granular leukocyte.

Metanephrons (मेटानेफरोन्स) भ्रूण-वृक्कांग का पिछला खण्ड। The posterior segment of the fetal renal organ.

Metaphase (मेटाफेस) मध्यावस्था, ऊतर-स्थिति। That period in karyokinesis during which the chromatin loops split in two.

Metaphysis (मेटाफाइजिस) लम्बी हड्डी का काण्ड एवं अधिवर्ध के बीच का चौड़ा भाग,अस्थिकॉण्ड--कोटि। The wide portion of a long bone and the region of the bone where growth occurs, it is located between diaphysis and epiphysis.

Metaphysitis (मेटाफाइजाइटिस) किसी हड्डी के अस्थिकॉण्ड कोटि का शोथ। Inflammation of the metaphysis of a bone.

Metaplasia (मेटाप्लेसिया) एक ऊतक का दूसरे ऊतक में बदलना। Conversion of one tissue into another.

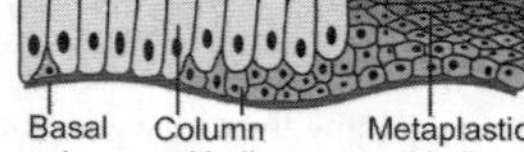

A model of squamous epithelial metaplasia

Metastasis (मेटास्टेसिस) रोग का किसी एक अंग से दूसरे अंग में स्थानान्तरण होना। Removal or tranfer of disease from one part of the body to another.

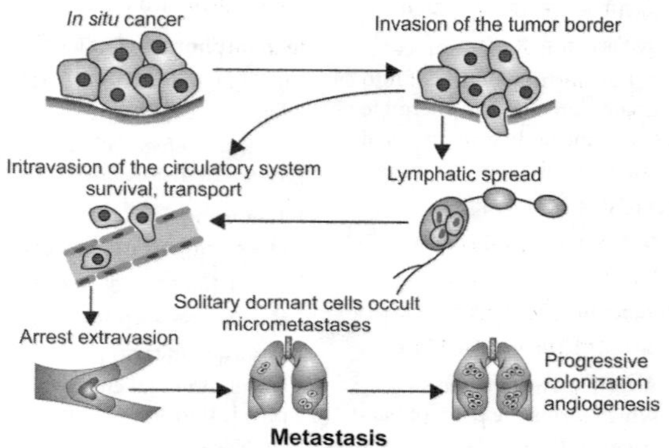

Metastasis

Metatarsus (मेटाटार्सस) पैर की हड्डियाँ जो उँगलियों और टखने के मध्य स्थित रहती है व जिसमें पैर के तलुवे की पाँच हड्डियाँ भी सम्मिलित है। The distal portion of the foot between the ankle and the toes including five metatarsal bones.

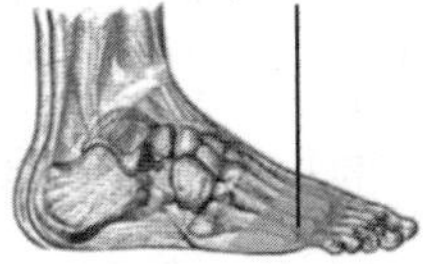

Metazoa (मेटाजुआ) सभी बहुकोशिकीय जन्तु। All multicellular animals.

Metazoonosis (मेटाजूनोसिस) एक जन्तु रोग जिसे अपनी अवधि पूर्ण करने के लिए एक पृष्ठवंशी एवं एक अपृष्ठवंशी परपोशी की आवश्यकता होती है। A zoonosis requiring both a vertebrate and an invertebrate host for completion of its course.

Metencephalon (मीटीन्सिफेलोन) अनुमध्य मस्तिष्क। The after brain or the caudal portion of the brain.

Meteorism (मीटीयोरिज्म) अफारा। Cavity.

Meter (मीटर) मैट्रिक प्रणाली में किसी वस्तु की लम्बाई चौड़ाई। A measuring unit of length in metric system of an object.

Methemoglobin (मीटहीमोग्लोबिन) आघात अथवा विषैले पदार्थो द्वारा हीमोग्लोबिन के फेरस लौह के फेरिक लौह में ऑक्सीकृत होने से बनने वाला एक यौगिक। A compound formed from hemoglobin by the oxidation of its ferrous iron to ferric iron by injury or toxic substance.

Methemoglobinemia (मीटहोमोग्लोबिनीमिया) मेटहीमोग्लोबिन-रक्तता। The presence of methemoglobin in the blood.

Metopic (मेटोपीक) ललाटीय। Relating to the forehead on inferior portion of the cranium.

Metopion (मीटोपियन) ललाट बिन्दु। Glabella.

Metoxeny (मीटोजेनी) जीवन चक्र को पूरा करने के लिए दो भिन्न पोशदों पर रहना। To live upon two different hosts to complete the life cycle.

Metratrophia (मीट्राट्रॉफिया) गर्भाशय-शोथ। Atrophy of the uterus.

Metrectasia (मीट्रेक्टेशेया) गर्भाशय से रहित गर्भाशय का विस्फारण। Dilatation of the nonpregnant uterus.

Metrectopia (मीट्रेक्टोपिया) गर्भाशय का विस्थापित हो जाना। Displacement of the uterus.

Metrelcosis (मीट्रेल्कोसिस) गर्भाशय में जख्म बन जाना। Ulceration of the uterus.

Metritis (मीट्राइटिस) गर्भाशय का शोथ। Inflammation of the uterus.

Metromalacia (मीट्रोमैलेशिया) गर्भाशय का कोमल हो जाना। Softening of the uterus.

Metropathia-hemorrhagica (मीट्रापैथिया-हीमोरैह्जिका) गर्भाशय से खून निकलना जो श्लेष्मिक कलाओं की अतिवृद्धि एवं डिम्बग्रंथि की पुटियों से संबद्ध होता है। Bleeding from the uterus associated with hypertrophy of the mucus membranes of the uterus and the ovarion cysts.

Metroptosis (मीट्रोप्टोसिस) गर्भाशय का नीचे की ओर विस्थापित हो जाना। Downward displacement or prolapse of the uterus.

Metrorrhagia (मीट्रोरैह्जिया) मासिक धर्म के अतिरिक्त अन्य किसी भी समय होने वाला गर्भाशय से रक्त स्राव। Uterine bleeding occurring at any time other than during the menstrual period.

Metrorrhea (मीट्रोरिह्या) अत्यधिक गर्भाशय-स्राव। Excessive uterine discharge.

Metrorrhexis (मीट्रोरैह्क्सिस) गर्भाशय का फट जाना। Rupture of the uterus.

Metrostaxis (मीट्रोस्टेक्सिस) गर्भाशय से लगातार रक्तस्राव होना। Blood oozing from the uterus.

MFD (एम.एफ.डी.) न्यूनतम घातक मात्रा। Minimum fatal dose.

MHD (एम.एच.डी.) न्यूनतम रक्तसंलायी मात्रा। Minimum hemolytic dose.

Miasmus (मिस्मस) विष दोष। Sycosis.

Micrencephaly (माइक्रेनसिफेली) मस्तिष्क का असामान्य रूप से छोटा होना। Abnormal smallness of the brain.

Micro (माइक्रो) सूक्ष्म, अल्प, लघु। Prefix meaning small.

Microadenoma (माइक्रोएडीनोमा) एक छोटा ग्रन्थ्यर्बुद जैसा कि अग्र पीयूश ग्रंथि का होता है। A very small adenoma, as that of the anterior pituitary gland.

Microanalysis (माइक्रोएनालाइसिस) किसी पदार्थ की बहुत ही सूक्ष्म मात्रा का रासायनिक विश्लेषण।

Chemical analysis of very small quantity of a material.

Microaneurysm (माइक्रोएन्यूरिज्म) सूक्ष्मदर्शी द्वारा दिखाई देने

वाला फुलाव। A microscopic aneurysm.

Microangiitis (माइक्रोएन्जाइटिस) बहुत छोटी रक्त वाहिनियों की सूजन। Inflammation of very small blood vessels.

Microangiopathy (माइक्रोएन्जियोपैथी) सूक्ष्म वाहिका विकृति। Thickening and reduplication of basement in blood vessels.

Microbe (माइक्रोब) रोगाणु, रोगोत्पादक जीवाणु। Disease producing bacterium, germs.

Microbicidal (माइक्रोबिसाइडल) जीवाणु नाशक। Destroying microbes.

Microbiology (माइक्रोबायोलॉजी) सूक्ष्म जीव-विज्ञान। Scientific study of the microorganisms.

Microbism (माइक्रोबिज्म) रोगाणुओं का संक्रमण। Infection of microbes.

Microblepharia (माइक्रोब्लेफेरिया) पलकें छोटी होना। Having abnormally small eyelids.

Microcoria (माइक्रोकोरिया) पुतली का छोटा होना। Smallness of the pupil.

Microcyte (माइक्रोसाइट) लघु लोहित कोशिका। An undersized red blood cell found in the anemic blood.

Microcytosis (माइक्रोसाइटोसिस) लघु लोहित कोशिका का ज्यादा पाया जाना। Presence of excessive number of microcytes in the blood.

Microfilaria (माइक्रोफाइलेरिया) फाइलेरिया रोग से पीड़ित व्यक्ति के रक्त में पाया जाने वाला फाइलेरिया कृमि का लार्वा से पूर्वस्थ। A prelarval form of filaria worms.

Microgamete (माइक्रोगैमेट) लघुयुग्मक, छोटा, अत्यधिक गतिशीत पुरूष युग्मक जो बड़े, अल्प गतिशीत स्त्री युग्मक को गर्भित करता है। The smaller male element in the conjugation of cells of unequal size.

Microgametocyte (माइक्रोगैमेटोसाइट) लघु युग्मकजनक। A cell that produces microgametes.

Microglia (माइक्रोग्लिया) सूक्ष्मतंत्रिकाबंध। The smallest neuroglial cell, the macrophage of brain and spinal cord. A types of neuronal support cell occuring in CNS of invertebrates and vertebrates that functions primarily as an immune cell.

Micrognathia (माइक्रोग्नेथिया) निचले जबड़े का असमान्य रूप से छोटा होना। Unusual smallness of the jaws especially the lower jaw.

Microgram (माइक्रोग्राम) 1 मिलीग्राम का हजारवॉ या एक ग्राम का

10 लाखवॉ भाग। μg or mcg 1000 of a miligram or 1 millionth part of a gram.

Microgyrus (माइक्रोगाइरस) मस्तिष्क का एक छोटा विकृत कर्णक। A small malformed gyrus of the brain.

Microlesion (माइक्रोलीजन) बहुत छोटी विक्षति। A very small lesion.

Microlithiasis (माइक्रोलिथिएसिस) किसी अंग में बहुत छोटी पथरियों का बनना। Formation of very small calculi in an organ.

Micromanipulation (माइक्रोमैनीपुलेशन) माइक्रोमैनीपुलेटर के द्वारा सूक्ष्मदर्शी में शल्य-क्रिया या विच्छेदन करना। To perform surgery or dissection or to administer injection, etc.

Micromastia (माइक्रोमैस्टिया) स्तनों का असामान्य रूप से छोटा होना। Abnormal smallness of the breasts.

Micrometer (माइक्रोमीटर) 1. एक मीटर का दस-लाखवां अथवा एक मिलीलीटर का हजारवां भाग। 2. सूक्ष्ममापी। 1. One million of a meter. 2. An instrument for measuring small distances.

Micron (माइक्रोन) एक मीटर का लाखवां भाग। A millionth part of a meter.

Micronutrient (माइक्रोन्यूट्रिएन्ट) एक पोशक जिसकी थोड़ी मात्राओं में ही लेने की आवश्यकता होती है। A nutrient required only in small amounts.

Microorganism (माइक्रोआरगेनिजम) सूक्ष्मजीव। A general term covering microscopic form, such as germs, viruses, etc.

Microphakia (माइक्रोफेकिया) ऑख के स्फटिकाभ लैन्स का असामान्य रूप से छोटा रहना। Abnormal smallness of the crystalline lens of the eye.

Microphobia (माइक्रोफोबिया) छोटी वस्तुओं अथवा रोगाणुओं से डर। Morbid fear of the small things or the germs.

Microphonia (माइक्रोफोनिया) कण्ड ध्वनि की कमजोरी। Weakness of the voice.

Micropipette (माइक्रोपिपेट) एक छोटा सा पिपेट जिससे तरल पदार्थो की छोटी-छोटी मात्राओं को मापने वाला। An extremely small pipette used for measuring small amounts of the fluid substances.

Microprobe (माइक्रोप्रोब) एक बहुत छोटी एशणी जिसका सूक्ष्मशल्यकर्म में प्रयोग किया जाता है।

A very small probe used in microsurgery.

Microprosopia (माइक्रोप्रोसोपिया) चेहरे का असामान्य रूप से छोटा होना। Abnormal smallness of the face.

Micropsia (माइक्रोपसिया) लघुदृशिता। A visual defect in which the objects are seen smaller in size.

Micropyle (माइक्रोपायेले) वह छिद्र जिसमें शुक्राणु प्रवेश करता है। अणुद्वारा। An opening in the ovum for the entrance of the spermatozoon.

Microradiography (माइक्रोरेडियोग्राफी) सूक्ष्मदर्शीय वस्तुओं का एक्स-रे चित्रण करना जिसमें एक्स-रे फिल्म बड़ी होती है। Radiography of the microscopic objects in which the X-ray films are enlarged.

Microscope (माइक्रोस्कोप) सूक्ष्मदर्शी यंत्र। An instrument for examining small objects.

Microscopic (माइक्रोस्कोपिक) 1. सूक्ष्मदर्शी संबंधी। 2. केवल सूक्ष्मदर्शी द्वारा दिखाई देने वाला। 1. Pertaining to the microscope. 2. Visible only by using the microscope.

Microscopy (माइक्रोस्कोपी) सूक्ष्मदर्शन। Examination the microscope.

Microsomia (माइक्रोसोमिया) बौनापन। Abnormal smallness of the body.

Microsporum (माइक्रोस्पोरम) कवकों का एक वंश जिसमें त्वचा, बालों या नाखूनों का रोग उत्पन्न होता है। A genus of fungi that cause disease of the skin, hair or nails.

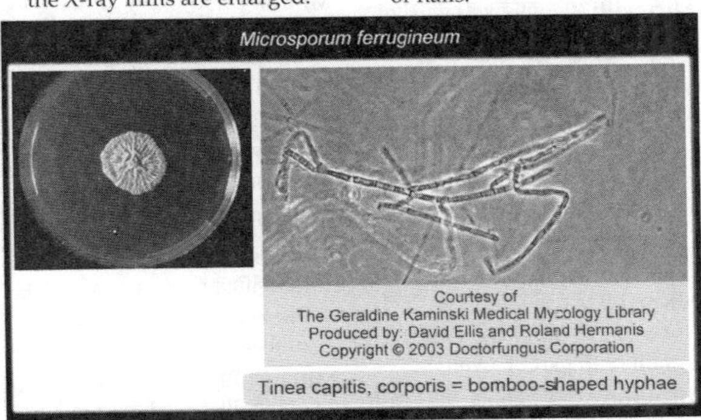

Microsporum

Microstomia (माइक्रोस्टोमिया) लघुमुखद्वार। Unusual smallness of the mouth.

Microtia (माइक्रोटिया) कर्णपाली का सामान्य रूप से बहुत छोटा होना। Abnormal smallness of the pinna of the ear.

Microtome (माइक्रोटोम) सूक्ष्मदर्शीय अध्ययन के लिए ऊतकों को पतले-पतले खण्डों में काटने वाला एक यंत्र। An instrument for cutting thin section of the tissues for microscopic study.

Microtonometer (माइक्रोटोनोमीटर) खून में ऑक्सीजन एवं कार्बनडाइ-ऑक्साइड की सांद्रता का पता लगाने वाला उपकरण। An instrument for measuring the partial pressure of gases in minute quantities of material.

Microvilli (माइक्रोविलाइ) कोशिका कलाओं की स्वतंत्र सतह से निकलने वाले सूक्ष्म प्रवर्ध जैसे–छोटी आँत की श्लेष्मिक कलाओं की कोशिकाओं पर पाये जाते है। Submicropic finger like-projections of cell membrane greatly increase cell surface area.

Microvolt (माइक्रोवोल्ट) एक वोल्ट का लाखवॉ भाग। μV. One millionth part of a volt.

Microwave (माइक्रोवेव) 1 मीमी तथा 30 सेमी के तरंगदैर्ध्य के बीच की तंरग। A wave between a wavelength of 1 mm to 30 cm.

Micturition (मिक्चुरीशन) मूत्र त्याग। Urination.

Midbrain (मिडब्रेन) मध्यमस्तिष्क। The mesencephalon.

Midget (मिडगेट) बौना। Dwarf.

Midgut (मिडगट) भ्रूणीय आंत का बीच का भाग। Middle portion of the embryonic intestine.

Midwife (मिडवाइफ) प्रसूति सहायक, दाई। A woman obstetrician.

Midwifery (मिडवाइफरी) प्रसूतिविधा, प्रसूतितंत्र। Obstetrics.

Migraine (माइग्रेन) आधे सिर का दर्द। A severe type of headache, often one-sided and sometimes accompanied by visual disturbances.

Mildew (मिल्डीव) फफूंदी, कवक। The common name for any one of a number minute fungi destructive to living plants, food, etc.

Miliaria (मिलियेरिया) स्वेद ग्रंथियों की वाहिनियों में अवरोध उत्पन्न हो जाने तथा स्वेद के रूक जाने से जलास्फोटों का बन जाना, स्वेदराजिका। A disorder of the sweat glands with obstruction of their ducts sudamina.

Miliary (मिलियेरिया) विकिरत, कंगु। Like millet-seeds as a miliary eruption.

Miliei (मिलियू) वातावरण। Environment.

Milium (मिलियम) नवजात शिशु के चेहरे एवं धड़ पर पिन के सिर के परिमाण की बनने वाली श्वेत पिटिका जो कुछ सप्ताहों में लुप्त हो जाती है। A minute whitish or yellowish papule on the skin caused by retention of fatty material or densely packed keratin.

Milk (मिल्क) दूध। The secretion of the mammary glands.

Milk fever (मिल्क फीवर) प्रसूति-काल में होने वाला ज्वर। Fever occurring during puerperal period.

Milk-teeth (मिल्कटीथ) प्रथम अथवा गिरने वाले दॉत। The first or deciduous teeth.

Milliequivalent (मिलीइक्वीवैलेन्ट) इसकी गणना मिलीग्राम प्रतिलीटर को रसायन की वैलेन्सी से गुणा करके तथा पदार्थ के अुण-भार से विभाजित करके की जाती है। A quantity equal to 10^{-3} of the equivalent weight of an element or compound.

Milligram (मिलीग्राम) एक ग्राम का हजारवॉ भाग। (mg) One thousandth part of a gram.

Millimeter (मिलीमीटर) एक मीटर का हजारवॉ भाग। (mm) One thousandth part of a meter.

Millimicrogram (मिलीमाइक्रोग्राम) एक ग्राम का एक अरबवॉ भाग। 10^{-9} gram. A nanogram. One billionth part of a gram.

Mimetic (मिमेटीक) कूट, मिथ्या। Imitative, false.

Mimicry (मिमीकरी) नकल उतारना। To imitate or simulate.

Min (मिन) बूंद, मिनट। Minim, minute.

Mind (माइन्ड) मन, चित्त। The organ of consciousness.

Mineral (मिनरल) खनिज, खान से निकलने वाला पदार्थ। A metabolic substance found in nature.

Mineralization (मिनरलइजेशन) ऊतकों में खनिजों का जमा होना। Deposition of minerals in the tissues.

Mineralocorticoid (मिनरलोकॉर्टिकॉयड) एड्रीनल कॉटेक्स के कॉर्टिकोस्टैरॉयड हॉर्मोनों के वर्गो में से एक वर्ग में से एक वर्ग जिसका संबंध वृक्कीय नालिकाओं की उपकला–कोशिकाओं में आयन परिवहन पर प्रभाव पड़ने के कारण जल व इलैक्ट्रोलाइट संतुलन के नियमन से होता है। सोडियम ठहर जाता है पोटेशियम शरीर से बाहर निकल जाता है। One of the steroids in the adrenal cortex that act principally on renal retention of sodium and excretion of potassium.

Minim (मिनिम) .06 मिलीमीटर, बूंद। A unit of fluid measure, about a drop or 1/60th of a dram.

Miosis (मियोसिस) पुतलियों का असामान्य रूप से संकुचित हो जाना। Abnormal contraction of the pupils.

Miotic (मायोटिक) पुतली को संकुचित करने वाला। Any agent causing miosis.

Mirror (मिरर) दर्पण, शीशा। A polished surface that forms optical images by reflection.

Miscarriage (मिस्केरियेज) गर्भपात, गर्भस्राव। Abortion, premature labor.

Misce (मिस्से) मिलाओं, मिश्रण करो। Mix, a direction placed on prescriptions.

Miscible (मिस्सीबिल) मिश्रित होने योग्य। Capable of being mixed.

Misogyny (मिसोगाइनी) स्त्रियों से घृणा करना। Aversion to women.

Misoneism (मिसोनीज्म) नये विचारों से नफरत करना। Aversion to new things or ideas.

Misopedia (मिसोपीडिया) बच्चों से नफरत करना। Aversion to children.

Mist (मिस्ट) धुंध। Filmy appearance before the eyes.

Mite (माइट) जू, सूक्षमकीट। A minute parasitic insect, the louse.

Miticide (माइटीसाइड) सूक्ष्म कीटनाशी, कुटष्कियों को मारने वाला पदार्थ। The substance who kills the mites.

Mitigate (माइटीगेट) शमन करना। Palliate.

Mitochondria (माइटोकॉण्ड्रिया) सूत्रकणिकाएँ। A double membrane cytoplasmic organelle, self-reproducing, present in cell cytoplasm of all living cells.

Mitogen (माइटोजन) कोशिका सूत्री विभाजन करने वाला पदार्थ। A substance that causes cell metosis.

Mitogenesis (माइटोजेनेसिस) कोशिका सूत्री विभाजन करना। To cause cell mitosis.

Mitosis (माइटोसिस) सूत्रीविभाजन, विषय कोशिका विभाजन। A complicated method of cell division occurring in specialized cells.

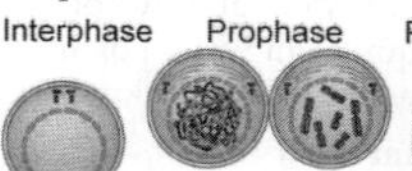
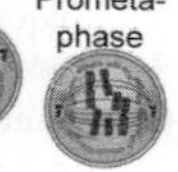
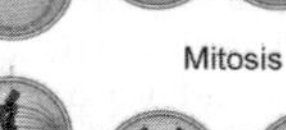
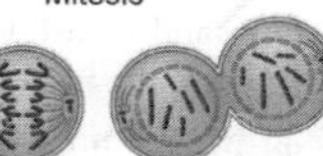
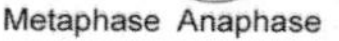

Mitral (माइट्रल) द्विकपर्दी। Denoting a structure resembling the shape of a headbond.

Mitral valve (माइट्रल वाल्व) हृदय का द्विमूल कपाट।
Bicuspid, value of the heart.

Mittelschmerz (माइटलस्कमर्ज) मासिक धर्मो के बीच एवं डिम्बोत्सर्जनके समय पेट में होने वाला दर्द। Intermenstrual pain especially at the time of evaluation.

Mixture (मिक्शचर) मिश्रण।
A mutual corporation, preparation or combination of several substances.

MLA (एम.एल.ए.) चिकित्सीय लाइब्रेरी एसोसियेशन। Medical library association.

MLD (एम.एल.डी.) न्यूनतम घातक मात्रा। Minimum lethal dose.

MMR (एम.एम.आर.) सामूहिक लघु एक्स-रे चित्रण। Mass miniature radiography.

Mnemonics (नीमोनिक्स) स्मृति बढ़ाने की तकनीक अथवा कोई उपकरण। The technique or an apparatus for improving the memory.

MO (एम.ओ.) चिकित्सा अधिकारी। Medical officer.

Moan (मोन) कराहना। To utter a sound expressive of suffering.

Mobility (मोबीलिटी) गतिशीलता। The quality of being movable.

Mobilization (मोबीलाइजेशन) गतिशील बनाने की क्रिया। The process of making movable.

Modality (मोडेलिटी) बहुलता। The condition of being better or worse, including various forms of sensations.

Mode (मोड) तरीका, प्रणाली। Custom, way.

Modiolus (मोडिल्यस) कर्णावर्तमध्याक्ष।
The axis of the cochlea of the ear.

Modulation (मोडूलेशन) रासायनिक या भौतिक वातावरण में परिवर्तन होने के कारण किसी वस्तु के कार्य अथवा स्थिति में अन्तर हो जाना। The changes that takes place in response to changes in the physical and chemical environment.

Mogilalia (मोगीलैलीया) हकलाना। Stuttering or stammering.

Mogiphonia (मोगीफोनिया) स्वर-ध्वनियाँ निकालने में कठिनाई। Difficulty in emitting vocal sounds.

Molar (मोलर) चबाने वाला। Any of the most posterior teeth in jaw.

Molarity (मोलारिटी) विलयन के प्रति लीटर में किसी विलेय के मोलों की संख्या।
To number of moles of a solute per liter of solution.

Molasses (मोलासेज) शीरा। The thick syrup drained from the sugar in the process of refining.

Mold (मोल्ड) साँचा, ढाँचा, फफूंदी। A cast, shape, mould, fungus which produces spores.

Molding (मोल्डिंग) प्रसव के दौरान भ्रूण के सिर की आकृति को प्रसव नली के अनुकूल बनाना। Shaping of the fetal head and adapting it to the birth canal during labor.

Mole (मोल) तिल। A brownish spot on the skin.

Molecular (मौलीकुलर) अणु संबंधी, आण्विक। Pertaining to molecules.

Molecule (मॉलीक्यूल) किसी पदार्थ की सूक्ष्मातिसूक्ष्म मात्रा। The smallest quantity of a substance.

Molluscum (मोलस्कम) त्वचा का कोई भी रोग जिसमें त्वचा पर कोमल, गोल अबुर्द बन जाते है। A skin disease that causes painless pink bumps on the skin. (Small raised lesions with dimple in center).

Momentum (मोमेन्टम) संवेग, गति प्रदान करने वाली शक्ति, बल। The quantity of the motion of the body obtained by multiplying its mass and velocity.

Monarthritis (मोनार्थ्राइटिस) एक अकेले जोड़ की सूजन। Inflammation of a single joint.

Mongolism (मोंगोलिज्म) मंगोलना। Down's syndrome.

Mongoloid (मोंगोलॉयड) 1. मंगोंल संबंधी। 2. मगौलकल्प।
1. Pertaining to Mangols.
2. Characterized by Mongolism.

Moniliasis (मोनीलिएसिस) किसी कवक का संक्रमण। Infection with any fungus of genus monillia.

Moniliform (मोनीलीफोर्म) माला अथवा गले के हार के समान। Resembling a necklace or string of beads.

Monillia (मोनीलिया) कवक कण्डिडा। Fungus candida.

Monitor (मॉनीटर) किसी स्थिति जैसे तापमान, रक्त चाप, ह्रदय गति आदि को निरन्तर नियंत्रित करना। To control constantly a condition, e.g. temperature, BP pulse, respiration.

Monoblast (मोनोब्लास्ट) एक केन्द्रक श्वेत कोशिका को उत्पन्न करने वाली कोशिका। An immature cell that develops into a monocyte.

Monobrachius (मोनोब्रेकियस) ऐसा भ्रूण जिसमें केवल एक बाँह होती है। The fetus with only one arm.

Monochromasy (मोनोक्रोमेसी) वर्णान्धता जिसमें सभी रंग भूरे

रंग के दिखाई देते है। Color blindness in which all colors appear to be of gray color.

Monochromatic (मोनोक्रोमेटिक) 1. पूर्ण वर्णान्धता से ग्रस्त व्यक्ति। 2. केवल एक रंग वाला। 1. Monochromat. 2. Having only one color.

Monocrotic (मोनोक्रोटिक) केवल एक नाड़ी तरंग का संकेत देने वाला जिसमें कोई खाँचा नहीं होता। Indicating a single pulse wave with no notches in it.

Monocular (मोनोकुलर) 1. केवल एक आँख को प्रभावित करने वाला। 2. केवल एक आईपीस से युक्त जैसे एकनेत्री सूक्ष्मदर्शी में होता है। 1. Pertaining to or affecting only one eye. 2. Having only one eye pixel as in a monocular microscope.

Monocyte (मोनोसाइट) एक केन्द्रक श्वेत कोशिका। A mono nuclear cell.

The elements of blood

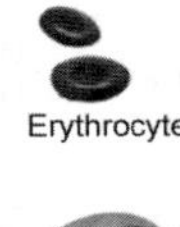

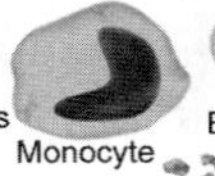

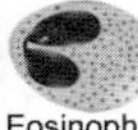

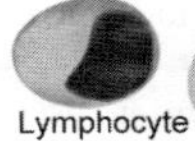

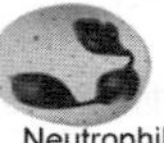

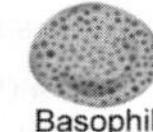

Monocytosis (मोनोसाइटोसिस) एक केन्द्रक श्वेत कोशिका बहुलता। Abnormal mono nuclear cell in the number of monocytes in the circulating blood.

Monomania (मोनोमेनिया) एकोन्माद, किसी एक ही वस्तु को पाने की सनक। Mania for a single object.

Monomorphic (मोनोमॉर्फिक) विकास की प्रत्येक अवस्था में एक ही रूप को धारण किए रहने वाला। Maintaining the same form throughout every stage of development.

Mononeucleosis (मोनोन्यूक्लियोसिस) एक केन्द्रक-श्वेत कोशिका। Presence of a large number of mononuclear leukocytes in the blood.

Mononeuritis (मोनोन्यूराइटिस) किसी अकेली नाड़ी का प्रदाह। Inflammation of a side nerve.

Monophasia (मोनोफेजिया) वाक्यखण्ड को बार-बार बोलने के सिवाय और कुछ भी बोलने में असमर्थता। Inability to speak anything except one word or phrase repeatedly.

Monophobia (मोनोफ्जोबिया) अकेलेपन से डर। A morbid fear of being left alone.

Monoplegia (मोनोप्लेजिया) केवल एक अंग का पक्षाघात होना। Paralysis of only one limb.

Monopus (मोनोपस) जन्म से ही एक पैर वाला। Having only one foot by birth.

Monorchid (मोनोर्किड) वह व्यक्ति जिसके केवल एक शुक्रग्रंथि होती है। An individual having only one testicle.

Monosaccharide (मोनोसैकेराइड) एक प्रकार की सामान्य चीनी, ग्लूकोज। A simple sugar that cannot be decomposed by hydrolysis.

Monoxide (मोनोक्साइड) ऐसा ऑक्साइड जिसके अणु में केवल एक ऑक्सीजन परमाणु होता है। Any oxide having only one atom of oxygen.

Monozygotic (मोनोजाइगोटिक) एकयुग्मज। Twins derived from a single fertilized ovum and so indentical twins.

Mons (मोन्स) उभार, शैल। A prominence.

Monster (मोन्स्टर) शिशु, राक्षस, एक बहुत विकृत भ्रूण। A grossly deformed fetus or infant.

Mood (मूड) चित्तवृति, भावदशा। The emotional state.

Morbid (मोर्बिड) रोगी, बीमार। Disease.

Morbidity (मोर्बिडिटी) विकृति, रूग्णता। A diseased state.

Morbilliform (मोर्बिलिफोर्म) खसरा जैसा, रोमान्तिकाभ। Resembling measles.

Morbus (मोर्बस) बीमारी। A disease or illness.

Morgue (मॉग) शवगृह। Mortuary.

Moria (मोरिया) पागलपन, मूर्खता। Dementia, foolishness.

Moribund (मोरीबण्ड) मरणासन्न। A dying state.

Mororeflex (मोरोरिफ्लेक्स) किसी उद्दीपन जैसे शिशु जिस बिस्तर पर लेटा हो उसे अचानक ढकने पर उत्पन्न उद्दीपन की अनुक्रिया में शिशुओं में दिखायी देने वाला एक प्रतिवर्त जिसमें वे अपनी बाहों को मोड़ते और फेलाते है जिसके पश्चात् बाँहों में आलिंगन करने वाली गति होती है। An infantile reflex where striking infants bed abduction and extension of arms.

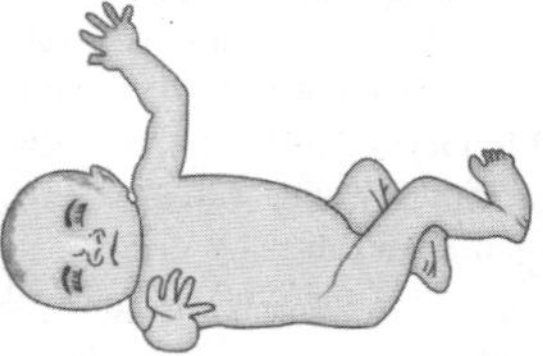

Morphea (मार्फीया) चमड़ी की दूर-दूर तक होने वाली कठोरता। A cutaneous lesion characterized by widespread sclerosis of the skin.

Morphia (मार्फीया) अफीम का सत। Morphine.

Morphogenesis (मॉर्फोजेनेसिस) अंगजनन। Development of the shape of the body, its parts or organs.

Morphologic (मॉर्फोलॉजिक) आकारिकी संबंधी। Relating to morphology.

Morphology (मॉर्फोलॉजी) जीवों के रूप एवं रचना का विज्ञान, आकारिकी। Science of the form and structure of lining things.

Mortal (मोर्टल) नष्ट होने वाला। Liable to death.

Mortality (मोर्टालिटी) मृत्यु। Death.

Mortar (मोर्टर) खरल। A laboratory vessel used for pulverizing.

Mortification (मॉर्टिफिकेशन) शरीर के मांस का सड़ना। Death of a part of the body, gangrene.

Mortuary (मोर्चरी) शवगृह। A room or building in which dead bodies are kept for hygienic storage or for examination, until burial or cremation.

Morula (मौरूला) कलल, डिम्बविभाजन में प्रथम ठोस गोलाकार आकृति। The mulberry mass of the ovum at a certain stage of cell segmentation.

Embryonic development–morula

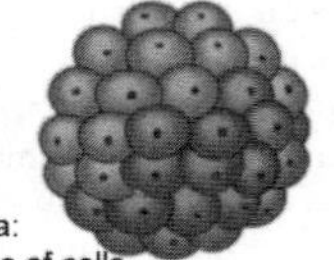

Morulation (मौरूलेशन) मौरूला का बनना। The formation of morula.

Mosquito (मॉस्क्यूटो) मच्छर। Blood sucking and disease transmitting insect as anopheles mosquito that transmits malaria.

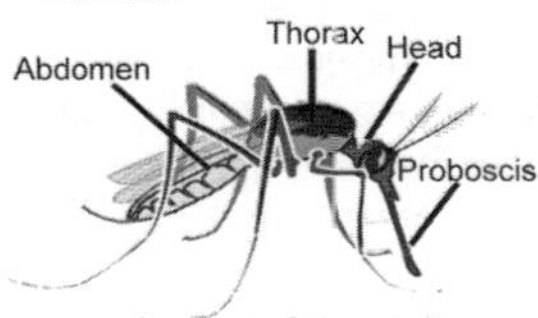

Anatomy of a mosquito

Mother's mark (मदर्स-मार्क) तिल, जन्म-चिन्ह। Nevus, a birth mark.

Motile (मोटाइल) स्वतःगतिशील। Able to move spontaneously.

Motility (मोटीलिटी) स्वतःगतिशीलता। Ability to move spontaneously.

Motion-sickness (मोशन सिक्नैस) कार, हवाई जहाज तथा पानी के जहाज आदि में यात्रा करने से जी घबराना, उल्टी होना, चक्कर आना। Nausea-vomiting and vertigo caused by traveling in the car, aeroplane, and ships, etc.

Motor (मोटर) गतिजनक। A part or center that induces movements as nerves or muscles.

Mottling (मोटलिंग) चितकबरा होना। The condition of being discolored.

Moulage (माऊलेज) 1. शरीर के किसी भाग का मोम अथवा प्लास्टिक का प्रतिरूप। 2. इस प्रकार के मॉडलो को ढालना। 1. A waxy or plastic model of some part of the body. 2. Molding of such models.

Mount (माऊन्ट) सूक्ष्मदर्शी-परीक्षण के लिए नमूनों की स्लाइड्स को तैयार करना। To prepare slides of the specimens for the microscopic examination.

Mourning (मौर्निंग) शॉक। Grief.

Mouth (माउथ) मुँह। The cavity which contains tongue and teeth.

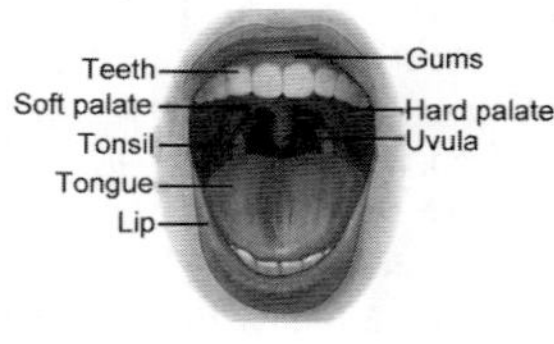

Mouthwash (माउथवॉश) मुँह धोने वाला घोल। A solution for washing the mouth.

Movement (मूवमेंट) गति, चाल। A motion, an action.

Mu (एमयू) मिलीमाइक्रोन का प्रतीक। Symbol for millimicron.

Muciferous (म्यूसीफेरस) श्लेष्मा पैदा करने वाला। Producing mucus.

Mucilage (म्यूसिलेज) गोंद, चेप। The solution of a gum in water.

Mucin (म्यूसिन) श्लेष्मरस, एक ग्लाइकोप्रोटीन जो श्लेष्मा का मुख्य घटक होता है। An albuminoid constituent of mucus.

Mucocele (म्यूकोसील) श्लेष्मपुटिका। Mucous tumor or polypus.

Mucoenteritis (म्यूकोएण्टीराइटिस) आँतों की श्लेष्मिक झिल्ली का प्रदाह। Inflammation of the mucous coat of the intestines.

Mucoid (म्यूकॉयड) श्लेष्मा से मिलता-जुलता। Resembling mucus or mucous tissue.

Mucor (म्यूकोर) एक प्रकार की फफूंदी जो कि एलर्जी का कारण हो सकती है। It is a fluffy white-gray fungus that may causes allergy to human's as mucor fungi.

Mucosa (म्यूकोसा) श्लैष्मिक झिल्ली। A mucous membrane.

Mucus (म्यूकस) श्लेष्मा। The viscid fluid secreted by mucous gland.

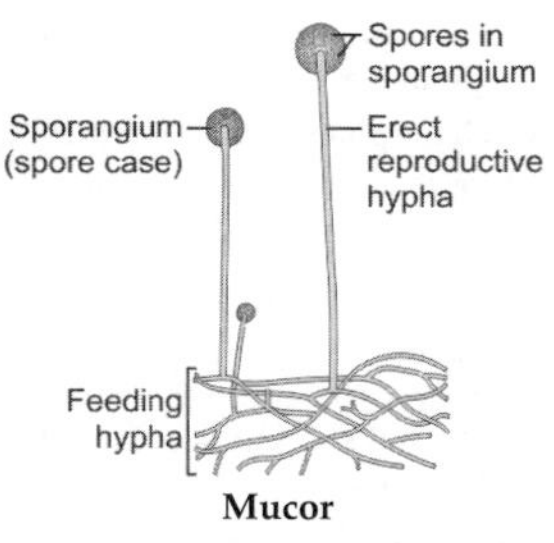

Mucor

Multi (मल्टी) अधिक का संकेत देने वाला। Prefixes indicating many or much.

Multifetation (मल्टीफीटेशन) दो से अधिक भ्रूण वाला गर्भ। A pregnancy more than two fetus.

Multigravida (मल्टीग्रेविडा) बहुप्रसूता। A woman who has borned many children.

Mummification (मम्मीफिकेशन) मृत भ्रूण का शुष्क होना या सिकुड जाना। The dessication of a tissue so that it resembles a mummy in color and texture.

Mumps (मम्पस) कर्णपूर्वग्रंथिशोथ। Inflammation of the parotid glands.

Musca domestica (मास्का डोमेस्टिका) घरेलू मक्खी। The common housesfly.

Musca volitantes (मास्का वोलिटेन्टस) आँखों के आगे चिनियं दिखाई देना। Spots before eyes.

Muscicide (मस्सीसाइड) मक्खियों को मारने वाला। Killing the flies.

Muscle (मसल) मांसपेशी। Musculus.

Muscle cramps (मसल क्रैम्पस) पेशियों के वेदनायुक्त अनैच्छिक संकुचन। Painful involuntary contractions of the muscles.

Mushroom (मशरूम) छत्रक। Umbrella-shaped fungus growing on decaying vegetable matter.

Musicomania (म्यूजिकोमेनिया) संगीत के लिए पागल बने रहना। Mania for music.

Mustard (मस्टर्ड) सरसों। Powder of mustard seeds used as counter irritant, rebefacient emetic, stimulant and condiment.

Mutagen (म्यूटेजन) उत्परिवर्तन। Any agent that causes production of a mutation.

Mutant (म्यूटेन्ट) उत्परिवर्ती, पैतृक लक्षणों से भिन्न। A cell which is the result of a genetic change.

Mutation (म्यूटेशन) भ्रूणपरिवर्तन। A change in presentation of a fetus.

Mutilation (म्यूटीलेशन) नष्ट करना। Destruction, meaning.

Mutism (म्यूटिज्म) गूंगापन। Inability to speak.

Myalgia (मायेल्जिया) पेशियों में दर्द होना। Pain in the muscle.

Myasthenia (मायस्थीनिया) पेशियों में कमजोरी हो जाना। Muscular debelity.

Mycetes (माइसिटीज) कवक। The fungi.

Mycetoma (माइसेटोमा) कवक के कवक जालों से बनी अबुर्द के समान सूजन। A tumorlike swelling of the fungal orycelia.

Mycobacterium (माइकोबैक्टीरियम) छोटे-छोटे लम्बे गोल दण्डाणु। Small slender rod bacteria containing gram-positive rods.

Mycology (माइकोलॉजी) कवक विज्ञान। Science of fungi.

Mycosis (माइकोसिस) कवकता। Any disease caused by a fungus.

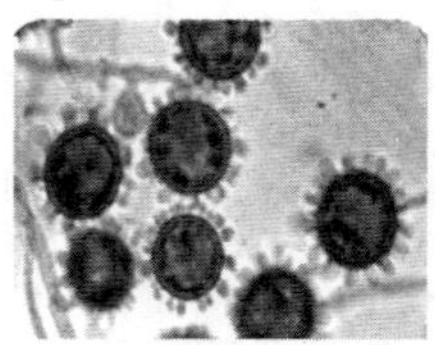

Mydriacis (मिडरिएसिस) आँखों की पुतलियां फैल जाना। Dilatation of the pupils.

Myelauxe (माइलौक्सी) सुषुम्ना रज्जु का असामान्य रूप से बढ़ जाना। Abnormal enlargement of the spinal cord.

Myelencephalon (माइलेनसिफालोन) भ्रूणीय पश्च मस्तिष्क का सबसे पिछला भाग जिससे मेड्यूला आब्लॉन्गेटा बनता है। The most posterior part of the embryonic hindbrain from which the medulla oblongata develops.

Myelin (माइलिन) वह श्वेत पदार्थ जो स्नायु मज्जा के आवरण का घटक होता है। An acute inflammation of the whole or of any part of the substance of the spinal cord.

Myelitis (माइलाइटिस) सुषुम्ना रज्जु अथवा अस्थि मज्जा का शोथ। Inflammation of the spinal cord or bone marrow.

Myelocele (माइलोसील) मेरूदण्ड में स्थित किसी फटन से सुषुम्ना रज्जु का बाहर निकल जाना। A form of spina bifida spinal cord protrusion.

Myelocyte (माइलोसाइट) प्राक्कणिका श्वेत कोशिका। The nucleus of a cell of gray matter.

Myelofibrosis (माइलोफाईब्रोसिस) अस्थिमज्जा एवं अस्थि गहवर के अंदर तन्तु-ऊतक का निर्माण होना। Formation of fibrous tissue in the bone marrow and cavity.

Myelogram (माइलोग्राम)

1. सुषुम्नारज्जु चित्रण द्वारा उपलब्ध एक्स-रे फिल्म। 2. अस्थि-मज्जा कोशिकाओं का विभेदक गणना। 1. X-ray film obtained by myelography.
2. Differential count of the bone marrow cells.

Myeloma (माइलोमा) मज्जार्बुद। A tumor of medullary substance.

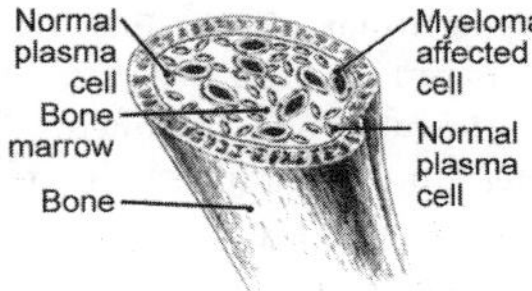

Myelomalacia (माइलोमैलेशिया) सुषुम्ना रज्जु का असामान्य रूप से कोमल हो जाना। Abnormal softening of the spinal cord.

Myelomeningocele (माइलोमैनिन्जोसील) मेरूरज्जुतानिका-हर्निया। Spinal bifida portion of cord and membranes protruding.

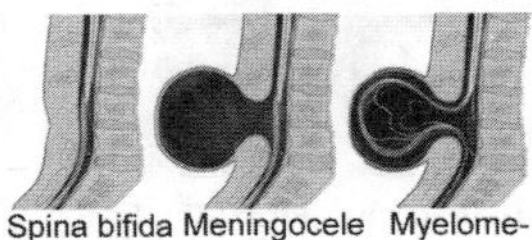

Myelopathy (माइलोपैथी) सुषुम्ना रज्जु का कोई भी रोग। Any disease of the spinal cord.

Myelopoiesis (माइलोपॅयसिस) अस्थि मज्जा अथवा इससे उत्पन्न होने वाली कोशिकाओं का बनना। Formation of bone marrow or the cells arising from it.

Myelopore (माइलोपोर) सुषुम्ना रज्जु में स्थित एक छिद्र। An opening in the spinal cord.

Myelorrhagia (माइलोरैइजिया) सुषुम्ना रज्जु में रक्तस्राव होना। Hemorrhage into the spinal cord.

Myerson's sign (मायरसन्स साइन) पार्किन्सन के रोग में, माथे या नासिका पुल पर थपथपाने पर प्रतिक्रिया स्वरूप आँखों का बार-बार मिचकाना। Inability to stop blinking on tapping the forehead as in Parkinson's disease.

Myiasis (मायेसिस) मक्खियों के लार्वों से उत्पन्न रोग। The disease caused by the maggots.

Myiodesopsia (माइयोडोसोप्सिया) आँखों के सामने धब्बों का दिखाई देना। The appearance of spots before the eyes.

Myocardial-infarction (मायोकार्डियल-इन्फार्कशन) दिल का दौरा। Death of myocardium usually due to coronary thrombosis or spasm.

Myocyte (मायोसाइट) पेशी कोशिका। A muscle cell.

Myodynamometer (मायोडाइनेमोमीटर) पेशीय शक्ति को मापने वाला एक उपकरण। An apparatus for measuring the muscular strength.

Myoepithelium (मायोइपिथिलियम) संकुचनशील उपकला-कोशिकाओं से बना ऊतक। Tissue made up of contractile epithelial cells.

Myoglobulin (मायोग्लोबुलिन) पेशियों में स्थित एक जमने योग्य ग्लोबुलिन। A coagulable globulin present in the muscles.

Myograph (मायोग्राफ) पेशीलेखी। An apparatus for making the tracing of muscular contractions.

Myography (मायोग्राफी) पेशीलेखन, किसी पेशीलेखी द्वारा पेशीय संकुचनों का अनुरेखण बनाने की क्रिया। The process of making tracings of muscular contraction by a myograph.

Myohemoglobin (मायोहीमोग्लोबिन) पेशी ऊतक में स्थित एक श्वसनीय वर्णक जो ऑक्सीजन वाहक के रूप में कार्य करता है। A respiration pigment present in the muscle tissue, which acts as an oxygen carrier.

Myolysis (माइलोलाइसिस) माइलिन का घुल जाना। Dissolution of myclin.

Myoma (मायोमा) पेशी-तत्व से निर्मित कोई रसौली। A tumor made up of the muscular element.

Myomalacia (मायोमैलेशिया) किसी पेशी का मुलायम हो जाना। Softening of a muscle.

Myomectomy (मायोमेक्टॉमी) गर्भाशय पेष्यर्बुदोच्छेदन। Removal of uterine myoma from abdominal section.

Myometrium (मायोमीट्रियम) गर्भाशय की पेशीय परत। Muscular layer of the uterus.

Myopathy (मायोपैथी) पेशी का कोई भी रोग। Any disease of the muscle.

Myope (मायोप) निकट दृष्टि। A short-sighted person.

Myopia (मायोपिया) दूर की चीज न दिखाई देने का रोग। Near-sightedness.

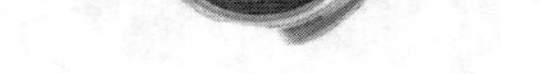

Myorrhaphy (मायोरैह्फी) किसी पेशी में टांके लगाना। Suture of a muscle.

Myosin (मायोसिन) पेशी-तन्तुक में स्थित एक प्रोटीन।

A protein present in the myofibril.

Myositis (मायोसाइटिस) पेशी के ऊतकों का प्रदाह। Inflammation of the muscular tissues.

Myospasm (मायोस्पाज्म) किसी पेशी की ऐंठन। Spasm of a muscle.

Myosuture (मायोसूचर) किसी पेशी में टांके लगाना। Stitching of muscles.

Myotonia (मायोटोनिया) किसी पेशी में तनावयुक्त ऐंठन होना। Tonic spasm of a muscle.

Myringa (मायरिन्गा) कान का पर्दा। The ear drum or tympanic membrane.

Myringitis (मायरिंगजाइटिस) कान के पर्दे का प्रदाह। Inflammation of the membrane tympani.

Myringoplasty (मायरिंजोप्लास्टि) कर्णपअहछेदक। A delicate instrument for incising the tympanic membrane.

Myringotomy (माइरिन्जोटॉमी) मध्यकर्ण कला में चीरा लगाना। To make an incision into the tympanic membrane.

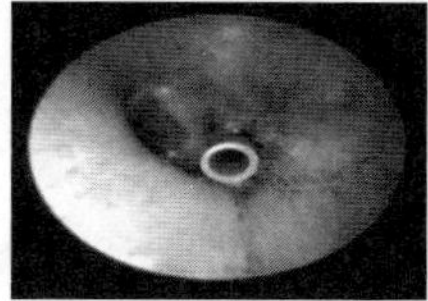

Myrmecia (मिर्मेसिया) गुबंद के आकार का अधिमांस। A dome-shaped wart.

Myster (माइस्टर) नाक। The nose.

Myxedema (मिक्सीडीमा) अवटु-अल्पक्रियता का नैदानिक संलक्षण या चिन्ह। Clinical syndrome of hypothyroidism.

Myxoid (मिक्सॉइड) श्लेष्मा से मिलता-जुलता। Resembling mucus.

Myxoma (मिक्सोमा) श्लेष्मार्बुद। A tumor composed of mucous connective tissue.

Myxopoiesis (मिक्सोपोइसिस) श्लेष्मोत्पादन। Mucus production.

Myxorrhea (मिक्सोरिह्या) श्लेष्मा का अत्यधिक रक्तस्राव होना। Excessive flow of mucus.

Myxosarcoma (मिक्सोसाकौमा) श्लेष्माबुर्द एवं सार्कोमा दोनों से बना मिश्रित अबुर्द। A mixed tumor composed of myxoma and sarcoma.

Myxosarcomatous (मिक्सोसार्कोमेटस) मिक्सोसार्कोमा से संबंधित अथवा उसकी प्रकृति वाला। Pertaining to or of the nature of myxosarcoma.

Myxoviruses (मिक्सोवाइरस) श्लेष्मविषाणु। Name for the influenza group of viruses.

N

N (एन) 1. नाइट्रोजन का रासायनिक प्रतीक। 2. सामान्य।

1. Chemical symbol for Nitrogen. 2. Normal.

Na (एन ए) सोडियम का रासायनिक प्रतीक। Chemical symbol for Sodium.

NaCl (एन.ए.सी.एल) सोडियम क्लोराइड। Sodium chloride.

NAD (एन.ए.डी.) कोई रोग नहीं। No any disease.

Nail (नेल) नाखून। The horny lamina covering the back of the terminal phalanx of each finger or toe.

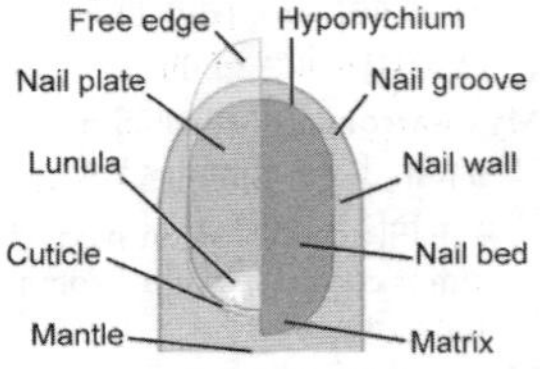

Naja (नजा) फनदार सर्प। A genus of venomous serpents, which includes cobras.

Naked (नेक्ड) नंगा। Unclothed.

Nano (नैनो) बौना। Dwarf.

Nanogram (नैनोग्राम) एक ग्राम का एक अरबवॉं भाग। One billionth part of a gram.

Nap (नैप) झपकी। A short sleep.

Nape (नेप) गर्दन। Nucha, scruff.

Narcissism (नारसिज्म) अपने आप में ज्यादा रूचिलेना। Self-love.

Narcolepsy (नार्कोलैप्सी) निद्रारोग, बार-बार सुस्ती छा जाने एवं सो जाने का एक जीर्ण रोग। A chronic condition of recurring attacks of drowsiness and sleepness.

Narcosis (नार्कोसिस) नशा, मादक वस्तुओं द्वारा उत्पन्न बेहोशी। Unconsciousness caused by narcotics.

Narcotic (नार्कोटिक) मादक अथवा नशीला पदार्थ। An opiate, anything induced sleep.

Narcotism (नार्कोटिज्म) 1. मादकता 2. मादक पदार्थो के सेवन का आदी होना। 1. Narcosis 2. Addiction to the use of narcotics.

Nasal reflex (नेजल रिफ्लेक्स) नासिक की श्लेष्मिक कला के क्षोभण के फलस्वरूप छीकें आना। Sneezing resulting from irritation of the mucous membrane of the nose.

Nascent (नेस्सेन्ट) नवजात। The newborn.

Nasion (नेजियोन) नासामूलबिन्दु। The middle point of the frontonasal suture.

Natal (नेटल) 1. जन्म सम्बन्धी। 2. नितंबों से सम्बन्धित। 1. Pertaining to the birth. 2. Pertaining to the buttocks.

Natality (नेटेलिटी) जन्म दर। Birth rate.

Nates (नेट्स) नितम्ब, कूल्हे। Buttocks.

Native (नेटिव) 1. स्वदेशीय। 2. स्वाभाविक 3. पैदाइशी। 4. प्राथमिक। 5. प्राकृतिक। 6. सहज। 1. Indigenous 2. Innate 3. Born 4. Original 5. Natural 6. Inherent.

Natriuresis (नेट्रीयूरेसिस) असामान्य मात्रा में सोडियम का मूत्र में विसर्जित होना। Excretion of abnormal amount of sodium in the urine.

Naturopathy (नेचुरोपैथी) प्राकृतिक चिकित्सा। Treatment by natural means like-heat, light, water, diet, etc.

Nausea (नौसिया) जी घबराना, मिचली। A desire to vomit, sickness of stomach.

Nauseant (नौसिएन्ट) जी मिचलाहट उत्पन्न करने वाला। Causing nausea.

Navel (नेवेल) नाभि। Umbillicus.

Navicula (नेवीकुला) एक छोटी नाव के आकार की रचना। A small boat-shaped structure.

Nearsight (नीयरसाइट) निकटदृष्टि। Myopia.

Nebula (नेबुला) धुंधलापन, धूमिल मूत्रता। Slight haziness on the cornea, a cloudy suspension in the urine.

Nebulization (नेबुलाइजेशन) 1. किसी द्रव को फुहार में बदलना। 2. औषधियों के छिड़काव से रोगों की चिकित्सा करना। 1. To convert a liquid into a spray. 2. Treatment of the disease by spray.

Nebulizer (नेबुलाइजर) तरल पदार्थ को सूक्ष्म कणों में बदलने वाला यंत्र। An atomizer.

Necator (नेकेटर) केंचुआ। A genus of nematode hookworm.

Neck (नेक) गर्दन। The part of the body between the head and trunk.

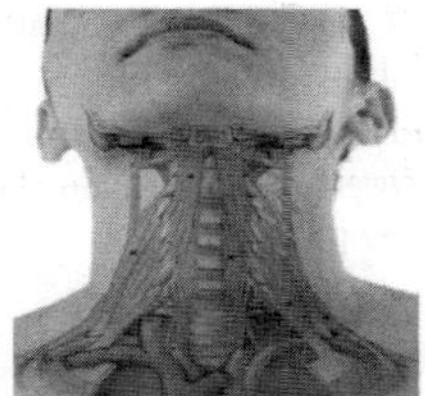

Necrobiosis (नेक्रोबायोसिस) किसी अंग की आणविक मृत्यु। Molecular death of a part.

Necrocytosis (नेक्रोसाइटोसिस) कोशिकाओं का मृत हो जाना एवं उनका विघटन होना। Death of the cells and their decomposition.

Necromania (नेक्रोमैनिया) मृत्यु की बहुत तमन्ना। Excessive desire for death or an interest in dead bodies.

Necromimesis (नेक्रोमाइमेसिस) मरे हुए होने का भ्रम। Delusion of being dead.

Necrophagous (नेक्रोफेगस) मरे हुए जीवों को खाकर जीवित रहने वाला। Living on dead bodies.

Necrophillia (नेक्रोफीलिया) मृतक के साथ संभोग करना। Sexual intercourse with dead body.

Necrophobia (नेक्रोफोबिया) शव को देखकर भयभीत होना। Morbid fear of a dead body.

Necropsy (नेक्रोप्सी) मृत-शरीर की जांच करना। The examination of dead-body.

Necrosis (नेक्रोसिस) परिगलन, अस्थिक्षय। Mortification of the body parts.

Necrotizing (नेक्रोटाइजिंग) परिगलनकारी। Causing necrosis.

Negativism (नेगेटिविज्म) ऋणात्मकता। An active refusal to cooperate.

Negri bodies (नेग्री बॉडीज) रेबीज से ग्रस्त व्यक्ति के मस्तिष्क की तंत्रिका कोशिकाओं में पाए जाने वाले सूक्ष्म कण। Minute particle found in the nerve cells of the brain of the person affected by rabies.

Neisseria (नाइसीरिया) जीवाणुओं का एक वंश जो ग्राम-निगेटिव गोलाणु होते है तथा सामान्यतः जोड़ों में पाये जाते है। A genus of bacteria which are gram-negative cocci and usually occur in pairs. There are two species of it causing disease in man—*Neisseria gonorrhoeae* which causes gonorrhea and *Neisseria meningitidis* which causes meningitis.

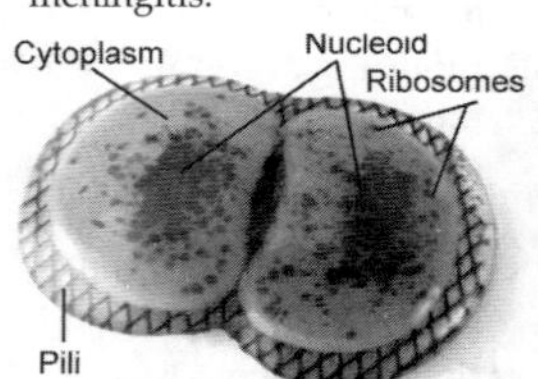

Neisseria gonorrhoeae (Bacterium)

Nematoda (निमैटोडा) फाइलम निमैथेल्मिनथीज का एक वर्ग जिसके अन्तर्गत गोल-कृमि एवं सूत्रकृमि आदि आते है। A class of phylum nemathelminthes that includes roundworms and threadworms, etc.

Neocerebellum (नियोसैरेबेलम) नवानुमस्तिष्क। The large lateral portion of the cerebellar hemisphere.

Neogenesis (नियोजेनेसिस) ऊतक का पुनर्जनन। Tissue regeneration.

Neologism (नियोलोगिज्म) नवशब्द, व्यर्थशब्द-रचना। A specially coined word, often meaningless.

Neomorphism (नियोमॉर्फिज्म) नवनिर्माण। New formation.

Neonate (नियोनेट) नवजात। A newborn baby up to 1 month old.

Neoplasia (नियोप्लेसिया) किसी अबुर्द का बनना। The formation of a neoplasm.

Neoplasm (नियोप्लाज्म) एक नवीन तथा असामान्य वृद्धि जो सुदम अथवा दुर्दम हो सकती है। Tumor or a new and abnormal growth which may be benign or malignant.

Neostriatum (नियोस्ट्रीटम) नवरेखीपिण्ड। The caudate nucleus and putamen considered together.

Neothalamus (नियोथेलेमस) नवचेतक। The lateral and dorsomedial nuclei of the thalamus.

Nephritis (नेफ्राइटिस) वृक्कशोथ। Inflammation of the kidney.

Nephrocalcinosis (नेफ्रोकेलसिनोसिस) वृक्ककैल्सीमयता। Multiple areas of calcification in the kidney substances.

Nephroid (नेफ्रोइड) गुर्दे जैसा, वृक्काभ। Resembling a kidney, kidney-shaped.

Nephromalacia (नेफ्रोमलेशिया) गुर्दो की कोमलता। A morbid softening of the kidneys.

Nephropathy (नेफ्रोपेथी) गुर्दो का रोग। Kidney disease.

Nephroptosis (नेफ्रोप्टोसिस) गुर्दे की निम्नाभिमुखी स्थान च्युति। Downward displacement of the kidney.

Nephropyosis (नेफ्रोप्योसिस) किसी वृक्क में पस पड़ जाना। Suppuration of a kidney.

Nephrosclerosis (नेफ्रोस्कलेरोसिस) गुर्दे का कठोर हो जाना। Hardening of the kidney.

Nephrosis (नेफ्रोसिस) वृक्क का कोई भी अशोथज रोग। Any non-inflammatory disease of the kidney.

Nephrotic-syndrome (नेफ्रोटिक सिण्ड्रोम) केशिकागुच्छ का एक रोग जिससे प्रोटीनमेह, सार्वदैहिक शोथ तथा अल्पएल्ब्युमिन रक्तता हो जाती है। A disease of the glomerulus that causes proteinuria, generalized edema and hypoalbumineria.

Nerve (नर्व) नाड़ी। A bundle of fibers, conveying the impulses of movement and sensation to and from the organs.

Nerve grafting (नर्व ग्राफ्टिंग) तंत्रिका आरोपण। Implantation of a piece of nerve-tissue into another nerve.

Nervimotion (नर्वीमोशन) तंत्रिका उद्दीपन की अनुक्रिया में गति होना। Movement in response to a nervous stimulus.

Nervine (नर्वीन) स्नायुजाल को प्रभावित करने वाली औषधि। A medicine which acts on the nerve.

Nest (नैस्ट) कोशिकाओं का एक पिण्ड जो चिड़िया के घोंसले के समान होता है। A mass of cells resembling a bird nest.

Nettle rash (नेटिल रैश) पित्ती उछलना। Urticaria.

Neuralgia (न्यूरेल्जिया) तंत्रिकाशुल। Pain in the nerve.

Neurarchy (न्यूरेर्की) शरीर के ऊपर तंत्रिका-तंत्र का प्रधानता। The domination of the nervous system over the body.

Neuraxon (न्यूरैक्सोन) अक्ष-तन्तु। Axon.

Neurectopia (न्यूरेक्टोपिया) तंत्रिका का विस्थापित हो जाना। Displacement or abnormal position of a nerve.

Neurectomy (न्यूरेक्टॉमी) तंत्रिका अपच्छेदन। The surgical removal of full or a part of a nerve due to any blockage in nerve.

Neurilemma (न्यूरीलेम्मा) किसी तंत्रिका तंतु को चारों ओर से बंद करने वाली एक पतली झिल्ली चादर। A thin membranes sheath enclosing a nerve fiber.

Neurilemmoma (न्यूरीलैमोम्मा) तंत्रिकाच्छदाबुर्द। A tumor of neurilemma.

Neuritis (न्यूराइटिस) तंत्रिका शोथ। Inflammation of nerve.

Neuroblastoma (न्यूरोब्लास्टोमा) तंत्रिका-कोशिका प्रसूअबुर्द। Malignant tumor arising in adrenal medulla from tissue of sympathetic origin.

Neurocytolysis (न्यूरोसाइटोलाइसिस) तंत्रिका कोशिकाओं का नष्ट होना। Destruction of the neurons.

Neurodermatitis (न्यूरोडर्माटाइटिस) भावात्मक गड़बड़ी के कारण उत्पन्न होने वाला त्वचा का शोथ जिसमें खुजली होती है। Inflammation of the skin itching caused by emotional disturbance.

Neuroepithelium (न्यूरोइपिथीलियम) तंत्रिका उपकला। Specialized epithelial structure forming the gustatory cells, olfactory cells, hair cells of inner ear, rods and cones of retina.

Neurofibril (न्यूरोफाइब्रिल) तंत्रिका तन्तु। Tiny fibrils in the cytoplasma of nerve cell body.

Neurofibroma (न्यूरोफाइब्रोमा) तंत्रिका तन्तु-अबुर्द, किसी तंत्रिका के संयोजी ऊतक का एक अबुर्द जो मुख में, फुफ्फुसावरणों अथवा आमाशय में उत्पन्न हो सकता है। Tumor of the connective tissue of a nerve, which may occur in the mouth, pleura or stomach.

Neurogenesis (न्यूरोजेनेसिस) तंत्रिकाजनन, तंत्रिका ऊतक का विकसित होना। Development of the nervous tissue.

Neurogenic (न्यूरोजेनिक) तंत्रिका ऊतक को बनाने वाला। Forming or originating from the nervous tissue.

Neuroglia (न्यूरोग्लिया) तंत्रिका बंध, संक्रमण के प्रति तंत्रिका तंत्र की प्रतिक्रिया में भी विशेष भाग लेता है। Supporting tissue of nervous system, includes astrocytes, microglia, Schwann cells, satellite cells, ependyma, etc. All except microglia are of ectodermal origin.

Neurogliomatosis (न्यूरोग्लायोमेटोसिस) तंत्रिका-तंत्र

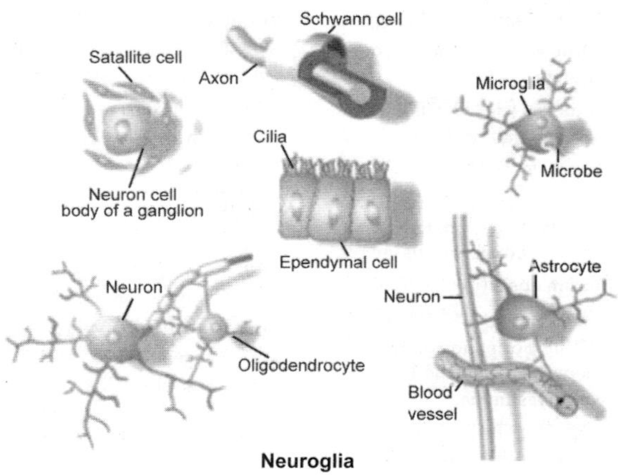

Neuroglia

में बहुत से तंत्रिका बंधाबुर्दों का बनना। Formation of multiple gliomas in the nervous system.

Neurohypophysis (न्यूरोहाइपोफाइसिस) मध्यवर्ती भाग सहित पीयूष ग्रंथि का पश्चज खण्ड। Posterior lobe of the pituitary gland including pars intermedia.

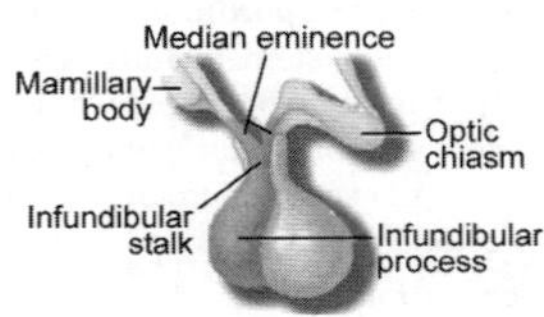

Neuroleptic (न्यूरोलैप्टिक) तंत्रिका-तंत्र पर क्रिया करने वाली औषधि। Drug acting on the nervous system.

Neurolysis (न्यूरोलाइसिस) तंत्रिकालयन, किसी तंत्रिका के चारो ओर के चिपकावों को अलग करना। Stretching of a nerve to relieve tension. Release of a nerve from fibrous tissue.

Neuromatosis (न्यूरोमेटोसिस) शरीर में बहुत से तंत्रिकाबुर्दों का बनना। Formation of multiple neuromas in the body.

Neuromyasthenia (न्यूरोमायस्थीनिया) मनोवेगी विकार के कारण होने वाली पेशीय दुर्बलता। Muscular weakness due to emotional disorder.

Neuron (न्यूरोन) तंत्रिका कोशिका। A nerve cell, consisting of cell body and its process, i.e. axons and dendrites.

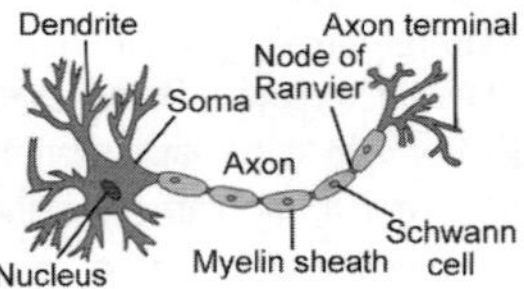

Neuronitis (न्यूरोनाइटिस) तंत्रिका कोशिका शोथ। Inflammation of the nerve cells.

Neuropathy (न्यूरोपैथी) तंत्रिका का कोई भी रोग। Any disease of the nerve.

Neurophonia (न्यूरोफोनिया) वाक् पेशियों के स्फुरण या उनमें ऐंठन हो जाने के फलस्वरूप उत्पन्न चिल्लाहट जिसे रोका नहीं जा सकता। A tic or spasm of the speech muscles resulting in uncontrollable cry.

Neurophysiology (न्यूरोफिजीयोलॉजी) तंत्रिका-तंत्र का शरीर क्रिया विज्ञान। Physiology of nervous system.

Neuroplegic (न्यूरोप्लेजिक) तंत्रिका-तंत्र का किसी रोग के कारण उत्पन्न पक्षाघात से सम्बन्धित। Pertaining to paralysis due to a disease of the nervous system.

Neuropore (न्यूरोपोर) तंत्रिका छिद्र। A small opening at the outerior extremity of the primary telencephalon.

Neuroradiology (न्यूरोरेडियोलॉजी) तंत्रिका-तंत्र का एक्स-रे परीक्षण। X-ray examination of the nervous system.

Neurorrhaphy (न्यूरोरैह्फी) किसी विभाजित तंत्रिका सिरों की सिलाई करना। Neurosuture, suturing of the ends of a divided nerve.

Neurosclerosis (न्यूरोस्क्लेरोसिस) किसी तंत्रिका-ऊतक का कठोर होना। Hardening of a nervous tissue.

Neurosis (न्यूरोसिस) विक्षिप्ति, पागलपन। An emotional disorder mania.

Neurosyphilis (न्यूरोसिफिलिस) केन्द्रीय तंत्रिका-तंत्र का सिफिलिस रोग। Syphilis of the central nervous system.

Neurotic (न्यूरोटिक) 1. विक्षिप्ति से सम्बन्धित। 2. विक्षिप्ति से पीड़ित। 3. अधीर व्यक्ति। 1. Pertaining to the neurosis. 2. Suffering from neurosis. 3. Nervous person.

Neurotmesis (न्यूरोमेसिस) तंत्रिकाविच्छेद। Nerve injury, complete loss of function of the nerve.

Neurotomy (न्यूरोटॉमी) किसी तंत्रिका को विभाजित करना। Division or dissection of a nerve.

Neurotransmitter (न्यूरोट्रान्समिटर) उत्तेजना से तंत्रिका के अंतिम सिरे पर मुक्त होने एक पदार्थ जैसे–एसिटाइलकोलीन जो अंतर्ग्रथनों एवं पेशीतंत्रिका-संगम पर तंत्रिका आवेगों के संचारण में भाग लेता है। Chemical substance released by stimulation of presynaptic neurone that excites or inhibits target cell, e.g. acetylcholine, dopamine, norepinephrine.

Neurotripsy (न्यूरोट्रिप्सी) एक तंत्रिका के ऑपरेटिंग पेराई। Operative chrusing of a nerve.

Neurotrophy (न्यूरोट्रॉफी) तंत्रिका पोषण। The nutritive influence of nerves.

Neutral (न्यूट्रल) उदासीन, क्रियाशून्य, नपुंसक। Possessing neither acidic nor basic properties, impotent.

Neutral point (न्यूट्रल पाइंट) pH पैमाने पर स्थित एक बिन्दु pH 7.0 जिस पर कोई विलयन प्रतिक्रिया में न तो अम्लीय और न ही क्षारीय होता है। pH 7.0, a point on the pH scale at which a solution is neither acidic nor alkaline in reaction.

Neutralization (न्यूट्रालाइजेशन) उदासीनीकरण, निराकरण। Rendering ineffective of any action, process or potential.

Neutrophil (न्यूट्रोफिल) उदासीनरागीकोशिका। A cell or histological element that is readily stained by neutral dyes.

Nevus (नीवस) जन्मचिन्ह, तिल। Birthmark, mole.

Niacin (नियासीन) निकोटिन अम्ल। Nicotinic acid.

Nicotin (नायकोटिन) तम्बाकु से प्राप्त एक विषैला क्षार। A poisonous alkaloid of tobacco.

Nidus (नाइडस) घोंसला, उद्गमकेन्द्र, उद्गम। A nest like structure, a focus of infection, a nucleus or origin of a nerve.

Night terror (नाइट टेरर) रात को डर लगना। A disorder allied to nightmares in which a child awakes screaming in fright.

Nightmare (नाइटमेयर) एक भयानक स्वप्न, दुःस्वप्न। A terrifying dream.

Nightsoil (नाइटसॉयल) मल। Feces.

Nigricans (नाइग्रीकेन्स) काला किया हुआ। Blackened.

Nikolsky's sign (निकोल्सकीज साइन) पेम्फीगस रोग (फफोले) का एक चिन्ह जिसमें त्वचा की बाह्य परत हल्की-सी रगड़ जाने अथवा जरा सी चोट लग जाने पर ही साफ हो जाती है। A sign of pemphigus in which the external laryer of the skin can be rubbed off by slight friction or injury.

Nipple (निपल) स्तन का अगला भाग, जहाँ से दूध बाहर निकलता

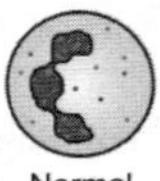
Normal

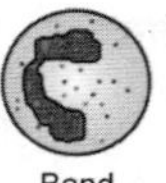
Band
Called into service in times of need

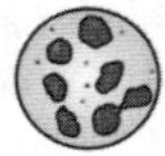
Hypersegmented
slowed DNA synthesis

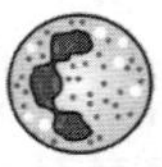
'Toxic' granulation/vacuolization think 'sepsis'

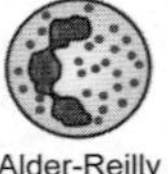
Alder-Reilly
Mucopoly-saccharidosis

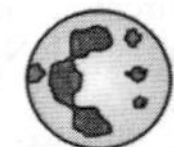
Döhle bodies
May-Hegglin; bad infections

Neutrophil

है। The conical eminence in center of each breast, containing the outlets of the milk ducts.

Nissl bodies (निज्ल बॉडीज) तंत्रिका कोशिकाओं के कोशिका कार्यों तथा पार्श्वतन्तुओं में कणिकाओं के रूप में पाया जाने वाला क्रोमोफिल पदार्थ जिनका सम्बन्ध प्रोटीन के निर्माण तथा चयापचय से होता है। Chromophil substance in the form of granules found in the cell bodies and dendrites of the neurons, concerned with protein synthesis and metabolism.

Nit (निट) लीख। The egg of the head louse attached to the human hair or clothing.

Nitrification (नाइट्रीफिकेशन) नाइट्रीकरण। The formation of nitrates especially due to the action of certain bacteria.

Nitrite (नाइट्राइट) नाइट्रस एसिड का कोई भी लवण नाइट्राइट रक्त वाहिनियों को विस्फारित करते है तथा रक्त-चाप को कम करते है अतः एमाइल नाइट्राइट का हृदशूल की चिकित्सा में प्रयोग किया जाता है। Any salt of nitrous acid, which can be used to dilate the blood vessels and reduce the blood pressure, hence any nitrites is used in the treatment of angina pectoris.

Nitroglycerin (नाइट्रोग्लिसरीन) ग्लिसरीन पर सलफ्युरिक एवं नाइट्रिक अम्लों की क्रिया से बनने वाला एक तैलीय, विस्फोटक, रंगहीन तरल जिसका वाहिका विस्फारक के रूप में विशेष रूप से हृदशूल में प्रयोग किया जाता है। An oily, explosive, colorless fluid formed by the action of sulfuric and nitric acids on glycerin, used as a vasodilator, especially in angina pectoris.

Nocardiosis (नोकार्डियोसिस) नोकार्डिया के संक्रमण के फलस्वरूप उत्पन्न रोग। The disease caused by the infection of nocardia

Nociceptive (नोसीसेप्टिव) मस्तिष्क के वेदनायुक्त उद्दीपनों से सम्बन्धित अथवा उन्हें संचारित करने में सक्षम। Pertaining to, or capable of transmitting the painful stimuli to the brain.

Nocturia (नॉक्चूरिया) रात्रि में ज्यादा मूत्र-त्यागना। Excessive urination at night.

Nocturnal emission (नॉक्युर्नल-एमिसन) स्वप्नदोष। Nightfall.

Nodal rhythm (नोडल रिद्म) हृदय-ताल जो आलिंद-निलय पर्व से उत्पन्न होता है। Cardiac rhythm arising from the atrioventricular node.

Nodding (नोडिंग) सिर की अनैच्छिक गतियां होना, बेमतलब सिर हिलाते रहना। Involuntary movements of the head.

Node (नोड) गांठ, गूमड़ी। A swelling or protuberance.

Nodule (नोड्यूल) छोटी-सी गांठ। A small node or excrescence.

Nomenclature (नोमेनक्लेचर) नामकरण, नामपद्धति। A system of technical names.

Nomogram (नोमोग्राम) सामान्य मानकलेख। The representing of correlations by graphs.

Nonabsorbable (नोनएब्जोरबेबल) शोषण के अयोग्य। That which is not capable of being absorbed.

Nonadherent (नोनएधेरेन्ट) न चिपकने वाला, अचिप्य। Not connected to adjacent organs.

Nonigravida (नोनीग्रेविडा) नवीं बार गर्भवती होने वाली स्त्री। Pregnant for the ninth time.

Nonocclusion (नॉनऑक्लूजन) ऐसी दशा जिसमें दाँत आपस में मिलने में सक्षम नहीं होते। The condition in which the teeth are not capable to make contact.

Nonresectable (नॉनरिसैक्टेबल) जिसे शल्यक्रिया द्वारा अलग न किया जा सकता है। Not removable by surgery.

Nonsense (नॉनसैन्स) मूर्ख। Foolish.

Nonviable (नोनवियेबल) जीने के अयोग्य, स्वतंत्र अस्तित्व वाला। Incapable of life, of independent existence.

Normoblast (नॉर्मोब्लास्ट) सामान्य आकार की रक्तकणिका। A blood corpuscle of normal size.

Normocyte (नॉर्मोसाइट) सामान्य लोहित कोशिका। A normoblast.

Normosthenuria (नॉर्मोस्थेनूरिया) सामान्य मात्रा में एवं सामान्य विशिष्ट गुरूत्व के मूत्र का उत्सर्जित होना। Excretion of urine in normal amount and of normal specific gravity.

Normotensive (नॉर्मोटैन्सिव) सामान्य तान, तनाव अथवा रक्त चाप वाला व्यक्ति। The person with normal tone, tension or blood pressure.

Nose (नोज) नाक। The organ of smell.

Nosocomial (नोसोकोमियल) किसी अस्पताल से सम्बन्धित अथवा उससे उत्पन्न होने वाला। Pertaining to or originating from a hospital.

Nosology (नोसोलॉजी) रोगों का वैज्ञानिक वर्गीकरण। The scientific classification of diseases.

Nosophobia (नोसोफोबिया) किसी बीमारी का रोगोत्पादक डर। Morbid fear of illness or a specific disease.

Nostalgia (नोस्टैल्जिया) खुशी और मामूली उदासी की भावना जब आप चीजों के अतीत में क्या हुआ के बारे में सोचते हैं। A feeling of pleasure and also slight sadness when you think about things that happened in the past.

Nostophobia (नोस्टोफोबिया) घर वापस जाने का रोगोत्पादक डर। Morbid fear of returning home.

Notalgia (नोटेल्जिया) पीठ में दर्द होना। Pain in the back.

Notch (नॉच) खांच, कटाव। A depression or indentation on the margin of a bone.

Notifiable (नोटीफॉयबल) सूचित करने योग्य। Worthy of notice.

Notochord (नोटोकॉर्ड) मेरूदण्ड, पृष्ठदण्ड। The primitive backbone.

Noxious (नोक्सियस) हानिकारक, क्षति पहुँचाने वाला। Harmful, injurious.

NPT (एन.पी.टी.) सामान्य दाब तथा तापमान। Normal pressure and temperature.

Nubile (न्यूबाइल) विवाह-योग्य। Fit for marriage.

Nucha (नुका) गर्दन का पिछला भाग। The back of the neck.

Nucleate (न्यूक्लीयेट) 1. केन्द्रक बनाना 2. केन्द्रक से युक्त। 1. To form a nucleus. 2. Having a nucleus.

Nucleolus (न्यूक्लीयोलस) उपकेन्द्रक, केन्द्रक के अंदर पाई जाने वाली छोटी कणिका। A small granule in the inferior of the nucleus.

Nucleus (न्यूक्लीयस) केन्द्रक। A mass of protoplasm.

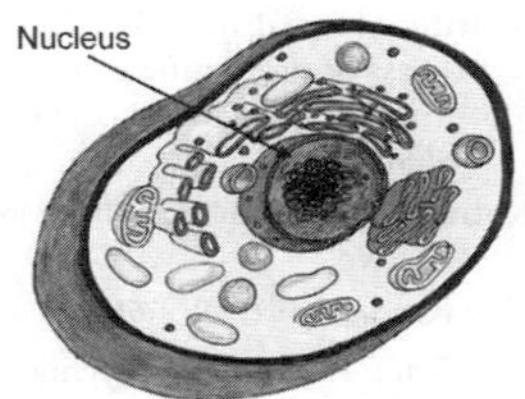

Nude (न्यूड) नंगा। Naked.

Nudism (न्यूडिज्म) 1. कपड़े उतारने की तीव्र इच्छा। 2. नंगा रहने की आदत। 1. Excessive desire for removing clothes. 2. A habit of living naked.

Nudophobia (न्यूडोफोबिया) नंगे रहने का विकृत डर। Morbid fear of being naked.

Nullipara (नलीपैरा) बांझ, अप्रसवा। A woman who has never borne a viable child.

Numb (नम्ब) अनुभूति। Lacking in feeling or in power to move as from child.

Nummular (न्यूमुलर) सिक्के के आकार का। Coin-shaped.

Nurse (नर्स) परिचारिका। One who takes care of the sick.

Nursery (नर्सरी) शिशुपालन गृह। Department of a hospital where the newborn are cared for.

Nutrient (न्यूट्रीएन्ट) पोषक। A nutritious substance.

Nutrition (न्यूट्रीशन) पोषण। The process of promoting growth, or repairing the losses of the system.

Nutritious (न्यूट्रीशियस) पौष्टिक। Nutritive.

Nux vomica (नक्स वोमिका) कुचला। The nuts of strychnos nux vomica from which strychnine is obtained.

Nyctalopia (निक्टालौपिया) रतौंधी, रात को दिखाई न देने का रोग। Night blindness.

Nyctophobia (निक्टोफोबिया) अंधकारभीति। A morbid fear of darkness.

Nympha (निम्फा) लघु भगोश्ठ। One of the labia minora.

Nympholepsy (निम्फोलैप्सी) उन्माद या पागलपन विशेष रूप से कामोत्तेजक प्रकार का। Frenzy, especially of erotic nature.

Nymphomania (निम्फोमैनिया) स्त्रियों में ज्यादा कामेच्छा होना। Excessive sexual desire in woman.

Nymphomaniac (निम्फोमैनियक) अत्यधिक कामेच्छा से ग्रस्त स्त्री। A woman affected by excessive sexual desire.

Nymphotomy (निम्फोटॉमी) भग्नशिश्निका में चीरा लगाना। To make an incision into the labia minora or clitoris.

Nystagmograph (निस्टैग्मोग्राफ) अक्षिदोलन में नेत्रगोलक की गतियों का अभिलेखन करने वाला एक उपकरण। An apparatus for recording the movements of the eyeball in nystagmus.

Nystagmography (निस्टैग्मोग्राफी) अक्षिदोलन का अभिलेखन करने की तकनीक। The techinque of recording nystagmus.

Nystagmoid (निस्टैग्मॉयड) अक्षिदोलन के समान। Similar to nystagmus.

Nystagmus (निस्टैग्मस) अक्षिदोलन, नेत्रकम्प। Oscillary movement of the eyeball.

Nyxis (निक्सीस) चुभन, छिद्र, परावेधन। Pricking, puncture, paracentesis.

O

O (ओ) ऑक्सीजन का रासायनिक प्रतीक। Chemical symbol for Oxygen.

O_2 (ओटू) ऑक्सीजन के आण्विक सूत्र का प्रतीक। Symbol for the molecular formula of oxygen.

O_3 (ओथ्री) ओजोन का प्रतीक। Symbol for ozone.

Oak (ओक) शाहबलूत, बॉज। A tree of genus.

Oat (ओट) एक अनाज, जई। A grain.

Oath (ओथ) कसम। A solemn attestation of affirmation.

Oatmeal (ओटमील) जई का आटा। A meal prepared from oats.

Obese (ओबेस) मोटा। Fatty.

Obesity (ओबेसिटी) मोटापा, स्थूलता। Corpulence, adiposity.

Obfuscation (ओबफसकेशन) 1. भ्रम पैदा करना 2. भ्रम। 1. To confuse 2. Confusion.

Object (ऑब्जेक्ट) 1. कोई भी वस्तु जिसका ज्ञानेन्द्रियों द्वारा ज्ञान हो सकता है। 2. उद्देश्य। 1. Anything perceptible by the sense organs. 2. Purpose.

Objective sign (ऑब्जैक्टिव साइन) रोगी में विद्यमान एक चिन्ह जिसे चिकित्सक द्वारा देखा या सुना जा सकता है। A sign present in the patient which can be seen, heard or felt by touch by the doctor.

Obligate (ऑबलिगेट) अविकल्प। Compelled to act in a given manner.

Oblique (ऑब्लीक) तिरछा, वक्र। Slanting.

Obliquity (ऑब्लीक्वीटी) निर्यक्ता, तिरछापन। The state of being slanting.

Oblongata (ऑब्लोंगेटा) मेरूमज्जा, ज्ञानेन्द्रिया। Medulla oblongata.

Obscure (ऑब्सक्योर) अस्पष्ट, दृष्टिगोचर होने में रूकावट डालना। Hidden or indistinct, to make less distinctor to hide.

Obsession (ऑब्सेसन) मनोद्वेग, प्रेतबाधा। The neurotic mental state of having an uncontrollable desire to dwell on an idea or an emotion, Possession on by a demon.

Obstetrics (ऑब्स्टेट्रिक्स) प्रसूति-विज्ञान। Medical specialty concerned with the care of a pregnant woman and her delivery.

Obstipation (ऑब्सटीपेशन) बहुत कब्ज होना। Severe constipation.

Obstruent (ऑब्स्ट्रएन्ट) मलरोधक, अवरोधक। That obstructs or prevents a normal discharge from the bowels obstructing.

Obtundent (ऑब्टुन्डेन्ट) एक पदार्थ जो शरीर पर जलन को कम करता है, एक नरम तैलीय पदार्थ। A substance which blunts irritation, usually some soft oily matter.

Obturator (ऑब्ट्यूरेटर) किसी गहवर में रूकावट डालने वाला। That obstructs a cavity or opening.

Occiput (ऑक्सीपट) सिर के पिछले भाग से संबंधित। Concerned with the back of the head, called occiput.

Occlusion (ऑक्लूजन) नाड़ीरोध, अंतरौध। The closure of the opening of a tube or duct.

Occult (ऑकल्ट) अस्पष्ट अथवा छिपा हुआ। Obscure or hidden.

Occult blood (ऑकल्ट ब्लड) खून का इतनी सूक्ष्म मात्रा में पाया जाना कि सिर्फ सूक्ष्मदर्शी परीक्षण द्वारा इसका पता लगाया जा सकता है। Blood present in such a minute quantity that it can be detected only by microscopic examination or chemical tests.

Occult therapy (ऑक्ल्ट थैरेपी) व्यावसायिक चिकित्सा। The use of occupation, usually manual for therapeutic or remedial purpose in mental and physical disorders.

Ochlophobia (ऑक्लोफोबिया) घनी आबादी वाले स्थानों का रोगात्पादक भय। Morbid fear of crowds or populated places.

Octan (ऑक्टेन) आठवें रोज आने वाला बुखार। Recurring every eighth day.

Oculentum (ऑकुलेन्टम) आँख का मरहम। Eye ointment.

Oculist (ऑकुलिस्ट) नेत्र-रोग विषेशज्ञ। Ophthalmologist.

Oculus dexter (ऑक्यूलस डेक्सटर) दाई आँख। The right eye.

Oculus sinister (ऑक्यूलस सिनिस्टर) बाई आँख। The left eye.

OD (ओ.डी.) प्रतिदिन, अतिमात्रा। Everyday, Overdose.

Odontia (ओडोन्टिया) 1. दन्तशूल 2. दातों की असामान्यता। 1. Odontalgia 2. Abnormality of the teeth.

Odontitis (ओडोन्टाइटिस) दन्त शोथ। Inflammation of a tooth.

Odontoblast (ओडोन्टोब्लास्ट) दंतकोशिकाप्रसू। A columnar cell forming dentin.

Odontocele (ओडोन्टोसील) दन्तडलूखल पुटी। An alveolodental cyst.

Odontoclasis (ओडोन्टोक्लोसिस) किसी दाँत का टूटना। The breaking of a tooth.

Odontoclast (ओडोन्टोक्लास्ट) दंतनाशक। A cell absorbing the root of the tooth.

Odontogenesis (ओडोन्टोजेनेसिस) दांतों का बनना। The formation of the teeth.

Odontoid (ओडोन्टॉयड) दांत जैसा। Like a tooth.

Odontology (ओडोन्टोलॉजी) दंतविज्ञान। Dentistry.

Odontoma (ओडोन्टोमा) दंत ऊतक का कोई भी अबुर्द। A tumor of the dental tissue.

Odontophobia (ओडोन्टोफोबिया) दांतो को देखने का विकृत डर। Fear of dentistry and receiving dental care.

Odor (ओडर) गंध। Smell.

Odorant (ओडोरैन्ट) कोई भी पदार्थ जो गंध-ज्ञान को उत्तेजित करता है। Any substance that stimulates the sense of smell.

Odoriferous (ओडोरीफेरस) किसी गंध से युक्त, सुगंधित। Having some smell, perfumed.

Odorless (ओडरलैस) गंधहीन। Without smell.

Odorous (ओडोरस) जिसनें कुछ गंध होती है। Having some smell.

Odynophagia (ओडाइनोफेजिया) निगलने पर दर्द होना। Painful swallowing.

Oikomania (ओइकोमैनिया) घर पर क्लेश रहने से उत्पन्न मानसिक विकार। A mental disorder created by unhappiness at home.

Ointment (ऑयन्टमैन्ट) मरहम। A medicated fatty soft substance for external application.

Olecranon (ओलीक्रेनन) कोहनी के जोड़ के पीछे अल्ना हड्डी का एक बड़ा प्रवर्ध, कूर्पर। A large projection of the ulna bone behind the elbow joint.

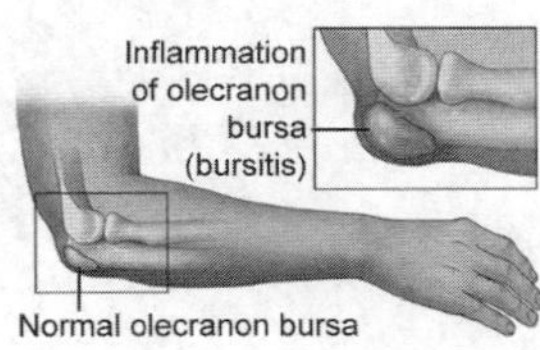

Oleic (ऑलिक) तेल से संबंधित। Pertaining to or produced by oil.

Oleogranuloma (ऑलियो ग्रेनुलोमा) तेलीय पदार्थों का अवत्वक इंजैक्शन लगाने के स्थान पर बनने वाला कणिकागुल्म। Granuloma formation at the site of injection of oily substances.

Olfaction (आलफैक्शन) 1. सूंघने की क्रिया 2. गंध का ज्ञान। 1. The act of smelling 2. The sense of smell.

Olfactometer (आलफैक्टोमीटर) गंध का ज्ञान करने की शक्ति का परीक्षण करने वाला एक उपकरण। An apparatus for testing the power of the sense of smell.

Olfactory tract (आलफैक्टरी ट्रेक्ट) घ्राण-कंद से पीछे मस्तिष्क से अग्र छिद्रयुक्त पदार्थ की ओर प्रसारित होने वाले तंत्रिका-तन्तुओं की पट्टी, जहां यह बढती है तथा घ्राण-रेखाओं में विभाजित हो जाती है। The tract that extends from olfactory bulb to the anterior perforated substance where it divides into olfactory strial.

Oligocholia (ओलिगोकोलिया) पित्त की कमी। Deficiency of bile.

Oligodendroglia (ओलिगोडैण्ड्रोग्लिया) केन्द्रीय तंत्रिका-तंत्र के तंत्रिकाबंध को बनाने वाली अतंत्रिका-कोशिकाएँ। The non neural cells forming the neuroglia of the central nervous system.

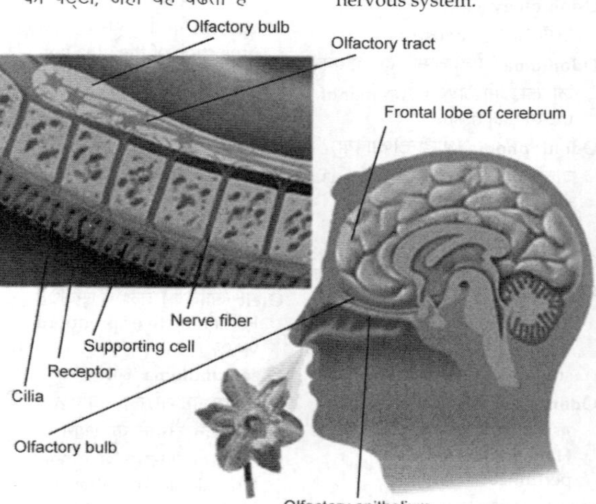

Olfactory tract

Oligodendroglioma (ओलिगोडैण्ड्रोग्लियोमा) प्रमस्तिष्क में उत्पन्न होने वाला अल्प-दन्द्रोनकोशिकाओं का बना एक दुर्दम अबुर्द। A malignant tumor consisting of oligodendrocytes occuring in the cerebrum.

Oligodipsia (ओलिगोडिप्सिया) प्यास कम लगना। Diminution of thirst.

Oligohydramnios (ओलिगोहाइड्रेम्नियोज) अल्प-उल्वोदकता। Abnormally small amount of amniotic fluid.

Oligomenorrhea (ओलिगोमैनोरीह्या) कभी-कभी मासिक धर्म होना। Scanty or infrequent menstruation.

Oligospermia (ओलिगोस्पर्मिया) अल्पशुक्राणुता। Deficiency of spermatozoa in the semen.

Oligotrophia, Oligotrophy (ओलिगोट्रॉफिया, ओलिगोट्रॉफी) अपर्याप्त पोषण। Insufficient nutrition.

Oliguria (ओलिगूरिया) पेशाब की कमी। Scantiness of urine.

Olive (ओलीव) जैतून। The olive tree or its fruits.

Omagra (आमेग्रा) कंधों का गठिया। Gout of the shoulders.

Omalgia (आमोल्जिया) कंधे में दर्द होना। Pain in the shoulder.

Ombrophobia (ओम्ब्रोफोबिया) बादलों की गड़गड़ाहट से डर। Morbid fear of storms, thundering clouds or rain.

Omentectomy (ओमेन्टेक्टॉमी) सम्पूर्ण वपा को काट कर निकाल देना। Excision of a portion or all of the omentum.

Omentopexy (ओमेन्टोपैक्सी) वपा स्थिरीकरण। Fixation of the omentum to the abdominal wall or adjacent organ.

Omentum (ओमेन्टम) पेट का पर्दा जो उदरस्थ आशयों को जठर के साथ जोड़ता है। A fold of peritoneum or serous covering of the bowels.

Omni Bihora (ओम्नी बाईहोर) प्रत्येक दो घण्टे पर। Every two hours.

Omni hora (ओमनी होर) प्रत्येक घण्टे पर। Every hour.

Omni mane (ओम्नी मेन) प्रति प्रातः। Every morning.

Omni nocte (ओम्नी नॉक्टे) रोज रात को। Every night.

Omnivorous (ओम्नीवोरस) हर प्रकार के भोजन पर जीवनयापन करने वाला। Living on food of all kinds.

Omohyoid (ओम्योइड) स्कन्धफलक एवं कण्ठिका सम्बन्धी। Pertaining to the scapula and the hyoid.

Omphalitis (ओम्फैलाइटिस) नाभिशोथ। Inflammation of the umbilicus.

Omphalocele (ओम्फैलोसील) नाभि हर्निया। Umbilical hernia.

Omphalotomy (ओम्फैलोटॉमी) जन्म के समय नाभि-रज्जु को काट देना। To cut the umbilical cord at birth.

Onanist (ओनानिस्ट) आत्मव्यभिचारी। One who is addicted to onanism.

Oncogenesis (ओन्कोजेनेसिस) अबुर्दों का बनना। The formation of tumors.

Oncology (ओन्कोलॉजी) अबुर्दों का अध्ययन। The study of tumors.

Oniomania (ओन्योमेनिया) खरीदारी करने का पागलपन। A morbid desire to buy everything.

Onlay (ओन्ले) किसी अंग की सतह पर लगाया जाने वाला निरोप। A graft applied on the surface of an organ.

Ontogeny (ओन्टोजेनी) जीवविकास का इतिहास। The history of individual development.

Onychia (ओनीकिया) नखषय्याकी सूजन जिसमें पस पड़ जाता है, जिससे नाखून गिर जाता है। Chronic inflammation of matrix of a nail.

Onychodystrophy (ओनीकोडिस्ट्रॉफी) किसी नाखून का कुविकास होना। Maldevelopment of a nail.

Onycholysis (ओनीकोलाइसिस) नाखषय्या से नाखून का ढीला होना अथवा उसका अलग हो जाना। Loosening or separation of a nail from the nailbed.

Onychomycosis (ओनीकोमाइकोसिस) नाखूनों का एक परजीवी रोग। A parasitic disease of the nails.

Oocyst (ऊसिस्ट) कोशिका को घेर कर रखने वाला आवरण। The envelope which surrounds the cell.

Oocyte (ऊसाइट) अपरिपक्व डिम्ब। An immature ovum.

Oogenesis (ऊजेनेसिस) अण्डे या डिम्ब का बनना तथा विकसित होना। Formation and development of the ovum.

Oogonium (ऊगोनियम) एक आद्य कोशिका जिससे कोई अपरिपक्व डिम्ब उत्पन्न होता है, डिम्बाणुप्रसूजनक। A primordial cell from which an oocyte arises.

Ookinete (ऊकिनेट) सक्रिय चलनिषित्तन-कोशिका। The actively motile fertilized cell.

Oophorrhaphy (ऊफोरैहफी) घ्रोणि भित्ति के साथ किसी विस्थापित डिम्बग्रंथि की सिलाई करना। Suturing of a displaced ovary to the pelvic wall.

Opaque (ओपेक) अपारदर्शी, धुंधला। Non-transparent, impervious to light.

Operation (ऑपरेशन) शल्यक्रिया, चीर-फाड़। Any surgical procedure, or operative technique.

Opercular (ओपरकुलर) ढकने वाली रचना से सम्बन्धित। Pertaining to a covering structure.

Operculitis (ओपरकुलाइटिस) आंशिक रूप से निकलने वाले दांतों के ऊपर स्थित मसूड़ों का शोथ। Inflammation of the gingiva over the partially erupted teeth.

Operculum (ओपरकुलम) पलक, ढक्कन, आवरण। A lid or cover.

Ophthalamia (ऑफ्थेल्मिया) आँख आना, आंख में दर्द, नेत्रशोथ। Inflammation of the eye.

Ophthalmic (ऑफ्थेल्मिक) नेत्र सम्बन्धी। Pertaining to the eye.

Ophthalmitis (ऑफ्थैल्माइटिस) आँख की सूजन। Inflammation of the eye.

Ophthalmodynamometry (ऑफ्थैल्मोडाइ-नेमोमेटरी) नेत्र रक्त दाब भित्ति। Use of an ophthalmodynamometer.

Ophthalmologist (ऑफ्थैल्मोलॉजिस्ट) नेत्र रोग विशेषज्ञ। Specialist in ophthalmology.

Ophthalmometer (ऑफ्थैल्मीटर) नेत्र की किरण-वक्रता या अपवर्तक शक्ति को मापने का यंत्र। An instrument used in ophthalmometry.

Ophthalmoplegia (ऑफ्थैल्मोप्लीजिया) नेत्र पेशियों का पक्षाघात। Paralysis of the eye muscles.

Ophthalmoscope (ऑफ्थैल्मोस्कोप) नेत्रदर्शी, दृष्टिपटलदर्शी। An instrument for examining the interior of the eye, especially the retina.

Opiate (ओपिएट) अफीम मिश्रित औषधि, निद्राकारी। A preparation of opium for producing sleep, it is commonly applied to any medicine capable of procuring sleep.

Opisthotonos (ओपिस्थोटोनस) शरीर का पीछे की ओर झुककर अकड़ जाना, धनुर्वात। Spasmodic bending backward of the body.

Opisthotonos in tetanus patient

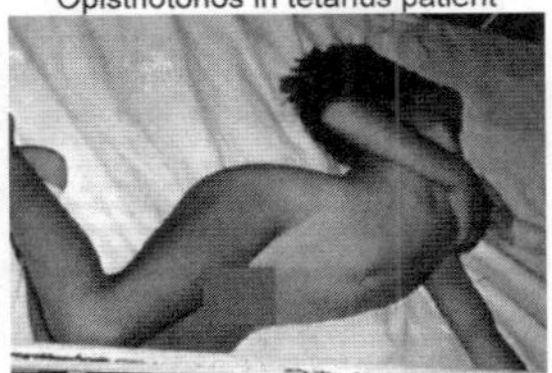

Opium (ओपियम) अफीम। The concrete juice of poppy.

Oppilative (ओपिलेटिव)

1. अवरोधक 2. मलावरोधक।

1. Obstructive 2. Constipation.

Oppression (ऑप्रेसन) श्वासावरोध। A sense of weight about the chest, abstracting respiration.

Opsoclonia, opsoclonus (ऑप्सोक्लोनिया, ऑप्सोक्लोनस) नैत्रों की अनैच्छिक, झटके के साथ होने वाली गतियाँ। Involuntary, non rhythmical, jerking movements of the eyes.

Opsonin (ऑप्सोनिन) रक्त सीरम में ऐसा पदार्थ जो जीवाणुओं एवं अन्य कोशिकाओं पर क्रिया करके उन्हें भक्षित किए जाने योग्य बना देता है। A substance present in blood that prepares bacteria for phagocytosis.

Optic (ऑप्टिक) नेत्र अथवा दृष्टि से संबंधित। Pertaining to the eye or the sight.

Optic chiasma (ऑप्टिक चियाज्मा) मस्तिष्क में दृष्टि-तंत्रिका तंतुओं का एक्स के आकार में पार-गमन। An 'X'-shaped crossing of the optic nerve fibers in the brain.

Opticokinetic (ऑप्टिकोकाइनेटिक) नेत्र की गति से संबंधित। Pertaining to the movement of the eye.

Optometer (ऑप्टोमीटर) दृष्टिमापी। An instrument for measuring refractive power of eye.

Optometry (ऑप्टोमीट्री) दृष्टि-सहायकों से दूर करना, दृष्टिमिति। Use of an optometer.

Orbicularis (ऑरबिक्यूलेरिस) वर्तुलपेशियाँ। A name given to muscles whose fibers encircle an orifice.

Orbit (ऑर्बिट) नेत्रगुहा, नेत्रकोटर। One of the two bony cavities in which the eyes are placed, orbit.

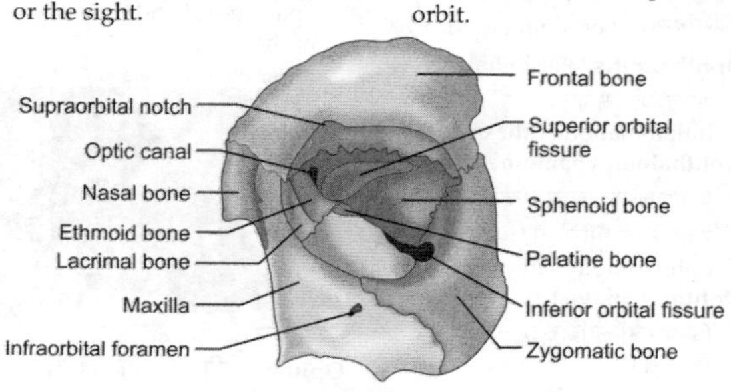

Orbit

Orchidopexy (ऑरचिडोपेक्सी) वृषणस्थिरीकरण। The suturing up of a testicle.

Orchitis (आर्काइटिस) शुक्रग्रंथि का शोथ। Inflammation of a testis.

Organelle (ऑर्गेनेल) किसी कोशिका की विषेश रचना जो किसी निश्चित काम को करती है, जैसे–माइटोकॉण्ड्रिया। Special structure of a cell, e.g. mitochondria.

Organic (ओरगेनिक) आंगिक कायिक। Relating to an organ.

Organic disease (आरगेनिक डिजीज) आंगिक रोग। A disease accompanied by demonstrable changes in the body.

Organism (ऑर्गेनिज्म) जन्तु अथवा पादप कोई भी जीवित वस्तु। Any living thing, animal or plant.

Organize (ऑर्गेनाइज) किसी आकारहीन अवस्था से किसी रचना अथवा अंग में विकसित होना। To develop from an amorphous state into a structure or organ.

Organum (ऑर्गेनम) अंग। Organ.

Orgasm (ऑर्गेज्म) लैंगिक चरमोत्कर्ष। The climax of sexual intercourse.

Orifice (ओरीफिस) द्वार, मुख। An opening or entrance.

Origin (ओरीजिन) उद्‌भव, उद्‌गम। The commencement, source or beginning.

Oropharynx (ओरोफेरिन्क्स) कोमल तालु एवं कण्ठच्छद के ऊपरी किनारे के बीच स्थित ग्रसनी का मध्य भाग। The middle part of the pharynx lying between the soft palate and upper margin of the epiglottis.

Orthochrometic (आर्थोक्रोमैटिक) सामान्य रूप से अभिरंजित हो जाना। Staining normally.

Orthodontics (ऑर्थोडोन्टिक्स) दाँतों के दोष को सुधारने सम्बन्धी विज्ञान। A branch of dentistry dealing, prevention and correction of irregularities of teeth.

Orthograde (ऑर्थोग्रेड) शरीर को सीधा करके चलने वाला जैसा कि आदमी चलता है। Walking the body up right as man walks.

Orthopedics (ऑर्थोपेडिक्स) विकलांग विज्ञान। Concerned with the bones, joints and other supporting tissues.

Orthophoria (ऑर्थोफोरिया) नेत्र अविघलन प्रवृत्ति। A tending of the visual lives in parallelism.

Orthopnea (ऑर्थोप्निया) बैठे होने अथवा खड़े होने की स्थिति के अतिरिक्त किसी भी। Difficult respiration relieved only in an upright position.

Orthoptics (ऑर्थोप्टिक्स) दोनों नेत्रों में दृष्टि-दोषों को ठीक करने का विज्ञान। The science of correcting the visual defect in both the eyes.

Orthostatic (ऑर्थोस्टेटिक) ऊर्ध्वस्थस्थितिज। Caused by the upright position.

Orthotics (ऑर्थोटिक्स) कृत्रिम अंग विज्ञान। The science concerned with the making and fitting of orthopedic appliances.

Orthotopic (ऑर्थोटॉपिक) किसी सामान्य स्थान में उत्पन्न होने वाला। Occurring in a normal place.

OS (ओ.एस.) बाई आँख। Left eye.

Os (औंस) मुँह, हड्डी, छिद्र। The mouth, bone, an opening into a hollow organ or canal.

Oscheoma (ऑस्कियोमा) अण्डकोश का कोई अबुर्द। A tumor of the scrotum.

Oscillation (ऑस्सीलेशन) कम्पन, थिरकन। A swimming or vibration.

Oscillopsia (ऑस्सीलोप्सिया) ऐसा दृष्टि संवेदना कि स्थिर वस्तुएँ आगे एवं पीछे को घूम रही है। Visual sensation that the fixed objects are moving forwards and backwards.

Osculation (ऑस्कुलेशन) चुम्बन, अधिस्पर्श। The act of kissing.

Osculum (ऑस्कुलम) एक छोटा-सा छिद्र। A small aperture.

Osmesis (औस्मेसिस) 1. गंध ज्ञान 2. सूँघने की क्रिया 1. The sense of smell. 2. The act of smelling.

Osmodysphoria (ओस्मोडिस्फोरिया) किसी प्रकार की गंध से घृणा होना। Aversion to certain odors.

Osmole (ऑस्मोल) परासरणीय दाब की एक इकाई जो विलेय पदार्थो की उस मात्रा के तुल्य होती है जो विलयन में वियोजित होकर कणों का एक मोल बनाती है। A unit of osmotic pressure equivalent to the amount of solute substances that dissociates in the solution to form one mole of particles.

Osmometer (ऑस्मोमीटर) परासरणमापी। Instrument for testing the sense of smell.

Osmophobia (ओस्मोफोबिया) गंध का विकृत भय। Morbid fear of odors.

Osmoreceptor (ऑस्मोरिसीप्टर) 1. अधश्चेतक में स्थित एक ग्राहक जो सीरम के परासरणीय दाब के प्रति संवेदनशील होता है। 2. मस्तिष्क में स्थित एक ग्राहक जो घ्राणीय उद्दीपनों के प्रति संवेदनशील होता है। परासणग्राही।

1. A receptor situated in the hypothalamus which is sensitive to the osmotic pressure of the serum. 2. A receptor situated in the brain which is sensitive to the olfactory stimuli.

Osmosis (ऑस्मोसिस) परामरण, प्रसरण। The passage of substance in solution through animal membranes.

Osmotic pressure (ऑस्मोटिक प्रेशर) दो भिन्न सांद्रता वाले विलयनों किसी अर्धपरागम्य झिल्ली द्वारा अलग किए जाने पर उत्पन्न होने वाला दाब। The pressure that develops when two solutions of different concentrations are separated by a semipermeable membrane.

Ossens (ऑसीन्स) हड्डी जैसा। Bony.

Ossicle (ऑसीकिल) छोटी हड्डी। Any small bone.

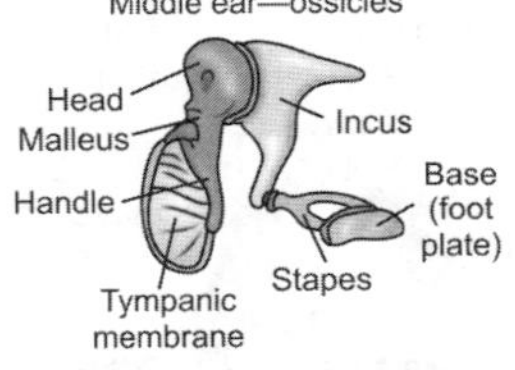

- They increase the amplitude of the vibrations 15–20 times because of leverage and the eardrum to oval window ratio
- Synovial joints between them

Ossification (ऑसीफिकेशन) हड्डी बनना। The formation of bony matter.

Osteitis (ऑस्टाइटिस) हड्डी की सूजन। Inflammation of a bone.

Osteoarthritis (ऑस्टियोआरथ्रराइटिस) जोड़ों के आस-पास की प्रदाह युक्त सूजन। Osteoarthrosis.

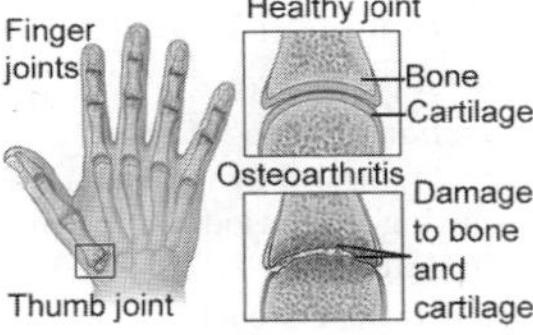

Osteoblast (ऑस्टियोब्लास्ट) हड्डी बनाने वाला तत्व। Cell concerned forming new bone material and repairing the old.

Osteoblastoma (ऑस्टियोब्लास्टोमा) वेदनायुक्त सुदम अबुर्द। A benign tumor of osteoblasts.

Osteochondral (ऑस्टियोकॉण्ड्रल) अस्थि एवं उपास्थि से सम्बन्धित। Pertaining to the bone and cartilage.

Osteochondritis (ऑस्टियोकॉण्ड्राइटिस) अस्थि एवं उपास्थि का शोथ। Inflammation of bone and cartilage.

Osteochondroma (ऑस्टियोकॉण्ड्रोमा) अस्थि एवं उपास्थि ऊतक दोनों से बना

एक सुदम अबुर्द। A bony and cartilaginous and cartilage.

Osteochondrosarcoma (ऑस्टियोकॉण्ड्रोसार्कोमा) किसी अस्थि में उत्पन्न काण्ड्रोसार्कोमा। Chondrosarcoma occurring in a bone.

Osteochondrosis (ऑस्टियोकॉण्ड्रोसिस) बच्चों में, वृद्धिकाल में अस्थिभवन केन्द्रों का ह्रास होना जिसके पश्चात पुनर्जनन हो जाता है। Degeneration of the ossification centers followed by regeneration during the period of growth in children.

Osteoclasia, Osteoclasis (ऑस्टियोक्लेसिया, ऑस्टियोक्लेसिस) किसी विकृति को ठीक करने के लिए शल्यकर्म द्वारा किसी हड्डी को तोड़ना। Surgical fracture of a bone to correct a deformity.

Osteoclast (ऑस्टियोक्लास्ट) वह कोशिका जो अस्थि-ऊतक का शोषण कर उसे छिन-भिन्न कर देती है। Cell which eliminates bone tissue not needed for skeletal strengh and efficiency.

Osteoclastoma (ऑस्टियोक्लास्टोमा) अस्थि-अवशोषीकोशिका अबुर्द। Giant cell tumor of bone.

Osteocopic (ऑस्टियोकोपिक) हड्डी में होने वाली तीव्र वेदना से सम्बन्धित। Pertaining to the severe pain in the bone.

Osteodystropia, Osteodystrophy (ऑस्टियोडिस्ट्रॉफिया, ऑस्टियोडिस्टॉफी) हड्डी का दोषपूर्ण विकास। Faulty growth of bone.

Osteofibroma (ऑस्टियोफाइब्रोमा) स्थितत्वबुर्द। A benign tumor of bony and fibrous tissues.

Osteogenesis Imperfecta (ऑस्टियोजेनेसिस इमपरफेक्टा) एक वंशागत विकार जिसमें अस्थियां असामान्य रूप से भंगुर होती है जो मामूली सी चोट लगने पर ही टूट जाती है। An inherited disorder marked by abnormally brittle bones which are broken readily with trivial injury.

Osteoid (ऑस्टीऑयड) हड्डी के समान। Resembling bone.

Osteolysis (ऑस्टीयोलाइसिस) हड्डी का नष्ट होना। Destruction of bone.

Osteoma (ऑस्टियोमा) हड्डी की रसौली। Any bone tumor.

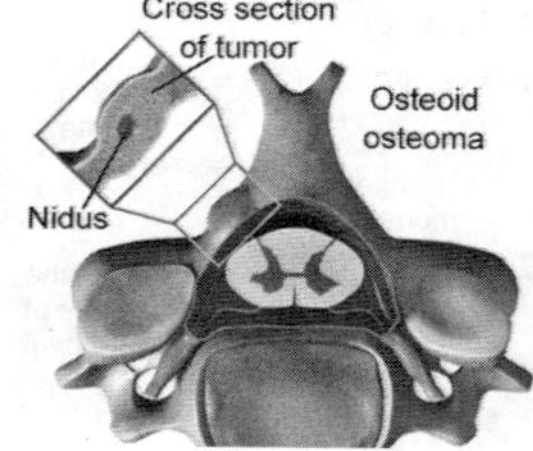

Osteomalacia (ऑस्टियोमलेसिया) हड्डियों का नरम पड़ जाना। A morbid softening of bones.

Osteomatosis (ऑस्टियोमेटोसिस) बहुत से अस्थ्यर्बुदों का बनना। Formation of multiple osteomas.

Osteometry (ऑस्टियोमेटरी) हड्डियों की माप लेना। Measurement of the bones.

Osteomyelitis (ऑस्टियोमाइलाइटिस) अस्थिमज्जा का प्रदाह। Inflammation commencing in the marrow of bone.

Osteopathy (ऑस्टियोपेथी) हड्डी का रोग। Any disease of bone.

Osteopoikilosis (ऑस्टियोपोइकिलोसिस) घनबिन्दुकित-अस्थिता। Mottled or spotted.

Osteoporosis (ऑस्टियोपोरोसिस) अस्थि सुषिरता। Absolute lose in quantity of bone tissue with enlarging marrow cavity and haversian spaces.

Osteopyesis (ऑस्टियोपाइसिस) किसी हड्डी के भीतर पस बन जाना। Suppuration occurring within a bone.

Osteosclerosis (ऑस्टियोस्कलेरोसिस) किसी हड्डी का कठोर हो जाना। Hardening of a bone.

Osteosis (ऑस्टियोसिस) अस्थि का गठन होना, बनना, हड्डीं ऊतको का निर्माण। Formation of bone and bony tissues.

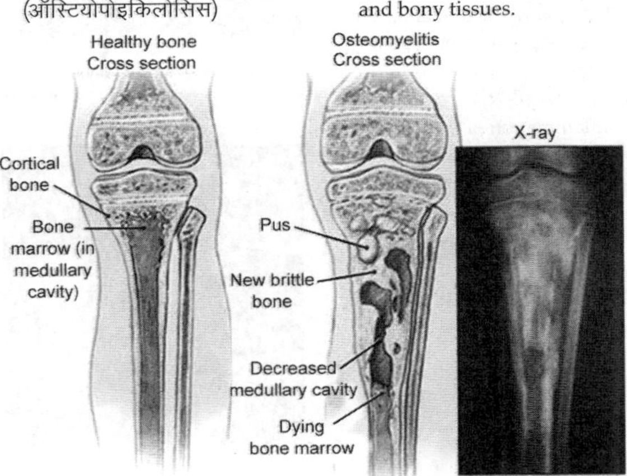

Osteomyelitis

Osteotome (ऑस्टियोटोम) हड्डी काटने वाला चाकू। A bone-saw.

Osteotomy (ऑस्टियोटोमी) हड्डी काटना। Division or cutting of a bone.

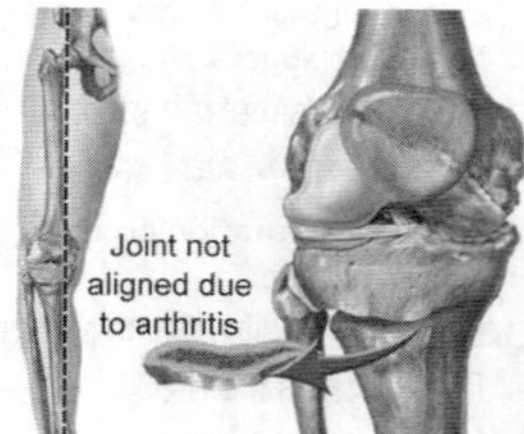

Osteotrophy (ऑस्टियोट्रॉफी) हड्डी का पोषण।Nutrition of the bone.

Ostium (ऑस्टियम) छिद्र, द्वार, मुख। The mouth of a tubular passage.

Otic (ओटिक) कान संबंधी। Pertaining to the ear.

Otitis (ओटाइटिस) कान की सूजन। Inflammation of the ear.

Otitis Externa (ओटाइटिस एक्सटर्ना) बाह्य कर्णशोथ। Inflammation of the external ear.

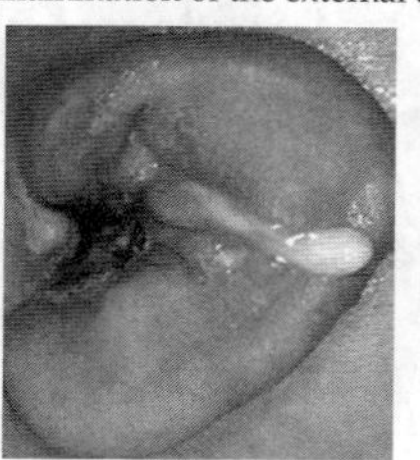

Otitis Interna (ओटाइटिस इन्टर्ना) अन्तःकर्ण का शोथ। Inflammation of the internal ear.

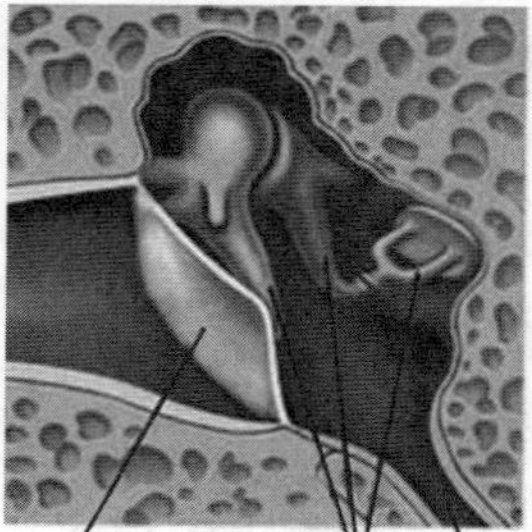

Otitis Media (ओटाइटिस मीडिया) कान के मध्य भाग का प्रदाह। Inflammation of the middle ear cavity.

Normal middle ear

Otitis media

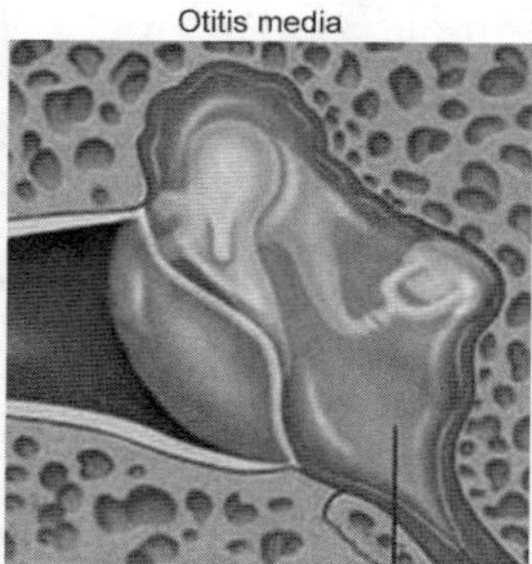

Otogenic (ओटोजेनिक) कर्णजनक। Having its origin in the ear.

Otolith (ओटोलिथ) कर्णपथरी। Stone in the ear.

Otology (ओटोलॉजी) कानों की बनावट, कर्ण रोग विज्ञान। The science which deals the structure, function and disease of the ear.

Otomycosis (ओटोमाइकोसिस) कर्णकवकता, कवक द्वारा उत्पादित बाह्य-कर्ण की अवस्था। The presence of or the condition caused by fungus in the external ear.

Otorrhagia (ओटोरैह्जिया) कान से खून बहना। Bleeding from the ear.

Otorrhea (ओटोरिह्या) कान से स्त्राव निकलना। Discharge from the ear.

Otoscope (ओटोस्कोप) कान का परीक्षण करने वाला एक उपकरण। An apparatus for examination of the ear.

Ototoxic (ओटोटॉक्सिक) श्रवण-अंगों पर विषैला प्रभाव रखने वाला। Having a toxic effect on the organs of hearing.

Oulitis (आऊलाइटिस) मसूड़ों की सूजन। Inflammation of the gums.

Ounce (औंस) आठ ड्राम, भार तथा तरल आयतन की एक माप। Eight drams, a measure of weight and fluid volume.

Ovalocyte (ओवेलोसाइट) एक अण्डाकार लाल रक्त कोशिका। An oval red blood cell.

Ovaltine (ओवेलटीन) एक पौष्टिक आहार। A proprietary food beverage.

Ovariocele (ओवेरियोसील) किसी डिम्बग्रंथि का हर्निया। Hernia of an ovary.

Ovariocyesis (ओवेरियोसाइसिस) डिम्बग्रंथि में गर्भावस्था का उत्पन्न होना। Pregnancy occurring in the ovary.

Ovary (ओवरी) अण्डाशय। One of the two generative glands in female containing the ova or the germ cell.

Oven (ओवेन) भट्टी। Furnace.

Overhydration (ओवरहाइड्रेशन) शरीर में तरलों का अधिक होना। An excess of fluids in the body.

Overresponse (ओवररैस्पोन्स) किसी उद्दीपन के लिए असामान्य रूप से तीव्र प्रतिक्रिया। An abnormally intense reaction to a stimulus.

Overriding (ओवराइडिंग) किसी टूटी हुई हड्डी के एक किनारे का दूसरी हड्डी के ऊपर को फिसलना। The slipping of one end of a fractured bone upon the other.

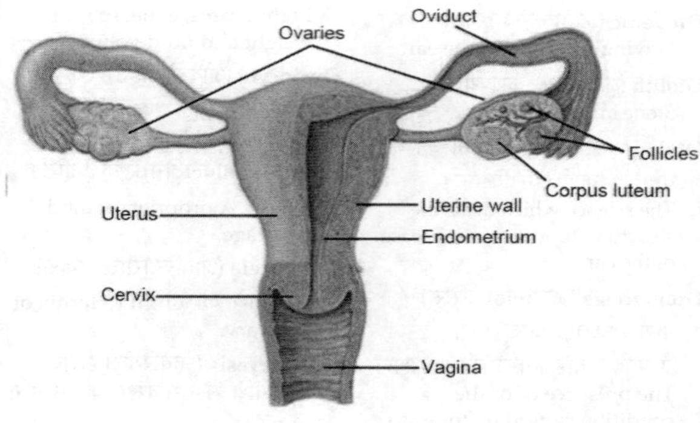

Ovary

Oviform (ओवीफोर्म) डिम्बाकार।
Egg-shaped, Oval.

Ovigerous (ओवीगेरस) डिम्ब उत्पन्न करने वाला।
Producing ova.

Oviparous (ओवीपैरस) अण्डे देने वाला। Bearing eggs.

Oviposition (ओवीपोजिशन) अण्डे देना। The laying of eggs.

Ovulation (ओव्यूलेशन) डिम्बक्षरण।
The maturation and escape of ova.

Ovum (ओव्यूम) डिम्ब, अण्डाणु।
The female reproduction cell.

Oxalate (ऑक्सेलेट) एक तिग्मीय पदार्थ।
A salt of oxalic acid.

Oxalosis (ऑक्जेलोसिस) कैल्सियम ऑक्जेलेट का शरीर के ऊतकों

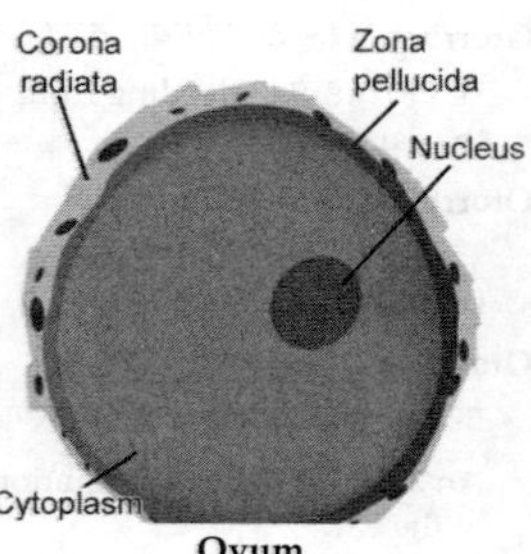

Ovum

विशेषकर गुर्दो में जमा होना।
Deposition of calcium oxalate in the body tissue, especially in the kidneys.

Oxaluria (ऑक्जेलूरिया) मूत्र में कैल्शियम ऑक्सैलेट विद्यमान रहना।
The presence of calcium oxalate in the urine.

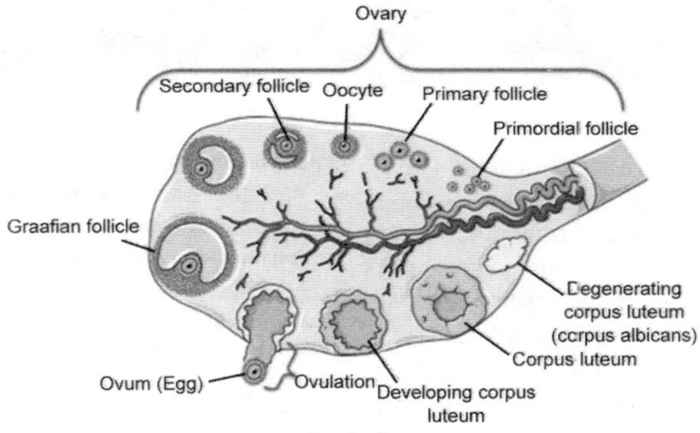

Ovulation

Oxidation (ऑक्सीडेशन) उपचयन, ऑक्सीकरण। The process of combining oxygen.

Oximeter (ऑक्सीमीटर) खून में ऑक्सीजन की मात्रा का पता लगाने वाला उपकरण। An apparatus for determining the amount of oxygen in the blood.

Oxycephalia (ऑक्सीसिफैलिया) एक ऊँची एवं नुकीली खोपड़ी धारण करने की दशा। The condition of having a high and pointed skull.

Oxygen (ऑक्सीजन) प्राणवायु। One of the gaseous elements which acts as a supporter of life and combustion.

Oxyhemoglobinometer (ऑक्सीहीमोग्लोबिनोमीटर) रक्त में ऑक्सीजन की मात्रा को मापने वाला एक उपकरण। An apparatus for measuring the amount of O_2 in the blood.

Oxyntic (ऑक्सीन्टिक) अम्लास्त्रावी, अम्लजनक। Rendering acid.

Oxyopia (ऑक्सीओपिया) दृष्टि की असामान्य तीक्षणता। Abnormal acuteness of vision.

Oxyphonia (ऑक्सीफोनिया) कण्ठ ध्वनि का असामान्य रूप से ऊँचा होना। An abnormally highpitch of the voice.

Oxytocia (ऑक्सीटोसिया) प्रसव शीघ्र होना। Rapid labor.

P

Pabular (पेबुलर) पोषण सम्बन्धी। Pertaining to the nourishment.

Pacemaker (पेसमेकर) कोई भी वस्तु जो किसी क्रिया के सम्पादित होने की दर एवं अनुक्रम को प्रमाणित करती है। दाँये आलिन्द में ऊर्ध्व महाशिरा के प्रवेश द्वार के निकट कोशिकाओं का एक समूह जिससे आवेग उठकर हृदय के दूसरे भागों में फैल जाते है, गतिप्रेरक, गतिचालक। Anything which affects the rate and rhythm of a process, the specialized cells in right atrium that generate impulse.

Pachyblepharosis (पैकीब्लेफेरोसिस) आँख की पलक की जीर्ण स्थूलता। Chronic thickening of the eyelid.

Pachyderma (पैकीडर्मा) त्वचा का असामान्य रूप से मोटा हो जाना, गजचर्मता। Abnormal thickening of the skin.

Pachyemia (पैकेमिया) रक्त गाढ़ा होना, रक्तघनता। Thickening of the blood.

Pachygnathous (पैकीग्नेथस) बड़ा जबड़ा धारण करने वाला। Possessing a large jaw.

Pachymeningitis (पैकीमेनिन्जाइटिस) दृढ़तानिका या ड्यूरामेटर का शोथ। Inflammation of the dura mater.

Pachyonychia (पैकीओनीकिया) नाखूनों का असामान्य रूप से मोटा हो जाना, स्थूलनखता। Abnormal thickening of the nails.

Pachyotous (पैकीओटस) मोटे कानों वाला। Having thick ears.

Pack (पैक) आर्द्रवस्त्रावेश्टन, आर्द्रवस्त्रावेश्टनोपचार। A moist blanket placed around the patients, wet pack.

Packed cells (पैक्ड सैल्स) प्लाज्मा से अलग हुई लाल रक्त कोशिकाएँ। RBC which have been separated from the plasma.

$PaCO_2$ (पीए सी O_2) धमनीय रक्त में कार्बन डाइऑक्साइड का आंशिक दाब। Partial pressure of carbon dioxide in the arterial blood.

Pad (पैड) कोमल गद्दी समान पिण्ड जो दबाव को कम करने अथवा शरीर के किसी अंग या भाग

को सहारा देने के लिए प्रयोग में लाया जाता है। Cushion of soft material used to apply pressure or support on an organ.

Paget's disease (पेजेट्स डिज़ीज) वृद्ध व्यक्तियों में अस्थियों का जीर्ण शोथ जिसके परिणामस्वरूप वे मोटी एवं कोमल हो जाती है तथा लम्बी हड्डियाँ मुड़ जाती है।
Chronic inflammation of the bones in old persons resulting in thickening and softening of bone and curving of the long bones.

Pain (पेन) दर्द, वेदना, शूल, पीड़ा। A sensation of discomfort, distress or suffering due to stimulation of specialized nerve endings.

Palate (पैलेट) मुख की छत, तालु, काकुद।
Roof of the mouth separating from nasal cavity.

Palatitis (पैलेटाइटिस) तालुशोथ। Inflammation of palate.

Palatonasal (पैलेटोनेजल) तालु एवं नासागुहा सम्बन्धी। Pertaining to the palate and nasal cavity.

Palatorrhaphy (पैलेटरैह्फी) तालुसीवन। Suture of a cleft palate.

Palilalia (पेलीलैलिया) किसी वाक्य को निरर्थक दोहराते जाना, निरर्थकपुनरूक्ति।
Constant repetition of a sentence, paliphrasia.

Palliate (पैलिएट) आराम पहुँचाना, रोगदमन। To relieve.

Pallidectomy (पैलिडेक्टॉमी) पाण्डुरगोलकोच्छेदन।
Surgical or cryogenic/laser destruction of globus pollidus.

Pallor (पेलर) पीलापन, पाण्डुता। Paleness.

Palm (पाम) हथेली, करतल। Anterior surface of hand from wrist to fingers.

Palmar reflex (पामर रिफ्लैक्स) शिशुओं में मुट्ठी बाँधने का प्रतिवर्त जो धीरे-धीरे गायब हो जाता है।

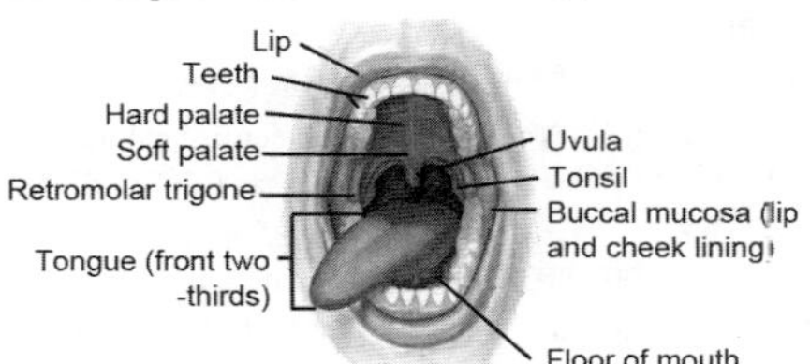

Palate

A grasping reflex in infants which gradually disappears.

Palpable (पैल्पेबिल) छू कर जिसका ज्ञान हो सके, परिस्पृश्य, परिस्पर्शन योग। Perceptible by touch.

Palpation (पैल्पेशन) परिस्पर्शन, संस्पर्शन। Examination by application of hand or fingers.

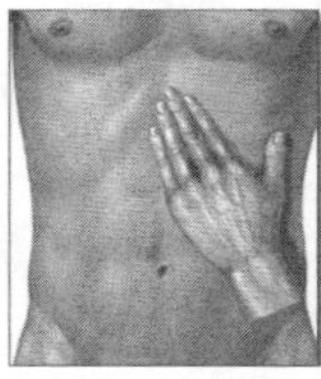

The examiner touches and feels the patient's body

Palpebra (पैल्पीब्रा) नेत्रच्छद, आँख की पलक। An eyelid.

Palpebral commisure (पैल्पीब्रल कमीशर) नेत्रच्छद-विदर के प्रत्येक सिरे पर आँख की पलकों का संयोजन। The corner of the eyelids at each end of the palpebral fissure.

Palpitation (पैल्पीटेशन) असामान्य रूप से तीव्र गति का तथा अनियमित हृदय स्पन्द जिसे रोगी महसूस करता है, धड़कन। Rapid throbbing pulsation of heart.

Palsy (पाल्सी) धात, अंगघात, पक्षाघात। Paralysis, loss of ability to act.

Palyp (पॉलिप) श्लेष्मिक कला से लटकने वाला वृन्तयुक्त एक अबुर्द जो अधिकतर नाक, गर्भाशय तथा मलाषय में पाया जाता है। पूर्वगक। A tumor with a pedicle hanging from the mucous membrane, usually found in the nose, uterus and rectum.

Pampiniform (पैम्पीनीफॉर्म) प्रतान या लता की भाँति घुमावदार, प्रतानाकार। Convoluted like a tendril.

Panangitis (पैनेन्जाइटिस) वाहिकास्तरशोथ। Inflammation of all the coats of a blood vessel.

Panarteritis (पैनार्टीराइटिस) धमनी की सम्पूर्ण संरचनाओं का प्रदाह, पूर्णधमनीशोथ। Inflammation of all the structure of an artery.

Panarthritis (पनार्थराइटिस) एक संयुक्त की सभी संरचनाओं की सूजन। Inflammation of all the structures of joint.

Pancaditis (पैनकाडाईटिस) पूर्णहृदयशोथ। Inflammation of the entire heart.

Pancolectomy (पैन्कोलैक्टॉमी) बड़ी आंत को पूरी तरह निकाल देना, पूर्णवृहदांत्रोच्छेदन। Excision of the entire colon.

Pancreas (पैन्क्रियाज) अग्नाशय, पाचकग्रन्थि, क्लोमग्रन्थि।The principal digestive gland situated below and behind the stomach.

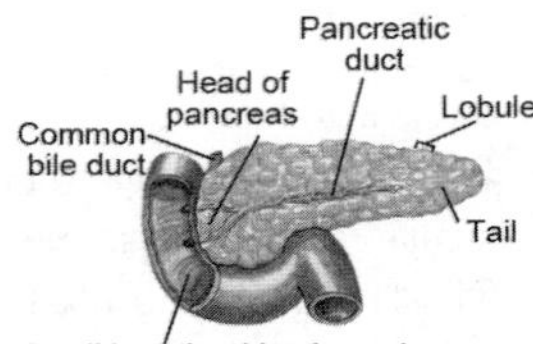

Pancreaticoduodenectomy (पैंक्रिअटिकोडुओडेनक्टोमी) अग्नाशयिक वाहिनी एवं ग्रहणी के बीच शल्य चिकित्सा के द्वारा एक मार्ग बनाना। A major surgical operation involving the removal of part of the pancreas and part of the stomach including the duodenum.

Pancreatin (पैन्क्रियाटिन) अग्नाशयरसनिर्मित एक खमीर, अग्नाशयजन्यकिण्व। A mixture of enzyme obtained from the pancreas.

Pancreatitis (पैन्क्रियाटाइटिस) पाचक ग्रन्थि का प्रदाह, अग्न्याशयशोथ। Inflammation of the pancreas.

Pancreatolith (पैन्क्रियाटोलिथ) अग्नाशय की पथरी। A stone of the pancreas.

Pancreatolysis (पैन्क्रियाटोलाइसिस) अग्नाशय-ऊतक का नष्ट होना। Destruction of the pancreatic tissue.

Pancytopenia (पैनसाइटोपीनिया) पूर्णरक्त-कोशिकाहीनता। Reduction of all the blood cells.

Pandemic (पैण्डेमिक) महामारी, सार्वलौकिक, देशान्तरगामी। A widespread epidemic.

Pandiculation (पैण्डीकुलेशन) अंगड़ाई, जम्हाई, कसमसाहट। Yawning the act of stretching the limbs.

Panencephalitis (पैनएन्सीफैलाइटिस) सम्पूर्ण मस्तिष्क का शोथ। Inflammation of the entire brain.

Panhyperemia (पैनहाइप्रीमिया) शरीर के किसी सम्पूर्ण अंग अथवा भाग में अतिरक्तता होना। Hyperemia of the entire organ or part of the body.

Panic (पैनिक) आतंक, भय, डर, भयभीत। Sudden anxiety, terror or fright.

Panniculitis (पैनीकुलाइटिस) अग्र उदरीय भित्ति के वसीय संयोजी ऊतक का शोथ। Inflammation of the fatty connective tissue of the anterior abdominal wall.

Pannus (पैन्स) नाखूना। Vascularization around cornea.

Pansinusitis (पैनसाइनुसाइटिस) सभी नासिका सम्बन्धित विवरों का शोथ। Inflammation of all the para nasal sinuses.

Panting (पैन्टिंग) शीघ्रगामी एवं छिछला श्वसन। Rapid shallow breathing.

PaO_2 धमनीय रक्त में ऑक्सीजन का आंशिक दाब। The partial pressure of oxygen in arterial blood.

Papilla (पैपिला) चूचुक के समान उभार, अंकुरक, फुन्सी, गूमड़ी, अक्षिबिम्ब। Small, nipple like elevation.

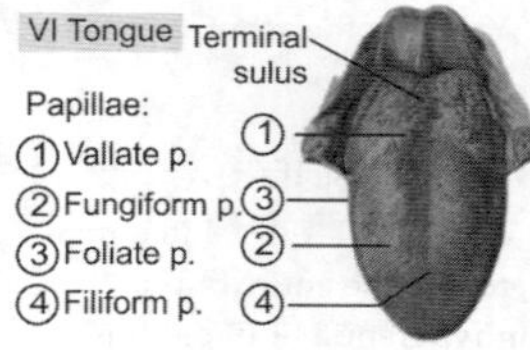

Papilledema (पैपिलीडीमा) दृष्टि-चक्रिका का शोथ। Edema of optic nerve head.

Papilliform (पैपिलीफोर्म) अक्षिबिम्ब के आकार का, अंकुराकार। Resembling papillae.

Papillitis (पैपिलाइटिस) दृष्टि-चक्रिका का शोथ, अंकुरकशोथ। Inflammation of the optic disk or a papilla.

Papilloma (पैपिलोमा) अंकुरकाबुर्द। A benign tumor of the epithelium.

Papillomatosis (पैपिलोमेटोसिस) बहुत से अंकुराकाबुर्दों का बनना। Formation of multiple papillomas.

Pappus (पैप्पस) दाढ़ी के प्रथम बारीक बाल जो गालों एवं ठुडढ़ी पर प्रकट होते है। The first downy beard hair on the cheeks and chin.

Papule (पैप्यूल) त्वचा पर एक छोटा, परिसीमित, ठोस उठा हुआ स्थान, पिटिका। Solid circumscribed elevation of skin.

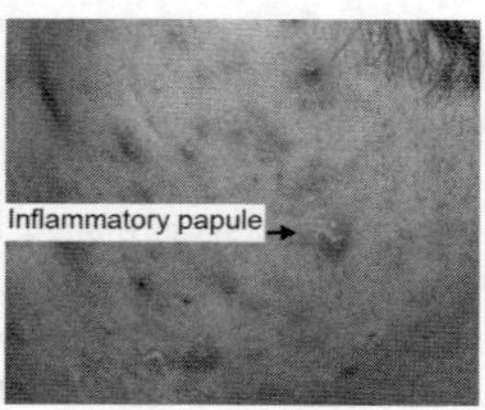

Papulosquamous (पैप्यूलोस्क्वामस) जो पिटिकीय एवं शल्कमय दोनों होता है। Presence of popular and scaly.

Parabionts (पैराबायोन्ट्स) संयोजन की अवस्था में रहने वाले दो प्राणी। Two individual living in the condition of parabiosis.

Paracentesis (पैरासेन्टेसिस) तरल को निकालने के लिए किसी गुहा का शल्यक्रिया द्वारा वेधन करना। Cavity puncture for drainage of fluid.

Paracentral (पैरासेन्ट्रल) केन्द्र के पास स्थित, पराकेन्द्रीय। Situated near the center.

Parachomatism (पैराक्रोमेटिज्म) रंगों को ठीक प्रकार से न पहचानना परन्तु वास्तविक वर्णान्धता नहीं होती। Defective color perception.

Paracidity (परैसिडिटी) असामान्य अम्लता। Abnormal acidity.

Paracrisis (पैराक्राइसिस) शरीर के स्रावों की कोई भी विकृति। Any abnormality of the body secretion.

Paradidymal (पेराडिडाइमल) परवृषण सम्बन्धी। Pertaining to the paradidymis.

Paraffin (पैराफिन) एक प्रकार का हल्का विरेचक, मृदुवसा। Hydrocarbon, derivative of petroleum.

Paraganglia (पैरागैन्गलिया) Paraganglion का बहुवचन। Plural of paraganglion.

Paraganglioma (पैरागग्लियोमा) परागण्डिकार्बुद। Pheochromocytoma.

Parakeratosis (पैराकेराटोसिस) त्वचा की असामान्य श्रृंगी वृद्धि। Abnormal horny growth of the skin.

Paralexia (पैरालैक्सिया) पढ़ कर बोलने की असमर्थता, उच्चारण-अक्षमता। Aphasic inability to read.

Parallax (पैरालैक्स) प्रेक्षक की स्थिति बदल जाने के कारण किसी वस्तु का विस्थापन होना, लम्बन। Displacement of object by change in observer's position.

Paralysis (पैरालाइसिस) पक्षाघात, अंगघात, घात, लकवा। Loss of muscular function usually due to nerve dysfunction.

(*i*) **Bell's Paralysis** (बैल्स पैरालाइसिस) मुखाघात, चेहरे का लकवा। Facial paralysis.

(*ii*) **Crossed Paralysis** (क्रॉस्ड पैरालाइसिस) एक ओर की भुजा तथा दूसरी ओर की टांग का पक्षाघात, विपरीतांगघात। Paralysis of an arm on one side and of a leg on the other.

Paralytic ileus (पैरालाइटिक इलियस) लकवाग्रस्त–आन्त्रावरोध, आँतों का पक्षाघात हो जाना जिसके कारण आँतों में रुकावट आती हैं। Paralysis with distention and obstruction of the intestines.

Paramagnetic (पैरामेग्नेटिक) चुम्बक के छोरों की ओर खिंच जाने में सक्षम। Anything attracted by a magnet.

Paramastitis (पैरामैस्टाइटिस) स्तन ग्रन्थि के चारों ओर की सूजन। Inflammation around the mammary gland.

Paramedian (पैरामीडियन) मध्य रेखा के पास। Close to the midline.

Paramedic (पैरामेडिक) रोगियों की आपातकालीन देख भाल में प्रशिक्षित एवं प्रमाणित व्यक्ति। A trained person to assist doctor.

Paramedical (पैरामेडिकल) पैराचिकित्साकर्मचारी, पैराचिकित्साकर्मी। Related to the medical science or practice of medicine such as laboratory technicians, etc.

Parametritis (पैरामीट्राइटिस) परागर्भाशय संयोजी ऊतकशोथ। Inflammation of the parametrium.

Parametrium (पैरामीट्रियम) गर्भाशय के चारों ओर का संयोजी ऊतक। The connective tissue sarrounding of uterus.

Paramnesia (पैराम्निसिया) अपस्मृति। Use of words without meaning or recall of events that never occurred.

Paramyotonia (पैरामायोटोनिया) पेशियों की दोषपूर्ण तानता, परापेशीतानता। Defective muscular tonicity.

Paranasal (पैरानेज़ल) नासा-गुहाओं के पास स्थित, परानासिक। Situated near the nasal cavities.

Paranoia (पैरानोइया) एक मानसिक विकार जिसमें उत्पीड़ित होने की भ्रान्ति हो जाती है। Paranoid schizophrenia.

Paranoid (पैरानॉयड) संविभ्रमी, चित्रविक्षेपी। Ideas of persecution, suspicious thinking.

Parapancreatic (पैरापैन्क्रियाटिक) अग्नाशय के पास स्थित। Situated near the pancreas.

Paraphasia (पैराफेजिया) शब्दों का अनुचित संयोग प्रयोग करता है, वाग्विकार, अपवाक। Misuse of spoken words or word combinations.

Paraphilia (पैराफीलिया) इस प्रकार के कार्यों के द्वारा जिनका सामाजिक रूप से निषेध है अथवा जिन्हें समाज स्वीकार नहीं करता या जीवविज्ञान के अनुसार जिन्हें उचित नहीं समझा जाता, लैंगिक स्वाभाविक प्रवृति को अभिव्यक्त करना। Expression of the sexual instinct by the acts socially prohibited, unacceptable or biologically undesirable.

Paraphimosis (पैराफाइमोसिस) किसी हुए शिश्नमुण्डच्छद का प्रतिगमन जो वापस नहीं हो सकता यह शिश्नमुण्ड को संकुचित करता है जिसमें दर्द होने लगता है और जो सूज जाता है। Retraction of the tight prepuce which cannot be returned and it constricts the glands penis which becomes painful and swollen.

Paraphrenitis (पैराफ्रेनाइटिस) मध्यपट के चारों ओर के ऊतकों का शोथ। Inflammation of the tissue around the diaphragm.

Paraplegia (पैराप्लीजीया) दोनों टाँगों सहित शरीर के निचले भाग में होने वाला पक्षाघात, अधरांगघात। Paralysis of the lower portion of the body including both legs.
(*i*) **Alcoholic Paraplegia** (एल्कोहॉलिक पैराप्लीजीया) अधिक शराब पीने से उत्पन्न अधरांगघात। Paraplegia occurring due to excessive use of alcohol.

Paraplegia Dolorosa (पैराप्लीजीया-डोलोरोसा) किसी अबुर्द के द्वारा पश्चज सुषुम्ना रज्जु एवं तंत्रिका मूलों पर दबाव पड़ने के कारण उत्पन्न अधरांगघात जिसमें दर्द बहुत होता है। Paraplegia due to pressure of a tumor on the posterior spinal cord and nerve roots which is extremely painful.

Parapleuritis (पैराप्लूराइटिस) फुफ्फुसावरणों एवं वक्ष का मृदु शोथ। Mild inflammation of the pleurae and the thorax.

Paraproctium (पैराप्रोक्टियम) मलाशय के चारों ओर का संयोजी ऊतक। The connective tissue around the rectum.

Pararthria (परार्थरिया) शब्दों को बोलने में कठिनई होना। Difficulty in utterance of the words.

Parasecretion (पैरासीक्रीशन) स्राव में कोई विकृति। An abnormality in the secretion.

Parasite (पैरासाइट) अन्य जीवों के अन्दर पलने वाले जीव, परजीवी। Animals which live in or on the bodies of other animal such as intestinal worms.

Parasitemia (पैरासाइटीमिया) रक्त में परजीवियों का पाया जाना, परजीवीरक्तता। The presence of parasite in the blood.

Parasiticide (पैरासाइटीसाइड) परजीवीनाशक। Destructive to parasite.

Parasitology (पैरासाइटोलॉजी) परजीवियों एवं परजीविता का वैज्ञानिक अध्ययन। The scientific study of the parasites and parasitism.

Parasitotrophic (पैरासाइटोट्रॉफिक) परजीवियों के प्रति आकर्षित। Having an attraction for the parasite.

Parasternal (पैरास्टर्नल) उरोस्थि के पास स्थित, पर उरोस्थिक। Situated near the sternum.

Parasympathetic nervous system (पैरासिम्पैथेटिक नर्वस सिस्टम) स्वचालित तंत्रिका-तंत्र का कपालत्रिकास्थि भाग जिसके

गण्डिका पूर्व तन्तु मध्य मस्तिश्क एवं मेडूला ऑब्लाँगेट में तथा सुषुम्ना रज्जु के त्रिकास्थि-भाग में स्थित केन्द्रकों से उत्पन्न होते है। The craniosacral portion of the autonomic nervous system its preganglionic fibers originate from the nuclei in the midbrain medulla oblongata and sacral portion of the spinal cord.

Parasympatholytic (पैरासिम्पैथोलाइटिक) परानुकम्पी तंत्रिका तंतुओं के लिए विनाशकारी अथवा उनके द्वारा आवेशों के परिसंचरण में अवरोध उत्पन्न करने वाला। Destructive to the parasympathetic nerve fibers or blocking the transmission of impulse by them.

Parasympathomimetic (पैरासिम्पैथोमाइमेटिक) शरीर के किसी भाग की परानुकम्पी तन्त्रिका के उद्दीपन से उत्पन्न प्रभाव के समान प्रभाव उत्पन्न करने वाला, परानुकम्पी-अनुकारी। Producing the effects similar to those produced by stimulation of the parasympathetic nerve of a part of the body.

Parasystole (पैरासिस्टोल) एक अस्थानिक हृदय-ताल। An ectopic cardiac rhythm.

Paratereseomania (पैराटेरीसीयोमैनिया) नवीन दृश्यों एवं विषयों के खोजने का उन्माद। Mania for investigating the new scenes and subjects.

Parathormone (पैराथोर्मोन) परावटु ग्रन्थियों का हार्मोन जो केल्सियम तथा फॉस्फोरस के चयापचय को नियन्त्रित करता है। Hormone of the parathyroid glands that regulates the calcium and phosphorus metabolism.

Parathyroid (पैराथॉइरॉइड) अवटुग्रन्थि के पिछले भाग में स्थित चार छोटी-छोटी ग्रन्थियाँ, परावटु। Four small endocrine glands lying close to or embedded in the posterior surface of the thyroid gland.

Paratrichosis (पैराट्राइकोसिस) बालों का विकृत हो जाना। Abnormality of the hair.

Paratyphoid fever (पैराटाइफॉयड फिवर) आंत्रिक ज्वर का एक मृदु रूप, परांत्रिक ज्वर। A variety of enteric fever but less severe and prolonged than typhoid.

Paraurethral (पैरायूरेथ्रल) मूत्रमार्ग के पास, परामूत्रमार्गी। Near the urethra.

Paravaginitis (पैरावैजिनाइटिस) योनि के चारों ओर के ऊतकों का शोथ। Inflammation of the tissue around the vagina.

Parazoon (पैराजून) परजीवी की भाँति अन्य जन्तु पर रहने वाला जन्तु। An animal living as parasite upon another animal.

Parenchyma (पैरेन्काइमा) किसी अंग के आवश्यक भाग जिनका सम्बन्ध अंग के कार्य करने से होता है और जो अंग की पीठिका या ढाँचे से भिन्न होते है, सार-ऊतक।
The essential parts of an organ that are concerned with its function and which are different from its stroma or framework.

Parenchymatitis (पैरेन्काइमेटाइटिस) सार-ऊतक का शोथ। Inflammation of the parenchyma.

Parent (पैरेन्ट) माता-पिता, अभिभावक। Father or mother, parents.

Parental (पैरेन्टल) पैतृक, माँ-बाप सम्बन्धी। Pertaining to the parents.

Paresis (पैरेसिस) हल्का अथवा अपूर्ण पक्षाघात, आंशिकघात, मृदुघात। Slight or incomplete paralysis.

Paresthesia (पैरेस्थीज़िया) एक विकृति अनुभूति जैसे सुन्न हो जाने, चुभने, झुनझुनी होने, जलने तथा शरीर पर कीड़े रेंगने आदि जैसी अनुभूति का होना। An abnormal sensation as numbness, pricking, tingling, burning and insect creeping on the body, etc.

Pareunia (पैरीयूनिय) मैथुन, सम्भोग। Coitus.

Parietal (पैराइटल) किसी गुहा की दीवारों का अथवा उनसे सम्बन्धित। Of or pertaining to the wall of a cavity.

Paripassu (पैरीपासु) एक ही समय पर अथवा एक ही गति से उत्पन्न होने वाला। Occurring at the same time or at the same speed.

Parity (पैरिटी) किसी स्त्री की कम से कम 20 सप्ताह तक गर्भवती रहने की क्षमता, प्रसविता। The ability of a woman to be pregnant up to minimum 20 weeks.

Parkinson's disease (पार्किनसन्स डिज़ीज) तंत्रिका तंत्र का एक जीर्ण रोग जिसमें कम्पन्न होते है पेशियाँ दुर्बल एवं कठोर हो जाती है और एक प्रकार की चाल हो जाती है। A chronic disease of the nervous system characterized by tremors, muscular weakness and rigidity and a peculiar gait.

Paronychia (पैरोनीकिया) हाथ की किसी अंगुली के नाखून के चारों ओर के किनारों के ऊतकों का शोथ। Witlow inflammation of the marginal tissue around a finger nail.

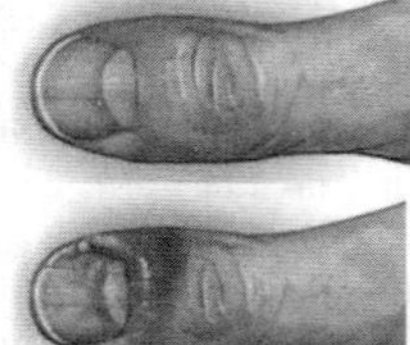

Healthy fingernail (top) Infected nail (bottom).

Paronychomycosis (पैरोनीकोमाइकोसिस) नाखूनों के आस-पास कवक का संक्रमण हो जाना। Fungus infection about the nails.

Paronychosis (पैरोनीकोकस) किसी नाखून का एक असामान्य स्थिति में वृद्धि करना। Growth of a nail in an abnormal position.

Parosmia (पैरॉस्मिया) घ्राण विकृति, परिवर्तित घ्राणसम्वेदना। Perverted sense of smell.

Parotid gland (पैरोटिड ग्लैण्ड) कर्णमूलग्रन्थि, कर्णपूर्णग्रन्थि। The salivary gland situated in front of and below the ear.

Parotitis (पैरोटाइटिस) कर्णपूर्ण ग्रन्थि की सूजन, कर्णपूर्णग्रन्थि शोथ। Mumps inflammation of the parotid gland.

Parous (पैरस) कम से कम एक बच्चे को जन्म देने वाली स्त्री, प्रजाता। Having borne at least one child.

Parovarium (पैरोवेरियम) पराडिम्बग्रन्थि। Vestigial remains of mesonephric tubules located in mesosalpinx between the ovary and fallopian tubes.

Paroxysm (पारौक्सिजम) किसी रोग के लक्षणों का अचानक पुनः उत्पन्न होना। Periodic recurrence of the symptoms of a disease.

Parthenogenesis (पार्थिनोजैनेसिस) अनिशेक जनन। Reproduction arising from unfertilized female eggs.

Particle (पार्टिकल) पदार्थ का एक बहुत ही छोटा टुकड़ा, कण। A very small piece or portion of anything.

Particulate (पार्टीकुलेट) कणों से बना हुआ। Composed of particles.

Parturient (पार्चुरिएन्ट) प्रसूता, प्रसवमाना। A woman who has recently given birth to a child.

Parturition (पार्चुरीशन) बच्चे को जन्म देने की क्रिया, प्रसूति प्रसव। Delivery of childbirth.

Parvule (पारव्यूल) गुलिका, कण, गोली। A granule or pellet.

Passary (पैसरी) गर्भाशय को थामने के लिए अथवा गर्भनिरोधक

साधन के रूप में योनि में रखा जाने वाला एक यंत्र। An instrument placed in the vagina to support the uterus or as a contraceptive device as diaphragm pessary.

Passion (पैशन) लैंगिक उत्तेजना के साथ होने वाली अतिभावुकता। Great emotion associated with sexual excitement.

Passivity (पैसिविटी) अन्य लोगों पर निर्भरता। Dependency on others.

Pasteurization (पैसच्युराइजेशन) रोगोत्पादक जीवाणुओं को ताप द्वारा नष्ट करने की प्रक्रिया, निर्जीवाणुकरण। The heating of milk to destroy disease causing germs named after Louis Pasteur its inventor.

Pastille (पैस्टाइल) चूसने वाली गोली। Lozenge or troche.

Past-pointing (पास्ट-प्वाइटिंग) अपनिर्देशन। A diagnostic point for brain disease.

Patella (पटेला) जानुका, जानुफलक, घुटने की चौड़ी हड्डी। A round sesamoid bone in front of knee, the knee cap.

Patellectomy (पटेलेक्टॉमी) जानुका-उच्छेदन। Excision of the patella.

Patency (पैटेन्सी) बिल्कुल खुला रहने की दशा, एकस्वत्व। The condition of being quite open.

Patent (पेटेन्ट) खुला अथवा अनवरूद्ध। Open or unobstructed.

Paternal (पेटरनल) पैतृक। Of pertaining to or inherited from the father.

Pathema (पैथीमा) रोगवस्था। Morbid condition.

Pathoanatomy (पैथोएनाटॉमी) रोगग्रस्त ऊतकों की शरीर रचना। Anatomy of the diseased tissue.

Pathogen (पैथोजन) कोइ रोगोत्पादक पदार्थ, रोगजन, विकृतिजन। Any disease producing agent.

Pathognomonic (पैथोग्नोमोनिक) किसी रोग के किसी चिन्ह अथवा लक्षण को प्रदर्शित करने वाला जिस पर रोग का निदान किया जा सकता है। Denoting a sign or symptom of disease on which the diagnosis can be made.

Pathologic (पैथोलॉजिक्ल) विकृतविज्ञान से सम्बन्धित। Pertaining to pathology.

Pathology (पैथोलॉजी) रोग के कारण, स्वभाव आदि से सम्बन्धित विज्ञान, रोगविज्ञान। The part of medicine which treats the cause, nature, etc. of a disease.

Pathophobia (पैथोफोबिया) बीमारी का डर, रोगभीति। A morbid fear of disease.

Pathophysiology (पैथोफिजियोलॉजी) विकारी-शरीरक्रिया। Derangement or alteration of function seen in disease.

Pathotropism (पैथोट्रॉपिज्म) रोगग्रस्त ऊतकों के प्रति औषधियों का आकर्षण। The attraction of drugs towards the diseased tissues.

Patient (पेशेन्ट) रोगी, बीमार। A sick person.

Patulous (पैचुलस) दूर-दूर तक फैला हुआ, खुला हुआ, फूला हुआ, विकृत। Spread apart, open, distended.

Pavor (पेवर) अत्यधिक भय, अतिभीति। Terror.

Peau D'orange (पीयू डी औरेंज) त्वचा की एक ऐसी दशा जिसमें यह संतरें के समान बन जाती है यह शोफयुक्त हो जाती है। The condition of the skin in which it becomes like orange, it becomes edematous.

Pectoral (पेक्टोरल) वक्षीय, अस्त्राणीय, वक्ष सम्बन्धी। Pertaining to the breast.

Pectoralis (पेक्टोरेलिस) छाती की पेशी, वक्षपेशी। The muscle of the breast.

Pectoriloquy (पेक्टोरिलोक्युई) वक्षध्वनि, परिश्रवणध्वनि। The distinct transmission of articulate speech to the ear on auscultation.

Pectus (पैक्टस) स्तन, वक्ष या छाती। Breast chest or thorax.

Pectus carinatum (पैक्टस कैरीनेटम) कपोतवक्ष, उन्नतोरोस्थिक। Pigeon chest, chicken breast.

Pectus excavatum (पैक्टस एक्सकेवेटम) कीपवक्ष। Funnel chest.

Pedal (पेडल) पाद सम्बन्धी, पदिक। Pertaining to the foot.

Pedatrophy (पेडाट्रॉफी) बच्चों में क्षयकारी रोग। A wasting disease in children.

Pederasty (पीडेरैस्टी) किसी पुरूष का किशोर के साथ गुदा-मैथुन करना। Sodomy, anal intercourse between a man and a young boy.

Pediatrics (पीडियाट्रिक्स) चिकित्सा-शास्त्र की वह शाखा जिसका सम्बन्ध बच्चों की देखभाल तथा उनके रोगों की चिकित्सा करने से होता है, बालरोग-विज्ञान। Pediatric, the branch of medical science which deals with the care and treatment of disease of the children.

Pedicle (पेडीकल) वृन्त। The stem attaching a new growth.

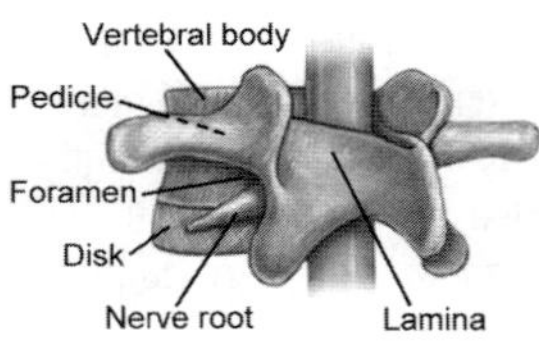

Pediculate (पेडीकुलेट) वृन्त या डण्ठल वाला, वृन्तमय। Having a pedicle.

Pediculosis (पेडीकुलोसिस) जुँओं से रोग हो जाना। Infestation with lice.

Pedicure (पेडीक्योर) पैरों की देखभाल करना। Care of the feet.

Pedionalgia (पेडीयोनैल्जिया) पैर के तलवे में तन्त्रिका-शूलपरक वेदना का होना। Neuralgic pain in the sole of the foot.

Pedodontics (पीडोडोन्टिक्स) शिशुदन्तचिकित्सा। Treating the teeth of the children.

Pedodontist (पीडोडोन्टिस्ट) शिशुदन्तचिकित्सक। A dentist who practices pedodontics.

Pedograph (पीडोग्राफ) कागज पर पाँव की छाप। An imprint of the foot on paper.

Peduncle (पेडन्किल) वृन्त, वतृक, बन्धन, रज्जु। A stalk like structure often acting as a support.

Peel (पील) छिलका। Bark.

Pejorative (पीज़ोरेटिव) बदतर बनने अथवा बनाने वाला। Becoming or making worse.

Pelage (पीलेज) शरीर का केश-जाल, लोम प्रणाली। The hair system of the body.

Peliosis (पीलियोसिस) चित्रता। Purpura.

Pellagra (पेलाग्रा) निकोटिनिक एसिड की कमी से होने वाला रोग जिसमें त्वकशोथ हो जाता है, दस्त आने लगते है तथा मनोभ्रंश हो जाता है। यह रोग विशेषकर उन लोगों में होता है जो केवल मक्का खाकर ही जीवित रहते है। A disease due to deficiency of nicotinic acid which is characterized by dermatitis diarrhea and dementia occurring mainly in the people who live upon maize only.

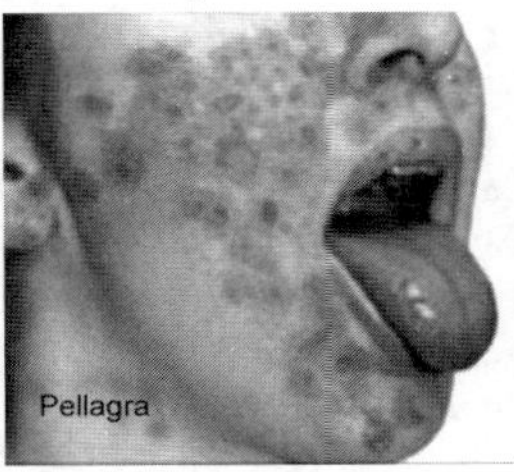
Pellagra

Pelotherapy (पिलोथिरैपी) शरीर पर कीचड़, मिट्टी का प्रयोग करके रोगों की चिकित्सा करना।

Treatment of the disease by the application of mud, clay, etc. on the body.

Pelvic girdle (पैल्विक गर्डिल) अनामी हड्डियों द्वारा बना चाप, श्रोणि-बन्ध। Arch formed by the innominate bones.

Pelvicaliceal (पैल्वीकैलीसियल) वृक्कीय श्रोणी एवं आलवालों से सम्बन्धित। Pertaining to the renal pelvis and the calyces.

Pelvimetry (पैल्वीमीट्री) श्रोणि की क्षमता एवं इसके व्यास को मापना, श्रोणिमिति। Measurement of the capacity and diameter of the pelvis.

Pelviperitonitis (पैल्वीपैरीटोनाइटिस) श्रोणि-पर्युदर्या का शोथ। Inflammation of the pelvic peritoneum.

Pelvis (पैल्विस) धड़ की निचली अस्थित रचना जो आगे तथा पार्श्व में कूल्हे की हड्डियों (इलियम, इस्कियम एवं प्यूबिस) एवं पीछे त्रिकास्थि और अनुत्रिक से मिलकर बनी होती है। गोणिका, श्रोणि। The lower bony structure of the trunk formed anteriorly and laterally by hip bones (ilium, ischium and pubis) and posteriorly by the sacrum and coccyx.

(*i*) **Android Pelvis** (एण्ड्रॉयड पैल्विस) पुंवत् श्रोणि। A masculine or funnel shaped pelvis, male type pelvis.

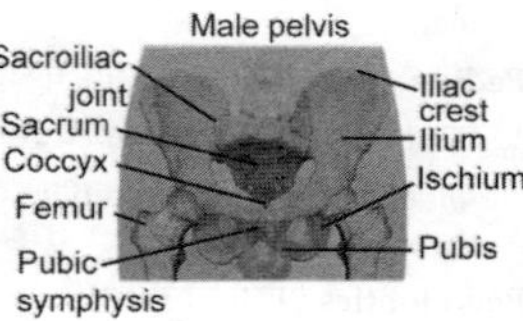

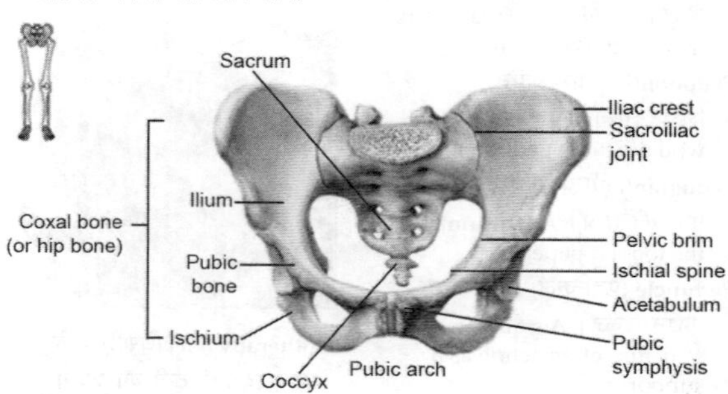

Pelvis

(*ii*) **Anthropoid Pelvis** (एन्थ्रोपॉयड-पैल्विस) एक स्त्री श्रोणिजो लम्बी एवं तंग होती है। A female pelvis which is long and narrow.

(*iii*) **Contracted Pelvis** (कॉन्ट्रेक्टेड-पैल्विस) संकुचित श्रोणि। A pelvis with less than normal measurements in any diameter.

(*iv*) **Cordate Pelvis** (कॉर्डेट पैल्विस) हृदय के आकार की श्रोणि ा। Heart-shaped pelvis.

(*v*) **Rachitic Pelvis** (रैकीटिक पैल्विस) रिकेट रोग से विकृत श्रोणि। The pelvis deformed from rickets.

Pelvisacral (पैल्वीसैक्रल) श्रोणि एवं त्रिकास्थि दोनों से सम्बन्धित। Pertaining to both the pelvis and the sacrum.

Pelvitherm (पैल्वीथर्म) योनि के द्वारा श्रोणि को गर्मी पहुँचाने के लिए एक उपकरण। An apparatus for applying heat to the pelvis through vagina.

Pemphigus (पेम्फीगस) पेम्फीगस नामक चर्म रोग, बिम्बिका, फफोला, छाला। A disease of the skin with an eruption of bullas.

Penetrance (पेनीट्रैन्स) वह दूरी जिसमें कोई वस्तु किसी वस्तु में घुसकर पार करती है। The extent to which something enters an object.

Penetrating (पेनीट्रेटिंग) किसी वस्तु की सतह में छेद करके उसमें प्रवेश करने वाला, वेधी। Entering an object by piercing its surface.

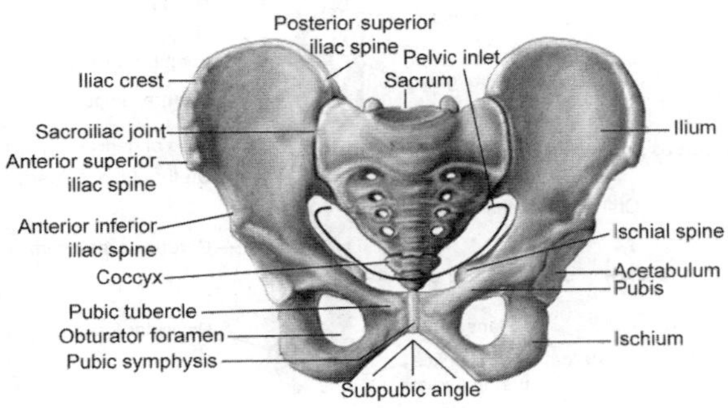

Anthropoid pelvis

Penicillium (पेनीसिलियम) कवकों का एक वंश जो रोटी, फल आदि पर नीले कवकच्छद (फफूँदी) के रूप में उग आते है। A genus of the fungi that grow on bread, fruit, etc. as blue molls.

Penis (पेनिस) शिश्न, लिंग। The male organ of copulation.

Penoscrotal (पेनोस्क्रोटल) शिश्न एवं वृषण सम्बन्धी। Pertaining to the penis and scrotum.

Pentadactyl (पेन्टाडैक्टाइल) प्रत्येक हाथ एवं पैर में पाँच अंगुलियाँ धारण करने वाला, पंचागुलिता। Possessing five digits in each hand and foot.

Pentavalent (पेन्टावैलेन्ट) पाँच की रासायनिक संयोजकता धारण करने वाला, पंचसंयोजी। Having a chemical valency of five.

Peotomy (पीयोटॉमी) लिंग को शल्यक्रिया द्वारा काट कर अलग कर देना। Surgical removal of penis.

Pepsin (पेप्सिन) जठर-रस का मुख्य एन्जाइम जो प्रोटीन को पेप्टोन तथा प्रोटीयोस में बदल देता है। The chief enzyme of the gastric juice which converts protein into peptones and proteoses.

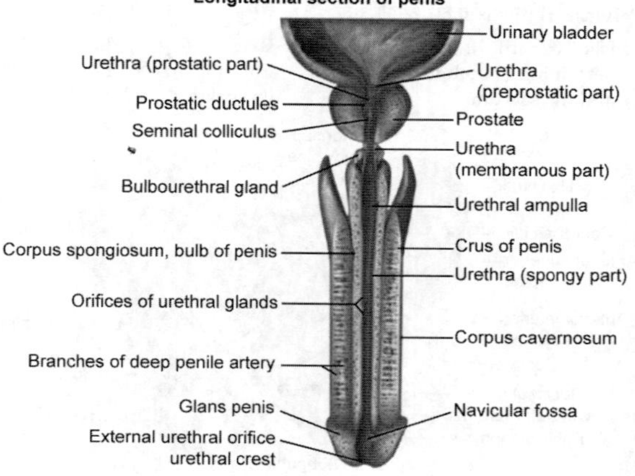

Penis

Pepsinogen (पेप्सिनोजन) पेप्सिन का पूर्वगामी। Precursor of pepsin.

Peptic ulcer (पेप्टिक अल्सर) आँत या पेट का फोड़ा अथवा घाव, उदरव्रण। Ulcer in the stomach or duodenum.

Peptone (पेप्टोन) नाइट्रोजनी यौगिक जो कुछ प्रोटीनों के ऊपर प्रोटीनसंलायी एन्जाइमों की क्रिया से उत्पन्न होते है। Nitrogenous compounds formed by action of proteolytic enzymes on certain proteins.

Per vias naturales (पर व्यास नेचुरल्स) प्राकृतिक मार्गों द्वारा। Through the natural ways.

Percept (परसेप्ट) देखी गई किसी वस्तु का मानसिक प्रतिबिम्ब, संवेदना। The mental image of an object seen.

Perception (परसैप्शन) प्रत्यक्ष ज्ञान, अवगम, बोध, अनुभूति। Receiving of an impression through the sense.

Perceptivity (परसैप्टीविटी) बोधगम्यता, अनुभूति क्षमता। Ability to receive impressions.

Percolate (पर्कोलेट) परिस्त्राव, रिसना। To subject, to percolation.

Percolator (पर्कोलेटर) परिस्रवण में प्रयोग में लाया जाने वाले एक उपकरण, परिस्रावित। An apparatus used in percolation.

Percussible (वर्कसीब्ल) परिताड़न द्वारा जिसका पता लगाया जा सके। Detectable by percussion.

Percussion (पर्कसन) शरीर के भीतर स्थित किसी संरचना की घनता, उसकी स्थिति एवं उसके परिमाण का पता लगाने के लिए शरीर के उस भाग को अंगुलियों के सिरों से पीटना।
The use of finger tips to tap the body directly or indirectly to determine position, size and consistency of underlying structure.

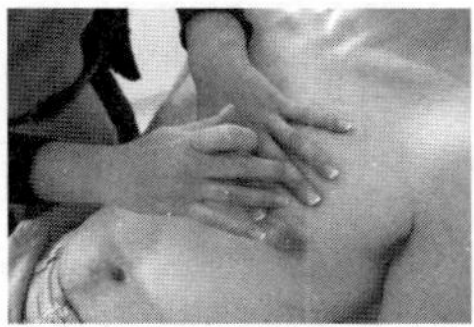

Percutaneous (परक्यूटेनियस) त्वचा के द्वारा, त्वचा प्रवेशी। Through skin.

Perforate (परफॉरेट) छेद करना, वेधना। To make holes.

Perforation (पर्फोरेशन) छेद करने की क्रिया। The process of making holes.

Perfusion (परफ्यूजन) किसी अंग अथवा ऊतक की रक्त पूर्ति करना। Supply of an organ/ tissue with blood.

Periadenitis (पैरीएडीनाइटिस) ग्रन्थि-ऊतकों का प्रदाह, परिलसीकापर्वशोथ। Inflammation of soft tissue surrounding the glands.

Perianal (पैरीएनल) गुदा के चारों ओर अथवा उसके पास, परिगुदीय। Surrounding the anus.

Periangiocholitis (पैरीएन्जियोकोलाइटिस) पित्त वाहिनियों के चारों ओर ऊतकों का शोथ। Inflammation of the tissue around the bile ducts.

Periarteritis (पैरीआर्टीराइटिस) धमनियों के बाहरी आवरण का प्रदाह, परिधमनीशोथ। Inflammation of the outer convering of the arteries.

Periarthric (पैरीआर्थिक) परिसन्धिक। Periarticular.

Periarthritis (पैरीआर्थ्राइटिस) किसी जोड़ के चारों के ओर के ऊतकों का शोथ। Inflammation of the tissue around a joint.

Periauricular (पैरीऑरीकुलर) बाह्य कर्ण के चारों ओर। Around the external ear.

Peribronchial (पैरीब्रोन्कियल) श्वासनली अथवा श्वासनलियों को चारों ओर से घेरने वाला। Surrounding a bronchus or bronchi.

Pericardial rub (पैरीकार्डियल) पुरोहृदीय क्षेत्र का परिश्रवण करने पर सुनाई देने वाली एक रगड़न की ध्वनि जो हृदयावरण की शोथयुक्त सतहों के आपस में रगड़ने से उत्पन्न होती है। A friction sound heard on auscultation of the precordial area when the inflamed surface of the pericardium rub against each other.

Pericardiectomy (पैरीक़ार्डियक्टॉमी) हृदयावरण के किसी भाग को काट कर निकाल देना, परिहृदुच्छेदन। Excision of a part of the pericardium.

Pericardiocentesis (पैरीकार्डियोसेन्टेसिस) शल्यक्रिया द्वारा हृदयावरण में छेद करना, परिहृदवेधन। Surgical perforation of the pericardium.

Pericardiopexy (पैरीकार्डियोपैक्सी) हृदय के रक्त की आपूर्ति बढ़ाने के लिए शल्यचिकित्सा द्वारा हृदयावरण को पास के किसी ऊतक से जोड़ दिया जाता है। To join the pericardium to an adjacent tissue to increase the blood supply to the heart by surgery.

Pericardiorrhaphy (पैरीकार्डियोरैह्फी) हृदयावरण में स्थित जख्म की सिलाई करना। Suture of a wound in the pericardium.

Pericardiosymphysis (पैरीकार्डियोसिम्फाइसिस)

अन्तरांगी एवं भित्तिक हृदयावरण के बीच आसंजन या चिपकाव हो जाना। Adhesion between the visceral and parietal pericardium.

Pericarditis (पैरीकार्डाइटिस) हृदय की झिल्ली का शोथ, हृदयावरणशोथ। Inflammation of pericardium.

Pericardium (पैरीकार्डियम) परिहृद, हृदयावरण। The fibroserous membrane covering the heart.

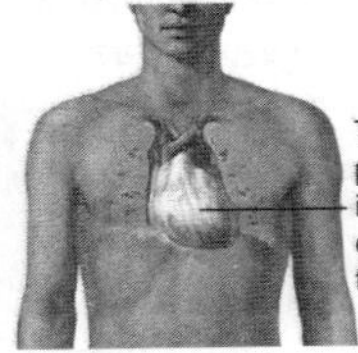

Pericecal (पैरीसीकल) सीकम या अन्धान्त्र के पास स्थित। Situated around the cecum.

Pericholecystitis (पैरीकोलीसिस्टाइटिस) पित्राशय के चारों ओर के ऊतकों का शोथ। Inflammation of the tissue around the gallbladder.

Perichondritis (पैरीकॉण्ड्राइटिस) पर्युपास्थिशोथ। Inflammation of the pericardium.

Perichondrium (पैरीकॉण्ड्रियम) पर्युपास्थि, उपास्थिआवरण, उपास्थ्यावरण। A membrane around a cartilage.

Pericolpitis (पैरीकोल्पाइटिस) योनि के चारों ओर के ऊतकों का शोथ। Inflammation of the tissues around the vagina.

Pericranium (पैरीक्रेनियम) कपाल का अस्थ्यावरण, परिकपाल। Periosteum of the skull.

Peridendritic (पैरीडैण्ड्राइटिक) किसी तंत्रिका कोशिका के पार्श्व तन्तु को चारों ओर घेरने वाला। Surrounding a dendrite of a nerve cell.

Peridural (पैरीड्यूरल) सुषुम्ना रज्जु के ड्यूरा मेटर या दृढ़तन्त्रिका के बाहर। Outside the dura mater of the spinal cord.

Perifalliculitis (पैरीफॉलीकुला. इटिस) रोम कूपों के चारों ओर का शोथ। Inflammation around the hair follicles.

Perigastric (पैरीगैस्ट्रिक) आमाशय के चारों ओर का। Surrounding the stomach.

Periglottis (पैरीग्लॉटिस) जीभ की श्लेष्मकला। The mucous membrane of tongue.

Perilaryngeal (पैरीलेरिन्जियल) स्वरयंत्र के आस-पास। Surrounding the larynx.

Perilenticular (पैरीलैन्टीकुलर) आँख के लैंस के चारों ओर। Around the lens of the eye.

Perimastitis (पैरीमेस्टाइटिस) किसी स्तन के चारों ओर के तन्तुमय ऊतक का शोथ। Inflammation of the fibrous tissue around a breast.

Perimetric (पैरीमीट्रिक) परिगर्भाशयऊति से सम्बन्धित। Pertaining to the perimetrium.

Perineal (पैरीनियल) मूलाधार से सम्बन्धित।
Pertaining to the perineum.

Perineorrhaphy (पैरीनियोरैह्फी) मूलाधार की सिलाई करना। Suture of the perineum.

Perineotomy (पैरिनियोटॉमी) मूलाधार छेदन।
To make an incision into the perineum.

Perinephric (पैरीनिफ्रिक) वृक्क के पास, परिवृक्कीय। Surrounding the kidney.

Perineum (पैरीनियम) श्रोणि-भूतल, एवं श्रोणि-बर्हिगम को घेरने वाली रचनाएँ।
The structures accruing the pelvic outlet and constituting pelvic floor.

Perineural (पैरीन्यूरल) किसी तंत्रिका के चारों ओर।
Around a nerve.

Perineurium (पैरीन्यूरियम) परितंत्रिका, तंत्रिकावरण।
A sheath investing a funiculus of a nerve fiber.

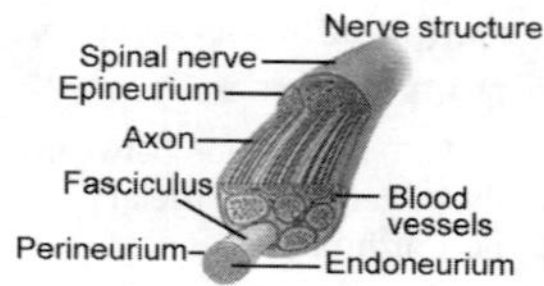

Period (पीरियड) मासिक धर्म, काल, अवधि। The menstruation, the time interval between two events.

(*i*) **Gestation Period** (जेस्टेशन पीरियड) गर्भावस्था-काल। Period of pregnancy (*ii*) **Incubation Period** (इनक्यूबेशन-पीरियड) रोगोद्भवन काल, उद्भवन काल। The period between implantation of a contagium and the appearance of a disease latent period. (*iii*) **Missed Period** (मिस्ड पीरियड) अपने संभावित समय पर मासिक-धर्म न होना। Absence of menstruation as its expected time.

(*iv*) **Safe Period** (सेफ पीरियड) आर्तव-चक्र या मासिक-चक्र में वह समय जब गर्भाधान नहीं हो सकता। The time during the menstrual cycle when conception is not possible.

Periodicity (पीरियोडीसिटी) निश्चित समयावकाशों के बाद पुनःउत्पन्न होना, आवर्तिता। Recurrence after definite intervals of time.

Periodontal (पैरीओडोन्टल) परिदन्तीय, दान्तों के चारों ओर का। Around teeth.

Periodontics (पैरिओडोन्टिक्स) दान्तों के समीपवर्ती ऊतकों के रोगों की चिकित्सा, परिदन्तोंपचार। Treatment of the disease of the tissue around the teeth.

Periodontitis (पैरीओडोन्टाइटिस) परिदनतशोथ। Inflammation of the periodontium.

Periodontium (पैरीओडोन्टियम) परिदन्त, दन्तावरण। A fibrous envelope of the cementum.

Periomphalic (पैरीओम्फेलिक) नाभि के चारों ओर अथवा उसके पास स्थित। Situated around or near the umbilicus.

Perionychia (पैरीयोनीकिया) किसी नाखून के चारों ओर का शोथ। Inflammation around a nail.

Perioperative (पैरीऑप्रेटिव) ऑपरेशन के समय के आस-पास। Paraoperative, around the time of operation.

Perioral (पैरीओरल) मुँह के चारों ओर। Circumoral, around the mouth.

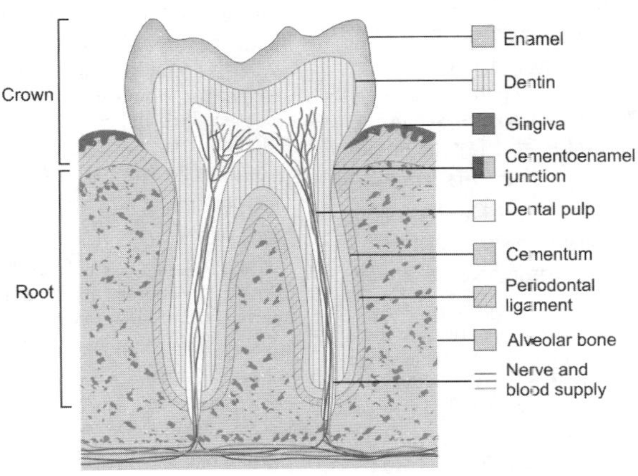

Periodontium

Periosteum (पैरीऑस्टियम) हड्डियों को ढक कर रखने वाली तन्तु-कला। A fibrous membrane investing bones.

Periostitis (पैरीऑस्टाइटिस) अस्थि-आवरक झिल्ली का प्रदाह, अस्थ्यावरण्यशोथ। Inflammation of the periosteum, a layer of connective tissue that surrounds bone.

Periovular (पैरीओव्यूलर) डिम्ब के चारों ओर। Around an ovum.

Peripatetic (पैरीपैटेटिक) एक स्थान से दूसरे स्थान को गति करने वाला। Moving from one place to another.

Periphakus (पैरीफेकस) नेत्र लैन्स के चारों ओर स्थित सम्पुट या कैप्सूल। The capsule surrounding the eye lens.

Peripheral nervous system (पैरीफ्रल नर्वस सिस्टम) तंत्रिका-तंत्र का केन्द्रीय तंत्रिका-तंत्र से बाहर का भाग जिसमें 12 जोड़ी कपालीय तंत्रिकाओं तथा 31 जोड़ी मेरूतंत्रिकाओं का समावेश होता है। The portion of the nervous system outside the central nervous system which consist of 12 pairs of the cranial nerves and 31 pairs of the spinal nerves.

Periphlebitis (पैरीफ्लेबाइटिस) शिरा की बाहरी झिल्ली का प्रदाह, परिशिराशोथ। Inflammation of the outer coat of a vein.

Periproctic (पैरीप्रोक्टिक) मलद्वार के चारो ओर। Around the anus.

Perisalpingitis (पैरीसैल्पिन्जाइटिस) डिम्ब वाहिनी के चारो ओर के ऊतकों का शोथ। Inflammation of the tissue around the fallopian tube.

Perisinous (पैरीसाइनुअस) किसी विवर के चारो ओर का। Surrounding a sinus.

Perisplanchnitis (पैरीस्प्लैंकनाइटिस) अन्तरांगों के चारों ओर के ऊतकों का शोथ। Inflammation of the tissue around the viscera.

Peristalsis (पैरिस्टैल्सिस) पुरःसरण, क्रमाकुंचन, लहर जैसी गति। Wavelike motion as of esophagus, stomach and intestines which keeps the food material moving.

Peristasis (पैरिस्टेसिस) शोथ की प्रारम्भिक अवस्था में रोगग्रस्त स्थान में रक्त प्रवाह में कमी हो जाना। The decrease in blood flow in the affected area in the early stage of inflammation.

Peristoma (पैरिस्टोमा) मुँह के चारों ओर का किनारा। The margin of a mouth.

Peritomy (पैरीटॉमी) स्वच्छमण्डल की परिधि के चारों ओर नेत्रश्लेष्मा में चीरा लगाना,

परिछेदन। To make an incision into the conjunctiva around the circumference of cornea.

Peritoneoclysis (पैरीटोनियोक्लाइसिस) इन्जैक्शन द्वारा तरल को पैरीटोनियम-गुहा में प्रविष्ट करना। To introduce the fluid into the peritoneal cavity by injection.

Peritoneopexy (पैरीटोनियोपैक्सी) पैरीटोनियम का स्थिरीकरण। Fixation of the peritoneum.

Peritoneoscope (पैरीटोनियोस्कोप) पर्युदर्यादर्शी, उदरावणदर्शी यंत्र। An instrument for performing laparoscopy.

Peritoneum (पैरीटोनियम) पर्युदर्या, उदरावरण। A thin smooth membrane that invest the whole internal surface of the abdomen and the organs contained in that cavity.

Peritonitis (पैरिटोनाइटिस) पैरीटोनियम की सूजन, उदरावरणशोथ। Inflammation of the peritoneum.

Peritonsillar (पैरीटॉन्सिलर) किसी टॉन्सिल के चारों ओर, परिगतुण्डिकीय। Around a tonsil.

Peritracheal (पैरीट्रेकियल) श्वास-प्रणाल के चारों ओर। Around the trachea.

Peritrichous (पैरीट्राइकस) एककोशिकाय जीवों का एक वर्ग जिनकी सम्पूर्ण सतह पर कशाभ या रोमक लगे होते है। A group of unicellular organisms having flagella or cilia over the entire surface.

Periurethral (पैरीयूरेथ्रल) मूत्रमार्ग के आस-पास स्थित, परिमूत्रपथीय। Situated around the urethra.

Perivaginal (पैरीवैजाइनल) योनि के चारों ओर, परियोनिक। Around the vagina.

Perivisceritis (पैरीविस्त्राइटिस) अंतरंगों को प्रभावित करने वाला प्रदाह, पर्यतरांगशोथ। Inflammation surrounding any viscus or viscera.

Perlingual (परलिंगुअल) जीभ के द्वारा, औषधियाँ देने की एक विधि। Through the tongue a method of administration of medicines.

Permeability (पर्मियेब्रिलिटी) पारगम्यता। The quality of being permeable.

Pernicious (पर्नीशियस) प्रणाशी, विनाशकारी। Fatal destructive.

Pernicious anemia (पर्नीशियस एनीमिया) प्रणाशी रक्ताल्पता, घातक अरक्तता, सांघतिक अरक्तता। Results from the inability of the bone marrow to produce normal red cells because of the deprivation of a protein released by gastric glands.

Pernio (पर्नियो) शीतदंश, बिवाई फटना। A chilblain, frostbite.

Perocormus (पेरोकोर्मस) ऐसा व्यक्ति, जिसका जन्म से धड़ विकृत होता है। An individual with a congenitally deformed trunk.

Peroneal (पेरोनियल) बहिर्जंघिकीय, बहिर्जंघिका सम्बन्धी। Pertaining to the fibula.

Peropus (पेरोपस) ऐसा व्यक्ति जिसके जन्म से ही पाद विकृत होते है। An individual with congenital deformed feet.

Peroral (परोरल) मुख द्वारा प्रयुक्त, मुखी। Administered through the mouth.

Perosseous (परोसियस) किसी हड्डी से होकर। Through a bone.

Personality (पर्सनैलिटी) व्यक्तित्व। The various mental attitude characteristics which distinguish a person.

Perspiration (पर्सपिरेशन) स्वेदन, स्वेद, पसीना। Sweating.

Pertusis (पर्टुसिस) काली खाँसी, कूकरखाँसी। Whooping cough.

Perversion (परवर्जन) सामान्य मार्ग से हट जाना, विपर्यास, उलट जाना। A turning away from the normal way.

Pervert (परवर्ट) सामान्य मार्ग से हटाना। To turn from the normal way.

Pervious (पर्वियस) प्रवेश्य, पारगम्य। Permitting penetration.

Pes (पेस) पद, पाद, पैर या पैर जैसा। A foot or foot like structure.

Pes cavus (पेस केवस) ऐसा पाद जिसमें असामान्य रूप से खोखला तलवा होता है। A foot with abnormally hollow sole.

Pes equines (पेस इक्वीनस) ऐसा पाद जिसमें ऐड़ी पृथ्वी से स्पर्श नहीं करती है ओर रोगी केवल अँगुलियां के सहारे ही चलता है। The foot in which heel does not touch the earth and the patient walks on toes only.

Pes equinovalgus (पेस इक्वीनोवैल्गस) ऐसा पाद जिसमें ऐड़ी ऊपर को उठी इुई एवं बाहर की ओर घूमी हुई होती है। Talipes equinovalgus, the foot in which the heel is elevated and turned outward.

Pes equinovarus (पेस इक्वीनोवेस) ऐसा पाद जिसमें ऐड़ी नीचे की ओर होती है तथा तलवा भूमि से ऊपर को उठा होता है, अन्तर्नतवाद। The foot in which heel remains downward and the sole is elevated from the earth.

Pest (पेस्ट) विनाशकारी कीट, बाधा, पीड़क। Destructive insect.

Pesticide (पेस्टीसाइड) विनाशक, जीवनाशी। Substances which kill pests.

Pestis (पेस्टिस) प्लेग। Plague.

Petechia (पेटीचिया) सूक्ष्म मात्रा में रक्त के मुक्त होने से त्वचा पर बना एक सूक्ष्म लाल धब्बा, रूधिरांक। Plural is petechiae a minute red spot on the skin due to escape of a small amount of blood.

Petechiae (पेटीची) पेटीचिया का बहुवचन। Plural of petechia.

Petit mal (पेटिट माल) मिर्गी का हल्का दौरा, मृदु-अपस्मार। Minor epilepsy in which the momentary loss of consciousness is characteristic.

Petrifaction (पैट्रीफैक्शन) कठोर पदार्थ अथवा पत्थर में परिवर्तित होने की क्रिया। The process of changing into hard substance or stone.

Petrissage (पेट्रीसाज) मालिश में गूँधना एवं पेशियों को दबाना। Kneading and pressing of the muscles in massage.

Petromastoid (पीट्रोमैस्टॉयड) अश्मकर्णमूल। The petrous and mastoid portions of the temporal bone.

Petrositis (पीट्रोसाइटिस) शंखास्थि के अश्माभ भाग का शोथ। Inflammation of the petrous portion of the temporal bone.

Petrous (पीट्रस) पत्थर के समान, अश्माभ। Petrosal, resembling stone.

Peyer's patch (पीयर्स पैच) लसीका पर्विकाओं का एक समूह जो मूख्य रूप से छोटी आँत के इलियम के कोलन के साथ संगन पर पाया जाता है। An aggregation of lymph nodules found chiefly in the ileum of the small intestine near its junction with the colon.

pH (पीएच) किसी पदार्थ की अम्लता अथवा क्षारता के डिग्री को व्यक्त करने वाला एक प्रतीक। A symbol for expressing the degree of acidity or alkalinity of a substance.

Phacocele (फैकोसील) नेत्र के अग्र कोष्ठ में स्फटिकाभ लैन्स का विस्थापन। Displacement of the crystalline lens into the anterior chamber of the eye.

Phacoemulsification (फैकोइमल्सीफिकेशन) मोतियाबिन्द की चिकित्सा की एक विधि। A method of treatment of cataract.

Phacoerysis (फैकोइराइसिस) चूशण द्वारा आँख के लैन्स को निकलना, लैन्सचूषण। Removal of the eye lens by suction.

Phacomalacia (फैकोमैलेसिया) आँख के लैन्स का कोमल हो जाना। Softening of the eye lens.

Phacosclerosis (फैकोस्क्लेरोसिस) नेत्र लैन्स का कठोर होना। Hardening of the eye lens.

Phacoscotasmus (फैकोस्कोटेस्मस) नेत्र लैन्स का धुँधला हो जाना। Clouding of the eye lens.

Phage (फेज़) जीवाणुभोजी। Eating bacteria.

Phagocyte (फेगोसाइट) भक्षककोशिका, भक्षकाणु, जीवणुभक्षी, जीवाणुनाशक। A white blood cell which destroys bacteria and tissue debris.

Phagocytosis (फगोसाइटोसिस) भक्षक कोशिका क्रिया। Ingestion and digestion of bacteria and foreign particles by phagocytes.

Phagophobia (फेगोफोबिया) खाने का रोगोत्पादक भय। Morbid fear of eating.

Phagosome (फैगोसोम) एक भक्षकोशिका में विद्यमान एक कला-परिबंध रिक्तिका जिसमें पचने वाली सामग्री होती है। A membrane bound vesicle in phagocyte containing the material to be digested.

Phakoma (फैकोमा) ट्यूबेरस स्क्लेरोसिस में रेटिना में कभी-कभी पाया जाने वाला एक सूक्ष्मदर्शी भूरा-सा सफेद अबुर्द। A microscopic grayish white tumor present occasionally in the retina in tuberous sclerosis.

Phalangette (फैलेन्जेट) किसी अँगुली की दूरस्थ अँगुल्यस्थि। The distal phalanx of a digit.

Phalanx (फैलेंक्स) हाथ अथवा पैर की किसी अँगुली की कोई हड्डी, अंगुल्यस्थि। Any bone of a finger or toe.

Phallagia (फैलेजिया) शिश्न में शूल होना। Pain in the penis.

Phallocompsis (फैलोक्ैम्पसिस) उत्थान के समय लिंग का वेदनायुक्त नीचे की ओर मुड़ जाना। Painful downward curvature of penis during erection.

Phallus (फैलस) लिंग, शिश्न। The penis.

Phaloid (फैलॉयड) किसी लिंग के समान। Like penis.

Phaneromania (फैनेरोमैनिया) नाखूनों को काटने अथवा नोचने, बाल, दाढ़ी, मूँछ, फुन्सी अथवा अधिमांस को खरोंचने या खींचने की प्रवृत्ति। A tendency for biting the nails or pricking, scratching or pulling a hair, beard, moustache, a pimple or wart.

Phanerosis (फेनेरोसिस) दृष्टिगोचर होने की क्रिया, व्यक्तता। The process of becoming visible.

Phantasy (फैन्टेसी) दिवास्वप्न, स्वैरकल्पना। A daydream or desire good for reality.

Phantom (फैन्टम) ऐसी वस्तु का आशय अथवा भ्रम होना जिसका कोई अस्तित्व नहीं होता। An apparition or illusion of something that does not exist.

Pharmaceutics (फार्मेस्युटिक्स) औषधि बनाने की विधि, औषधि निर्माण विज्ञान। Pertaining to the art of preparing or using, dispending of drugs and dosage.

Pharmacodynamics (फार्मेकोडाइनामिक्स) भेशजक्रिया विज्ञान। The science that relates to the action of the drugs.

Pharmacognasy (फार्मेकोग्नोसी) औषध-प्रकृति विज्ञान। The science of natural drugs and their properties.

Pharmacology (फार्मेकोलॉजी) औषधियों का वैज्ञानिक अध्ययन, भेषजगुणविज्ञान। The science of drugs in all their relations.

Pharmacomania (फार्मेकोमैनिया) औषधियाँ लेने अथवा देने की तीव्र इच्छा होना। Uncontrollable desire for taking or giving the medicines.

Pharmacy (फार्मेसी) भेषजी, वह स्थान जहाँ औषधियों का निर्माण किया जाता है। The act of preparation and dispensing drug.

Pharyngalgia (फैरिन्जैल्जिया) ग्रसनी या गले में दर्द होना, ग्रसनीपीड़ा। Pharyngodynia pain in the pharynx.

Pharyngismus (फैरिन्जिस्मस) ग्रसनी में पेशियों की ऐंठन होना, ग्रसनी आकर्ष। Spasm of the muscles in the pharynx.

Pharyngitis (फैरिन्जाइटिस) ग्रसनीशोथ, गलकोषप्रदाह। Inflammation of the pharynx.

Pharyngoamygdalitis (फैरिन्जोएमाइग्डेलाइटिस) गले एवं टॉन्सिल की सूजन। Inflammation of the pharynx and tonsil.

Pharyngography (फैरिन्जोग्राफी) किसी एक्स-रे अभेद्य पदार्थ को निगलने के पश्चात् ग्रसनी का एक्स-रे परीक्षण करना। X-ray examination of the pharynx after ingestion of a radiopaque substance.

Pharyngoparalysis (फैरिन्जोपैरालाइसिस) ग्रसनी की पेशियों का पक्षाघात होना, ग्रसनीघात। Paralysis of the muscles of the pharynx.

Pharyngoplasty (फैरिन्जोप्लास्टी) प्लास्टिक सर्जरी द्वारा गले की मरम्मत करना। Repair of the pharynx by plastic surgery.

Pharyngorrhea (फैरिन्जोरिह्या) ग्रसनी से श्लेष्मा स्राव होना। Mucus discharge from the pharynx.

Pharyngostenosis (फैरिन्जोस्टेनोसिस) ग्रसनी का तंग होना। Narrowing of the pharynx.

Pharynx (फैरिंक्स) ग्रसनी, गलकोष, वायु के लिए नासा-गुहाओं के पीछे से स्वरयंत्र तक तथा भोजन के लिए मुख से ग्रासनली तक पेशीकलामय मार्ग। A muscle membranous passage for air behind the nasal cavities to the larynx and for food mouth to esophagus.

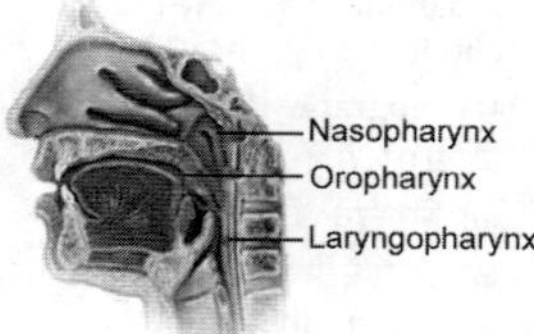

Phase (फेज) विकास की कोई अवस्था, प्रावस्था। A stage of development.

Phasphaturia (फॉस्फेचूरिया) मूत्र में फॉस्फेटों का अधिक पाया जाना, फॉस्फेटमेह।
An excess of phosphates in the urine.

Phasphopenia (फॉस्फोपीनिया) शरीर में फॉस्फोरस की कमी हो जाना। Deficiency of phosphorus in the body.

Phenodynamics (फीनोडाइनामिक्स) सांस लेने की यान्त्रिकाविधि। The mechanism of breathing.

Phenol (फीनोल) दर्शव, प्रांगविक अम्ल, कार्बोलिक अम्ल, फेनिक एसिड। Carbolic acid, a powerful antiseptic widely used as a 1 in 20 solution phenic acid.

Phenomenon (फीनोमेनन) लक्षण, घटना क्रम, घटनाचक्र। A symptom, an occurrence of any short in relation to a disease.

Phenotype (फीनोटाइप) समलक्षणी, ऐसे व्यक्ति जिनमें भिन्न पैत्रिकता होते हुए भी समान लक्षण मिलते है। Persons of like characteristics though of different heredity.

Pneumoarthrography (न्यूमोआरथ्रोग्राफी) भेदक माध्यम के रूप में सन्धि में वायु अथवा गैस का इन्जैक्शन लगाकर सन्धि का लिया गया एक्स-रे चित्र। X-ray film of a joint after an injection of air or gas into the joint as contrast medium.

Phial (फॉयल) काचकूपिका, लघुकूपी, छोटी शीशी। A small glass bottle, a vial.

Philtrum (फिलट्रम) ओष्ठरवात। The vertical groove in the middle of the upper lip.

Phimosis (फाइमोसिस) शिश्नमुण्डच्छद के छिद्र का संकुचित हो जाना जिससे यह शिश्नमुण्ड के ऊपर नहीं खीचा जा सकता, निरूद्ध प्रकाश। Constriction of the orifice of the prepuce preventing it from being drawn over the glans penis.

Phlebalgia (फ्लेबैल्जिया) किसी शिरा में उठने वाला दर्द। Pain arising from a vein.

Phlebectomy (फ्लेबेक्टॉमी) किसी शिरा को काट कर हटा देना, शिरा-उच्छेदन। Excision of a segment of a vein, venectomy.

Phlebectopia (फ्लेबेक्टोपिया) किसी शिरा की असामान्य स्थिति। Abnormal position of a veins.

Phlebitis (फ्लेबाइटिस) शिराशोथ, शिराप्रदाह। Inflammation of a vein.

Phlebogram (फ्लेबोग्राम) शिरालेख, शिराचित्र।
A radiograph of venous system.

Phlebography (फ्लेबोग्राफी) शिराओं की रचना एवं उनके कार्य का अध्ययन, शिराचित्रण। Study of the structure and function of the veins.

Phlebolith (फ्लेबोलिथ) किसी शिरा में स्थित पथरी, शिराश्मरी। A calculus in a vein.

Phleborrhagia (फ्लेबोरैह्जिया) किसी शिरा से रक्तस्राव होना। Bleeding from a vein.

Phlebosclerosis (फ्लेबोस्क्लेरोसिस) किसी शिरा की भित्तियों की तन्तुमय कठोरता, शिराकाठिन्य। Fibrous hardening of the walls of a vein.

Phlebostenosis (फ्लेबोस्टेनोसिस) शिरा का संकुचित होना। Constriction of a vein.

Phlebotome (फ्लेबोटोम) शिरा में चिरा लगाने वाला एक यंत्र, शिरोछेदक। An instrument for incising a vein.

Phlegmasia (फ्लेग्मेसिया) शोथ या सूजन। Inflammation.

Phlegmon (फ्लेग्मोन) संयोजी ऊतक का तीव्र विस्तृत शोथ, शोथव्रण। A cute diffuse inflammation of the connective tissue.

Phlyctenula (फ्लाइक्टेनुला) सुक्ष्मक्षुद्रकोष, छोटा-सा फफोला या छाला। A minute vesicle or phlyctenule.

Phlyctenulosis (फ्लाइक्टेनुलोसिस) बहुत से सूक्ष्मक्षुद्रकोषों का बनना। Formation of numerous phlyctenules.

Phobia (फोबिया) किसी भी वस्तु का विकृत अथवा रोगोत्पादक भय या उससे अत्यधिक घृणा होना, भीति। Morbid fear of or a version to an object.

Phonal (फोनल) वाणी सम्बन्धी। Pertaining to the voice.

Phonation (फोनेशन) ध्वनन, ध्वनि-निस्सारण, ध्वनि-उच्चारण, शब्दोच्चार। The emission of vocal sound.

Phonetics (फोनेटिक्स) ध्वनि विज्ञान। The study of vocal sound.

Phono receptor (फोनो रिसेप्टर) ध्वनिग्राही। A receptor for sound stimuli.

Phonocardiogram (फोनोकार्डियोग्राम) हृदय ध्वनियों का रेखाचित्र अभिलेख बनाना, हृद्ध्वनिलेख। The graphic record of heart sound.

Phonophobia (फोनोफोबिया) आवाजों अथवा शोरगुल का विकृत भय। Morbid fear of the sound or noise.

Phonophoresis (फोनोफोरेसिस) किसी ऊतक में किसी औषधि को त्वचा के जरिए समावेषित कराने के लिए अल्ट्रासाउण्ड का प्रयोग करना। Use of ultrasound to enhance the topically applied drugs into tissue.

Phosphate (फॉस्फेट) फॉस्फोरिक अम्ल का एक लवण। A salt of phosphoric acid.

Phosphorism (फॉस्फोरिज्म) फॉस्फोरस से उत्पन्न जीर्ण विषाक्तता। Chronic poisoning from phosphorus.

Photalgia (फोटेल्जिया) प्रकाश से दर्द होना जैसे आँख में, दीप्ति नेत्रशूल। Pain produced by light as in the eye.

Photism (फोटिज्म) किसी वस्तु के सुनने, उसके चखने, सूँघने अथवा त्वचा द्वारा उसके स्पर्श के प्रभाव से दृष्टि-संवेदना का उत्पन्न होना। Visual sensation produced by the effect of something heard, tasted, smelled or felt by touch.

Photobiotic (फोटोबायोटिक) प्रकाश में जीवित रहने वाला, प्रकाशजीवी। Living only in the light.

Photocoagulation (फोटोकोगुलेशन) प्रकाश-स्कन्दन। Light energy used to coagulate tissue proteins as in retinal detachment or diabetic proliferating retinopathy.

Photodermatitis (फोटोडर्माटाइटिस) अल्ट्रा-वॉयलेट प्रकाश के कारण त्वचा का शोथ। Skin allergy due to ultraviolet light.

Photoerythema (फोटोइरीद्मा) प्रकाश द्वारा उत्पन्न त्वकरिक्तमा। Erythema of the skin produced by light.

Photogen (फोटोजन) ऐसा सूक्ष्मजीव जिससे प्रकाश की चमक निकलती है। A microorganism that produce luminescence.

Photokinetic (फोटोकाइनेटिक) प्रकाश के उद्दीपन से प्रतिक्रिया करने वाला जिससे उसकी गतियों में परिवर्तन हो जाता है। Reacting with alteraction in movement to stimulus of light.

Photomania (फोटोमैनिया) रोशनी के लिए पागल बने रहना, प्रकाशोन्माद। Mania for light.

Photometer (फोटोमीटर) प्रकाश की तीव्रता के मापने का यंत्र, प्रकाशमापी। An instrument for measuring the intensity of light.

Photomicrography (फोटोमाइक्रोग्राफी) सूक्ष्म-दर्शीफोटोग्राफ। Photograph of an object under microscope.

Photophobia (फोटोफोबिया) प्रकाश का असामान्य रूप से सहन न होना, प्रकाशभीति। Abnormal intolerance of light.

Photopsia (फोटोप्सिया) प्रकाशभास, प्रकाशानुभूति। Subjective sensation of light photopsy.

Photoptometer (फोटोप्टोमीटर) किसी वस्तु को देखने के लिये आवश्यक प्रकाश की न्यूनतम मात्रा को मापने वाला एक उपकरण। An instrument for measuring the smallest amount of light to make an object visible.

Photoreception (फोटोरिसैप्शन) प्रकाश का ज्ञान होना। Perception of light.

Photoreceptor (फोटोरिसैप्टर) प्रकाश के प्रति संवेदनशील एक संवेदी तंत्रिका अन्त। A sensory nerve ending sensitive to light.

Photoretinitis (फोटोरेटिनाइटिस) तीव्र प्रकाश में अनावृत होने से उत्पन्न दृष्टिपटल की सूजन। Inflammation of the retina due to exposure to intense light.

Photosensitive (फोटोसैंन्सीटिव) प्रकाशसुग्राही। Sensitive to light.

Photosensitizer (फोटोसैन्सीटाइज़र) वह पदार्थ जो प्रकाश से संयुक्त होकर शरीर में सुग्राहिता प्रतिक्रिया उत्पन्न करता है। A substance in which combination with light causes sensitivity reaction in the body.

Photosynthesis (फोटोसिन्थेसिस) प्रकाश-संश्लेषण। The process by plants combine water and trapped carbon dioxide to produce carbohydrates.

Phototherapy (फोटोथिरैपी) प्रकाश के प्रति अनावृत करके रोग की चिकित्सा करना। Treatment of disease by exposure to light.

Phototropism (फोटोट्रॉपिज्म) किसी जीव अथवा पौधे की प्रकाश की ओर घूम जाने अथवा गति करने की प्रवृति। The tendency of an organism or a plant to turn or move toward the light.

Phren (फ्रेन) मस्तिष्क, मध्यपट। The mind and diaphragm.

Phrenemphraxis (फ्रेनेम्फ्रेक्सिस) मध्यच्छद-तंत्रिका संदलन। Crushing of the phrenic nerve.

Phrenic (फ्रेनिक) मस्तिष्क से सम्बन्धित, मध्यच्छदीय। Pertaining to the diaphragm or to the mind.

Phrenicotomy (फ्रेनिकोटॉमी) शल्यक्रिया द्वारा फ्रेनिक तंत्रिका को विभाजित करना। Surgical division of the phrenic nerve.

Phrenitis (फ्रेनाइटिस) मस्तिष्क का प्रदाह। Inflammation of the brain.

Phrenodynia (फ्रेनोडाइनिया) मध्यपट में दर्द होना। Pain in the diaphragm.

Phrenoptosis (फ्रेनोप्टोसिस) मध्यपट का नीचे की ओर विस्थापित हो जाना। Downward displacement of the diaphragm.

Phthisic (थाइसिक) यक्ष्माग्रस्त, क्षयग्रस्त, तपेदिक से पीड़ित। Concerning pulmonary tuberculosis.

Phylum (फाइलम) जन्तु अथवा पादप जगत का एक प्राथमिक विभाग जो किसी वर्ग से अगला ही ऊँचा विभाग होता है। संघ। A primary division of the animal or plant kingdom next high than a class.

Physiatrist (फिजियाट्रिस्ट) भौतिक चिकित्सा विज्ञान का विशेषज्ञ। A specialist in physiatrics.

Physical (फिज़िकल) भौतिक, शारीरिक। Relating to the physic or the body.

Physician (फिजिशियन) चिकित्सक, कायचिकित्सक। One who treats disease or patients.

Physicist (फिज़िसिस्ट) चिकित्सक, वैद्य। A physician.

Physics (फिज़िक्स) भौतिक विज्ञान, भौतिकी, भौतिकशास्त्र। The science of inorganic matters and its forces.

Physiocopyrexia (फिज़ियोकोपाइरैक्सिया) भौतिक विधियों द्वारा उत्पन्न किया गया कृत्रिम ज्वर। Artificial fever produced by physical means.

Physiological (फिजियोलॉजिकल) शरीर के कार्य से सम्बन्धित, शरीर क्रियात्मक। Concerning body function.

Physiology (फिजियोलॉजी) शरीर क्रिया विज्ञान, शरीरवृत्ति। The science of the function of the body.

Physique (फ़िज़ीक) शारीरिक गठन। Body constitution.

Physometra (फाइसोमीट्रा) गर्भाशय-गुहा में वायु या गैस का पाया जाना, वायु-गर्भाशयता। Air or gas in the uterine cavity.

Pica (पिका) किसी विशेष प्रकार के भोजन की इच्छा, दोहद। Desire for extraordinary articles of food.

Picomole (पिकोमोल) एक मोल का दस खरबवॉ भाग। One trillionth of a mole.

Pigeon breast (पिजीयोन ब्रेस्ट) कपोतवक्ष। Sternum projecting forward due to ricket or childhood respiratory obstruction.

Pigment (पिग्मैन्ट) शरीर में स्थित कोई भी रंजन द्रव्य, वर्णक, रंजक। Any coloring matter in the body.

Pigmented (पिग्मैंटेड) वर्णकयुक्त। Colored by deposit of pigments.

Piitis (पाइटिस) मृदुतानिकाशोथ। Inflammation of the pia mater.

Piles (पाइल्स) एक अकेला अर्श (बवासीर), बाल। A single hemorrhoid, the hair.

Pili (पाइली) रोम, केश, बाल। Hair.

Piliation (पिलिएशन) बालों का बनना व विकसित होना। Formation and development of hair.

Piliform (पिलीफार्म) बालों के समान। Like hair.

Pill (पिल) औषधि का एक छोटा-सा गोलाकार अथवा अण्डाकार पिण्ड जिसे निगल लिया जाता है। A small globular or oval mass of medicine to be swallowed or chewed.

Pillar (पिलर) स्तम्भ। A supporting column.

Pillion (पिलीयोन) एक अस्थायी कृत्रिम पैर। A tempcrary artificial leg.

Piloerection (पाइलोइरैक्शन) बालों का खड़ा होना। Erec:ion of hairs.

Pilomotor (पाइलोमोटर) बालों को हिलाने-डुलाने वाला। Causing movements of the hairs.

Pimelitis (पाइमेलाइटिस) वसीय ऊतक का शोथ। Inflammation of the adipose tissue.

Pimelosis (पाइमेलोसिस) वसामयता, वसापजनन। Adiposis fatty degeneration.

Pimple (पिम्पिल) फुन्सी, पुटिका, मुँहासा। A small pustule, boil or papule.

Pineal body (पीनियल बॉडी) मस्तिष्क में महासंयोजिका की पट्टिका के नीचे एक थैली में

स्थित एक छोटी, चीड़ के शंकु के आकार की, ग्रन्थि के समान रचना। It is a small gland like structure in the brain shaped like a pine cone situated in a pocket below the splenium of corpus callosum.

Pinealoma (पीनियालोमा) पीनियल काय का एक अबुर्द जो कालपूर्व यौवनारम्भ से सम्बन्धित होता है। A tumor of the pineal body which is associated with precocious puberty.

Pineocytoma (पीनियोसाइटोमा) मस्तिष्क की पीनियल ग्रन्थि का एक दुर्दम अबुर्द। A malignant tumor of the pineal gland of the brain.

Pinguecula (पिंग्युइकुला) कन्दी नेत्रश्लेष्मा पर स्वच्छमण्डल के भीतरी एवं बाहय किनारों पर स्थित एक सुदम, पीलापन लिए हुए, तिकोना धब्बा। A benign yellowish triangular spot and the bulbar conjunctiva on the inner and outer margins of the cornea.

Pink disease (पिंक डिजीज) शिशुशाखावेदना। Acrodynia.

Pinna (पिना) कर्णपाली अथवा कान का सिर से बाहर का भाग। The auricle or external ear.

Pinocytosis (पिनोसाइटोसिस) अवशोषी कोशिकता। The imbibitions of liquids by cells.

Pinworm (पिनवर्म) सूत्र कृमि। Threadworm enterobius vermicularis.

Pisiform (पिज़ी फोर्म) मटर के आकार का, चणकाकार। Pea shaped.

Pit (पिट) गड्ढा-गर्त। Depression.

Pitch (पिच) ध्वनि की तीव्रता का गुण। The quality of intensity of sound.

Pitting (पिटिंग) गड्ढों का बनना जैसा कि चेचक में देखा जाता है। The formation of pits as seen in smallpox.

Pituitary gland (पिट्युटरी ग्लैण्ड) पीयूषिका-ग्रन्थि। The principal gland of internal secretion located under the middle of lower surface of the brain.

Pityriasis (पिटीरिएसिस) एक चर्मरोग, चमड़ी का एक पपड़ीदार उद्भेद। A scaly eruption of the skin.

Pityriasis rosia (पिटीरिएसिस रोजीया) गुलाबी लाल तुषाभशक्लन। Rose red scaly patches.

Pityriasis rubra pilaris (पिटीरिएसिस रूब्रा पिलेरिस) सार्वदैहिक उपशल्कित त्वकशोथ। General exfoliative dermatitis.

Pivot (पाइवट) एक खूँटा जिस पर कोई वस्तु घूमती है। A pillar on which something revolves.

Placebo (प्लेसीबो) रोगी की औषधि के लिए माँग की संतुष्टि के लिए दिया जाने वाला एक निष्क्रिय पदार्थ, कूट-भेषज। An inactive substance given to satisfy the patient's demand for medicine.

Placenta (प्लेसेन्टा) अपरा, गर्भनाल, जरायुनाल। The special organ which nourishes the unborn.

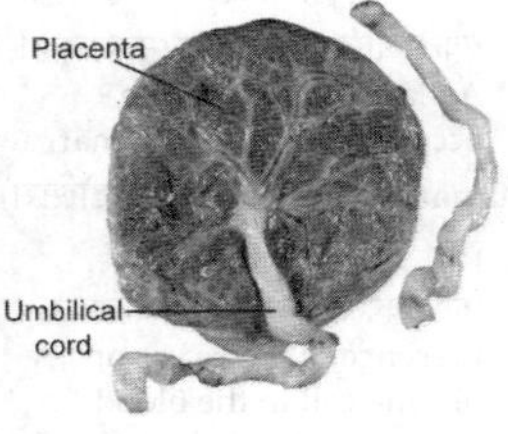

(*i*) **Cordiform Placenta** (कॉर्डीफोर्म प्लेसेन्टा) हृदय के आकार का अपरा। Heart shaped placenta (*ii*) **Retained placenta** (रिटेन्ड प्लेसेन्टा) प्रसव की द्वितीय अवस्था के पश्चात् दो घण्टे तक बाहर न निकलने वाली अपरा, अनिर्गत अपरा। Placenta not expelled for two hours after the second stage of labor. (*iii*) **Trilobate placenta** (ट्राइलोबेट प्लेसेन्टा) अपरा जिसमें तीन खण्ड होते है। A placenta with three lobes.

Placenta previa (प्लेसेन्टा प्रीविया) सम्मुखी अपरा। Presentation of the placenta before the fetus.

Placental soufflé (प्लेसेन्टल सफिल) परिश्रवण करने पर गर्भावस्था में रक्त परिसंचरण के कारण अपरा के ऊपर सुनाई देने वाली ध्वनि। Sound heard over the placenta in pregnancy on auscultation due to circulation of blood.

Placentitis (प्लेसेन्टाइटिस) अपराशोथ। Inflammation of the placenta.

Plagiocephaly (प्लेजियोन्सिफेली) असममितशीर्षता। Irregular closure of cranial suture resulting in deformed skull.

Plague (प्लेग) ताऊन। A severe epidemic caused due to rat infection.

(*i*) **Hemorrhagic plague** (हेमरैहजिक प्लेग) रक्तस्रावी प्लेग। The hemorrhagic form of bubonic plague.

Plane (प्लेन) तल, कोमल तल। A smooth surface.

(*i*) **Median plane** (मीडियन प्लेन) लम्बान में शरीर के बीच से होकर आगे से पीछे की ओर गुजरने वाला तल जो शरीर को दाँयें एवं बाँयें दो अर्द्ध भागों में विभाजित करता है, मध्यम तल। The plane passing longitudinally through the middle of the body front to back dividing it into right and left halves.

(*ii*) **Transverse plane** (ट्रान्सवर्स प्लेन) शरीर या भुजाओं के लम्ब अक्ष के अनुलम्ब एक तल।

A plane perpendicular to the long axis to the body or limbs.

Planoconcave (प्लेनोकॉनकेव) एक ओर सपाट तथा दूसरी ओर नातेदार हो, समतलावतल। Plane on one side and concave on the other.

Planoconvex (प्लेनोकॉनवैक्स) जो एक ओर सपाट तथा दूसरी ओर उन्नतोदर होता है, समतलोत्तल। Plane on one side and convex on the other.

Planta (प्लान्टा) पादतल, पैर का तलवा। The sole of the foot.

Plantalgia (प्लान्टेल्जिया) पैर के तलवे में दर्द होना। Pain in the sole of the foot.

Plantaris (प्लान्टेरिस) पैर की प्रसारक पेशी, जंघा-उपपिण्डिका। An extensor muscle of the foot.

Plaque (प्लाक) चकता, सपाट स्थान। Any patch or flat area.

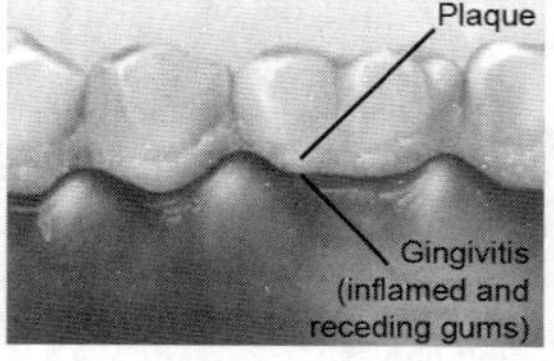

Plasma (प्लाज्मा) प्लाविका, रक्त का सरिम या द्रव अंश, रक्तरस। The serum or liquid portion of the blood plasma.

Plasmacyte (प्लाज्मासाइट) प्लाविककोशिका, प्लाज्मा कोशिका। Plasma cell, plasmocyte.

Plasmacytoma (प्लाज्मासाइटोमा) अस्थि मज्जा में उत्पन्न होने वाला एक प्लाज्मा कोशिका मज्जाबुर्द। A plasma cell myeloma occurring in the bone marrow.

Plasmacytosis (प्लाज्मासाइटोसिस) रक्त में अधिक प्लाज्मा कोशिकाओं का पाया जाना। Presence of an excess of plasma cell in the blood.

Plasmapheresis (प्लाज्माफेरेसिस) प्लाविकाहरण। Similar to plasma exchange.

Plasmodium (प्लोज्मोडियम) मलेरिया को उत्पन्न करने वाला जीव, मलेरिया परजीवी जो मनुष्य की लाल रक्त कोशिकाओं में रहता है। The causative organism of malaria, the malarial parasite which live in RBC of man.

Plasmogamy (प्लाज्मोगैमी) कोशिकाओं का संयोजन। The fusion of cells.

Plasmoptysis (प्लाज्मोप्टाइसिस) किसी कोशिका से कोशिका द्रव्य

का मुक्त होना। Escape of the cytoplasm from a cell.

Plasmoschisis (प्लाज्मोस्काइसिस) कोशिका का चिर जाना। The splitting of a cell.

Plaster (प्लास्टर) पट्टी, पलस्तर। A substance used in medical practice being made to adhere to the surface of the body.

Plastic surgery (प्लास्टिक सर्जरी) शरीर की रचनाओं की मरम्मत के लिए किया जाने वाला ऑपरेशन, शल्यचिकित्सा। Operation performed for repair of body structure.

Plate (प्लेट) एक पतली, चपटी संरचना अथवा शरीर का कोई भाग। A thin flattened structure or part of the body.

Platelet (प्लेटलेट) बिम्बाणु। Thrombocyte.

Platycephaly (प्लेटीसिफैली) सिर का चौड़ा होना। Widening of the head.

Platyglossal (प्लेटीग्लौसल) चौड़ी एवं चपटी जीभ वाला। Having a broad and flat tongue.

Platyopic (प्लेटीयोपिक) बहुत चौड़े चेहरे वाला। Having a very broad face.

Platyrrhine (प्लेटीराहइने) वह व्यक्ति, जिसकी नाक बहुत चौड़ी होती है। Having a very wide nose.

Pleocytosis (प्लीयोसाइटोसिस) अनुमस्तिष्क मेरूद्रव्य में लिम्फोसाइटों की वृद्धि होना। Increase of lymphocytes in the cerebrospinal fluid.

Pleomorphism (प्लीयोमॉर्फिज्म) किसी जीव के जीवन चक्र में एक से अधिक रूपों का उत्पन्न होना, बहुरूपता। The occurring of more than one forms in the life cycle of an organism.

Pleonosteosis (प्लीयोनोस्टीयोसिस) हड्डियों का असामान्य रूप से अस्थिभवन बढ़ जाना। Abnormally increased ossification of bones.

Plessesthesia (प्लेसेस्थीसिया) परिस्पर्शनीय परिताड़न। Palpatory percussion.

Plethora (प्लेथोरा) अधिक रक्त के द्वारा रक्त वाहिनियों का फूल जाना। Distention of blood vessels by an excess of blood.

Plethysmography (प्लेथिस्मोग्राफी) रक्तसंचार-मापन। Use of plethysmograph.

Pleura (प्लूरा) फुफ्फुसावरण, फेफड़े की झिल्ली। Lining membrane of the thorax covering also the lungs.

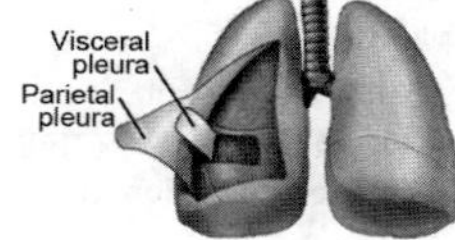

Pleuralgia (प्लूरैल्जिया) फेफड़े की झिल्ली का दर्द, फुफ्फुसावरणशूल। Pain in the intercostal muscle.

Pleurisy (प्लूरिसी) फुफ्फुसावरण शोथ। Inflammation of the pleura.

Pleurocentrum (प्लूरोसेन्ट्रम) कशेरूका के केन्द्रक का पार्श्विक आधा भाग। The lateral half of the centrum of a vertebra.

Pleurodynia (प्लूरोडाइनिया) अन्तरापर्शुकी पेशियों में दर्द होना, पार्श्व-वेदना। Pain occurring in the intercostals muscles.

Pleurolysis (प्लूरोलाइसिस) शल्यक्रिया द्वारा फुफ्फुसावरण को उसके चिपकावों से अलग करना। Surgical separation of pleura from its adhesions.

Pleuropericarditis (प्लूरोपेरीकार्डाइटिस) हृदयावरणशोथ के साथ फुफ्फुसावरणशोथ। Plexitis with pericarditis.

Pleurorrhea (प्लूरोरिह्या) फुफ्फुसावरण से तरल का स्रावित होना। Discharge of fluid from the pleura.

Pleurotomy (प्लुरोटॉमी) फुफ्फुसावरण में चीरा लगाना। To make an incision into the pleura.

Plexiform (प्लैक्सीफोर्म) जालरूप, जालिकारूप। Resembling a plexus.

Pleximeter (प्लैक्सीमीटर) परिताड़न के दौरान शरीर की सतह पर रखी जाने वाली प्लेट जो परिताड़न करने वाली अँगुली अथवा हथौड़े की चोट को सहन करती है। A disk held over the surface of the body during percussion which bears the stroke of the processing finger or hammer.

Plexitis (प्लैक्साइटिस) जालिका शोथ। Inflammation or irritation of plexus.

Plexus (प्लैक्सस) जल, जालिका, जालक, स्नायुजाल, नाड़ीजाल, तन्तुजाल। A network of the nerve or vessel.

Pliability (प्लीयाबिलिटी) आसानी से मुड़ जाने अथवा ऐंठ जाने की क्षमता। Capability of being bent or twisted easily.

Plica (प्लीका) वली, पुटक, झुर्री, तह। A fold.

Plicate (प्लीकेट) तह किया हुआ। Folded.

Plication (प्लीकेशन) वलीकरण। The stitching of folds in the walls of an organ to reduce its size.

Pliers (प्लायर्स) जम्बू, प्लास। Pincers.

Ploidy (प्लॉयडी) किसी कोशिका में गुणसूत्रों के समूह की संख्या। The number of chromosome sets in a cell.

Plug (प्लग) किसी पदार्थ का कोई पिण्ड जो किसी छिद्र को बन्द कर देता है। A mass of a material that obstructs an opening.

Plumbism (प्लम्बिज्म) जीर्ण लेड विषाक्तता, सीसात्यय। Chronic lead poisoning.

Plummer-Vinson Syndrome (प्लमर–विनसन सिण्ड्रोम) अधिकतर स्त्रियों में लगभग 40 वर्ष की आयु में उत्पन्न होने वाला एक रोग जिसमें लोह अल्पताजन्य रक्ताल्पता हो जाती है, निगलने में कठिनाई होती है तथा नाखून चम्मच के आकार के हो जाते है। A condition occurring mostly in women at the age of about 40 years characterized by iron deficiency anemia, difficulty in swallowing and spooning of the nails.

Plumose (प्लमोस) पंख जैसी वृद्धि से युक्त। Having feathery growth.

Pluripara (प्लूरीपैरा) वह स्त्री जिसने दो से अधिक बच्चों को जन्म दिया हो, बहुप्रसवा। A woman who has borne more than two children.

Pluripotent (प्लूरीपोटेन्ट) बहुशक्तिक। Having the capacity to affect more than one organ or tissue.

Plutomania (प्लूटोमेनिया) रईस होने की भ्रान्ति। Delusion of being rich.

Pneumalithiasis (न्यूमोलिथिएसिस) फेफडों में पथरियों का बनना। Formation of calculi in the lungs.

Pneumatics (न्यूमेटिक्स) भौतिक-शास्त्र की एक शाखा जिसका, सम्बन्ध वायु अथवा गैसों से होता है। A branch of physics dealing with the air and gases.

Pneumatization (न्यूमेटाइजेशन) ऊतक में, विशेषकर शंखास्थि के कर्णमूल वाले भाग में वायुपूरित कोशिकाओं अथवा गुहाओं। The formation of air filled cells or cavities in the tissue especially in the mastoid portion of temporal bone.

Pneumatized (न्यूमेटाइज्ड) वायु से भरा हुआ। Filled with air.

Pneumatocele (न्यूमेटोसील) फेफड़े की एक वायु-पुटी। An air cyst of the lung.

Pneumatosis (न्यूमेटोसिस) शरीर के किसी भाग में गैस का अधिक जमाव होना। वायुपुटिता। Morbid accumulation of gas in any part of the body.

Pneumaturia (न्यूमेच्यूरिया) पेशाब के साथ हवा निकलना, वायुमेह। The passage of flatus with urine.

Pneumobulbar (न्यूमोबल्बर) फेफड़ों एवं मस्तिष्क के मेडुला आब्लॉगेटा में स्थित श्वसन-केन्द्र से सम्बन्धित। Pertaining to the lungs and the respiratory center situated in the medulla oblongata of the brain.

Pneumocholecystitis (न्यूमोकीलीसिस्टाइटिस) पित्ताशयशोथ जिसमें पित्ताशय में गैस भरी होती है। Inflammation of the gallbladder with gas in it.

Pneumococcidal (न्यूमोकॉक्कसाइडल) न्यूमोकॉक्कसों को नष्ट करने वाला। Destroying pneumococci.

Pneumococcus (न्यूमोकॉक्कस) क्लोमगोलाणु। A coccal bacterium arranged characteristically in pairs.

Pneumoconiosis (न्यूमोकोनियोसिस) फुफ्फु-सधूलिमयता, फेफड़ों की तन्तुमयता। Dust disease, fibrosis of the lungs caused by long continued inhalation of dust in industrial occupations.

Pneumocystography (न्यूमोसिस्टोग्राफी) मूत्राशय में वायु अथवा गैस प्रविष्ट करके उसका एक्स-रे परीक्षण करना। X-ray examination of the urinary bladder after introducing air or gas into it.

Pneumoderma (न्यूमोडर्मा) त्वचा के नीचे स्थित वातस्फीति। Emphysema under the skin.

Pneumodilation (न्यूमोडायलेशन) फुफ्फुस-विस्फार, फेफड़ों का फैलाव। Dilation or dilatation of the lungs.

Pneumoencephalogram (न्यूमोएन्सिफैलोग्राम) मस्तिष्कवाय की चित्रण द्वारा उपलब्ध मस्तिष्क की एक्स-रे फिल्म, मस्तिष्कवाय की चित्र। X-ray film of the brain obtained by pneumoencephalography.

Pneumogalactocele (न्यूमोगैलेक्टोसील) स्तन अबुर्द जिसमें दूध एवं गैस होती है। A tumor of the breast containing milk and gas.

Pneumogastric (न्यूमोगेस्ट्रिक) फेफड़ों एवं आमाशय से सम्बन्धित, फुफ्फुसजठरीय। Pertaining to the lungs and stomach.

Pneumohemopericardium (न्यूमोहिमोपैरिकार्डियम) हृदयावस्था में वायु अथवा गैस तथा रक्त का इकट्ठा होना। Air or gas and blood in the pericardium.

Pneumohydrometra (न्यूमोहाइड्रोमीट्रा) गर्भाशय में गैस तथा पानी इकट्ठा हो जाना। The accumulation of gas and water in the uterus.

Pneumohydrothorax (न्यूमोहाइड्रोथौरेक्स) फुफ्फुसावरणी गुहा में तरल के साथ वायु अथवा गैस का इकट्ठा हो जाना। Air or gas with fluid in the pleural cavity.

Pneumomalacia (न्यूमोमैलेशिया) फेफड़े का असामान्य रूप से कोमल हो जाना। Abnormal softening of the lung.

Pneumomediastinum (न्यूमोमीडियास्टाइनम) मध्यस्थानिक के ऊतकों में वायु या गैस का पाया जाना जो किसी रोग के कारण हो सकती है अथवा नैदानिक उद्देश्य से इन्जैक्शन द्वारा प्रविष्ट की गई होती है, वातमध्यस्थानिका। Presence of air or gas in the tissues of the mediastinum which may be due to some disease or introduced by injection for diagnostic purpose.

Pneumomelanosis (न्यूमोमेलानोसिस) फुफ्फुसधूलिमयता में फेफड़ों में दिखाई देने वाली वर्णकता। Pigmentation of the lungs seen in pneumoconiosis.

Pneumonectasia (न्यूमोनेक्टेसिया) वायु से फेफड़ों का फूल जाना। Distention of the lungs with air.

Pneumonectomy (न्यूमोनेक्टॉमी) फेफड़ा काटकर हटाना, फुफ्फुसोच्छेदन। Excision of lung.

Pneumonia (निमोनिया) फेफड़ों का प्रदाह, फुफ्फुस शोथ। Inflammation of the lungs.

(*i*) **Aspiration Pneumonia** (एस्पिरेशन निमोनिया) चूषण फुफ्फुसपाक। Due to the inspiration of irritant substance into the lung.

(*ii*) **Bronchial Pneumonia** (ब्रोन्कियल निमोनिया) श्वसन प्रणाली का संक्रमण। An infection of the respiratory system that effects the bronchial tubes.

(*iii*) **Hypostatic Pneumonia** (हाइपोस्टेटिक निमोनिया) अधःस्थितिक फुफ्फुसपाक। A kind occurring in the weak or aged affecting the lower posterior portions of the lung.

(*iv*) **Interstitial Pneumonia** (इन्टरस्टिशियल निमोनिया) अन्तरालीय फुफ्फुसपाक। That marked by the increase of interstitial connective tissue.

(*v*) **Lobar Pneumonia** (लोबर निमोनिया) फुफ्फुसीय लोब का संक्रमण। Pneumonia involving one or more lobes of the lungs.

(Inflammation of pulmonary lobe).

Pneumonocyte (न्यूमोनोसाइट) फेफड़ों की एक वायुकोष्ठीय कोशिका। An alveolar cell of the lungs.

Pneumonopexy (न्यूमोनोपैक्सी) किसी फेफड़े को शल्यक्रिया द्वारा वक्ष-भित्ति से संलग्न करना। Surgical attachment of a lung to the chest wall.

Pneumonorrhaphy (न्यूमोनोरैह्फी) फेफड़े में टॉका लगाना। Suture of the lung.

Pneumoperitoneum (न्यूमोपैरीटोनियम) वायुपर्युदर्या, उदरावरण में वायु अथवा गैस विद्यमान रहना। Air or gas in the peritoneal cavity.

Pneumoradiography (न्यूमोरेडियोग्राफी) फुफ्फुसवायुचित्रण। Radiographic examination of the lungs after injection of air.

Pneumotaxic (न्यूमोटैक्सिक) श्वसन-गति को नियमित करने वाला, श्वास-नियामक। Regulating the respiratory rate.

Pneumothorax (न्यूमोथौरेक्स) फुफ्फुसावरणीय गुहा में वायु अथवा गैस का इकट्ठा हो जाना। A collection of air or gas in the pleural cavity.

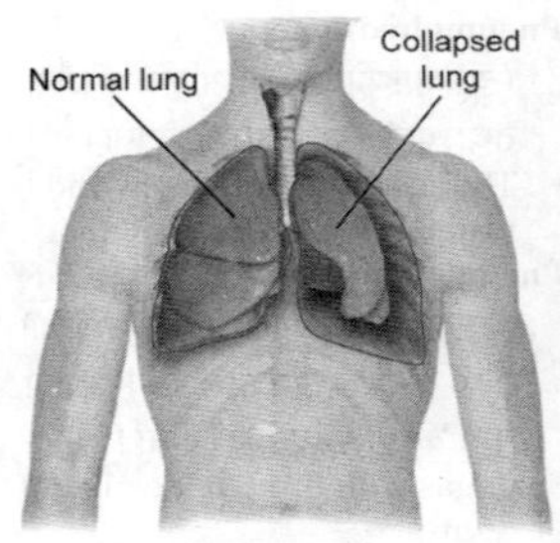

Pneumotyphus (न्यूमोटाइफस) टाइफॉयड ज्वर के साथ न्यूमोनिया हो जाना। Typhoid fever with pneumonia.

Podagra (पोडेग्रा) पैर का गठिया या पैर के अँगूठे में गाउथ का दर्द होना, पादवात। Gout of foot, gouty pain in the big toe.

Podiatrist (पोडियाट्रिस्ट) पाद-चिकित्सा विज्ञान। Chiropodist.

Podobromidrosis (पोडोब्रोमीड्रोसिस) पादों से बदबूदार पसीना निकलना। Offensive sweating from the feet.

Podocyte (पोडोसाइट) पादकोशिका। A special type of epithelial cell lining the glomeruli.

Podogram (पोडोग्राम) पदललचित्र, पादतलचित्र, पैर के तलवे की छाप। The imprint of the sale of the foot.

Podology (पोडोलॉजी) पादचिकित्सा-विज्ञान, पाद चिकित्सा का अध्ययन करना। The study of anatomy and physiology of foot.

Poikilocyte (पॉयकिलोसाइट) अस्वाभाविक आकार की लोहितकोशिका, विषमलोहित-कोशिका। Red blood cell of abnormal shape.

Poikiloderma (पॉयकिलोडर्मा) त्वचा का एक रोग जिसमें त्वचा में वर्णकता, वाहिकास्फीति, रक्तचित्रिता, कण्डू (खुजली) हो जाती है तथा अपक्षय हो जाता है। A condition of the skin characterized by pigmentation telangiectasia, purpura, punitus and atrophy.

Poikilothermy (पॉयकिलोथर्मी) शरीर का ऐसा तापमान होना जो वातावरण के तापमान के अनुसार घटता बढ़ता है।

The condition of having a body temperature which varies according to that of the environment.

Poikilothrombocyte (पॉयकिलोथ्रॉम्बोसाइट) असामान्य आकृति की बिम्बाणु कोशिका। A platelet cell of abnormal shape.

Point (प्वाइन्ट) एक सूक्ष्म-सा धब्बा, बिन्दु या किसी वस्तु का तेज सिरा। A minute spot, sharp end of an object.

(*i*) **Boiling Point** (बॅायलिंग प्वाइन्ट) वह तापमान जिस पर कोई द्रव उबल जाता है। Temperature at which a liquid boils. (*ii*) **McBurney's Point** (मैकबर्नीज़ पाइन्ट) दॉयें अग्र ऊर्ध्व श्रोणिफलक कंटक एवं नाभि के बीच की रेखा पर कंटक से ½ से 2 इंच दूर स्थित एक बिन्दु। A point ½ to 2 inches from the right anterior superior iliac spine on the line between this spine and the umbilicus.

Poison (पॉयजन) विष, गरल, कालकूट, जहर। A toxic agent.

Poison ivy (पॉयजन आईवी) सिरपेंची विषमता, सिरपॅचीविश। Skin irritation due tc toxic oils in this wild plant.

Poison oak (पॉयजन ओएक) बलूत विषण्णता, बलूत विष। Skin irritation due to toxic oils in this common wild plant.

Polar (पोलर) ध्रुवीय, ध्रुव सम्बन्धी। Pertaining to a pole.

Polioclastic (पोलियोक्लास्टिक) तंत्रिका-तंत्र के धूसर द्रव्य को नष्ट करने वाला। Destroying the gray matter of the nervous system.

Polioencephalitis (पोलियोएन्सिफैलाइटिस)

मस्तिष्क के धूसर द्रव्य का शोथज रोग, पोलियोमस्तिष्क शोथ। Inflammation disease of the gray matter of the brain.

Poliomyelitis (पोलियोमायलाइटिस) बच्चों में मुख्यतया 2 से 5 वर्ष की आयु में होने वाला सुषुम्ना रज्जु के धूसर द्रव्य का तीव्र विषाणु शोथ। An acute viral inflammation of the gray matter of the spinal cord accruing in children chiefly between 2 to 5 years of age.

Poliosis (पोलियोसिस) पालित्य, बालों का भूरापन। Grayness of the hair.

Pollen (पोलेन) पराग, पुष्परज, रोग। The male cell of certain plant distributed by the wind.

Pollex (पौलेक्स) हस्तांगुश्ठ, हाथ का अँगुठा। The thumb.

Polyadenitis (पोलीएडीनाइटिस) बहुत-सी ग्रन्थियों की सूजन। Inflammation of many gland.

Polyadenosis (पोलीएडीनोसिस) बहुत सी ग्रन्थियों का विकार। Disorder of many glands.

Polyangitis (पोलीएन्जाइटिस) बहुत सी रक्त वाहिनियों का शोथ। Inflammation of many blood vessels.

Polyarteritis nodosa (पोलीआर्टीराइटिस नोडोसा) छोटी धमनियों का षोथ, पर्विल बहुधमनीषोथ। Inflammation of the small arteries with formation of small aneurysms.

Polyarthritis (पोलीआर्थराइटिस) कई जोड़ो की सूजन, बहुसंधिशोथ। Inflammation of several joints.

Polyblennia (पोलीब्लेनिया) श्लेष्मा का अत्यधिक स्रावित होना। Excessive secretion of mucus.

Polycheiria (पोलीकीरिया) दो से अधिक हाथों वाला। Having more than two hands.

Polychromasia (पोलीक्रोमेसिया) बहुवर्णकता। Quality of being stainable with various stains.

Polychromatophilia (पोलीक्रोमेटोफीलिया) बहुत से अभिरंजकों द्वारा अभिरंजित होने का गुण, बहुवर्णरागिता।

The quality of being stainable with various stains.

Polyclinic (पोलीक्लीनिक) सर्वोपचारगृह, सामान्य-चिकित्सालय। A hospital where all kinds of disease and injury are treated, a general hospital.

Polycoria (पोलीकोरिया) किसी आँख में एक से अधिक पुतलियों का पाया जाना। Presence of more than one pupil in an eye.

Polycystic (पोलीसिस्टिक) बहुत-सी पुटियों से बना हुआ, बहुपुटीय। Composed of many cysts.

Polycythemia (पोलीसाइथीमिया) रक्त में लाल रक्त कोशिकाओं की संख्या बढ़ जाना। An increase in the number of RBC in the blood.

Polydactylism (पोलीडैक्टाइलिज्म) हाथ अथवा पैर में अधिसंख्य अँगुलियों का पाया जाना। The presence of supernumerary fingers or toes.

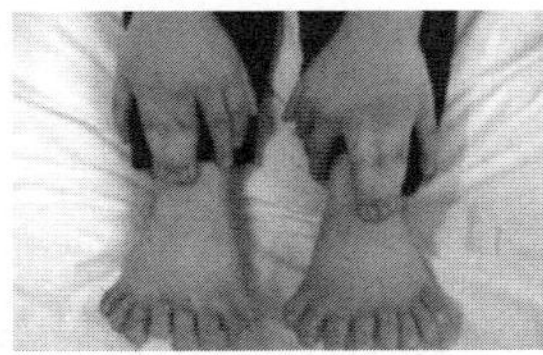

Polydipsia (पोलीडिप्सिया) अत्यधिक प्यास लगना। Excessive thirst.

Polydystrophy (पोलीडिस्ट्रॉफी) संयोजी ऊतकों की बहुत सी जन्मजात विकृतियों का पाया जाना। Presence of numerous congenital abnormalities of the connective tissue.

Polyemia (पोलीमिया) रक्त की अत्यधिक बढ़ी हुई मात्रा। Abundance of blood, abnormal increase of the mass of the blood.

Polygenic (पोलीजेनिक) बहुत से विभिन्न जीनों से सम्बन्धित अथवा उनके द्वारा उत्पन्न। Pertaining to or caused by several different genes.

Polygraph (पोलीग्राफ) बहुस्पन्दलेखी, बहुलेखी। An instrument which records pulses simultaneously.

Polyhydramnios (पोलीहाइड्रेम्नियोज़) उल्वकोष में उल्व-तरल का बढ़ जाना। An excessive of amniotic fluid in the amniotic sac.

Polymastia (पोलीमैस्टिया) दो से अधिक स्तनों का पाया जाना, बहुस्तनता। The presence of more than two breast.

Polymastigote (पोलीमैस्टीगोट) बहुत से कषाभों से युक्त। Having many flagella.

Polymenorrhea (पोलीमेनोरिह्या) असामान्य रूप से बार-बार होने वाला मासिक धर्म, बहुआर्तव। Abnormally frequent menstruation.

Polymyalgia Rheumatica (पोलीमायेल्जिया रूमेटिका) आमवातज बहुपेष्यार्ति, आमवाती बहुपेष्यर्ति। A syndrome occurring in elderly people comprising of a crippling ache in the shoulders.

Polymer (पॉलीमर) बहुलक। A substance of high molecular.

Polymerization (पॉलीमिराइजैशन) बहुलीकरण। A reaction in which a molecular weight product is produced by successive additions.

Polymorph (पोलीमॉर्फ) एक बहुरूपीकेन्द्रक श्वेत रक्त कणिका। A polymorphonuclear leukocyte.

Polymorphism (पोलीमॉर्फिज्म) बहुत से रूपों में उत्पन्न होने का गुणए बहुरूपता। The quality of occurring in many forms.

Polymorphonuclear (पोलीमॉर्फोन्यूक्लियर) ऐसे केन्द्रक वाला जिसमें कई खण्ड होते है। Having a nucleus consisting of several lobes.

Polymyositis (पोलीमायोसाइटिस) अनेक पेशीयों का प्रदाह, बहुवेषीशोथ। Inflammation of many muscles at a time.

Polyneuralgia (पोलीन्यूरौल्जिया) कई तंत्रिकाओं में तंत्रिकार्ति का होना। Neuralgia in several nerves.

Polyneuropathy (पोलीन्यूरोपैथी) बहुतंत्रिका-विकृति। A disease affecting many nerves.

Polyneuroradiculitis (पोलीन्यूरोरेडीकुलाइटिस) सुषुम्ना गण्डिकाओं, तंत्रिका मूल एवं परिसरीय तंत्रिकाओं का शोथ। Inflammation of the spinal ganglia nerve roots and peripheral nerves.

Polyonychia (पोलीओनीकिया) अधिसंख्य नाखूनों का पाया जाना। The presence of supernumerary nails.

Polyopsia (पोलीओप्सिया) एक ही वस्तु के एक से अधिक प्रतिबिम्ब दिखाई देना। Visual perception of more than one image of the same object.

Polyorchidism (पोलीऑर्काइडिज्म) दो से अधिक शुक्रग्रन्थियों का पाया जाना। Presence of more than two testes.

Polyostotic (पोलीऑस्टोटिक) बहुत सी हड्डियों से सम्बन्धित। Pertaining to many bone.

Polyotia (पोलीऑटिया) दो से अधिक कानों का पाया जाना। The presence of more than two ear.

Polypectomy (पॉलिपैक्टॉमी) पुर्वंगक को काट कर हटाना। Surgical removal of a polyp.

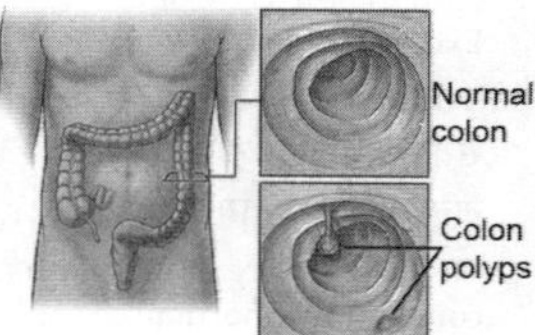

Polypeptide (पोलीपेप्टाइड) एक पेप्टाइड जिसमें दो से अधिक अमीनों अम्ल होते है। A peptide containing more than two amino acids.

Polyphagia (पोलीफैजिया) खाना बहुत खाना, अतिभक्षण। Excessive eating of food.

Polypharmacy (पोलीफार्मेसी) एक ही समय में दी जाने वाली बहुत-सी औषधियों का नुस्खा, बहुभेषजी। Prescription of many drugs given at a time.

Polyphrasia (पोलीफ्रेजिया) अत्यधिक बात बनाना। Excessive talkativeness.

Polyphyletic (पोलीफाइलेटिक) बहुद्भवी। Derived from more than one source.

Polyplegia (पोलीप्लेजिया) असंख्य पेशियों का पक्षाघात, बहुपेशीघात। Paralysis of several muscles.

Polyploidy (पोलीप्लॉयडी) समजात गुणसूत्रों के दो सैटों से अधिक धारण करना। Possession of more than two set of homologus chromosomes.

Polyporous (पोलीपोरस) बहुत से छिद्रो वाला। Having many pores.

Polyposis (पोलीपोसिस) बहुत से पॉलिपों का बनना, पॉलिपमयता, बहुपुर्वंगकता। The formation of numerous polyps.

Polypotrite (पॉलिपोट्राइट) पॉलिपो को कुचलने वाला यंत्र। An instrument for crushing the polyps.

Polyptychial (पोलीपटाइकियल) कई परतों में व्यवस्थित। Arranged in several layers.

Polyrrhea (पोलीरिह्या) तरल का अत्यधिक स्राव। Excessive secretion of fluid.

Polyscellia (पोलीसीलिया) दो से अधिक पैरों का पाया जाना। The presence of more than two legs.

Polyserositis (पोलीसीरोसाइटिस) बहुसीर-मीकलाशोथ। General inflammation of the serous membrane.

Polysocchoride (पोलीसैकेराइड) एक प्रकार का कार्बोहाइड्रेट जिसका जलअपघटन होने पर साधारण शुगर के दो से अधिक अणु बनते है। A type of carbohydrate which upon hydrolysis yields more than two molecules of simple sugar.

Polysomus (पोलीसोमस) एक से अधिक शरीर वाला भ्रूण। A fetus having more than one body.

Polystichia (पोलीस्टाइचिया) किसी पलक में बालों का दो तथा अधिक पंक्तियों में पाया जाना। Presence of two or more rows of eyelashes on a lid.

Polytendinitis (पोलीटैण्डीनाइटिस) बहुकण्डराशोथ Inflammation of several tendons.

Polythelia (पोलीथिलिया) एक से अधिक चुचूक होना, बहुचूचुकता। Having more than one nipple.

Polyuria (पोलीयूरिया) मूत्र-त्याग अधिक होना, बहुमूत्रता। Excessive excretion of urine.

Polyvalent (पोलीवैलेन्ट) हाइड्रोजन के दो से अधिक परमाणुओं के साथ संयुक्त होने में सक्षम, बहुसंयोजक। Multivalent capable of combining with more than two atoms of hydrogen.

Pompholyx (पोम्फोलिक्स) पादचर्मस्फोट, हस्तचर्मस्फोट। Vesicular skin eruption on the feet or hands.

Pomphus (पोम्फस) फफोला या छाला। Blister.

Pontile (पोन्टाइल) पोन्स बेरोलाइ से सम्बन्धित। Pertaining to pons varolii.

Pontobulbar (पोन्टोबल्बर) पोन्स एवं मेडुला ऑब्लॉगेटा से सम्बन्धित। Pertaining to the pons and medulla oblongata.

Popliteal (पोप्लीटियल) घुटने के पष्च क्षेत्र से सम्बन्धित, जनुपृष्ठीय। Pertaining to the posterior region of the knee.

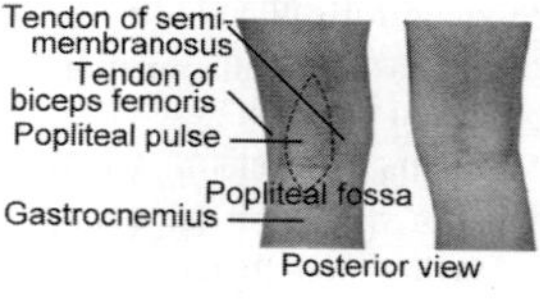

Posterior view

Popliteus (पोप्लीटियस) घुटने के पीछे की पेशी। The popliteal muscle.

Pore (पोर) एक छोटा-सा छेद अथवा खाली स्थान, रोमकूप, लोमरन्ध्र। Porus a small opening or empty space.

Porencephalous (पोरेन्सिफैलस) सुषिरमस्तिष्कता से सम्बन्धित। Pertaining to porenephalia.

Porencephaly (पोरेन्सिफैली) मस्तिष्क में पुटियों अथवा गुहाओं का बनना जिनका सम्बन्ध अक्सर किसी पर्श्विक निलय से होता है। सुषिरमस्तिष्कता। Development of the cysts or cavities in the brain usually communicating with a lateral ventricle.

Porphyrin (पोर्फाइरिन) जीवद्रव्य में उत्पन्न होने वाला हिमोग्लोबिन तथा पर्णहरित से उपलब्ध श्वसनीय वर्णकों का आधार बनाने वाला नाइट्रोजनयुक्त कार्बनिक यौगिकों के वर्ग में से कोई भी एक। Nitrogen containing organic compounds obtained from hemoglobin and chlorophyll.

Porphyrinuria (पोर्फाइरीनूरिया) मूत्र में अधिक पोर्फाइरिन का उत्सर्जित होना, पोर्फाइरिनमेह। Increased excretion of porphyrin in the urine.

Porta (पोर्टा) तंत्रिकाओं एवं वाहिनियों का प्रवेश/प्रवाह करने का स्थान, प्रतिहार, द्वार। Point of entry for nerves and vessels.

Portal circulation (पोर्टल सर्कुलेशन) पोर्टल शिरा तथा यकृती शिरा द्वारा यकृत में होने वाला रक्त परिसंचरण। The circulation of blood in liver via portal vein and hepatic vein.

Portal system (पोर्टल सिस्टम) प्रतिहार-प्रणाली, प्रतिहार-जाल।

Four large veins two mesenteric one and plenic and one gastric.

Portal vein (पोर्टल वैन) प्रतिहारी शिरा। One conveying blood into the liver.

Portography (पोर्टोग्राफी) पोर्टल शिरा में किसी रेडियोअपारदर्शक पदार्थ का इन्जैक्शन लगाकर उसका एक्स-रे परीक्षण करना। X-ray of portal vein after injection of contrast.

Position (पोज़ीशन) शरीर का आसन या उसकी स्थिति, दशा। Manner in which the body of patient is put.

(*i*) **Fowler's Position** (फाऊलर्स पोजीशन) ऐसी स्थिति जिसमें रोगी का पलंग का सिरहाना 18 से 20 इंच तक फर्श से ऊपर उठा दिया जाता है तथा साथ ही घुटनों को भी उठा दिया जाता है। Position in which head of the patient's bed is raised 18–20 inches above the floor with the knees also elevated. (*ii*) **Horizontal Position** (हॉरीजॉन्टल पोज़ीशन) अधिपृष्ठ-स्थिति जिसमें पाद प्रसारित हो जाते है। Dorsal position with the feet extended. (*iii*) **Lithotomy Position** (लिथोटॉमी पोज़ीशन) ऐसी स्थिति जिसमें रोगी कमर के सहारे लेटता है, जाँघों को पेट के ऊपर तथा पैरों को जाँघों के ऊपर आकुचित कर लेता है। The position in which the patient lies on the back with the thighs flexed on the abdomen and the legs on the thighs. (*iv*) **Prone position** (प्रोन पोज़ीशन) ऐसी स्थिति जिसमें रोगी चेहरा नीचे को करके लेटा होता है। Position in which the patient lies with the face downward.

Post traumatic (पोस्टट्रोमेटिक) किसी चोट के लगने के बाद। Following an injury.

Postadolescence (पोस्टएडोलेसैन्स) किशोरावस्था या यौवनारम्भ के बाद का काल।
The period after adolescence or puberty.

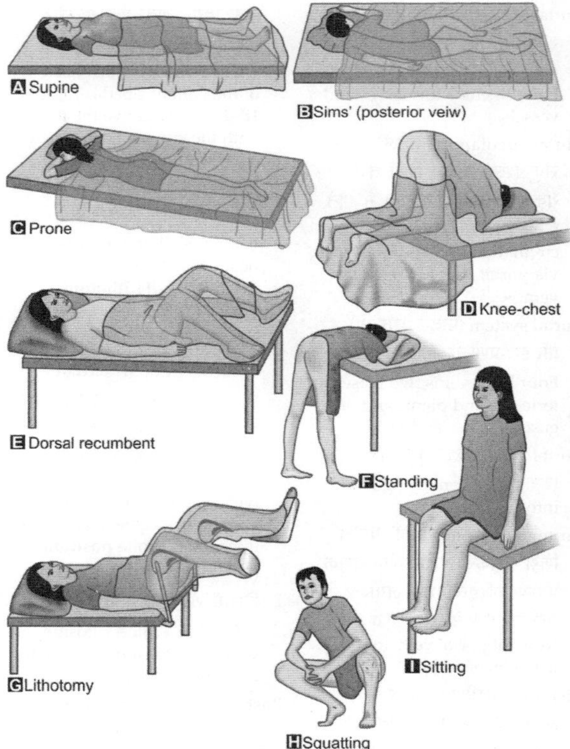

Positions

Postauricular (पोस्टऑरीकुलर) कर्णपाली या बाह्य कर्ण के पीछे स्थित अथवा वहाँ पर किया गया कोई ऑपरेशन। Situated or operation performed behind the auricle of the ear.

Postcardiotomy (पोस्टकार्डियोटॉमी) ओपन हार्ट सर्जरी के बाद का

काल। The period following open heart surgery.

Postcibal (पोस्टसाइबल) खाने के बाद उत्पन्न होने वाला, भोजनोत्तर। Accruing after eating.

Postclimacteric (पोस्टक्लाइमैक्ट्रिक) रजोनिवृत्ति के पश्चात् उत्पन्न होने वाला। Accruing after the menopause.

Postcoital (पोस्टकॉयटल) लैंगिक संसर्ग के पश्चात् उत्पन्न होने वाला। Happening after sexual intercourse.

Posterior (पोस्टीरियर) पीठ अथवा पीछे की ओर निर्देशित अथवा वहाँ पर स्थित, पश्च। Situated at back or behind dorsal.

Posteroanterior (पोस्टीरोएन्टीरियर) पीछे से आगे को दर्शाने वाला शब्द। The word indicating from back towards the front.

Posteromedial (पोस्टीरोमीडियल) पीठ एवं मध्यवर्ती तल की ओर। Towards the back and the midian plane.

Postfebrile (पोस्टफैब्राइल) किसी ज्वर के बाद उत्पन्न होने वाला, ज्वरोत्तर। Accruing after a fever.

Posthemorrhagic (पोस्टहीमोरहेजिक) रक्तस्राव के पश्चात् उत्पन्न होने वाला। Accruing after hemorrhage.

Posthitis (पोस्थाइटिस) अग्रच्छद का शोथ, शिष्नम। Inflammation of the foreskin.

Posthypnotic (पोस्टहिप्नोटिक) निद्रावस्था के पश्चात्। Following hypnotic state.

Postmature (पोस्टमेच्योर) गर्भावस्था के 42 सप्ताह के बाद उत्पन्न होने वाले शिशु से सम्बन्धित। Infant born after 42 week of gestation.

Postmortem (पोस्टमॉर्टम) मृत्यु के पश्चात् उत्पन्न होने वाला अथवा किया गया, मरणोत्तर। Accruing or performed after death.

Postnatal (पोस्टनेटल) जन्म के पष्चात् उत्पन्न होने वाला, प्रसवोत्तर, जन्मोत्तर। Accruing after birth.

Postoral (पोस्टोरल) मुख के पश्च भाग में। In the posterior part of the mouth.

Postpartum (पोस्टपार्टम) बच्चे के जन्म के पश्चात् उत्पन्न होने वाला। Accruing after childbirth.

Postpoludal (पोस्टपैल्युडल) मलेरिया ज्वर के पश्चात उत्पन्न होने वाला। Accruing after malaria fever.

Postprandial (पोस्टप्रैण्डियल) खाने के बाद, भोजनोत्तर। After a meal.

Poststenotic (पोस्टस्टेनोटिक) किसी संकुचित स्थान से दूर स्थापित या उत्पन्न होने वाला। Distal to a stenosed site.

Postulate (पोस्चुलेट) एक अनुमान या विचार, अभिधारणा। Supposition or view.

Postural (पोस्चुरल) स्थितिज, स्थिति सम्बन्धी, आसन। Pertaining to the posture.

Postural hypotension (पोस्चुरल हाइपोटैन्शन) खड़े रहने की स्थिति में रक्तचाप का कम हो जाना।
Decrease in blood pressure in standing position.

Posture (पोश्चर) शरीर की स्थिति, आसन। Attitude or position of the body.

Postvaccinal (पोस्टवैक्सीनल) चेचक का टीका लगाने के पश्चात् उत्पन्न होने वाला, टीकोत्तर। Accruing after vaccination for smallpox.

Potable (पोटेबिल) पेय, पीने योग्य। Suitable for drink.

Potash (पोटाश) लकड़ी की राख से प्राप्त एक क्षार पदार्थ। An alkaline substance obtained from wood ashes.

Potassium (पोटेशियम) शरीर में पाया जाने वाला अन्य तत्वों से संयुक्त एक खनिज तत्व। A mineral element found in combination with other elements in the body.

Potency (पोटेन्सी) सामर्थ्य, शक्ति या क्षमता जैसे किसी पुरूष की सम्भोग करने की क्षमता। Strength power, ability to perform sexual intercourse in case of male.

Potent (पोटेन्ट) शक्तिशाली। Powerful highly effective.

Potentiate (पोटेन्शियेट) शक्तिशाली बनाना।
To strengthen.

Potentiator (पोटेन्शियेटर) ऐसी औषधि जो दूसरी औषधियों के साथ मिलकर उन्हें शक्तिशाली बनाती है। A drug which in combination with other drugs makes them more powerful.

Potion (पोशन) किसी तरल औषधि की बड़ी खुराक, घूँट।
A large dose of a liquid medicine.

Pott's disease (पॉट्स डिज़ीज) कशेरूकाओं का क्षय रोग। Tuberculosis of vertebra.

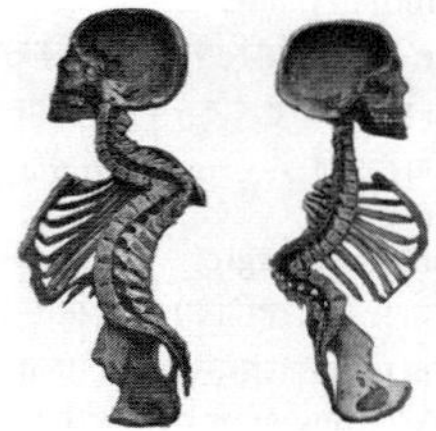

Pott's Fracture (पॉट्स फ्रैक्चर) फिब्यूला हड्डी के निचले सिरे तथा टिबिया के मध्यवर्ति गुलन का अस्थि भंग होना जिससे पॉव बाहर के ओर विस्थापित हो जाता है। Fracture of medial malleolus of tibia with lower end of fibula causing outward and backward dislocation of foot.

Pott's Paralysis (पॉट्स पैरालिसिस) क्षय रोग एंव कशेरूका सन्धिशोध के दबाब के कारण शरीर के निचले भाग का पक्षाघात। Paralysis of the lower part of the body due to pressure on the spinal cord as the result of tuberculosis spondylitis.

Pouch (पॉउच) जेब के समान गुहा अथवा कोश या थैली। Any pocket or sac.

Poultice (पुल्टिस) उपनाह, प्रलेप, लेई। Counter irritant preparation in the form of plaster.

Pox (पॉक्स) एक सांसर्गिक विस्फोटक रोग जैसे चेचक, स्फोट। Pustular lesion.

Practice (प्रेक्टिस) वृत्ति, व्यवसाय। The exercise of any professional practice.

Prandial (प्रेण्डियल) भोजन सम्बन्धी। Pertaining to a meal.

Praxis (प्रेक्सिस) कार्य या सक्रियता, अभ्यास। Act or activity practice.

Preagonal (प्रीएगोनल) मृत्यु के कष्ट से ठीक पहले। Immediately before death agony.

Preaxial (प्रीएक्सियल) किसी भुजा अथवा शरीर के अक्ष के सामने स्थित, पुरोक्ष। Situated in front of the axis of a limb or of the body.

Precancerous (प्रीकैन्सरस), एक वृद्धि अथवा विकृतिजन्य प्रक्रिया जो दुर्दम बनने के लिए प्रवृत होती है। कैन्सरपूर्व। A growth or a pathological process tending to become malignant.

Precava (प्रीकेवा) ऊर्ध्व महाशिरा। Superior vena cava.

Precipitate (प्रेसीपिटेट) अवक्षेप, प्रक्षेप, निस्साद, तलछट। A substance separated by precipitation.

Precipitin (प्रेसीपिटिन) किसी घुलनशील एन्टिजन जो अधिकतर एक प्रोटीन होता है, की विद्यमानता से बनी एक एण्टीबॉडी। An antibody formed due to presence of a soluble antigen usually a protein.

Precocity (प्रीकोसिटी) शारीरिक अथवा मानसिक विकास का

कालपूर्व विकास, कालपूर्वपक्वता। Premature development of physical or mental traits.

Precognition (प्रीकॉग्नीशन) ज्ञानेन्द्रियों से परे ज्ञान द्वारा यह पूर्व जानकारी हो जाना की कोई घटना होने वाली है। Prior knowledge that an event will occur through extrasensory perception.

Preconscious (प्रीकॉन्शियस) जो चेतनावस्था में न हो परन्तु शीघ्र ही फिर से चेतनावस्था में आ सकता है।
Not present in consciousness but able to be recalled readily into it.

Precordium (प्रीकार्डियम) हृदय के ऊपर स्थित वक्ष-प्रदेश, पुरोहृद। The area of chest overlying the heart.

Precornu (प्रीकोर्नू) मस्तिष्क के पार्श्विक निलय का अग्र श्रृंग। Anterior horn of the lateral ventricle of the brain.

Precursor (प्रीकर्सर) वह जो दूसरे से पहले होता है जैसे कोई चिन्ह या लक्षण अथवा ऐसा पदार्थ जिससे दूसरा, सामान्यतः अधिक सक्रिय पदार्थ बनता है, पूर्वगामी। Something that occurs before another as a sign or symptom or a substance from which another usually more active substance is formed.

Prediabetes (प्रीडायबिटीज़) मधुमेह प्रकट होने से पहले। Potential disposition to diabetes mellitus.

Predisposing (प्रीडिस्पोजिंग) रोग के प्रति प्रवृत्ति या ग्राहकत्व प्रदर्शित करने वाला, प्रवर्तनपूर्व। Showing a tendency or susceptibility to the disease.

Predisposition (प्रीडिस्पोजीशन) रोग के प्रति सुग्राह्यता, रोग प्रवणता। A tendency or susceptibility to the disease.

Pre-eclampsia (प्री-एक्लैम्पसिया) गर्भहेतुक विषरक्तता जिसकी विशिष्टताएँ उच्च रक्तचाप, एल्ब्यूमिनमेह एवं पैरों पर शोथ होना है, प्राकगर्भाक्षेपक।
A toxemia of pregnancy characterized by hypertension albuminuria and edema of the legs.

Pre-eruptive (प्री-इरप्टिव) किसी विस्फोट से पूर्व। Before an eruption.

Preganglionic (प्रीगैंग्लियोनिक) गण्डिकापूर्व। In front of a ganglion.

Pregnancy (प्रीग्नैन्सी) गर्भावस्था, सगर्भता।
The condition of having a developing embryo or fetus in uterus.

(*i*) **Abdominal Pregnancy** (एब्डोमिनल प्रेग्नैन्सी) उदर गुहा में

अस्थानिक गर्भावस्था। Extrauterine pregnancy. (*ii*) **Ectopic Pregnancy** (एक्टोपिक प्रेग्नैन्सी) गर्भाशय के बाहर होने वाली गर्भावस्था। Pregnancy occurring outside the uterus. (*iii*) **Tubal Pregnancy** (ट्यूबल प्रेग्नैन्सी) किसी डिम्ब वाहिनी में उत्पन्न होने वाली अस्थानिक सगर्भता। Ectopic pregnancy accruing within a fallopian tube.

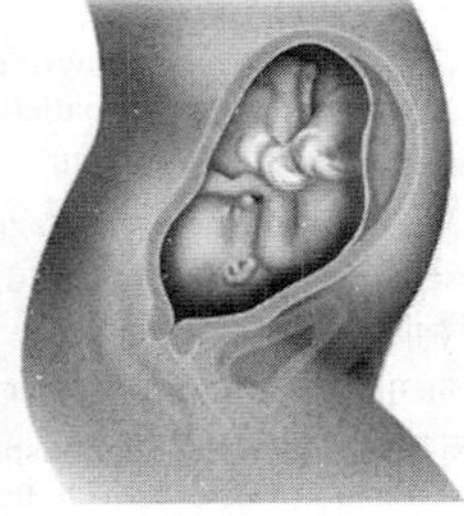

Prehemiplegic (प्रीहेमीप्लीजिक) अर्द्धांगघात के आरम्भ होने से पूर्व उत्पन्न होने वाला। Accruing before the onset of hemiplegia.

Preictal (प्रीइक्टल) किसी आघात अथवा अवक्षेप के तुरन्त ही पहले उत्पन्न होने वाला। Accruing just before a stroke or convulsion.

Preleukemia (प्रील्यूकीमिया) ल्यूकीमिया के विकसित होने से पूर्व अस्थि मज्जा की दुश्क्रिया की एक अवस्था। A stage of bone marrow dysfunction prior to the development of leukemia.

Premature (प्रीमेच्योर) पूर्ण विकसित होने से पूर्व, अपरिपक्व, असमय, कालपूर्व। Before full development.

Premature infant (प्रीमेच्योर इन्फैन्ट) ऐसा शिशु जो जन्म के समय पूर्णतया विकसित नहीं हुआ होता है ओर इसका वजन 2500 ग्राम या इससे कम होता है। An infant who is not fully develop at birth and its weight is 2500 gms or less.

Premenarchal (प्रीमेनार्कल) प्रथम मासिक धर्म से पूर्व। Prior to the first menstrual period.

Premenstrual tension syndrome (प्रीमैन्सट्रुअल टैन्शन सिण्ड्रोम) ऋतुस्त्राव या मासिक धर्म के आरम्भ होने से कुछ दिन पूर्व उत्पन्न होने वाला एक संलक्षण। A syndrome accruing several days prior to the onset of menstruation.

Premolar (प्रीमोलर) रदनक एवं चर्णवक दाँतों के बीच उत्पन्न होने वाले स्थायी दाँतों में से एक। One of the permanent teeth accruing between canine and molar.

Premorbid (प्रीमोर्बिड) रोग उत्पन्न होने से पूर्व उत्पन्न होने वाला। Accruing prior to the development of disease.

Preneoplastic (प्रीनियोप्लास्टिक) किसी अबुर्द के बनने से पहले। Before the formation of a tumor.

Prepatellar bursitis (प्रीपटेलर बर्साइटिस) पटेला हड्डी के सामने श्लेषपुटी का शोथ। Inflammation of the bursa in front of the patella bone.

Preprandial (प्रीप्रेण्डियल) भोजन से पहले। Before meal.

Prepubescent (प्रीप्यूबेसेन्ट) यौवनारम्भ से ठीक पहले के समय से सम्बन्धित। Pertaining to the period just before puberty.

Prepuce (प्रीप्यूस) शिश्नमुण्ड के आगे की त्वचा अथवा उसके ऊपर त्वचा की तहः शिश्न-मुण्डच्छद। The foreskin or fold of skin over the glans penis.

Preputiotomy (प्रीप्यूटियोटॉमी) निरूद्धप्रकाश को मुक्त करने के लिए शिश्नमुण्डच्छद को चीरना। To incise the prepuce of penis to relieve phimosis.

Prepyloric (प्रीपाइलोरिक) आमाशय के जठरनिर्गम या पाइलोरस के आगे या पहले। Anterior to or before the pylorus of stomach.

Prerenal (प्रीरीनल) वृक्क के सामने स्थित। In front of the kidney.

Presbyacusis (प्रेस्बायक्यूसिस) जरा-वधिरता। Sensory neural deafness of old age.

Presbyopia (प्रेस्बायोपिया) जरादूरदृष्टि। Farsightedness in old age.

Prescribe (प्रेस्क्राइब) औषध-निर्देशन, नुस्खा लिखना।
To indicate the medicine to be administered.

Prescription (प्रिस्क्रिप्शन) नुस्खा, औषधपत्र। The formula written by a physician for his patient.

Presenile (प्रीसेनाइल) कालपूर्व वृद्धावस्था। Premature old age.

Presentation (प्रीजेन्टेशन) प्रस्तुति, स्थिति या भ्रूण के लम्ब अक्ष का माता के लम्ब अक्ष के साथ सम्बन्ध। Lie or the relationship of the long axis of fetus to that of the mother.

(*i*) **Brow Presentation** (ब्रो प्रेजेन्टेशन) प्रसव में भ्रूण की भौंहों या माथे की प्रस्तुति, भाल प्रस्तुति। Presentation of brow of the fetus in labor.

(*ii*) **Cephalic Presentation** (सिफैलिक प्रेजेन्टेशन) भ्रूण के सिर के किसी भी भाग की प्रस्तुति।
Presentation of any part of the head of the fetus.

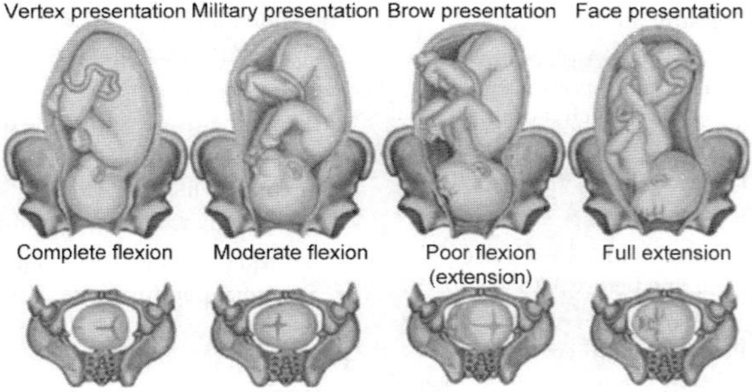

Presentation

(*iii*) **Funic Presentation** (फ्यूनिक प्रेजेन्टेशन) प्रसव में नाभि-रज्जु की प्रस्तुति। Presentation of the umbilical cord in labor.

Preservative (प्रिज़र्वेटिव) औषधियों अथवा खाद्य पदार्थों को खराब होने से बचाने के लिए उनमें मिलाया जाने वाला एक पदार्थ। A substance which is added to medicines or food materials to prevent them from spoiling.

Pressoreceptive (प्रेसोरिसीप्टिव) दाब उद्दीपनों के प्रति संवेदनशील। Sensitive to pressure stimuli.

Pressure (प्रेशर) दबाव, फैलाव, खिंचाव, तनाव अथवा भार से पड़ने वाला बल या दाब। Stress or force exerted by compression, expansion, pulling, tension or weight.

(*i*) **Capillary pressure** (कैपिलरी प्रेशर) रक्त कोशिकाओं के अन्दर का रक्त दाब। Blood pressure in the blood capillaries.

(*ii*) **Parital pressure** (पार्शिय प्रेशर) किसी मिश्रित गैस के घटकों में से प्रत्येक घटक द्वारा पड़ने वाला दाब। Pressure exerted by each of the components of a mixed gas. (*iii*) **Pulse pressure** (पल्स प्रेशर)

प्रकुचन एवं अनुशिथिलन के दाबों का अन्तर, नाड़ी दाब। The difference between the systolic and diastolic pressure.

(*iv*) **Thredy pulse** (थ्रेडी पल्स) क्षीण नाड़ी। A weak, usually rapid and scarcely perceptible pulse.

Pressure point (प्रेशर पॉइन्ट) दाब-बिन्दु। A place at which an artery passes over a bone against which it can be compressed to stop bleeding.

Preterm (प्रीटर्म) गर्भावस्था के 37वें सप्ताह से पहले उत्पन्न होने वाला, अकाल प्रसव। Occurring before 37th week of pregnancy.

Prevalence (प्रीवैलेन्स) किसी निर्दिष्ट आबादी में किसी विशेष समय पर विद्यमान किसी विशिष्ट रोग के रोगियों की कुल संख्या। The total number of cases of specific disease present in given population at a certain time.

Prevention (प्रीवेन्शन) रूकावट। Obstruction.

Preventive medicine (प्रीवेन्टिव मेडिसिन) चिकित्सा-शास्त्र की वह शाखा जिसका सम्बन्ध शारीरिक एवं मानसिक रोगों की रोकथाम से होता है। The branch of medical science concerned with the prevention of physical and mental disease.

Prevertebral (प्रीवर्टीब्रल) किसी कशेरूका के सामने, पूर्वकशेरूकीय। In front of a vertebra.

Prevesical (प्रीवैसाइकल) मूत्राशय के सामने स्थित। Located in front of the urinary bladder.

Previable (प्रीवॉयबल्) उस भ्रूण से सम्बन्धित जो गर्भाशय से बाहर जीने योग्य नहीं होता। Pertaining to a fetus unable to survive outside the uterus.

Priapism (प्रियापिज्म)। लिंग का निरन्तर बना रहने वाला असामान्य वेदनायुक्त उत्थान। Persistent abnormal painful erection of the penis.

Prickle cell (प्रिकिल सेल) दण्डाकार प्रवधों से युक्त एक कोशिका। A cell with rod shaped processes.

Prickly heat (प्रीकली हीट) गर्मी के मौसम में त्वचा पर निकलने वाला लाल-लाल दाने जिनमें खुजली आती है। घमौरी। Red cutaneous eruption with itching seen in hot weather.

Primary amputation (प्राइमरी एम्पुटेशन) शोथ के आरम्भ होने से पहले किया जाने वाला अंगोंच्छेद। Amputation performed before the onset of inflammation.

Primigravida (प्राइमीग्रेविडा) पहली बार गर्भवती होने वाली स्त्री, प्रथमसगर्भा। A woman pregnant for the first time.

Primipara (प्राइमीपैरा) प्रथम बार प्रसव होने वाली स्त्री, प्रथमप्रसवता। A woman giving birth to her first child.

Primitive (प्राइमिटिव) प्राथमिक, प्रारम्भिक, भ्रूणीयया आद्य। First in point of time, original.

Primordium (प्राइमोर्डियम) किसी अंग या बनावट की मूल अवस्था। An organ or structure in its earliest state.

Principle (प्रिन्सिपिल) रासायनिक मिश्रण, तत्व, सिद्धान्त, नियम, घटक। A chemic compound, a theory a constituent.

Privacy (प्राइवेसी) गुप्तता, एकान्त स्थान। Secrecy, lonely place.

Proactivator (प्रोएक्टीवेटर) किसी सक्रियकारक का पूर्वगामी। A precursor of an activator.

Proantithrombin (प्रोएन्टीथ्रॉम्बिन) रक्त प्लाज्मा या सीरम में विद्यमान एक पदार्थ जो हिपैरिन कि क्रिया द्वारा एन्टीथ्रॉम्बिन में परिवर्तित होता है। A substance present in the blood plasma or serum which is converted into antithrombin through the action of heparin.

Probang (प्रोबैन्ग) एक पतली, लचीली छड़ जिससे श्वयंत्र में दवाई लगाई जाती है। A device to apply medicines in larynx.

Probe (प्रोब) किसी जख्म-नासूर अथवा मार्ग की गहराई तथा उसकी दिशा का पता लगाने वाला एक लम्बा, पतला यंत्र, एशणी। A long slender instrument for exploring the depth and direction of a wound sinus or passage.

Process (प्रोसेस्) क्रिया की विधि, प्रक्रिया, किसी ऊतक से उत्पन्न होने वाला एक प्रक्षेपण या अतिवृद्धि। The steps or method of action, a projection or outgrowth of tissue.

Procheilon (प्रोकीलॉन) ऊपरी होंठ के केन्द्र में स्थित एक उभार। Prominence in the center of the upper lip.

Procidentia (प्रोसीडैन्सिया) पूर्ण भ्रंश विषेषक गर्भाशय का पूर्ण भ्रंश, गभाशयपूर्णभ्रंश। A complete prolapse especially of the uterus.

Proconvertin (प्रोकनवर्टिन) स्कन्दन कारक सातवां। Coagulation factor 7.

Procreate (प्रोक्रिएट) जन्मदेना, जनना, पैदा करना। To beget, to produce by the sexual act.

Proctalgia (प्रोक्टैल्जिया) गुदा के चारों ओर तथा मलाशय में दर्द होना, मूलान्त्रशूल। Pain around the anus and in rectum.

Proctatresia (प्रोक्टेट्रेसिया) गुदा की छिद्र युक्त न होना। Imperforate of the anus.

Proctitis (प्रोक्टाइटिस) मलाशयशोथ। Inflammation of the rectum.

Proctoclysis (प्रोक्टोक्लाइसिस) किसी तरल को मलाशय में धीरे-धीरे बूँद-बूँद करके प्रविष्ट करना। Introduction of a fluid into the rectum slowly drop by drop.

Proctocolitis (प्रोक्टोकोलाइटिस) मलाशय एवं कोलन का शोथ। Inflammation of the rectum and colon.

Proctocystotomy (प्रोक्टोसिस्टोटॉमी) मलाशय से गुजरकर मूत्राशय में चीरा लगाना। To make an incision into urinary bladder through the rectum.

Proctodynia (प्रोक्टोडाइनिया) मलद्वार अथवा मलांत्र का दर्द। Pain in the anus or rectum.

Proctology (प्रोक्टोलॉजी) गुदारोगविज्ञान। Branch of medicine dealing with disease of rectum, colon and anus.

Proctophobia (प्रोक्टोफोबिया) मलाशय के रोग से पीड़ित होने का विकृत भय। Morbid fear of suffering from rectal disease.

Proctoptosis (प्रोक्टोप्टोसिस) मलाशय का भ्रंश। Prolapse of the rectum.

Proctorrhea (प्रोक्टोरिह्या) गुदा या मलद्वार से श्लेष्मिक स्राव निकलना। Mucous discharge from the anus.

Proctoscopy (प्रोक्टोस्कोपी) मलाशय का निरीक्षण करना, मलाशयदर्शन। Inspection of the rectum with a proctoscope.

Proctosigmoidoscopy (प्रोक्टोसिग्मॉयडोस्कोपी) मलाशय-अवग्रहान्त्रदर्शी द्वारा मलाशय एवं अवग्रहान्त्र का नेत्र परिक्षण करना। Visual examination of the rectum and sigmoid colon by proctosigmoidoscope.

Proctostasis (प्रोक्टोस्टेसिस) कब्ज हो जाना। Constipation.

Procursive (प्रोकर्सिव) आगे को भागने के लिए उद्यत। Tending to run forward.

Prodromal (प्रोड्रोमल) किसी रोग की प्रारम्भिक अवस्था से सम्बन्धित, पूर्व-रूपी। Pertaining to the initial stage of a disease.

Prodrome (प्रोड्रोम) किसी रोग की शुरूआत का संकेत देने वाला एक लक्षण। A symptom indicating the onset of a disease.

Proenzyme (प्रोएन्जाइम) किसी एन्जाइम का एक निष्क्रिय पूर्वगामी। Zymogen, an inactive precursor of an enzyme.

Proerythroblast (प्रोइरिथ्रोब्लास्ट) प्राक्लाहित कोशिकाप्रसू। Pronormoblast.

Profluvium lactis (प्रोफ्लूवियम लैक्टिस) दूध का अत्यधिक बहना। Excessive flow of milk.

Profunda (प्रोफण्डा) गहराई में स्थित, गम्भीर। Deeply seated.

Progenitor (प्रोजेनाइटर) पूर्वज। An ancestor.

Progeny (प्रोजनी) सन्तान, संतति। Offspring.

Progeria (प्रोजैरिया) बचपन में कालपूर्व वृद्धावस्था का उत्पन्न होना, कालपूर्व जरा। Premature old age accruing in childhood.

Progestational (प्रोजेस्टेशनल) गर्भपूर्व। Before or favoring pregnancy.

Progesterone (प्रोजेस्टेरोन) पीत पिण्ड, अधिवृक्क प्रान्तस्था तथा अपरा से मुक्त होने वाला एक स्टैरॉयड हार्मोन। A steroid harmone liberated by corpus luteum adrenal cortex and placenta.

Progestin (प्रोजेस्टिन) कृत्रिम रूप से तैयार एक औषधि जिसका गर्भाशय पर प्रोजेस्टेरोन के समान प्रभाव होता है। A synthetic drug having the progesterone like effect on the uterus.

Proglottid (प्रोग्लोटिड) फीताकृमि के खण्डों में से एक देहखण्ड। One of the segments of a tapeworm.

Prognathism (प्रोग्नेथिज्म) एक या दोनो जबड़ों का असामान्य प्रक्षेपण (उभार), उद्गत-हनुता। Abnormal projection of one or both jaw.

Prognosis (प्रोग्नोसिस) पूर्वानुमान, प्राग्ज्ञान, फलानुमान, भावीफल। A forecast as to the probable result of an attack of a disease.

Progressive (प्रोग्रेसिव) प्रगामी, वर्धमान। Going forward.

Prohormone (प्रोहॉर्मोन) किसी हॉर्मोन का कोई पूर्व गामी। A precursor of a harmone.

Proinsulin (प्रोइन्सुलिन) अग्नाशय की बीटा कोशिकाओं में उत्पन्न होने वाला इन्सुलिन का एक पूर्वगामी। A precursor of insulin produced in the beta cells of the pancreas.

Projectile Vomiting (प्रोजैक्टाइल–बोमीटिंग) ऐसी उल्टी जिसमें आमाशय के पदार्थ बलपूर्वक बाहर को फेंक दिए जाते है जो रोगी से कुछ दूर जाकर गिरते हैं। Vomiting in which contents of the stomach are ejected forcibly, which fall down at a little distance from the patient.

Projection (प्रोजेक्शन) आगे को फेंकने की क्रिया, तीक्ष्ण, उभार, प्रक्षेपण। The process of throwing forward, sharp, prominence.

Prolabium (प्रोलैबियम) ऊपरी होंठ का बीच का उठा हुआ भाग। The prominent central portion of the upper lip.

Prolactin (प्रोलैक्टिन) पीयूष ग्रन्थि का एक हार्मोन जो दुग्ध निर्माण को उत्तेजित करता है, स्तनप्रेरक। A hormone of the anterior pituitary gland which stimulates the milk formation.

Prolapse (प्रोलैप्स) शरीर के किसी अंग अथवा भाग का नीचे खिसकना, भ्रंश, स्थानच्युति। A falling down of downward displacement of an organ or part of the body.

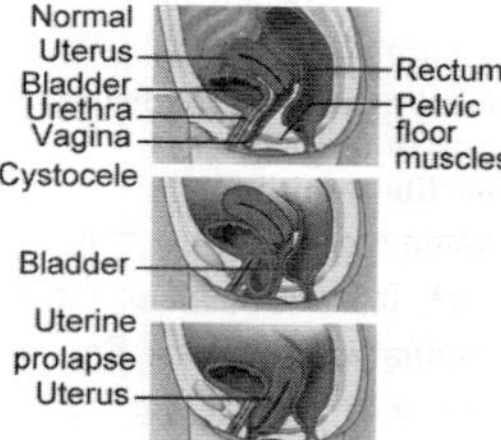

Proliferate (प्रोलीफ्रेट) जनन द्वारा एक ही रूप वालों की वृद्धि करना, आत्मपुनर्जनन करना। To increase by reproduction of the same forms.

Prolific (प्रोलीफिक) अबन्धक, उपजाऊ, प्रजननशील। Fertile, reproductive.

Promegakaryocyte (प्रोमेगाकैरियोसाइट) महामूललोहित कोशिका का एक पूर्वगामी। A precursor of megakaryocyte.

Prometaphase (प्रोमेटाफेज़) कोशिका के सूत्रीविभाजन की अवस्था जिसमें केन्द्रकीय कला विघटित हो जाती है तथा तारक केन्द्रक कोशिका के ध्रुवों तक पहुँचते है जबकि गुणसूत्र संकुचित होते रहते है। The stage of mitosis in which the nuclear membrane disintegrates and the centrioles reach the poles of the cell, which the chromosomes continue to contract.

Prominence (प्रोमीनेन्स) उत्सेध। An elevation.

Promonocyte (प्रोमोनोसाइट) एक केन्द्रक कश्वेत कोशिका का एक पूर्वगामी। A precursor of monocyte.

Promontory (प्रोमोन्टरी) एक उभरा हुआ प्रवर्ध या भाग, प्रोतुंग। A projecting process or part.

Pronation (प्रोनेशन) अलिन्दतल का नीचे को मुड़ना। Turning the ventral surface downwards.

Prong (प्रोंग) शंक्वाकार जैसे किसी दाँत की मूल। Conical such as the root of a tooth.

Pronormoblast (प्रोनॉर्मोब्लास्ट) लाल रक्त कोशिका का सर्वप्रथम पूर्वगामी। The earliest precursor of the RBC.

Propagate (प्रोपेगेट) प्रजनन करना या उत्पन्न करना। To reproduce or generate.

Prophase (प्रोफेज़) सूत्रीविभाजन प्रकार के कोशिका विभाजन की प्रथम अवस्था, पूर्वावस्था। First stage of the cell division of the mitosis type.

Prophylaxis (प्रोफाइलैक्सिस) रोगनिरोध, रोगरोधक चिकित्सा। The preventive treatment.

Proprioception (प्रोप्रायोसैप्शन) शरीर के आसन एवं उसकी गति से अवगत रहना तथा शरीर के सम्बन्ध में वस्तुओं की स्थिति, उनके भार तथा प्रतिरोध की जानकारी होना। The awareness of posture and movement of the body and the knowledge of position, weight and resistance of objects in relation to the body.

Proprioceptor (प्रोप्रायोसैप्टर) प्रग्राहक। Receptors responsible for body position and equilibrium.

Proptosis (प्रोप्टोसिस) नेत्रगोलक का आगे की ओर फैलना। Forward protrusion, especially of an eyeball.

Proptotic (प्रोप्टोटीक) नीचे की ओर विस्थापन से सम्बन्धित। Pertaining to proptosis.

Prosection (प्रोसैक्शन) शरीर रचना सम्बन्धी रचना को प्रदर्शित करने के लिए पहले से सोच-विचार कर किया जाने वाला व्यवच्छेदन। Preplanned dissection for demonstrating the anotomic structure.

Prosector (प्रोसैक्टर) व्यवच्छेदन को सम्पन्न करने वाला व्यक्ति। The person who performs dissection.

Prosencephalon (प्रोसेन्सीफैलॉन) भ्रूणीय अग्रमस्तिष्क। Embryonic forebrain.

Prosopagnosia (प्रोसोपैग्नोसिया) चेहरों को पहचानने में असमर्थता यहाँ तक कि अपना चेहरा भी नहीं पहचाना जाता। Inability to recognize the faces, even one's own face.

Prosoplasia (प्रोसोप्लेसिया) कोशिकाओं का रूपान्तरण जब तक वे उच्च कार्य करने वाली कोशिकाओं में विकसित नहीं हो जाती है। The transformation of cells until they develop into the cell with higher function.

Prosopoplegia (प्रोसोपोप्लीजीया) चेहरे का पक्षाघात। Facial paralysis.

Prosoposchisis (प्रोसोपोस्काइसिस) चेहरे की जन्मजात फटन या दरार। Congenital fissure of the face.

Prosopothoracopagus (प्रोसोपोथौरेकोपेगस) दो जुड़वाँ भ्रूण जो चेहरे से वक्ष तक जुड़े होते है।
Two conjoined fetuses joined from the face to thorax.

Prosopotocia (प्रोसोपोटोसिया) बच्चे के जन्म के समय चेहरे की प्रस्तुति। Face presentation during childbirth.

Prostaglandins (प्रोस्टेग्लैण्डिनस) शरीर में असंतृप्त वसीय अम्लों से बनने वाला वसीय अम्ल व्युत्पन्नों का एक वर्ग।
A group of fatty acid derivatives, synthesized in the body from unsaturated fatty acids.

Prostate (प्रोस्टेट) पुरूष में मूत्राशय की गर्दन एवं मूत्रमार्ग को चारों ओर से घेरने वाली तीन खण्ड वाली एक ग्रन्थि जो वाहिनियों द्वारा मूत्रमार्ग के प्रोस्टेट वाले भाग में खुलती है।
A three lobed gland surrounding the neck of the urinary bladder and urethra in the male, which opens into the prostatic portion of urethra through ducts.

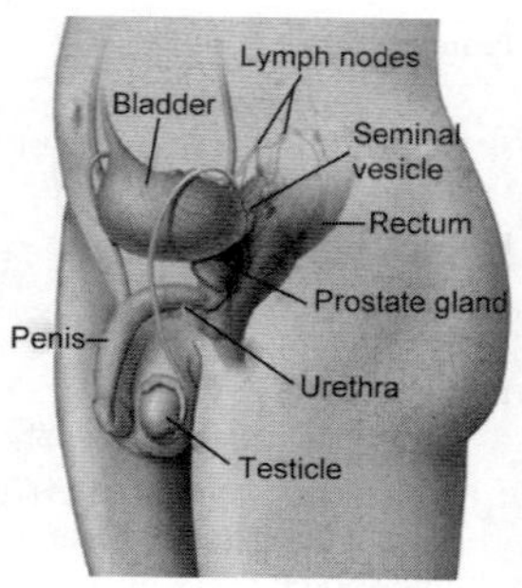

Prostatelcosis (प्रोस्टेटेल्कोसिस) प्रोस्टेट ग्रन्थि में जख्म बन जाना। Ulceration of the prostate gland.

Prostatism (प्रोस्टेटिज्म) प्रोस्टेट ग्रन्थि का कोई भी रोग जिससे मूत्राशय से मूत्र के बहने में अवरोध उत्पन्न हो जाता है। Any condition of the prostate gland interfering with the flow of urine from the urinary bladder.

Prostatitis (प्रोस्टेटाइटिस) प्रोस्टेट ग्रन्थि की सूजन। Inflammation of the prostate gland.

Prosthesis (प्रोस्थेसिस) कृत्रिम अंग, नकली अंग। An artificial part or organ.

Prosthetic (प्रोस्थेटिक) कृत्रिम अंगों अथवा कृत्रिम-अंग विज्ञान से सम्बन्धित।
Pertaining to prosthesis or prosthetics.

Prosthetist (प्रोस्थेटिस्ट) कृत्रिमांगविज्ञानी। One skilled in constructing and fitting prosthesis.

Prostration (प्रोस्ट्रेशन) अवसाद, अवसन्नता। Extreme nervous exhaustion.

Protanopia (प्रोटोनोपिया) लाल वर्णान्धता। Red color blindness.

Protease (प्रोटीयेस) एक प्रोटीनविघटनकारी एन्जाइम। A Protein-splitting enzyme.

Protein (प्रोटीन) जटिल कार्बनिक यौगिकों के वर्ग में से कोई भी एक जो वृद्धि एवं विकास के लिए आवश्यक है। Complex organic compounds which are essential for growth and development.

Proteinogenous (प्रोटीनोजीनस) प्रोटीन उत्पन्न करने वाला। Producing protein.

Proteinosis (प्रोटीनोसिस) अधिक प्रोटीन का ऊतकों में जमा हो जाना, प्रोटीनमयता। Accumulation of excess of protein in the tissue.

Proteinuria (प्रोटीनूरिया) मूत्र में प्रोटीन का पाया जाना, प्रोटीनमेह, अन्नसारमेह। Protein in the urine.

Proteolysis (प्रोटीयोलाइसिस) प्रोटीनलयन, प्रोटीन-अपघटन। The breaking down of proteins into simpler substance.

Proteopepsis (प्रोटीयोपेप्सिस) प्रोटीनों का पाचन। The digestion of protein.

Proteus (प्रोटियस) यह ग्राम-निगेटिव, विकल्पी, वातनिरपेक्षी, खमीरण करने वाले आन्त्रीय दण्डाणुओं का एक वंश होता है जो ऑतों में तथा मल पदार्थो में पाया जाता है और प्रोटिन का विघटन करता है। It is a genus of gram-negative, facultative, anaerobic, fermenting enteric bacilli, found in the intestines and fecal matter causing protein decomposition.

Prothrombin (प्रॉथ्रोम्बिन) स्कन्दन कारक दूसरा। Coagulation factor II.

Prothrombinase (प्रोथ्रोम्बिनेस) रक्त स्कन्दन में एक महत्वपूर्ण एन्जाइम। An enzyme important in the coagulation of blood.

Prothrombinemia (प्रोथ्रॉम्बिनीमिया) रक्त में प्रोथ्रॉम्बिन का पाया जाना। Presence of prothrombin in the blood.

Prothymocyte (प्रोथाइमोसाइट) थाइमस ग्रन्थि में टी-कोशिका का एक पूर्वगामी। A precursor of T-cell in the thymus gland.

Protistologist (प्रोटिस्टोलॉजिस्ट) एककोशिकीय जीवों का अध्ययन करने वाला व्यक्ति। One who studies the unicellular organisms.

Protocol (प्रोटोकॉल) किसी रोगी के परीक्षण, किसी प्रयोग अथवा पोस्टमार्टम परीक्षण पर तैयार की गई प्रारम्भिक टिप्पणियाँ। The original notes made on examination of a patient, on an experiment or at postmortem examination.

Protoduodenum (प्रोटोड्योडिनम) ड्योडिनम का ऊपरी आधा भाग। The upper half of the duodenum.

Proton (प्रोटोन) किसी परमाणु की नाभि का धनात्मक पूरित भाग। A positively charged particle in the atom.

Protoplasia (प्रोटोप्लेसिया) ऊतक का प्राथमिक निर्माण। The primary formation of tissue.

Protoplasm (प्रोटोप्लाज्म) कोशिकाओं तथा ऊतकों का सजीव पदार्थ, जीवद्रव्य। The living matter of cells and tissues.

Protoporphyrinuria (प्रोटोपोर्फाइरिनूरिया) मूत्र में प्रोटोपोर्फाइरिन का पाया जाना। Presence of protoporphyrin in the urine.

Protovertebra (प्रोटोवर्टिब्रा) आधपृष्ठवंश में आद्य कशेरूका। Primitive vertebra in the notochord.

Protozoa (प्रोटोजुआ) प्रजीवाणु, शुक्राणु, बीजाणु। A class of unicellular animal organism.

Protozoacide (प्रोटोजुआसाइड) एककोशिकीय जन्तुओं के लिए विनाशकारी। Destructive to protozoa.

Protozoology (प्रोटोजूलॉजी) एककोशिकिय जन्तुओं का अध्ययन। Study of the protozoa.

Protractor (प्रोट्रेक्टर) जख्मों से बाह्य पदार्थो को बाहर निकालने वाला एक यंत्र। An instrument for removing foreign bodies from wounds.

Protrude (प्रोट्रयूड) आगे को निकालना या बढ़ाना, उभारना। To project or to extend.

Protuberance (प्रोट्यूबेरैन्स) गाँठ के समान उठा हुआ भाग, प्रोद्वर्ध। A prominent part like a knob.

Provitamin (प्रोविटामीन) एक निश्क्रिय पदार्थ जो शरीर में पहुँच कर किसी विटामिन में रूपान्तरित हो जाता है। An inactive substance which can be transformed in the body to a vitamin.

Prurigo (प्रूराइगो) त्वचा पर तेज खाज मारते छोटे-छोटे दाने, कण्डूपिटिक। A chronic papular skin disease with intense itching.

Pruritus (प्रूराइटस) खुजली, कण्डू। Itching.

Pruritus Ani (प्रूराइटस एनाइ) मलद्वार की खुजली, गूदकण्ड। Itching of the anus.

Pruritus Hiemalis (प्रूराइटस हाइमेलिस) जाड़े के मौसम में होने वाली। Itching accruing in winter season.

Psammoma (सेम्मोमा) मस्तिष्क का एक छोटा-सा अबुर्द जिसमें कैल्सियमी कण मौजूद रहते है। A small tumor of the brain containing calcareous particles.

Psammotherapy (सेम्मोथिरैपी) रेत का प्रयोग करके रोगों का चिकित्सा करना। Treatment of the disease by application of sand.

Psammous (सेम्मस) रेतीला, किरकिरा। Sandy, Gritty.

Pseudacousma (स्यूडेकाऊज्मा) ध्वनियों का मिथ्या बोध होना। Flase perception of sounds.

Pseudagraphia (स्यूडेग्राफिया) स्वतंत्र रूप से लिखने में अक्षमता परन्तु शब्दों की नकल करने की क्षमता। Inability to write independently but ability to cope the words.

Pseudarthrosis (स्यूडाथ्रोसिस) किसी अस्थिभंग के पश्चात जो जुड़ा नहीं होता, बनने वाली मिथ्यासन्धि, कूटसन्धि। A false joint developing after a fracture that has not united.

Pseudoamenorrhea (स्यूडोएमैनोरिह्या) कूट-अनार्तव। Flase amenorrhea.

Pseudo-angina (स्यूडोएनजाइना) कूट-हृदयशूल। मानसिक विचार से उत्पन्न होने वाले लक्षण जो हृदयशूल के समान होते है। A nervous disorder approximative angina consisting of chest pain or breast pain.

Pseudoblepsia (स्यूडोब्लेप्सिया) मिथ्या अथवा काल्पनिक दृष्टि। False or imaginary vision.

Pseudobulbar (स्यूडोबलबर) कूटमेरू-शीर्षघात। किसी भी प्रकार के मस्तिष्क संबंधी विकारो के कारण चेहरे पर किसी भी प्रकार की क्रियाओं को नियंत्रित नही कर पाना। Inability to control facial movements (such as chewing and speaking) caused by neurological disorder.

Pseudocele (स्यूडोसील) मस्तिष्क में पाँचवा निलय। Fifth ventricle in the brain.

Pseudochromidrosis (स्यूडोक्रोमीड्रोसिस) पसीना

निकलने के बाद उसका रंगीन दिखाई देना। Appearance of the sweat colored after it is excreted.

Pseudocyesis (स्यूडोसाइसिस) मिथ्या गर्भावस्था। False pregnancy.

Pseudocyst (स्यूडोसिस्ट) एक विस्फारण जो पुटी के समान होता है। A dilatation resembling a cyst.

Pseudodementia (स्यूडोडिमैन्शिया) ऐसी दशा जिसमें मनोभ्रंश के समान अपने चारों ओर की कोई सुध नहीं रहती परन्तु बुद्धि में कोई नहीं होती। A state of indifference to the environment resembling dementia but without impairment of intelligence.

Pseudodipsia (स्यूडोडिप्सिया) मिथ्या प्यास जिसमें पानी पीने से संतुष्टि नहीं होती। False thirst in which there is no satisfaction by drinking water.

Pseudoedema (स्यूडोइडीमा) त्वचा का फुलाव जो शोफ के समान होता है। Puffiness of the skin resembling edema.

Pseudofracture (स्यूडोफ्रैक्चर) कुछ प्रकार की अस्थिमृदुता में एक्स-रे में दिखाई देने वाली विकैल्सीभवन की एक रेखा। A line of decalcification seen in X-ray in certain types of osteomalacia.

Pseudogout (स्यूडोगाउट) जीर्ण सन्धिशोथ जिसमें क्रिस्टल कैल्सियम पाइरोफॉस्फेट डिहाइड्रेट होते है। Joint pain resembling gout but caused by calcium pyrophosphate dihydrate crystals.

Pseudohermaphrodite (स्यूडोहर्मेफ्रोडाइट) ऐसा व्यक्ति जिसमें कूट-उभय लिंगता हो, कूट-उभयलिंगी। An individual with pseudohermaphroditism.

Pseudohypertrophy (स्यूडोहाइपरट्रॉफी) कूट-अतिवृद्धि। Increase in size of an organ or part of the body due to overgrowth of unimportant tissue.

Pseudohypoparathyroidism (स्यूडोहाइपोपैराथाइरॉडिज्म) एक अनुवांशिक रोग जो अल्पपरावटुता के समान होता है, परन्तु जो पैराथाइरॉड हार्मोन की कमी से होने के बजाय उसके प्रत्युत्तर देने में निष्फल हो जाने के कारण होता है। A hereditary disease resembling hyperthyroidism, but caused by failure to response rather than the deficiency of parathyroid hormone.

Pseudojaundice (स्यूडोजॉण्डिस) त्वचा का पीलापन जो कामला या जॉण्डिस के कारण नहीं बल्कि

रक्त के परिवर्तनों के कारण होता है। Yellowness of the skin, which is not caused by jaundice, but by blood changes.

Pseudomania (स्यूडोमेनिया) कूट-उन्माद, कूट-विक्षिप्ति। Feigned insanity.

Pseudomembrane (स्यूडोमेम्ब्रेन) कूट-कला, अयथार्थ झिल्ली। A false membrane.

Pseudomenstruation (स्यूडोमेंस्ट्रुएशन) गर्भाशय से रक्तस्त्राव होना परन्तु जो अन्तर्गर्भाशयकला या एण्डोमीट्रियम में होने वाले सामान्य परिवर्तनों के साथ नहीं होता। Bleeding from the uterus but not accompanied by the usual changes in the endometrium.

Pseudomonas (स्यूडोमोनास) गतिशील, ग्राम-नेगेटिव, वातापेक्षी दण्डाणुओं का एक वंश जिनसे पीले व नीले वर्णक बनते है। A genus of motile, gram-negative, aerobic bacilli, some of which produce yellow and blue pigment.

Pseudoparalysis (स्यूडोपैरालाइसिस) कूट-अंगछात। False paralysis.

Pseudoparasite (स्यूडोपैरासाइट) परजीवी के समान कोई भी वस्तु। Anything resembeling a parasite.

Pseudoparesis (स्यूडोपैरेसिस) कूट-आंशिकछात। The condition simulating paresis which is due to hysteria.

Pseudopodium (स्यूडोपोडियम) किसी एककोशिकीय जन्तु जैसे अमीबा अथवा श्वेत रक्त कोशिका के कोशिकाद्रव्य का अस्थी बहिःसरण जो चलने एवं भोजन कणों को निगलने का कार्य करता है, कूटपाद। A temporary protrusion of the cytoplasm of a protozoon such as an ameba, or a white blood cell, serving for locomotion and engulfing the food particles.

Pseudorickets (स्यूडोरिकेट्स) वृक्कीय बालास्थिविकार। Renal rickets.

Pseudosmia (स्यूडोस्मिया) बिना उद्दीपन के गन्ध की अनुभूति होना। The sensation of odor with stimulus.

Pseudotuberculosis (स्यूडोट्यूबरकुलोसिस) कूटयक्ष्मा। A condition simulating tuberculosis.

Psittacosis (सीट्टेकोसिस) शुष्क रोग, पक्षियों को होने वाला एक संक्रामक रोग। Parrot fever, an infectious disease of birds.

Psoas (सोआस) कटि-प्रदेश की दो पेशियों में से एक। One of two muscles of the loins.

Psoas abscess (सोआस एब्सेस) सोआस मेज़र मेशी के आवरण में स्थित एक ठण्डा फोड़ा, कटि–विद्रधि। A cold abscess in the sheath of psoas major muscle.

Psoriasis (सोरीयासिस) एक जीर्ण त्वचा रोग जिसमें बारीक-बारीक शुष्क चाँदी के समान शल्कों से ढकी हुई, थोड़ी उठी हुई, चमकीली लाल पिटिकाएँ अथवा चकते बन जाते है। विचर्चिका, अपरस। A chronic skin disease marked by the formation of slightly elevated bright red papules or plaques covered with fine, dry silvery scales.

In general, psoriasis can be classified as:

Mild	Moderate	Severe
only a few patches, less than 3% of the skin surface	3 to 10% of the skin surface	More than 10% of the skin surface

Psychataxia (साइकेटैक्सिया) ध्यान केन्द्रित करने में असमर्थता। Inability to concentrate.

Psyche (साइकी) दिमाग। The mind.

Psychiatry (साइकियाट्री) मनोरोगविज्ञान, मनोविकारविज्ञान। The study diagnosis, prevention and treatment of mental disease.

Psychoactive (साइकोएक्टिव) मस्तिष्क अथवा व्यवहार को प्रभावित करने वाला जैसे कोई औषधि। Affecting the mind or behavior, such as a drug.

Psychoanalysis (साइकोएनालाइसिस) मनो-विश्लेषण, मनोगहन। A division of psychiatry that involves prolonged exploration of the patient's personality.

Psychodynamics (साइकोडाइनामिक्स) मानव व्यवहार एवं प्रेरणा का वैज्ञानिक अध्ययन। Scientific study of human behavior and motivation.

Psychogenesis (साइकोजेनेसिस) मानसिक विकास। Mental development.

Psychogenic (सोइकोजेनिक) मनोजात, मानसिक, आधिज। Arising from the mind.

Psychograph (साइकोग्राफ) रोगी के व्यक्तित्व विशेषकों का रेखाचित्र द्वारा अभिलेखन किये जाने के लिए एक चार्ट। A chart for recording graphically the patient's personality traits.

Psychokinesis (साइकोकाइनेसिस) मस्तिष्क में किसी विचार के उत्पन्न होने से सक्रिय अथवा भावावेगी हो जाना। To become active or emotional caused by a thought originated in the mind.

Psycholagny (साइकोलैग्नी) कल्पना मात्र या विचार आने से ही लैंगिक उत्तेजना होना। Psychic or mental masturbation, sexual excitement by imagination only.

Psychologist (साइकोलॉजिस्ट) मनोविज्ञान, मनोरोगविशेषज्ञ। A specialist in psychology.

Psychometry (साइकोमीट्री) मानसिक क्षमता की माप लेना, मनोभित्ति। The measurement of mental ability.

Psychoneurosis (साइकोन्यूरोसिस) मनस्तंत्रिका-विक्षिप्ति, मनोविक्षिप्ति। Mental neurosis.

Psychopathy (साइकोपैथी) कोई भी मानसिक रोग। Any mental disease.

Psychopharmacology (साइकोफार्मेकोलॉजी) मानसिक विकारों पर औषधियों की क्रिया का अध्ययन। The study of the action of drugs on mental disorders.

Psychophysiologic (साइकोफिजियोलॉजिक) मस्तिष्क के शरीरक्रियाविज्ञान से सम्बन्धित। Pertaining to psychophysiology.

Psychoplegic (साइकोप्लीजीक) मानसिक दुर्बलता उत्पन्न करने वाला। Causing mental weakness.

Psychosexual (साइकोसैक्सुअल) लिंग के मानसिक अथवा भावावेगी पहलुओं से सम्बन्धित। Pertaining to the psychic or emotional aspects of sex.

Psychosis (साइकोसिस) मनोविक्षिप्ति, पागलपन। A specific mental illness arising in the mind itself.

Psychosomatic (साइकोसोमैटिक) मस्तिष्क एवं शरीर के सम्बन्ध से सम्बन्धित। Pertaining to the relationship of the mind and body.

Psychotherapeutic (साइकोथिराप्यूटिक) मनश्चिकित्सा से सम्बन्धित। Pertaining to psychotherapy.

Psychotherapy (साइकोथिरैपी) रोगों विशेषकर मानसिक रोगों की मनोवैज्ञानिक चिकित्सा। Psychological treatment of the disease, especially the mental disease.

Psychotropic (साइकोट्रॉपिक) मस्तिष्क पर प्रभाव डालने वाला। Exerting an effect on the mind.

Psychrophile (साइक्रोफाइल) कम तापमान पर सबसे अच्छी वृद्धि करने वाला जीव। An organism growing best at low temperature.

Psychrophobia (साइक्रोफोबिया) ठण्ड से घृणा होना अथवा उसका विकृत भय। A version to or morbid fear of cold.

Pterygium (टेरीजियम) कन्दी नेत्रश्लेष्मता की त्रिभुजाकार मोटाई जो आन्तर नेत्रकोण से स्वच्छमण्डल तक फैली होती है। A triangular thickening of the bulbar conjunctiva extending from inner canthus to the cornea.

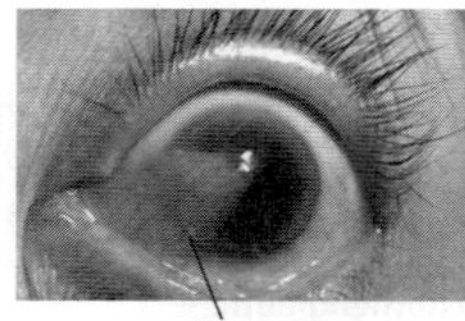

Pterygium

Pterygoid (टेरीगॉयड) पंख जैसा, पक्षाभ। Alate, wing shaped.

Pterygopalatine (टेरीगोपैलाटाइन) पक्षाभ प्रवर्ध एवं तालव हड्डी से सम्बन्धित, पक्षाभतालुज। Pertaining to the pterygoid process and the palate bone.

Ptomaine (टोमैनी) खाद्य, भोजन, आहार। The food.

Ptosis (टोसिस) किसी अंग का नीचे को लटक अथवा गिर जाना जैसे पक्षाघात होने से आँख की ऊपरी पलक का नीचे को झुक जाना, वर्त्मपात। Dropping of an organ, as of the upper eyelid from paralysis.

Ptyalagogue (टायलागौग) लालावर्धक, लारवर्धक। Sialogogue.

Ptyalin (टॉयलीन) लार, लाला। Any amylolytic ferment of saliva.

Ptyalism (टायलिज्म) लार अधिक बनना, अतिलालास्रावता। Excessive secretion of saliva.

Ptyalith (टायलिथ) लार ग्रन्थि में स्थित पथरी। A calculus in a salivary gland.

Ptyalocels (आयलोसील) लार ग्रन्थि का पुटीय अबुर्द। Cystic tumor of the salivary gland.

Ptyalorrhea (टायलोरीह्या) अत्यधिक लार बहना। Excessive flow of saliva.

Ptysis (टायसिस) थूकना अथवा थूक का मूख से बाहर को फेंक दिया जाना। Spitting or ejection of saliva from the mouth.

Pubarche (प्यूबार्के) 1. यौवनारम्भ की शुरूआत 2. जघन रोमों का प्रथम बार प्रकट होना। 1. Beginning of puberty. 2. First appearance of the pubic hair.

Puberty (प्यूबर्टी) जीवन का वह काल जिसमें किसी लिंग का व्यक्ति जनन के सक्षम हो जाता है। यह लड़कों में 13 से 15 तथा

लड़कियों में 9 से 16 वर्ष की आयु होती है जब उनके द्वितीयक लैंगिक लक्षण विकसित होने आरम्भ हो जाते है। The period of life during which the person of their sex becomes capable of reproduction. It is 13 to 15 years of age in boys and 9 to 16 in girls, when their secondary sexual characters begin to develop.

Pubescence (प्यूबेसैन्स) यौवनारम्भ पर पहुँचना। The act of approching puberty.

Pubis (प्यूबिस) जघनास्थि, जांघ के बाल। Pubic bone, the mons veneris.

Puborectal (प्यूबोरैक्टल) जघनास्थि एवं मलाशय से सम्बन्धित। Pertaining to the pubic bone and rectum.

Pudenda (प्यूडेन्डा) बाह्य जननांग विशेषकर महिला के। External genitalia especially of female.

Puerile (प्यूराइल) बचपन अथवा बच्चों से सम्बन्धित। Pertaining to childhood or children.

Puerperal (प्यूरपीरल) प्रसूतिकाल अथवा प्रसूता से सम्बन्धित, प्रासूतिक। Pertaining to the puerperium or a puerpera.

Puerperal Sepsis (प्यूरपीरल सैप्सिस) प्रसूति-काल में उपद्रव के रूप में जननांगी पथ में उत्पन्न होने वाला कोई भी संक्रमण। Infection of genital tract in the puerperium.

Puerperium (प्यूरपीरियम) बच्चे के पैदा होने के बाद तथा अपरा एवं झिल्लियों के निकल जाने के बाद का 42 दिन का समय जिसमें गर्भाशय अपने सामान्य परिमाण में लौट आता है।
The period of 42 days following childbirth and expulsion of the placenta and membranes during which the uterus returns to its normal size.

Pulmometry (पल्मोमीटरी) फेफड़े की क्षमता का पता लगाना। Determination of the capacity of the lungs.

Pulmonary (पल्मोनरी) फेफड़ों से सम्बन्धित। Pertaining to the lungs.

Pulmonitis (पल्मोनाइटिस) फेफड़े का प्रदाह। Inflammation of the lungs.

Pulp (पल्प) गूदा, मज्जा। The soft part of the fruit.

Pulpitis (पल्पाइटिस) किसी दन्त-मज्जा का शोथ। Inflammation of a dental pulp.

Pulsate (पल्सेट)
अनुक्रम में स्पन्दन करना या धड़कन। To throb or beat in rhythm.

Pulsation (पल्सेशन) क्रमबद्ध स्पन्द जैसे हृदय का, एक धड़कन, स्पन्दन। The rhythmic beat, as of the heart; a throb.

Pulse (पल्स) नाड़ी, नब्ज, नाड़ीस्पन्द। The beat or throbbing of the heart and arteries, usually felt at the wrist above the ball of the thumb pulses.

(*i*) **Aternating pulse** (आल्टरनेंटिंग पल्स) नाड़ी जिसमें बारी-बारी से एक दुर्बल एवं एक शक्तिशाली स्पन्दन होता है। The pulse in which there is alternate weak and strong.

(*ii*) **Collapsing pulse** (कोलैप्सिंग पल्स) दुर्बल नाड़ी जो तुरन्त ही एवं पूर्णत्या लुप्त हो जाती है, निपाती नाड़ी। Weak pulse which subside quickly and completely.

Pulverization (पल्वेराइज़ेशन) किसी पदार्थ को कुचल कर पाउडर बनाने की क्रिया, चूर्णन। The crushing of a substance to powder.

Pump (पम्प) उदांचिका, पिचकारी। An apparatus for drawing liquids from a reservoir.

Punched out (पंच्ड आउट) स्पष्ट कटे हुए गोल किनारों से युक्त जो किसी बर्मे या छेद करने वाले यंत्र से बनाये गये छिद्र के समान प्रतीत होता है। With clear cut circular edges, appearing as hole made by a punch or boring instrument.

Punctate (पंक्टेट) बहुत सूक्ष्म छिद्रों या गड्ढों से चिन्हित, कर्बुरित। Dotted marks with very minute holes or depressions.

Punctio (पंक्षियो) छेद करना या चुभोना। The act of puncturing or pricking.

Puncture (पंक्चर) किसी तेज नुकीले औजार से बना छेद या जख्म। A hole or wound made by a sharp pointed instrument.

Pungent (पन्जैन्ट) तीखा या तेज जैसी कोई गन्ध या स्वाद। Acrid or sharp, as an odor or taste.

Pupil (प्यूपिल) आँख के परितारिका या उपतारा के केन्द्र में स्थित संकुचनशील छिद्र जिसके द्वारा प्रकाश आँख में प्रवेश करता है, तारा, पुतली। The contractile opening in the center of iris of eye through which light enters the eye.

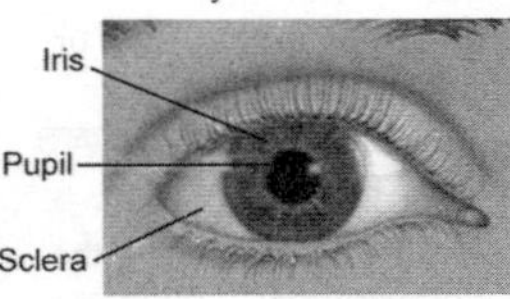

Pupillary reflex (प्यूपिलरी रिफ्लैक्स) पुतली पर प्रकाश डालने पर इसका संकुचित हो जाना।

Contraction of the pupil by light throwing upon it.

Pupillometer (प्यूपिलोमीटर) पुतली के व्यास को मापने वाला एक उपकरण। An apparatus for measuring diameter of the pupil.

Pupilloplegia (प्यूपिलोप्लेज़िया) पुतली की धीमी प्रतिक्रिया होना। Slow reaction of the pupil.

Purgative (पर्गेटिव) विरेचक, रेचक, दस्तावर। Causing watery evacuation of the intestinal contents.

Purge (पर्ग) किसी विरेचक का प्रयोग करके दस्त लाना। To evacuation the bowels by means of a purgative.

Puriform (प्यूरीफार्म) पस या मवाद के समान, पूयाभ। Resembling pus.

Purkinge fibers (पर्किन्जी फाइबर्स) ये हृदय में हिज की पूलिका से उत्पन्न होने वाले बहुत बड़े तन्तु होते है और निलयों में प्रवेश कर जाते है। ये हृदय आवेग को आलिन्दो से निलयों में संचालित करते है। These are very large fibers originating from the bundle of His in the heart and enter the ventricles. They conduct the cardiac impulse from the atria to the ventricles.

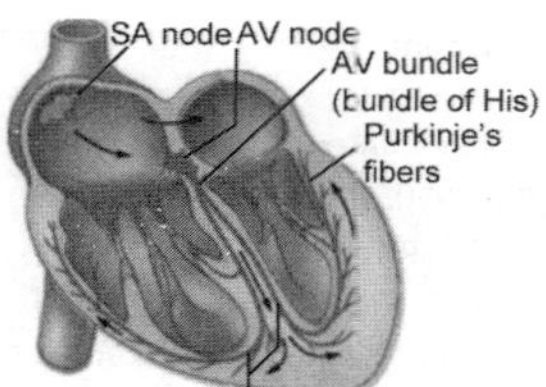

Purpura (परप्यूरा) रक्तचित्रता या परप्यूरा त्वचा, श्लेष्मिक कलाओं, जोड़ों, आन्तरिक अंगों तथा अन्य ऊतकों में रक्तस्राव होता है। Purpura is hemorrhage into the skin, mucous membranes joints, internal organs and other tissue. (*i*) **Rheumatic Purpura** (रिहयूमेटिका-परप्यूरा) जोड़ों के दर्द के साथ सम्बद्ध रक्तचित्रिता। Purpura associated with joint pains.

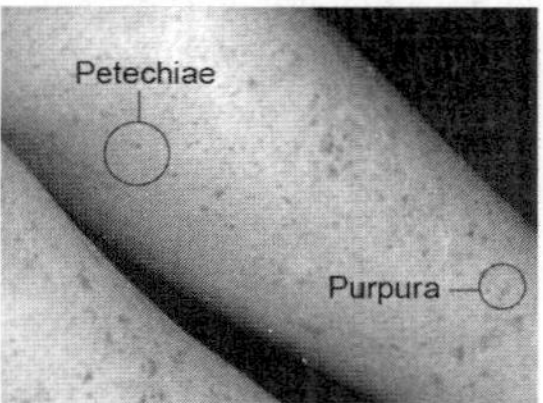

Purpuric (परप्यूरिक) रक्तचित्रिता से सम्बन्धित, उसके समान या उससे पीड़ित। Pertaining to, resembling or suffering from purpura.

Purulent (पुरूलैन्ट) सपूय, पीतयुक्त, मवादयुक्त। Consisting of pus like matter.

Pus (पस) शोथ का द्रव उत्पाद जो एक पतले तरल, प्रोटीन पदार्थो, श्वेत रक्त कोशिकाओं तथा कोशिकीय मलबे से बना होता है एवं साधारण पीलापन लिए होता है, पस, मवाद, पूय। Liquid product of inflammation composed of a thin fluid, protein substance, white blood cells and cellular debris, generally yellowish in color.

Pus cells (पस सैल्स) मवाद में पाई जाने वाली मृत श्वेत रक्त कोशिकाएँ। Dead leukocytes found in pus.

Pustule (पुस्तुले) पूयस्फोटिका, फुंसी। A small elevated pus containing lesion of the skin.

Putrefaction (प्यूट्रीफेक्शन) जन्तु पदार्थ विशेषकर प्रोटीनों का जीवाणुओं अथवा कवकों द्वारा विघटन जिससे दुर्गन्धित यौगिक जैसे अमोनिया हाइड्रोजन सल्फाइड उत्पन्न होते है, पूतीभवन। Decomposition of animal matter, especially proteins by bacteria of fungi with the production of foul-smelling compounds such as amonia, hydrogen sulfide.

Putrefy (प्यूट्रीफाइ) सड़ना। To undergo putrefaction.

Putrescence (प्यूट्रीसैन्स) सड़ान्ध, पूतीभवन। Decay; rottenness.

Pyarthrosis (प्यारथ्रोसिस) किसी सन्धि गुहा में पस बन जाना, पयूसन्धि। Pus in a joint cavity.

Pyelitis (पायलाइटिस) वृक्कीय गोणिकाशोथ। Inflammation of the renal pelvis.

Pyelocystitis (पायलोसिस्टाइटिस) वृक्कीय श्रोणि एवं मूत्राशय का शोथ। Inflammation of the renal pelvis and the urinary bladder.

Pyelogram (पायलोग्राम) गवीनी अथवा मूत्रनली तथा वृक्कीय श्रोणि की एक एक्स-रे फिल्म। An X-ray film of the ureter and renal pelvis.

Pyelolithotomy (पायलेलिथोटॉमी) पथरियों को निकालने के लिए वृक्कीय श्रोणि में चीरा लगाना। To incise the renal pelvis for removal of calculi.

Pyelonephritis (पायलोनैफ्राइटिस) वृक्क एवं इसकी श्रोणि का शोथ। Inflammation of the kidney and its pelvis.

Pyeloplasty (पायलोप्लास्टी) प्लास्टिक सर्जरी द्वारा वृक्कीय श्रोणि की मरम्मत करना। Repair of the renal pelvis by plastic surgery.

Pyelostomy (पायलोस्टॉमी) वृक्कीय श्रोणि में शल्यक्रिया द्वारा एक

छिद्र बनाना। Surgical formation of an opening into the renal pelvis.

Pyemesis (पायमेसिस) पस या मवाद की उल्टी होना। Vomiting of pus.

Pyemia (पायमिया) रक्त में पस बनाने वाले जीवों की विद्यमानता से उत्पन्न एक प्रकार की पूतिजीवरक्तता जिसमें द्वितीयक स्थलान्तरणीय प्रकार के बहुत से फोड़े बन जाते है। पूयरक्तता। A form of septicemia due to presence of pus forming organism in the blood, forming multiple abscesses of secondary metastatic nature.

Pyencephalus (पायेनासिफैलस) मस्तिष्क का फोड़ा जिसमें पस पड़ गया हो। Brain abscess with suppuration.

Pygal (पाइगल) नितम्बों से सम्बन्धित। Pertaining to the buttocks.

Pygmy (पिग्मी) बौना। Dwarf.

Pyknocyte (पिक्नोसाइट) एक छोटी सूचिकार लाल रक्त कोशिका। A small needle-shaped RBC.

Pyknocytosis (पिक्नोसाइटोसिस) रक्त में छोटी सूचिकार लाल रक्त कोशिकाओं का बढ़ जाना। An excess of pyknocytes in the blood.

Pyknosis (पिक्नोसिस) केन्द्रकसंघनन, श्यान-केन्द्रता। A condensation and reduction in size of the cell or its nucleus.

Pylephebitis (पायलेफ्लेबाइटिस) पोर्टल शिरा का शोथ। Inflammation of the portalvein.

Pylethrombosis (पायलेथ्रॉम्बोसिस) पोर्टल शिरा की घनास्त्रता। Thrombosis of the portal vein.

Pylon (पाइलॉन) एक अस्थायी कृत्रिम टाँग। A temporary artificial leg.

Pylorectomy (पाइलोरेक्टॉमी) शल्यक्रिया द्वारा पाइलोरस को काट कर अलग कर देना। Surgical removal of the pylorus.

Pyloric antrum (पाइलोरिक एन्ट्रम) आमाशय के जठरनिर्गमीय भाग का प्रथम भाग। The first part of the pyloric portion of the stomach.

Pyloric stenosis (पाइलोरिक स्टिनोसिस) जठरानिर्गम की सिकुड़न। Contraction of the pylorus.

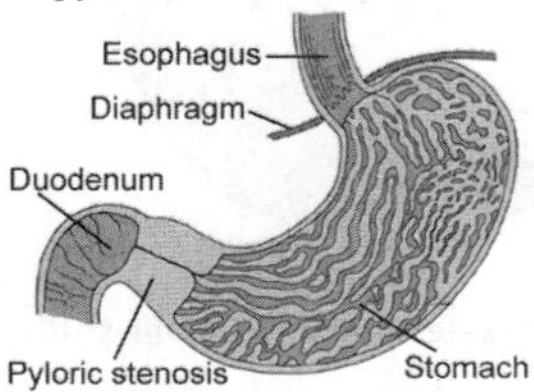

Pylorodiosis (पाइलोरोडायोसिस) पाइलोरस का चौड़ा हो जाना। Dilatation of the pylorus.

Pylorodudenitis (पाइलोरोड्योडीनाइटिस) पाइलोरस एवं ड्योडिनम की श्लेष्मकला का शोथ। Inflammation of the pyloric and duodenal mucosa.

Pyloroplasty (पाइलोरोप्लास्टी) प्लास्टिक सर्जरी द्वारा पाइलोरस की मरम्मत करना। Repair of the pylorus by plastic surgery.

Pylorospasm (पाइलोरोस्पाज्म) पाइलोरस का ऐंठ जाना, जठरनिर्गमाकर्ष। Spasm of the pylorus.

Pylorotomy (पाइलोरोटॉमी) पाइलोरस में चीरा लगाना। Incision of the pylorus.

Pylorus (पाइलोरस) आमाशय का निचला भाग जो ड्यूडिनम में खुलता है, जठर निर्गम। The lower portion of the stomach opening into the duodenum.

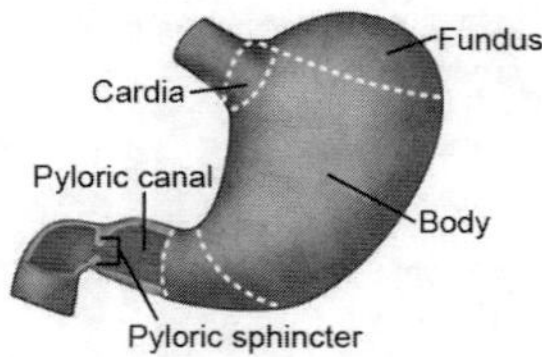

Pyocele (पायोसील) पस का संचय जैसा की वृषण या अण्डकोश में हो जाता है। A collection of pus, as in the scrotum.

Pyochezia (पायोचीज़िया) मल में पस का पाया जाना। Pus in the feces.

Pyocolpos (पायोकोल्पोस) योनि में पस का इकट्ठा हो जाना। Accumulation of pus in the vagina.

Pyoderma (पायोडर्मा) कोई भी सपूय त्वचा रोग। Any suppurative skin disease.

Pyogenic (पायोजेनिक) पूतिजनन सम्बन्धी। Pertaining to the formation of pus.

Pyometra (पायोमीट्रा) गर्भाशय के भीतर पस इकट्ठा होना, पूयगर्भाशयता। Accumulation of pus within the uterus.

Pyonephritis (पायोनेफ्राइटिस) वृक्क का सपूय शोथ। Purulent inflammation of the kidney.

Pyoovarium (पायोओवेरियम) किसी डिम्बग्रन्थि का फोड़ा। Abscess of an ovary.

Pyopericardium (पायोपैरीकार्डियम) हृदयावरण में पस बनना। Pus formation in the pericardium.

Pyoperitonitis (पायोपैरीटोनाइटिस) पैरीटोनियम का सपूय शोथ। Purulent inflammation of the peritoneum.

Pyophysometra (पायोफाइज़ोमिट्रा) गर्भाशय में मवाद एवं गैस का

संचित होना। Accumulation of pus and gas in the uterus.

Pyopneumopericardium (पायोन्यूमोपैरीकार्डियम) हृदयावरण में पस तथा वायु या गैस का होना। Pus and air or gas in the pericardium.

Pyopneumothorax (पायोन्यूमोथोरैक्स) फुफ्फुसावरणी गुहा में मवाद तथा वायु या गैस की विद्यमानता। Presence of pus and air or gas in the pleural cavity.

Pyopyelectasis (पायोपाइलेक्टेसिस) मवाद से वृक्कीय श्रोणि का चोड़ा हो जाना। Dilatation of the renal pelvis with pus.

Pyorrhea (पायोरिह्या) मवादयुक्त पदार्थ का स्रावित होना, पूयस्राव। A discharge of purulent mater.

Pyosalpingitis (पायोसैल्पिन्जाइटिस) डिम्ब वाहिनी की मवाद से युक्त सूजन। Purulent inflammation of the fallopian tube.

Pyosalpinx (पायोसैल्पिंक्स) डिम्ब वाहिनी में पस का संचित होना। Accumulation of pus in the fallopian tube.

Pyosis (पायोसिस) पूयरचना, पीब अथवा मवाद का बनना, पूयर्निमाण।
The formation of pus.

Pyotorrhea (पायोटीरिह्या) कान से मवाद बहना। Discharge of pus from the ear.

Pyramid (पिरामिड) एक नुकीली अथवा शंक्वाकार रचना, पिरामिड। A pointed or conical structure as renal pyramid.

Pyrenemia (पाइरीनीमिया) रक्त में केन्द्रक-युक्त लाल रक्त कोशिकाओं का पाया जाना। Presence of nucleated red blood cells in the blood.

Pyrexia (पाइरैक्सिया) ज्वर या बुखार। Fever.

Pyriform (पाइरीफार्म) नाशपती के आकार का। Shaped like a pear.

Pyrogen (पाइरोजन) कोई भी पदार्थ जो ज्वर उत्पन्न करता है, ज्वरोत्पादक। Any substance producing fever.

Pyrolysis (पाइरोलाइसेस) तापमान के बढ़ जाने पर कार्बनिक पदार्थ का विघटन होना। Decomposition of organic matter when the temperature rises.

Pyropuncture (पाइरोपंक्चर) गर्म सूईयों से बधन करके शरीर के किसी भाग के रोग की चिकित्सा करना। Treatment of disease of a part of the body by puncturing with hot needles.

Pyrosis (पाइरोसिस) आमाशय में पीड़ा होना। Burning in epigastrium and lower chest.

Pyuria (पाइयूरिया) मूत्र में पस का पाया जाना। Presence of pus in the urine.

Q

Q (क्यू.) मात्रा, तादाद, कूलम्ब का प्रतीक। Quantity, symbol for Coulomb.

QD (क्यू.डी.) प्रतिदिन। Every day.

Q Fever (क्यू. फिवर) हर चौथे दिन प्रकट होने वाला बुखार, चतुर्थक ज्वर। Acute infection disease caused by *Coxiella burnetii* a rickettsial organism, characterized by fever, sweating, myalgia.

QI (क्यू.आई.) अधिकतम उतना जिससे कोई प्रसन्न रहता हो। As much as one please.

QS (क्यू.एस.) अधिक से अधिक उतना जिससे पूर्ण संतुष्टि हो। As much as suffices.

Quack (क्वैक) मिथ्या चिकित्सक, कुर्वध, नीमहकीम। A person who pretends to have knowledge and skills of medicine.

Quadrangular (क्वाड्रेन्गुलर) चार कोणों वाला, चतुष्कोण। Having four angles.

Quadrangular Lobe (क्वाड्रेन्गुलर लोब) चतुष्कोणीय खण्ड। A region forming the superior portion of each cerebellar hemisphere.

Quadrangular Membrane (क्वाड्रेन्गुलर मैम्ब्रेन) चतुष्कोणीय कला। The upper portion of the elastic membrane of the larynx.

Quadrant (क्वाड्रेन्ट) 1. किसी वृत्त का एक चौथाई भाग। 2. चार एक से, जैसे उदर की सतह के भागों में से एक। 1. One fourth part of a circle. 2. One of the four corresponding parts, as the surface of abdomen.

Quadrantanopia (क्वाड्रेन्टेनोपिया) एक चौथाई दृष्टि-क्षेत्र में दृष्टिदोष या अन्धता का उत्पन्न हो जाना। Defective vision or blindness in one fourth of the visual field.

Quadrate lobe (क्वाड्रेट लोब) पाइलोरस एवं ड्योडिनम के सम्पर्क में रहने वाला यकृत का एक छोटा खण्ड। A small lobe of the liver lying in contact with the pylorus and duodenum.

Quadriceps (क्वाड्रीसेप्स) चार सिर वाला जैसे कोई क्वाड्रीसेप्स पेशी होती है, चतु:शिरस्क। Four-headed, as a quadriceps muscle.

Quadridigitate (क्वाड्रीडिजीटेट) किसी हाथ अथवा पाँव में केवल चार अंगुलियाँ धारण करने वाला। Having only four fingers on a hand or four toes on a foot.

Quadrigeminus (क्वाड्रीजेमिनस) चार भागों से बना हुआ। Consisting of four parts.

Quadrilocular (क्वाड्रीलॉकुलर) चार कोष्ठों अथवा गुहाओं से युक्त। Having four chambers or cavities.

Quadriplegia (क्वाड्रीप्लीजिया) चारों भुजाओं का पक्षाघात हो जाना, चतुरंगघात। Paralysis of all the four limbs.

Quadrisection (क्वाड्रीसैक्शन) चार भागों में विभाजित होना। Division into four parts.

Quadrivalent (क्वाड्रीवैलेन्ट) चार की रासायनिक वैलेन्सी से युक्त। Having a chemical valency of four.

Quadruped (क्वाडरूपेड) चार पैरों वाला, चौपाया, चतुष्पादी। A four footed animal.

Quadruplet (क्वाडरूप्लेट) एक जन्म से उत्पन्न होने वाले चार बच्चों में से एक, चतुर्ज। One of four children born at one birth.

Quantivalence (क्वान्टीवैलेन्स) हाइड्रोजन परमाणुओं की वह संख्या जिसके साथ कोई तत्व या मूलक संयुक्त होगा। The number of hydrogen atoms with which an element or radical will combine.

Quantum libet (क्वान्टम लाइबेट) अधिक से अधिक जितनी इच्छा हो। As much as desired.

Quarantine (क्वारेन्टाईन) किसी सांसर्गिक रोग के प्रारम्भ होने से लोगों को पब्लिक से अलग रखने की अवधि। संगरोध। Period

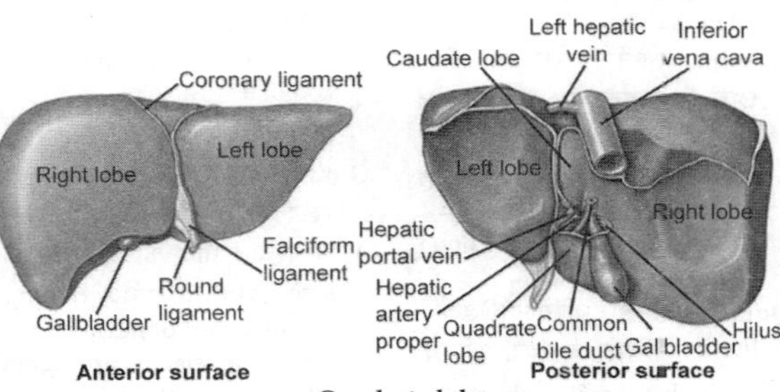

Quadrate lobe

of isolation of the persons from public, from the onset of contagious disease.

Quartan (क्वार्टन) हर चौथे दिन होने वाला जैसे मलेरिया ज्वर होता है, चतुर्थक। Occurring every fourth day, as malarial fever.

Quartisect (क्वार्टीसैक्ट) चार भागों में काटना। To cut into four parts.

Quenching (क्विंचिंग) बुझाना या किसी गर्म वस्तु जैसे किसी गर्म धातु को ठण्डा करना। To extinguish or to cool a hot object as a hot meal.

Quickening (क्विकनिंग) गर्भाशय में महसूस की जाने वाली भ्रूण की प्रथम गति। First movement of the fetus felt in the uterus.

Quick lime (क्विक लाइम) अनबुझा चूना। Unslaked lime.

Quiescence (क्वाइसैन्स) शान्ति। Silence, calmness.

Quinine (क्वीनीन) सिन्कोना की छाल से उत्पन्न एक कडुवा श्वेत रवेदार एल्कालॉयड जिसका मलेरिया में प्रयोग किया जाता है। A bitter white crystalline alkaloid derived from cinchona bark, used in malaria.

Quinsy (क्विंन्सी) परिगलतुण्डिका विद्रधि, टॉन्सिल के चारों ओर का फोड़ा। Peritonsillar abscess.

Quintan (क्विंनटान) प्रत्येक पाँचवे दिन पुनः उत्पन्न होने वाला जैसे कोई बुखार होता है। पंचक। Recurring every fifth day as a fever.

Quintuplet (क्विन्टूप्लेट) एक जन्म से उत्पन्न होने वाले पाँच बच्चों में से एक। One of five children born at one birth.

Quiver (क्विवर) कांपना। Shiver.

Quotid (क्योटिड) नित्य, हर रोज। Daily.

Quotidian (क्योटीडियन) रोज होने वाला जैसे मलेरिया बुखार। Occurring daily, as malarial fever.

Quotient (क्योशिएन्ट) विभाजन के द्वारा उपलब्ध संख्या। A number obtained by division.

QV (क्यू.वी.) 1. जितना अधिक से अधिक आप चाहते है।

2. जिसे देखो।

1. Quantum viz. as much as you like.

2. Quod vide, which see.

Q wave (क्यू वेव) किसी इलैक्ट्रोकार्डियोग्राम की पी तंरग के पश्चात् नीचे की ओर जाने वाली अथवा ऋणात्मक तंरग। A downward or negative wave of an electrocardiogram following the P wave.

R

R (आर) 1. दांई, श्वसन, रौंटजन 2. कार्बनिक रेडिकल का रासायनिक प्रतीक।

1. Right, respiration, Röntgen.

2. Chemical symbol for organic radical.

Ra (आरए) रेडियम का रासायनिक प्रतीक। Chemical symbol for Radium.

Rabbetting (रेबैटिंग) किसी टूटी हुई हड्डी के टेढ़े-मेढ़े किनारों का आपस में सट जाना। Interlocking of the jagged margins of a fractured bone.

Rabid (रैबिड) जलातंकग्रस्त, पागल। Pertaining to or affected with rabies.

Race (रेस) जाति। A class of animals or individual having common somatic inherited characteristics.

Rachial (रैकियल) मेरूदण्ड सम्बन्धी। Spinal.

Rachilysis (रैकीलाइसिस) कशेरूका दण्ड की पार्श्विक वक्रता को खिंचाव एवं दबाव दोनों से ठीक करना। Correction of the lateral curvature of the vertebral column by combined traction and pressure.

Rachiometer (रैकियोमीटर) कशेरूका-दण्ड की किसी वक्रता को मापने वाला एक यंत्र। An instrument for measuring a curvature of the vertebral column.

Rachischisis (रैकिस्चाइसिस) मेरूनलिकाविदर। Spina-bifida.

Rachitis (रेकाइटिस) अधिवक्रता, रिक्केट। Ricked, Inflammatory disease of the vertebral column.

Raclage (रैक्लेज) किसी कोमल वृद्धि को नष्ट करके रगड़कर साफ करना। Destruction and removal of a soft growth by scraping or rubbing.

Rad (राड) रेडिएशन अवशोषित मात्रा। Radiation absorbed dose.

Radiant (रेडिएन्ट) उज्जवल, चमकदार। Shining or glowing brightly.

Radiate (रेडिएट) बिखराना, विकीर्ण होना। To spread out in all directions from a center.

Radiation (रेडियेशन) विकिरण, बिखराव। The invisible energy rays given off by X-ray, radium and other chemicals when exposed to radioactivity.

Radical (रेडिकल) मूलक, जड़ अथवा मूल सम्बन्धी। Pertaining to the root or origin.

Radical treatment (रेडिकल ट्रीटमैन्ट) रोग का पूरी तरह सफाया करने के लिए की जाने वाली चिकित्सा जो सामान्यतया रेडिकल शल्यचिकित्सा होती है जैसे पूर्ण गर्भाशयोच्छेदन। The treatment given for absolute cure which is usually a radical surgery, e.g. total hysterectomy.

Radicle (रेडिकल) तंत्रिकामूल, शिरामूल। Any one of the smallest branches of a vessel or nerve.

Radiculitis (रेडिकुलाइटिस) तंत्रिका मूलों का शोथ। Inflammation of the spinal nerve roots.

Radioactive (रेडियोएक्टिव) विकिरण ऊर्जा को निकालने वाला, रेडियोधर्मी। Capable of emitting radiant energy.

Radioactivity (रेडियोएक्टीविटी) विकिरणशीलता। Capability of a substance to emit rays, or particles from its nucleus.

Radiobiology (रेडियोबायोलॉजी) विज्ञान की वह शाखा जिसका सम्बन्ध प्रकाश, अल्ट्रावायेलेट एवं आयनीकृत विकिरण के जीवित ऊतकों या जीवों के ऊपर होने वाले प्रभावों के अध्ययन से है। Branch of biology dealing effects of ionizing radiation on living organisms.

Radiodermatitis (रेडियोडर्माटाइटिस) एक्स-रे अथवा रेडियो सक्रिय तत्वों के प्रति अनावृत होने से उत्पन्न त्वक्शोथ। Dermatitis caused by exposure to X-ray or radioactive elements.

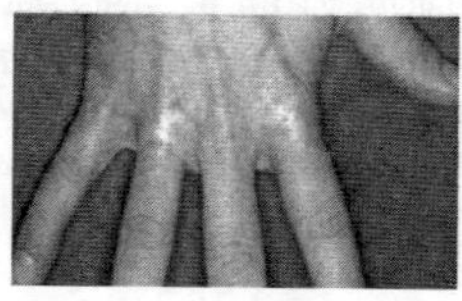

Radiograph (रेडियोग्राफ) विकिरणचित्र। The finished printed X-ray picture.

Radioimmunoassay (रेडियोइम्यूनोऐसे) यह पदार्थो विशेषकर एण्टीजन एवं एण्टीबॉडी की सान्द्रता का पता लगाने वाली एक संवेदनशील निर्धारण विधि है। A method for determining concentration of substances particularly protein bound hormones to the range of picograms.

Radioimmunodiffusion (रेडियोइम्यूनोडिफ्यूजन) रेडियोआइसोटोपयुक्त एण्टीजन का प्रयोग करके एण्टीजन-

एण्टीबॉडी के आपसी कार्य का अध्ययन करना। Study of the antigen-antibody interaction by use of radioisotope labeled antigens.

Radioimmunoelectrophoresis (रेडियोइम्यूनोइलैक्ट्रोफोरेसिस) रेडियोआइसोटोपयुक्त एण्टीजन अथवा एण्टीबॉडी के प्रयोग द्वारा विद्युतकण संचलन होना। Electrophoresis by the use of radioisotope labeled antigens or antibody.

Radioiodine (रेडियोआयोडीन) आयोडीन का रेडियोसक्रिय आइसोटोप जिसका थाइरॉयड ग्रंथि के रोगों के निदान एवं चिकित्सा में प्रयोग किया जाता है। Radioactive isotope of iodine used in the diagnosis and treatment of the disease of thyroid gland.

Radioisotopes (रेडियोआइसोटोपस) तत्वों के रेडियोसक्रिय रूप। Radioactive forms of elements.

Radiologist (रेडियोलॉजिस्ट) विकिरण विज्ञान में विशेषज्ञ। Specialist in radiology.

Radiolucency (रेडियोलूसैन्सी) विकिरण-ऊर्जा के लिए अर्द्धपारदर्शकता। Semitransparency to radiant energy.

Radiolucent (रेडियोलूसैन्ट) विकिरण-ऊर्जा के लिए अर्द्धपारदर्शकता। Semitransparent to radiant energy.

Radiometer (रेडियोमीटर) 1. एक्स-रे की मात्रा का अंदाज लगाने वाला। 2. ऐसा यंत्र जिसमें विकिरण ऊष्मा तथा प्रकाश के सीधे यांत्रिक शक्ति में बदल दिया जा सकता है। 1. An instrument measuring the emission of X-ray. 2. An instrument in which radiant heat and light may be directly converted into mechanical energy.

Radiomimetic (रेडियोमाइमेटिक) विकिरण के प्रभावों को उत्पन्न करने वाला। Producing the effects similar to those of radiation.

Radionecrosis (रेडियोनेक्रोसिस) विकिरण में अनावृत हो जाने पर ऊतकों का नष्ट हो जाना। Destruction of the tissues by exposure to radiation.

Radiopaque (रेडियोपेक) एक्स-रे अथवा अन्य प्रकार के विकिरण के लिए अभेद्य। Impenetrable to the X-ray or other forms of radiation.

Radiopelvimetry (रेडियोपैल्वीमीट्री) एक्स-रे चित्रण द्वारा घ्रोणि की माप लेना। Measurement of the pelvis by radiography.

Radioresistant (रेडियोरेजिस्टैन्ट) विकिरण की क्रिया का

प्रतिरोधक जैसे कोई अर्बुद होता है जो विकिरण से चिकित्सा करने पर नष्ट नहीं हो सकता। Tumors that cannot be destroyed by radiation and hence are radio resistant.

Radiotherapist (रेडियोथिरापिस्ट) विकिरण चिकित्सा का विशेषज्ञ। Specialist in radiotherapy.

Radiotherapy (रेडियोथिरैपी) विकिरण चिकित्सा। The treatment of diseases by application of radiation, ultraviolet or other forms of radiations.

Radium (रेडियम) बहुत सूक्ष्म मात्राओं में पाया जाने वाला एक विकिरणशील धात्विक तत्व जिससे एल्फा, बीटा, गामा किरणें निकलती है। A radioactive metallic element found in very small quantities, emitting alpha, beta, and gamma rays.

Radius (रेडियस) त्रिज्या, बहिःप्रकोष्ठिका। The bone on the outer side of the forearm.

Radix (रेडिक्स) जड़, मूल। The root.

Rage (रेग) हिंसक, क्रोध। Violent anger.

Rale (राल) आगन्तुक ध्वनि, फेफड़े की बुदबुद करती हुई आवाज। Rattle or rhoncus, a bubbling sound heard in the branchi in disease.

Ramulus (रेमुलस) अंतिम विभाजन। A small branch or terminal division.

Ramus (रैमस) प्रशाखा, शिरा या नाड़ी की शाखा। A branch of an artery vein or nerve.

Rancid (रेन्सिड) विशेष रूप से वसीय पदार्थ के विघटन से पैदा दुर्गन्धयुक्त या बदबूदार अथवा अप्रिय स्वाद। Offensive or having disagreeable taste from decomposition, especially of the fatty substance.

Ranula (रैनुला) जीभ के नीचे उत्पन्न रसौली या गिल्टी। A tumor under the tongue.

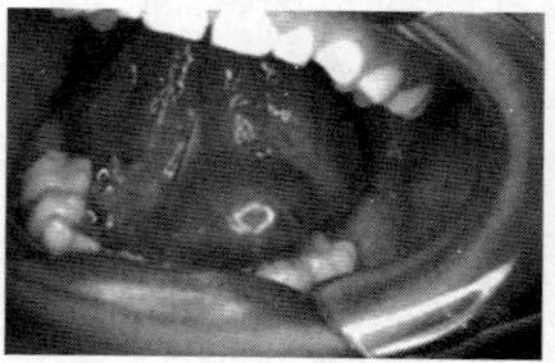

Rape (रेप) बलात्कार। Intercourse by force.

Raphe (रैफी) संधिरेखा, सीवनी। A seam, suture.

Rarefaction (रेयरीफैक्शन) विरलीकरण, विरलन। An act or process of making a substance less dense.

Rash (रैश) विस्फोट, दाना। An eruptive on the skin.

Rate (रेट) दर। A record of the measurement of an event or process in terms of its relation to some fixed standard.

Ratio (रेशियो) अनुपात। An expression of the relationship of one quantity to another.

Rational (रैशनल) युक्तिसंगत, तर्कसंगत। Reasonable, opposed to empiric.

Rattle (रैट्ल) परिश्रवण करने पर सुनाई देने वाली ध्वनि। A sound or rale heard on auscultation.

Rave (रेव) बेहुदी बातें करना जैसे प्रलाप में की जाती है। To talk irrationally, as in delirium.

Ray (रे) किरण, प्रकाशरेखा। A line of light or heat proceeding from a luminous point.

Raynaud's disease (रेनॉयड डिजीज) अँगुली की धमनियों की दौरे के रूप में प्रकट होने वाली ऐंठन। Paroxysmal spasm of the digital arteries producing pallor or cyanosis of fingers or toes and occasionally resulting in gangrene.

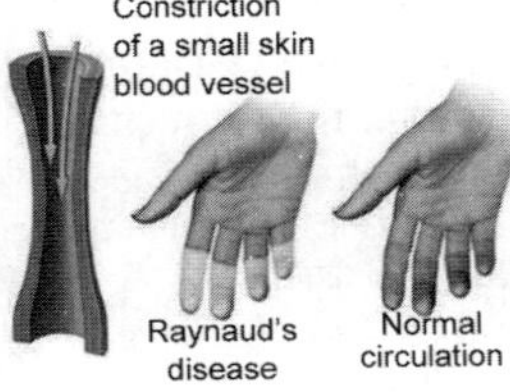

Reaction (रिएक्शन) प्रभाव। Effect.

Reactivate (रिएक्टीवेट) पुनः क्रियाशील या सक्रिय करना। To render active again.

Reagent (रीएजेन्ट) प्रतिक्रियाशील द्रव्य अथवा शक्ति। An agent capable of producing a chemical reaction.

Receptor (रिसेप्टर) ग्राहक, ग्राही। Sensory afferent nerve-endings capable of receiving and transmitting stimulation.

Recess (रिसेस) एक छोटा गड्ढा अथवा गुहा, दरी। A small depression or cavity.

Recipe (रिसीपी) नुस्खालेखन में 'लीजिये' के निर्देशार्थ प्रयुक्त संकेत चिन्ह। The caption of a prescription, which means take symbol R.

Recipient (रेसीपिएन्ट) आदाता, वह व्यक्ति जो दाता से कुछ विशेषकर रक्त, ऊतक अथवा अंगों आदि को प्राप्त करता है। The person who receives some things from a donor, especially blood, tissues or organs, etc.

Reciprocal (रेसीप्रोकल) परस्पर बदलने योग्य। Interchangeable.

Reciprocate (रेसीप्रोकेट) आगे-पीछे चलना, अदल-बदल करना। To walk forward and backward, to interchange.

Recover (रिकवर) पुनः प्राप्त करना जैसे किसी बीमारी के पश्चात् पुनः स्वास्थ्य लाभ प्राप्त करना। To regain as health after an illness.

Recovery room (रिकवरी रूम) उपलब्धि कक्ष। Area provided with equipment and nursing needed to care for patient's immediately after surgical operation.

Recrudescent (रीक्रूडीसैन्ट) किसी बीमारी के पश्चात् पुनः सक्रिय हो जाना। Becoming active again after an illness.

Recruitment (रीक्रुइटमैन्ट) 1. किसी उद्दीपन के लम्बे समय तक रहने पर यद्यपि इसकी शक्ति में परिवर्तन नहीं होता, किसी प्रतिवर्त क्रिया में धीरे-धीरे वृद्धि होकर उसका अधिकतम हो जाना। 2. श्रवण विज्ञान में, ध्वनि की तीव्रता में थोड़ी सी वृद्धि हो जाने पर इसका एकदम से बहुत तेज हो जाना।
1. Gradual to a maximum in a reflex action when a stimulus is prolonged, even though strewing of the stimulus is not changed. 2. In audiology, excessively rapid in the loudness of sound caused by a slight in its intensity.

Rectal crisis (रैक्टल क्राइसिस) मलोत्सर्ग के समय ऐंठन होना तथा मलाशय वेदना। Tenesmus and rectal pain.

Rectal reflex (रैक्टल रिफ्लैक्स) मलोत्सर्ग की सामान्य इच्छा। The normal desire for defecation.

Rectified (रेक्टीफाइड) शुद्ध किया गया, शोधित। Made more pure or stronger.

Rectifier (रेक्टीफायर) विद्युत में एक आल्टरनेटिंग करन्ट को डाइरैक्ट करन्ट में बदलने वाला एक उपकरण। In electricity, an apparatus for changing an alternate current into a direct current.

Rectocele (रैक्टोसील) मलाशयभ्रंश। Herniation of a part of the rectum into vagina.

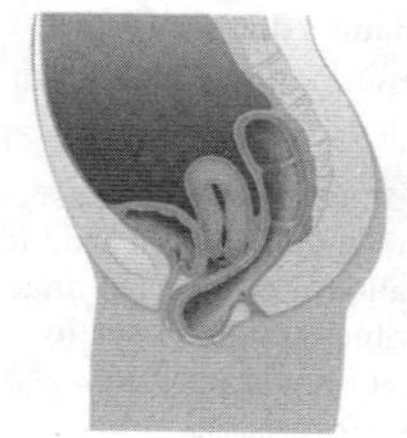

Rectoclysis (रैक्टोक्लाइसिस) मलाशय में धीरे-धीरे तरल को प्रविष्ट करना। To introduce slowly the fluid into rectum.

Rectopexy (रैक्टोपेक्सी) मलाशयस्थिरण। Fixation of the rectum.

Rectosigmoid (रैक्टोसिग्मॉयड) मलाशय का ऊपरी एवं सिग्मॉयड कोलन का अंतिम भाग। Upper part of the rectum and terminal part of the sigmoid colon.

Rectourethral (रैक्टोयूरेथ्रल) मलाशय एवं मूत्रमार्ग से संबंधित अथवा इनसे सम्बन्ध स्थापित करने वाला। Pertaining to or communicating the rectum and urethra.

Rectouterine (रैक्टोयूटेराइन) मलाशय एवं गर्भाशय सम्बन्धी। Pertaining to the rectum and uterus.

Rectovaginal (रैक्टोवेजाइनल) मलाशय एवं योनि सम्बन्धी। Pertaining to the rectum and vagina.

Rectovesical (रैक्टोवेसिकल) मलाशय एवं मूत्राशय सम्बन्धी। Pertaining to the rectum and bladder.

Rectum (रेक्टम) मलाशय। The termination of the intestines at the fundament so called, the outlet being termed as anus, the lower part of the large intestine.

Recumbent (रीकम्बेन्ट) लेटने वाला। Lying down.

Recuperation (रीकूपरेशन) पुनः स्वास्थ्य लाभ। Return to health.

Recurrence (रीकरैन्स) पुनरावृत्ति। A return, relapse.

Recurrent (रीकरन्ट) पुनरावर्ती। Relapsing.

Recurved (रिकर्वड) पीछे की ओर मुड़ी हुई। Bent backward.

Red cross (रैड क्रॉस) श्वेत पृष्ठभूमि पर बना लाल रंग का एक क्रॉस जो चिकित्सा सम्बन्धी व्यक्ति अथवा संस्था का अंतर्राष्ट्रीय मान्यता प्राप्त एक चिन्ह होता है। A cross of red color on white background, which is an internationally recognized sign of medical person or institution.

Redox (रीडॉक्स) ऑक्सीकरण एवं अपचयन के लिये संयुक्त शब्द। Combined word for oxidation and reduction.

Reduce (रिड्यूस) 1. घटाना। 1. To weaken. 2. अपचयन करना। 2. To decompose.

Referred pain (रेफर्ड पेन) अपने उद्‌गम के स्थान से दूर स्थानों पर महसूस किया जाने वाला दर्द जैसे एन्जाइना पैक्टोरिस का बायीं भुजा में महसूस होने वाला दर्द। Pain felt in the areas distant from its point of origin, e.g. pain of angina pectoris felt in the left arm.

Reflect (रिफ्लैक्ट) 1. प्रतिबिम्ब डालना 1. To throw back the image. 2. चिंतन करना। 2. To think over the matter.

Reflection (रिफ्लैक्शन) परावर्तन, पीछे की ओर मुड़ना। A bending back, throwing back a ray of light or radiant energy from surface.

Reflex (रिफ्लैक्स) प्रतिवर्त, परावर्तित क्रिया। An involuntary response in which a stimulus is received by a nerve transmitted and finally translated into muscular activity—all in a fraction of seconds reflected or thrown back.

Reflux (रिफ्लक्स) पीछे की ओर बहना। A backward flow.

Refraction (रिफ्रैक्शन) परावर्तन, वक्रीकरण। The behavior of light rays passing from mediums of different densities.

Refractive power (रिफ्रैक्टिव पावर) डिग्री जितना कोई पारदर्शक वस्तु प्रकाश की किरणों को सीधे मार्ग से घुमा देती है। The degree to which a transparent object deviates the rays of light from a straight path.

Refractometer (रिफ्रैक्टोमीटर) नेत्रापवर्तन मापने का यंत्र। An instrument for measuring refraction of the eye.

Refractometry (रिफ्रैक्टोमीटरी) लैन्सों की अपवर्तनी शक्ति को मापना। Measurement of the refractive power of lenses.

Refrigerant (रेफ्रीजरैन्ट) तापहर, ठण्डा करने अथवा बुखार कम करने वाला। Cooling and reducing fever.

Refrigeration (रेफ्रीजरेशन) ठण्डा होना। The process of cooling.

Regeneration (रीजेनेरेशन) ह्रास के विपरीत, पुनरूद्भवन जनन, मरम्मत, पुनःवृद्धि अथवा ऊतकों का पूर्वावस्था में पहुँचना। Opposite to degeneration reproduction, repair, regrowth or restoration of the tissues.

Regimen (रेजीमेन) आहारविधान। The methodic use of food, also called diet regimen.

Regressive (रिग्रेसिव) प्रत्यागमनशील। Retreating.

Regurgitation (रिगर्गीटेशन) खाद्य अथवा पेय पदार्थो का आमाशय से मुँह के द्वारा वापस आना। Return of food or drink from the stomach.

Rehabilitation (रिहेबीलिटेशन) पुनरूत्थान, पुनर्वास। Restoration to the best possible functioning state after serious illness or injury.

Rehydration (रीहाइड्रेशन) ऐसे व्यक्ति में जिसमें से पानी निकल चुका है, मुख से अथवा इन्जैक्शन

द्वारा पुनः तरल पहुंचाना। Restoration of fluid orally or by injection in a person who has been dehydrated.

Reimplantation (रीइमप्लान्टेशन) निष्कासित अंग को पुनः जोड़ना। Replacement of a part that has been removed from the body.

Reinfection (रीइन्फैक्शन) पुनः संक्रमण। Infection a second time.

Rejection (रिजैक्शन) 1. अस्वीकृति 2. पोषद की कोशिकाओं की रोगक्षम प्रतिक्रिया द्वारा निरोपित ऊतक का नष्ट होना। 1. Refusal. 2. Destruction of the grafted tissue by immune reaction of cells of the lost.

Relapse (रिलैप्स) पुनरावृत्ति, आवृति। The return of a disease soon after convalescence.

Relapsing fever (रिलैप्सिंग फीवर) पुनरावर्ती ज्वर। Epidemic remittent, billions remittent, mild yellow fever, etc.

Relax (रिलैक्स) ढीला करना, तनाव कम करना अथवा मानसिक दबाव व चिंता से मुक्त होना। To loose, to lose tension or to get rid of mental stress or anxiety.

Relaxant (रिलैक्सेन्ट) तनाव कम करना। That which reduces tension.

Relieve (रिलीव) आराम पहुँचाना। To provide relief.

Remedy (रेमिडी) उपचार, प्रतिकार। Cure for a disease.

Remission (रेमीसन) विच्छेद, तीव्रता का ह्रास। A lessening in severity, the period of abatement in fever.

Remittent fever (रेमीटैन्ट फीवर) ऐसा ज्वर जो बारी-बारी से उतर जाता तथा फिर चढ़ जाता है परन्तु सामान्य नहीं होता। A fever which alternately abates and returns but the temperature does not come to normal.

Remote (रीमोट) दूराध, सुदूर। The more distant.

Ren (रीन) गुर्दा। Kidney.

Reniform (रेनीफार्म) गुर्दे के आकार का। Kidney-shaped.

Renin (रेनिन) मूत्रपिण्ड में पाया जाने वाला एक पदार्थ। An enzyme, found only in the kidney cortex.

Rennet (रेनेट) जमा हुआ दूध। A gastric ferment curdling milk.

Rennin (रेनिन) दूध को दही में बदलने वाला पदार्थ। Milk curdling enzyme of gastric juice.

Renography (रीनोग्राफी) गुर्दे का एक्स-रे परीक्षण करना। Radiography of the kidney.

Repellent (रीपीलैन्ट) दूर हटा देने वाला अथवा अलग कर देने वाला। Capable of driving off or repelling.

Replication (रीप्लीकेशन) प्रतिकृति। Refolding or duplication of a part.

Reposition (रीपोजिशन) नियोजन, पुनर्स्थापन। Replacement of a part.

Repositor (रीपोजिटर) पुनः स्थायी। An instrument for replacing a part.

Repression (रीप्रैशन) दमन, उपशमन। Suppression.

Reproduce (रीप्रोड्यूज) संतान उत्पन्न करना। To produce offspring.

Reproduction (रीप्रोडक्शन) सन्तानोपत्ति। Regeneration.

Repulsion (रिपल्सन) 1. आकर्षण के विपरीत 2. पीछे को खींचने की क्रिया 3. अलग करने के लिए किसी के द्वारा दूसरे पर लगाया गया बल।
1. Opposite to attraction.
2. The act of pulling back.
3. The force exerted by some body on another to cause separation.

Research (रिसर्च) अनुसंधान।
A critical investigation.

Resect (रिसैक्ट) काट देना। To cut off; to excise a segment of a part.

Resection (रिसैक्शन) काटकर निकाल फेंकना। Surgical excision.

Resectoscope (रिसैक्टोस्कोप) मूत्रमार्ग से होते हुए प्रोस्टेट ग्रंथि को निकालने वाला यंत्र। An instrument for resection of prostate through urethra.

Reserve (रिजर्व) 1. भविष्य के प्रयोग के लिये शेष को रोके रखना अथवा शेष रूका हुआ जैसे अम्ल के उदासीनीकरण के लिये उपलब्ध शरीर का सुरक्षित क्षार संचिति। 2. किसी व्यक्ति का अपनी संवेदनाओं एवं विचारों पर आत्म-संयम।
1. To hold or which is held back for future use, as alkali reserve of the body available for neutralization of acid.
2. Self-control of one's feelings and thoughts.

Reservoir (रिजर्वायर) 1. तरलों के संचयन के लिये एक स्थान।
2. किसी रोगोत्पादक जीव के लिये एक वैकल्पिक अथवा निष्क्रिय वाहक।
1. A place or cavity for storage of fluids. 2. An alternate or passive carries of a disease-producing organism.

Resident (रेजीडैन्ट) एक चिकित्सा-शास्त्र का स्नातक एवं लाइसेन्सशुदा कायचिकित्सक

जो किसी अस्पताल में चिकित्सा में आगे ट्रेनिंग ले रहा हो। A medical graduate and licensed physician obtaining further training in medicine in a hospital.

Residual (रेजिडुअल) अवशिष्ट, अवशेषांगी। Remaining after a disease or any injury, as residual debility.

Residue (रेजिड्यू) अवशिष्ट, अवशेष, बाकी, शेष। Remainder; rest, that which remains, residue.

Residue free diet (रेजिडयू फ्री डाइट) सेल्युलोज अथवा रूक्षांश मसे रहित भोजन। Diet out cellulose or roughage.

Resilience (रेजिलियेन्स) लचीलापन। Elasticity.

Resin (रेजिन) राल, सर्जास, यक्षधूप। A mixture of complex organic substances which can occur naturally or be manufactured synthetically.

Resistance (रेसिस्टैन्स) प्रतिरोध। Power of resisting, a passive force exerted in opposition to another and active force.

Resolution (रेजोलयूशन) शमन, विभेदन, विघटन, अवशोषण। Disappearance of a tumor or inflammation by a gradual process, without suppuration, decomposition, absorption.

Resolve (रिजोल्व) 1. सानान्य अवस्था में वापिस पहुँचना। 2. विघटित होना। 1. To subside or to return to normal. 2. To decompose.

Resonance (रेजोनैन्स) अनुकम्पन, प्रतिनाद। A sound heard on percussing the chest or on ausculting chest during speech.

Resorb (रीजार्ब) पुनःअवशोषित करना। Absorb (something) again.

Resorbant (रीजार्बेन्ट) असामान्य पदार्थ जैसे रक्त के थक्को के अवशोषण को प्रोत्साहित करने वाला। Promoting the absorption of abnormal matter as blood clots.

Resorption (रीजार्प्शन) पुनःशोषण, पुनर्ग्रहण। To reabsorbed.

Respiration (रैस्पिरेशन) सांस, श्वसन। The act of breathing, inhaling and exhaling air by the lungs.

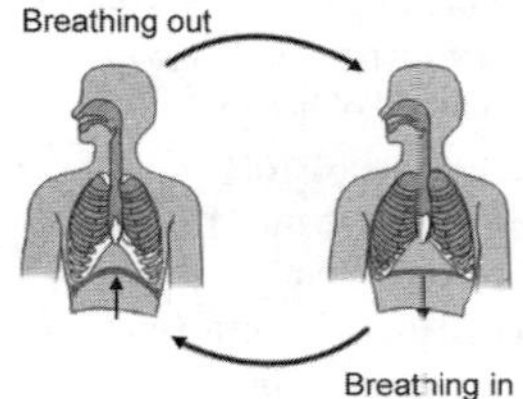

Respirator (रैस्पिरेटर) कृत्रिम श्वास देने वाला उपकरण, श्वासयंत्र। An apparatus for giving artificial respiration.

Respiratory quotient (रैस्पिरेट्री कुयोशिएन्ट) साँस के साथ निकाली गई वायु में कार्बन डाइऑक्साइड की मात्रा को साँस के साथ खींची गई ऑक्सीजन की मात्रा से विभाजित करने पर प्राप्त परिणाम जो सामान्यतया 0.9 होता है। The result of dividing the amount of carbon dioxide in expired air by the amount of O_2 inhaled, which is normally 0.9.

Response (रेस्पोन्स) अनुक्रिया। An action or movement due to the application of a stimulus.

Restitution (रेस्टीट्यूशन) पहली अवस्था में लौटना। A return of a former state.

Restless (रेस्टलेस) व्याकुल, बेचैन। Agitated mentally.

Restoration (रेस्टोरेशन) प्रत्यावर्तन, आरोग्यलाभ। Recovery or renewal of health.

Resuscitate (रीससाइटेट) पुनर्जीवित करना। To perform resuscitation.

Retardation (रिटार्डेशन) मन्दता, अवरूद्धता, विलंबन। Delay; hinderance.

Retch (रेच) उल्टी के लिए अनैच्छिक प्रयास। Involuntary attempt to vomit.

Retching (रेचिंग) उबकाई। An unsuccessful attempt at vomiting.

Rete (रेटी) जाली, जाल। A network of nerve fibers.

Retention (रिटेन्शन) रूकावट, अवरोधक। Stopping of natural, discharge, as of urine, etc.

Retention cyst (रिटेन्शन सिस्ट) ग्रंथि की वाहिनी के बंद हो जाने के कारण ग्रंथि में स्त्राव के रूक जाने से उत्पन्न पुटी। Cyst caused by retention of secretion in a gland, due to closure of duct of the gland.

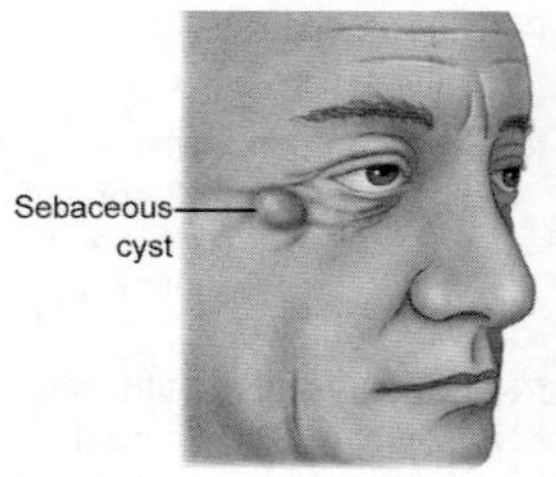

Retention enema (रिटेन्शन एनीमा) पोषण उपलब्ध कराने हेतु, श्लेष्मित कला को औशधियुक्त करने अथवा संज्ञाहरण उत्पन्न करने के लिए रोक लिया जाने वाला एनीमा। Enema to be retained to provide nourishment, medicate the mucous membrane or to produce anesthesia.

Reticulocyte (रेटिकुलोसाइट) एक अपरिपक्व लाल रक्त कोशिका जिसमें कणिकाओं तथा सूत्रों का एक जाल होता है, जाल लोहितकोशिका।
An immature red blood cells containing a network of granules or filaments.

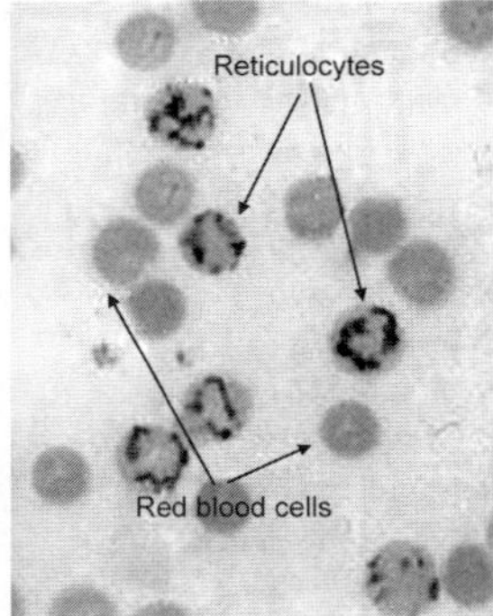

Reticulocytosis (रेटिकुलोसाइटोसिस) परिसंचरण करने रक्त में जाललोहित कोशिकाओं का संख्या में बढ़ जाना। An excess of reticulocytes in the circulating blood.

Reticuloendothelium (रेटिकुलोएण्डोथीलियम) जालीय अन्तःकला प्रणाली का ऊतक। Tissue of the reliculoendothelial system.

Reticulosarcoma (रेटिकुलोसार्कोमा) लसीका एवं अन्य ग्रंथियों की जालीय अन्तःकला में उत्पन्न होने वाली वृहत एककेन्द्रकश्वेत कोशिकाओं से बना एक दुर्दम अर्बुद।A malignant tumor composed of large monocytic cells originating in the reticuloendothelium of the lymph and other glands.

Retifera (रेटिफेरा) गोलाकृमि। A roundworm.

Retina (रेटिना) दृष्टिपटल।
The innermost or the third layer of the eyeball on which image of an object is formed.

Retinaculum (रेटिनाकुलम) उपबंधनी।
A band holding back a part.

Retinitis (रेटिनाइटिस) नेत्रपटल प्रदाह। Inflammation of the retina.

Retinoblastoma (रेटिनोब्लास्टोमा) बच्चों में उत्पन्न होने वाला रेटीना का एक दुर्दम अर्बुद, दृष्टिपटल प्रसूअर्बुद। A malignant tumor of the retina, occurring in children.

Retinol (रेटिनोल) विटामिन ए1 स्तनपायी में पाया जाने वाला एक प्रकार का विटामिन ए।
Vitamin A1, a form of Vitamin A found in mammals.

Retinopathy (रेटिनोपैथी)
दृष्टिपटल-विकृति। Any disease of the retina.

Retinoscopy (रेटिनोस्कोपी)
दृष्टिपटल दर्शन। The objective method of determining eye refraction by the character of reflected images. Observation of the retina.

Retort (रिटार्ट) आसवन क्रिया के लिए प्रयुक्त किया जाने वाला शीशे का बर्तन, कांचपत्र।
A vessel with a long neck in distillation.

Retractile (रिट्रैक्टाइल) पीछे को खिंच जाने योग्य। Capable of being drawn back.

Retraction (रिट्रेक्शन) पीछे की ओर खींचने की क्रिया। The act of drawing back.

Retractor (रिट्रेक्टर) प्रतिकर्षक, घाव की चमड़ी पीछे खींचने वाली एक चिमटी। An instrument for drawing back the lip of the wound.

Retro (रेट्रो) 'प्रति' के रूप में प्रयुक्त उपसर्ग। The 'per' occurring in loanwards from Latin meaning 'backwards'

Retroflexed (रेट्रोफ्लेक्सड) पीछे की ओर झुका हुआ। Bent backward.

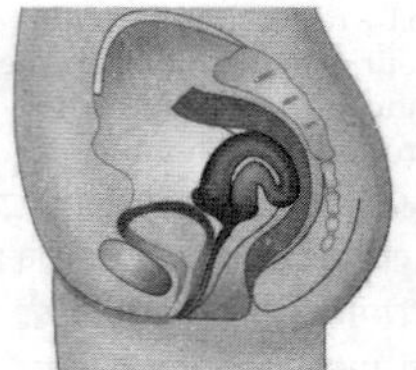
Retroflexed uterus

Retrograde (रेट्रोग्रेड) पश्चगामी, प्रतिगामी। Recoding or going backward.

Retrograde amnesia (रेट्रोग्रेड एम्नेसिया) हाल ही की घटनाओं को भूल जाना परन्तु बीती घटनाओं को याद करना। To forget the recent events but to remember the past ones.

Retroposition (रेट्रोपोजिशन) पीछे की ओर विस्थापन। Backward displacement.

Retropulsion (रीट्रोपल्सन) पीछे की ओर चलना। Driving or turning back.

Retrospection (रीट्रोस्पेक्शन) बीते हुए दिनों की याद में ही डूबा रहना। Morbid dwelling in the past.

Retrovirus (रीट्रोवाइरस) कुल का कोई भी विषाणु।
Any virus of the family retroviridae.

Reunion (रीयूनियन) दुबारा जुड़ना। Joining again.

Revaccination (रीवेक्सीनेशन) दुबारा या बार-बार टीका लगाना। Second or repeated vaccination.

Reversal (रिवर्सल) परिवर्तन, उत्क्रमण। A turning in the opposite direction.

Reversion (रिवर्जन) परावर्तन, मूल रूप से वापस जाना। A return to the original type.

RFA (आर.एफ.ए.) भ्रूण की दाई ललाट-अग्रज स्थिति। Right fronto-anterior fetal position.

RFP (आर.एफ.पी.) भ्रूण की दाई ललाट-पश्चज स्थिति। Right fronto-posterior fetal position.

RFT (आर.एफ.टी.) भ्रूण की दाई ललाट-अनुप्रस्थ स्थिति। Right fronto-transverse fetal position.

RH (आर.एच.) मुक्त करने वाला हार्मोन। Releasing hormone.

Rhabdophobia (रेह्ब्डोफोबिया) स्टिक से पीटे जाने का विकृत भय। Morbid fear of being beaten up by a rod or stick.

Rhabdovirus (रेह्ब्डोवाइरस) दण्डाकार आर एन ए विषाणुओं के किसी वर्ग में से कोई एक जिनमें से रेबीज विषाणु संक्रमित जन्तु से मनुष्य में संचारित होकर रेबीज रोग उत्पन्न करता है। Any of a group of rod shaped RNA viruses of which rabies virus is transmitted to man from the infected animal and cause rabies.

Rhagades (रेह्गेड्स) चमड़ी या श्लैष्मिक झिल्लियों की फटन। A fissure or chap in the skin or mucous membrane.

Rhagadiform (रेह्गेडीफॉर्म) दरार पड़ गई हो। Fissured.

Rhage, rhagia (रेह्ज, रेह्जिया) प्रत्यय जिनका अर्थ खून बहना अथवा अति स्त्राव है। Suffixes which mean bleeding or profuse discharge.

Rheology (रीह्योलॉजी) स्त्रावविज्ञान, धाराविज्ञान। The study of the deformation and flow of material.

Rheumatic fever (रूमेटिक फीवर) आमवातज्वर।

Disease usually occurs in children and young adults and is characterized by fever, pain in and around joints and strep throat.

Rheumatoid (रिह्यूमेटॉयड) जोड़ों का दर्दनाक प्रदाह तथा सूजन। An acute disease with painful inflammation and swelling of one or more joints often with endocarditis.

Rheumatoid arthritis (रिह्यूमेटॉयड आर्थ्राइटिस) जोड़ों की सूजन जिसमें जकड़ाहट होती है, दर्द होता है तथा उपास्थियों में अतिवृद्धि हो जाती है जिससे जोड़ों में पंगु बनाने वाली विरूपता उत्पन्न हो जाती है। Inflammation of the joints with stiffness and pain and hypertrophy of the cartilages causing crippling deformity of the joints.

Rheumatology (रिह्यूमेटोलॉजी) आमवात रोग का वैज्ञानिक अध्ययन। The science or the study of rheumatic disease.

Rhexis (रैह्क्सिस) किसी अंग अथवा रक्त वाहिनी का फट जाना। The rupture of an organ or of a blood vessels.

Rh factor (आर.एच. फैक्टर) खून की विशेष अवस्था जिसकी महत्ता का अंकन सगर्भता के दौरान किया जाता है। A characteristic of blood which is important in pregnancy.

Rhin (राह्इन) नाक। Nose.

Rhinalgia (राह्इनैल्जिया) नाक में दर्द होना। Pain in the nose.

Rhinencephalon (राह्इनैन्सिफैलॉन) मस्तिष्क का घ्राणी खण्ड। The olfactory lobe of the brain.

Rhinism (राह्इनिज्म) नाक की आवाज में बोलना। To speak in the nasal voice.

Rhinitis (राह्इनाइटिस) नासिका की श्लेष्मिक कला का प्रदाह। Inflammation of the mucous membrane of the nose.

Rhinologist (राह्इनोलॉजिस्ट) नासा-रोगों का विशेषज्ञ। A specialist in nasal disease.

Rhinomiosis (राह्इनोमायोसिस) शल्यक्रिया द्वारा नासिका के परिमाण को घटाना। Surgical reduction in size of the nose.

Rhinopathy (राह्इनोपैथी) नासिका का कोई भी रोग। Any disease of the nose.

Rhinophyma (राह्इनोफाइमा) नाक की चमड़ी बढकर कठोर हो जाना। Nodular enlargement of the skin of the nose.

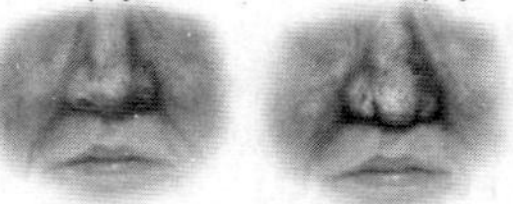

Rhinoplasty (राह्इनोप्लास्टी) नाक की प्लास्टिक सर्जरी करना। Plastic surgery of the nose.

Rhinorrhea (राह्इनोरिह्या) नासिका से पतला जल के समान स्त्राव होना। Thin watery discharge from the nose.

Rhinoscopy (राह्इनोस्कोपी) नासिकादर्शन। The examination of the nasal fossas.

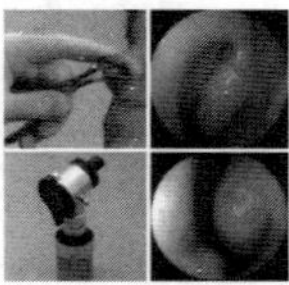

Rhinostenosis (राह्इनोस्टेनोसिस) नासिका-मार्गो में अवरोध उत्पन्न

हो जाना। Obstruction of the nasal passage.

Rhinovirus (राइनोवाइरस) कुल के विषाणुओं का एक वंश जिससे ठण्ड लग जाने का रोग होता है। A genus of viruses belonging to the family pricornaviridae that causes common cold.

Rhizo (राइजो) एक उपसर्ग जिसका अर्थ जड़ या मूल होता है। A prefix meaning root.

Rhizotomy (राइजोटॉमी) किसी तंत्रिका मूल का विभाजन। Division of transection of a nerve root.

Rhodopsion (रोह्डोप्सिन) विजुअल पर्पिल, रेटिना की शलाकाओं में स्थित एक बैंगनी लाल रंग का प्रकाशसुग्राही वर्णक जो प्रकाश द्वारा विरंजित होकर पीला हो जाता है जिससे रेटिना के संवेदी तंत्रिका तंत्र उत्तेजित हो जाते है। Visual purple, a purple red, photosensitive pigment in the rational rods which is bleached by light to yellow stimulating the retinal sensory nerve endings.

Rhombencephalon (रोह्म्बेन्सिफैलॉन) पश्चमस्तिष्क। Hind brain.

Rhomboid (रोह्म्बॉयड) हीरे के आकार जैसा। Diamond-shaped.

Rhoncal, Rhonchial (रॉन्कल, रॉन्कियल) कण्ठ की खड़खड़ाहट। A rattling in the throat.

Rhus (रस) पौधों की एक जाति। A genus of shrubs.

Rhythm (रिद्म) ताल, अनुक्रम। A measured periodic movement.

Rib (रिब) पसली। One of the bones enclosing the chest.

Riboflavin (रिबोफ्लेविन) विटामिन 'बी' कॉम्प्लेक्स का एक घटक। A constituent of vit 'B' complex, found generally in green vegetables, liver, kidneys, wheat germ, milk, eggs and cheese.

Rice-waterstool (राइस-वाटरस्टूल) हैजाजनित दस्त। The stool of Asiatic cholera.

Ricin (राइसिन) एरण्ड की फलियों से प्राप्त होने वाला अन्नसार। A toxic albuminoid from castor-oil bean.

Rickets (रिकेट्स) हड्डियों का टेढापन, बालास्थिविकार। A constitutional disease of childhood, marked by the cell-growth of the bones, deficiency of earthy matter, deformities and changes in the liver and the spleen.

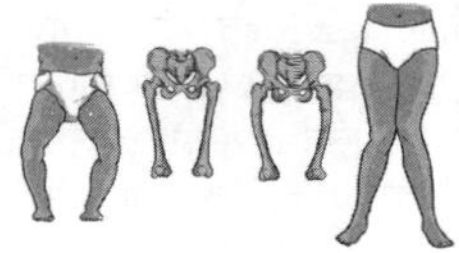

Rider's bone (राइडर्स बोन) घुड़सवारों की टांगों की पेशियों में होने वाली अस्थिरचना। A bony formation in the leg-muscles from riding.

Ridge (रिज) कटक। A linear elevation.

Riedel's lobe (राइडल्स लोब) यकृत का जिह्वा की आकृति का प्रवर्ध। Tongue-shaped projection of the liver.

Rigidity (रिजिडिटी) अकड़न, कठोरता अथवा लचीलेपन का अभाव। Stiffness, hardness or conflexibility.

Rigor (राइगर) 1. ठण्ड लगना 2. कठोरता। 1. Chill 2. rigidity.

Rim (रिम) किनारा। A border or edge.

Rima (रिमा) रेखाछिद्र, विदर। A slit or fissure, or narrow elongated opening between two symmetric parts.

Ring (रिंग) छल्ला, अंगूठी। A circular opening.

Ringworm (रिंगवार्म) दाद, चमड़ी का एक कवक रोग। A fungus infection of the skin, hair and nails.

Rinne's test (राइन्स टैस्ट) अस्थि चालन द्वारा होने वाली ध्वनि की वायु चालन द्वारा होने वाली ध्वनि से तुलना करने का एक परीक्षण। A test for comparing between the hearing through bone conduction and through air conduction.

RMA (आर.एम.ए.) पंजीकृत चिकित्सक सहायक। Registered medical assistant.

RMP (आ.एम.पी.) पंजीकृत चिकित्सक। Registered medical practitioner.

RN (आर.एन.) पंजीकृत परिचारिका। Registered nurse.

RNA (आर.एन.ए.) राइबोन्यूक्लिक एसिड। Ribo nucleic acid.

RNC (आर.एन.सी.) प्रमाणित पंजीकृत परिचारिका। Registered nurse certified.

Robust (रोबस्ट) ह्रष्ट-पुष्ट। Of strong constitution.

Rock-fever (रॉक फीवर) एक तरह का ज्वर जो कि संक्रमित जानवरो के दूध व मांस के सेवन करने से होता है। (सर्वप्रथम व ज्यादातर माल्टा द्वीप में होता है)। A highly contagious zoonosis caused by ingestion of unsterilized milk or meat from injected animals. (Known as Malta fever)

Rock-salt (रॉक साल्ट) सेंधा-नमक। Comman salt found in masses or beds.

Rodent (रोडैन्ट) स्तनी वर्ग एवं रोडेन्शिया गण का एक जन्तु जैसे चूहा, गिलहरी तथा गिनी-पिग

आदि जो कुतर कर भोजन ग्रहण करता है।An animal of the class mammalia and of the order rodentia such as rat, squirrel and guinea pig, etc. that takes food by gnawing.

Rodenticide (रोडेन्टीसाइड) कुतरकर खाने वाले जन्तुओं को मारने वाला। Killing rodents.

Roentgen (रैंटजन) एक्स अथवा गामा-विकिरण की अंतर्राष्ट्रीय इकाई। The international unit of X or Y radiation.

Roentgenism (रैंटजेनिज्म) एक्स-रे का गलत इस्तेमाल करने से उत्पन्न रोग। The disease caused by mixture of X-ray.

Roentgenology (रैंटजीनोलॉजी) एक्स-रे अध्ययन। Radiology.

ROM (आर.ओ.एम.) गति-प्रसार। Range of motion.

Romberg's sign (रोमबर्गस साइन।) खड़े हो कर पावों को पास-पास लाकर आँखों को बंद करने पर शरीर का संतुलन बनाये रखने में असमर्थता तथा नीचे गिरने की प्रवृति।
Inability to maintain the body balance and tendency to fall down while standing the eyes closed and the feet close together.

Rongeur (रॉन्गियर) हड्डी के छोटे–छोटे टुकड़ों को निकालने वाला एक यंत्र। An instrument for removing small pieces of bone.

Root canal (रूट कैनाल) किसी दन्त मूल की मज्जा गुहा। Pulp cavity of root of a tooth.

ROP (आर.ओ.पी.) दांयी पश्चकपाल के पीछे।
Right occipito posterior.

Rosacea (रोजेसिया) गुलाबी मुहासे। A skin disease which shows on flush areas of the face.

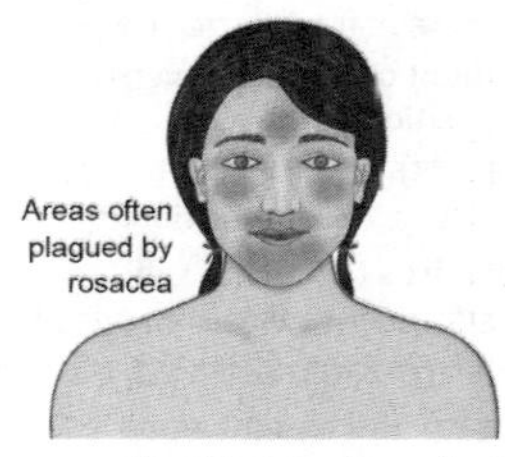

Rosary (रोजरी) माला के दानों की डोरी के समान संरचना।
A structure resembling a string of beads.

Roseola (रोजीयोला) 1. कोई भी गुलाबी रंग का त्वचा विस्फोट।
2. असंक्रामी स्फोट।
1. Any rose-colored skin rash.
2. Exanthema subitum

Rose rash (रोज रेश) गुलाबी दाना, लाल खसरा। Scarlet-rash, roseola.

Rosette (रोजेट) 1. गुलाब के समान स्तवक। 2. मलेरिया परजीवी

प्लाज्मोडियम मलेरी अपनी परिपक्व अवस्था में।
1. Resembling a rose.
2. Malarial parasite plasmodium malariae in its mature phase.

Rostellum (रोजेस्टलम) छोटी चोंच। A small beak.

Rostral (रोस्ट्रल) चोंच के समान, सिर की ओर। Resembling a beak; towards the head.

ROT (आर.ओ.टी.) भ्रूण की दायीं पष्चकपालीय अनुप्रस्थ स्थिति। Right occipitotransverse position of the fetus.

Rot (रोट) सड़ना, विगलन, क्षय। Decay, decomposition.

Rotavirus (रोटावाइरस) कुल के आर.एन.ए. विषाणुओं का एक वर्ग जिससे सर्वाधिक शिशुओं एवं छोटे बच्चों में दस्त आने लगते है। A group of RNA viruses belonging to the family reoviridace that causes mostly diarrhea in infants and small children.

Rotula (रोट्यूला) घुटने की चौड़ी हड्डी। The knee-pan or patella.

Roughage (रफेज) रूक्षांश, रेशा, अनाज का चोकर आदि। Coarse food containing much indigestible vegetable fiber composed of cellulose.

Round ligament (राउण्ड लिगामैन्ट) गोलबंधन। Ligamentum teres hepatis.

RPh (आर.पीएच.) पंजीकृत भेषज। Registered pharmacist.

RPO (आर.पी.ओ.) 1. विकिरण सुरक्षा अधिकारी। 2. दायाँ पष्चतिर्यक।
1. Radiation protection officer.
2. Right posterior oblique.

Rub (रब) घीसना, घर्षण। Friction encountered in moving one body over another.

Rubedo (रूबेडो) त्वचा की अस्थायी लालिमा। Temporary redness of the skin.

Rubefacient (रूबीफेशिएन्ट) रक्तिमकारी। An agent that reddens the skin.

Rubella (रूबेला) जर्मन रोमान्तिका अथवा खसरा। Infections fever of childhood, resembling mild measles, german measles, lasting for one day.

Rubeola (रूबीयोला) 1. खसरा 2. रूबेला। 1. Measles
2. Rubella.

Rubeosis-iridis (रूबीयोसिस-आइराइडिस) परितारिका या उपतारा की अग्रज सतह पर नयी रक्त वाहिनियों का बनना। Formation of new blood vessels on the anterior surface of the iris.

Rubigo (रूबीगो) जंग। Rust.

Rubor (रूबर) रक्तिमा, लाली। Erythema, Redness.

Ructus (रूक्टस) डकार, उबकाई। The belching of wind from the stomach.

Rudiment (रूडीमैन्ट) मूलांग, आद्यावशेष। A small incompletely developed structure which has been more fully developed in the embryo.

Ruga (रूगा) झुर्री, एक सिकुड़न। A crease, wrinkle or fold.

Rugose, Rugous (रूगोस, रूगस) बहुत सी सिकुड़ने अथवा झुर्रीदार। Having many creases or wrinkles.

Rugosity (रूगोसिटी) झुर्रिया पड़ना। The condition of being in wrinkles.

RUL (आर.यू.एल.) फेफड़े का दायाँ ऊपरी खण्ड। Right upper lobes of the lung.

Rum (रम) गन्ने की शराब। Spirit distilled from sugarcane.

Rum fits (रम फिट्स) पुराने शराबी का शराब पीना छोड़ देने पर मिर्गी के समान दौरे पड़ना। Occurrence of epileptic form convulsions following withdrawal of chronic use of alcohol.

Rumination (रूमीनेशन) निगले हुए भोजन का पुनर्चर्वण। Remastication of swallowed food.

Rump (रम्प) कूल्हे, नितम्ब। Buttocks.

Rundown (रनडाउन) दुर्बल, क्षीण। Weak, debilited.

Rupia (रूपिया) उपदंश का पपड़ीदार विस्फोट, फफोले, याज। Ulcer's that develop in late secondary syphilis and are covered with yellowish or brown crusts.

Rupture (रपचर) फटन, विदर, छिद्र। A break of any organ or soft part.

RUQ (आर.यू.क्यू.) दायाँ ऊर्ध्ववर्ती चतुर्थांश। Right upper quadarant.

Rush (रश) शक्तिशाली क्रमाकुंचन गति। Strong peristaltic movement.

Rut formation (रट फोर्मेशन) वातावरण में रूचि का अभाव केवल एक ही वस्तु पर ध्यान केन्द्रित रखना। Lack of interest in the environment, fixing the mind upon a single object.

Ryle's tube (राइल्स ट्यूब) आमाशय से पदार्थों को निकालने के लिये उपयोग की जाने वाली रबर की एक नली। A rubber tube used for withdrawing the contents of the stomach.

S

S (एस) आधा, बायाँ। Semis (half), sinister (left).

Sabulous (सेबुलस) रेतीला अथवा किरकिरा। Sandy or gritty.

Sac (सैक) थैली। A bag like organ or structure.

Saccades (सैक्केड्स) एक वस्तु को देख कर दूसरी वस्तु के देखने पर दोनों नेत्रों में एक साथ उत्पन्न होने वाली अनियन्त्रित झटका देने वाली गतियाँ। Involuntary jerky movements of both eyes occurring simultaneously on changing them from viewing one object to another.

Saccate (सैकेट) कोशीय, कोश सम्बन्धी। Relaxing to a sac.

Saccharide (सैकेराइड) शर्कराओं सहित कार्बोहाइड्रेटों की श्रृंखला में से कोई एक। One of a series of carbohydrates, including the sucroses.

Saccharin (सैकेरिन) एक कृत्रिम उत्पाद जो शुगर से 300 से 500 गुना मीठा होता है और किसी वस्तु को कृत्रिम रूप से मीठा बनाने के लिए प्रयुक्त किया जाता है, कोलतार शक्कर। A synthetic product, 300 to 500 times as sweet as sugar, used as artificial sweetener.

Saccharogalactorrhea (सैकेरोगेलेक्टोरिह्या) दुध में अत्यधिक शुगर का स्रावित होना। Excessive secretion of sugar in the milk.

Saccharolytic (सैकेरोलाइटिक) शुगर को खण्डित करने के सक्षम, शर्करालयी। Capable of splitting up sugar, glycolysis.

Saccharose (सैकेरोज़) ईख से निर्मित शर्करा, इक्षुशर्करा। Cane-sugar; sucrose.

Saccular (सैक्कुलर) कोश के आकार का, थैलीनुमा। Shaped like a sac.

Sacculation (सैक्कुलेशन) एक या अधिक लघुकोशों का बनना। Formation of a sac or sac.

Saccule (सैक्यूल) लघु कोश। A small sac.

Sacrad (सैक्राड) सैक्रम की ओर। Towards the sacrum.

Sacral plexus (सैक्रल प्लेक्सस) सेक्रमी तंत्रिकाओं का जाल जिससे आसन-तंत्रिका या शियाटिक नर्व निकलती है। Network of sacral nerves from which sciatic nerve originates.

Sacralgia (सैक्रेल्जिया) सैक्रम में दर्द होना, त्रिकास्थिशूल। Pain in the sacrum.

Sacrococcygeal (सेक्रोकॉक्सीजियल) सैक्रम तथा कॉक्सिक्स से संबन्धित, त्रिकानुत्रिकीय। Pertaining to the sacrum and coccyx.

Sacrocoxiitis (सैक्रोकॉक्साइटिस) त्रिकानुत्रिक संधिशोथ। Inflammation of the sacrococcygeal joint.

Sacroiliitis (सैक्रोइलियाइटिस) त्रिकश्रोणि-फलकीय सन्धिशोथ। Inflammation of the sacroiliac joint.

Sacrotomy (सैक्रोटॉमी) सैक्रम के निचले भाग में चीरा लगाना। To make an incision into the lower portion of the sacrum.

Sacrum (सैक्रम) कॉक्सिक्स के ठीक ऊपर पाँच कशेरूकाओं के आपस में जुड़ जाने से बनी एक त्रिकोनी हड्डी जो कशेरूका-दण्ड का आधार होती है तथा कॉक्सिक्स के साथ मिलकर वास्तविक श्रोणि की पश्च सीमा का निर्माण करती है, त्रिक या त्रिकास्थि। A triangular bone made up of five fused vertebral just above the coccyx, which is the base of the vertebral column and with the coccys, from the posterior boundary of the true pelvis.

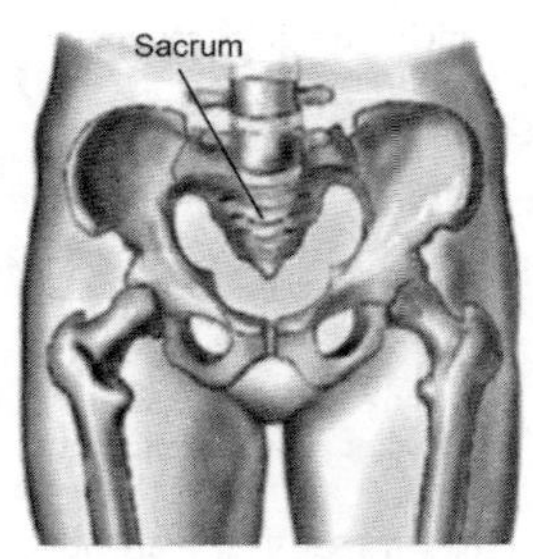

Saddle (सैड्ल) घोड़े पर सवारी करने वाली सीट से मिलती-जुलती संरचना जैसे कृत्रिम दन्तावली का आधार होता है। The structure resembling a seat used to ride a horse, e.g. the base of an artificial denture.

Saddle area (सैड्ल एरिया) नितम्बों, मूलाधार तथा जंघाओं का भाग जो घोड़े पर चढ़ने पर काठी के सम्पर्क में आती है। The portion of the buttocks, perineum and thighs that come in contact with the seat of the saddle.

Saddle joint (सेड्ल जॉइन्ट) अवतलोत्तर सन्धि। A concavo-convex articulation.

Saddle nose (सैड्ल नोज़) ऐसी नासिका जिसका सेतु या पुल दबा हुआ होता है जो जन्मजात सिफिलिस का एक चिन्ह है। A nose with a depressed bridge which is a sign of congenital syphilis.

Sadism (सैडिज्म) दूसरों को मानसिक अथवा शारीरिक वेदना पहुँचा कर लैंगिक आनन्द की प्राप्ति होना, परपीड़ाकामुकता। The derivation of sexual pleasure from inflicting mental or physical pain on others.

Sadist (सैडिस्ट) परपीड़न्कामुकता को करने वाला।
One who practise sadism.

Sadness (सैडनेस) उदासी। An emotion/feeling of dejection and melancholy.

Sadomasochism (सैडोमेज़ोचिज्म) परपीड़नकामुकता एवं परपीड़ितकामुकता देने से सम्बन्धित लैंगिक आनन्द। Sexual pleasure related to both sadism and masochism.

Sagging (सैगिंग) झोलदार। Bulging in a downwards direction.

Sagittal (सैजिटल) अग्रपश्च सीवन की दशा अथवा अग्रपश्च तल में स्थित। Situated in the direction of sagittal suture or anteroposterior.

Sagittal sulcus (सैजीटल सल्कस) ऊर्ध्ववर्ती अग्रपष्चज विवर के खाँचा। Groove for superior sagittal sinus.

Sago (सैगो) साबूदाना। A starchy substance prepared from various palms.

Salacious (सैलासियस) कामातुर। Lustful.

Saline (सैलाइन) लवण या नमक से युक्त अथवा उससे सम्बन्धित, लवणीय नमकीन। Containing or pertaining to salt, salty.

Salinometer (सैलाइनोमीटर) किसी घोल में नमक की मात्रा मापने का यंत्र, लवणमापी। An instrument for measuring the quantity of a salt in a solution.

Saliva (सैलाइवा) लार-ग्रन्थियों का एन्जाइम युक्त स्राव जो भोजन नम बनाता है, लार, लाला, थूक। The enzyme containing secretion of the salivary gland, which moistens food.

Salivant (सैलीवैन्ट) लार के बहाव को उद्दीप्त करने वाला, लारोत्पादक, लारजन्य। Stimulating the flow of saliva.

Salivary glands (सैलावरी ग्लैण्ड्स) मुख की ग्रन्थियाँ जिनसे लार स्रावित होती है। कर्णपूर्व, अवअधोहनुज एवं अवजिह्वी—तीन प्रकार की लार ग्रन्थियाँ होती है जिनमें से प्रत्येक जोड़े में होती है, लार-ग्रन्थियाँ। The glands of the mouth which secret saliva. There are three types of salivary glands—parotid, submandibular and sublingual salivary glands, each in pair.

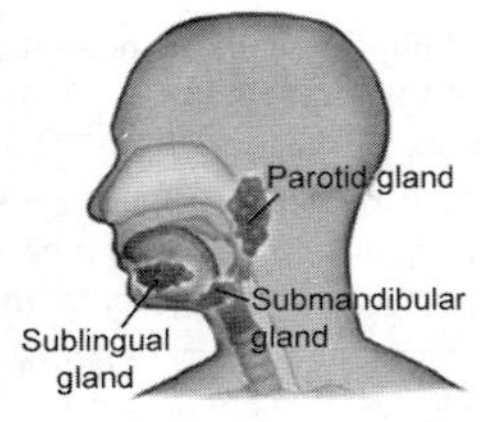

Salivator (सैलाइवेटर) लार पैदा करने वाला पदार्थ। An agent causing salivation.

Salk vaccine (साल्क वैक्सीन) मृत पोलियोमायलाइटिस विषाणुओं से युक्त एक वैक्सीन जो पोलियोमायलाइटिस के प्रति रोगक्षमता उत्पन्न करने के काम आती है, पोलियोरोधी टीका। A vaccine containing killed poliomyelitis viruses, used to produce immunity against poliomyelitis.

Sallow (सैलो) त्वचा की पीलापन, पाण्डु वर्ण। Yellowish color of the skin.

Salmonellosis (साल्मोनेलोसिस) साल्मोनैला वंश के जीवाणुओं का संक्रमण। Infection with bacteria genus Salmonella.

Salpingectomy (सैल्पिंजैक्टॉमी) शल्यक्रिया द्वारा किसी डिम्बवाहिनी को काट कर अलग कर देना। Surgical removal of the fallopian tube.

Salpingitis (सैल्पिंजाइटिस) डिम्ब वाहिनी अथवा श्रवणीय नली का शोथ। Inflammation of the fallopian or auditory tube.

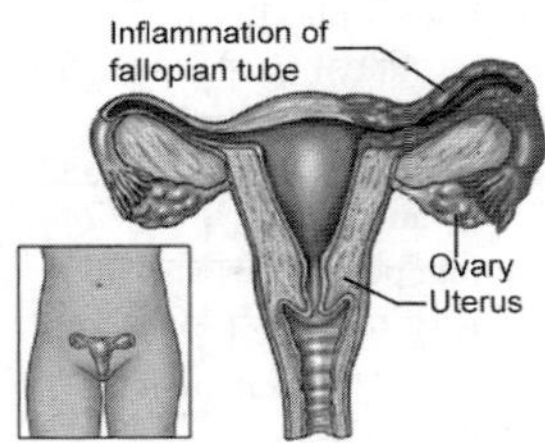

Salpingocele (सैल्पिंजोसील) डिम्ब वाहिनी का बहिःसरण। Hernia of the fallopian tube.

Salpingography (सैल्पिंजोग्राफी) किसी रेडियोअपारदर्शक पदार्थ का इन्जैक्शन लगाने के पश्चात डिम्ब वाहिनियों का एक्स-रे परीक्षण करना। X-ray examination of the fallopian tubes after injection of a radiopaque substance.

Salpingolysis (सैल्पिंजोलाइसिस) किसी डिम्ब वाहिनी के भीतर के चिपकावों को शल्यक्रिया द्वारा अलग कर देना। Surgical separation of the adhesion in a fallopian tube.

Salpingo-oophorectomy (सैल्पिंजो-ऊफोरेक्टॉमी) किसी डिम्ब वाहिनी एवं किसी डिम्ब

ग्रन्थि को शल्यक्रिया द्वारा काट कर निकाल देना। Salpingo-ovariectomy, excision of a fallopian tube and an ovary.

Salpingo-oophoritis (सैल्पिंजो-ऊफोराइटिस) किसी डिम्ब वाहिनी एवं डिम्ब ग्रन्थि का शोथ। Inflammation of a fallopian tube and an ovary.

Salpingopexy (सैल्पिंजोपैक्सी) किसी डिम्ब वाहिनी का स्थिरीकरण। Fixation of a fallopian tube.

Salpingoplasty (सैल्पिंजोप्लास्टी) प्लास्टिक सर्जरी द्वारा डिम्ब वाहिनी की मरम्मत करना। Repair of the fallopian tube by plastic surgery.

Salpingorrhaphy (सैल्पिंजोरैह्फी) किसी डिम्ब वाहिनी की सिलाई करना अथवा उसमें टाँकें लगाना। Suture of a fallopian tube.

Salpingoscope (सैल्पिंजोस्कोप) नासाग्रसनी एवं यूस्टेशियन नली का परीक्षण करने वाला एक यंत्र। An instrument for examining the nasopharynx and eustachian tube.

Salpingostomy (सैल्पिंजोस्टॉमी) किसी अवरूद्ध डिम्ब वाहिनी में अथवा निकासी के लिए एक छिद्र बनाना, डिम्बवाहिनी-छिद्रीकरण। To make an opening into an occluded fallopian tube, or for drainage.

Salpingotomy (सैल्पिंजोटॉमी) किसी डिम्ब वाहिनी में चीरा लगाना। To make an incision into a fallopian tube.

Salpinx (सैल्पिंक्स) डिम्ब वाहिनी अथवा यूस्टेशियन नली। The fallopian or Eustachian tube.

Salt (साल्ट) सोडियम क्लोराइड या साधारण नमक, लवण। Sodium chloride or common salt.

Saltatory (साल्टेटरी) उछल-कूद करने अथवा नाचने वाला। Marked by leaping or dancing.

Salting-in (साल्टिंग-इन) लवणन, नमक में बदलना। A conversion into salt.

Salting-out (साल्टिंग आउट) लवणक्षेपण, नमकविहीन करना। Making free from salt.

Salubrious (सॉल्यूब्रियस) स्वास्थ्यकर। Promoting health or wholesome.

Salutary (सॉल्यूटरी) स्वास्थ्यप्रद, आरोग्यकारी। Healthful, promoting health, wholesome.

Sample (सैम्पल) प्रतिदर्श, नमूना। A specimen.

Sanatorium (सेनेटोरियम) क्षयरोगचिकित्सालय। A special hospital for the treatment of tubercular patients.

Sand (सैन्ड) बालुका, बालु, रेत, सिकता। Minute fragments of stone.

Sandfly fever (सैन्डफ्लाई फिवर) बालु-मक्षिका ज्वर। Fever caused due to sandfly.

Sane (सेन) स्वस्थचित्त का। Of sound mind.

Sanguicolous (सैग्वीकोलस) रक्त में रहने वाला जैसे कोई परजीवी। Living in the blood, as a parasite.

Sanguine (सैंग्वीन) 1. रक्त से सम्बन्धित अथवा रक्त युक्त। 2. प्रफुल्ल, प्रसन्न। 1. Pertaining to, or consisting of blood. 2. Cheerful.

Sanguineous (सैग्वीनियस) रक्तिम, रक्त सम्बन्धी, रक्त से पूर्ण। Bloody, pertaining to blood, plethoric, full of blood.

Sanguinopurulent (सैग्वीनोपूरूलैन्ट) रक्त एवं पस से सम्बन्धित अथवा उन्हें धारण करने वाला। Pertaining to, or containing blood and pus.

Sanies (सेनीज) पतला रक्तपूतिस्राव, पतली रक्त-मिश्रित पीब बहना। A thin, often blood stained purulent discharge from wounds on sores, hence sanious.

Sanitary (सेनीटरी) स्वास्थ्यवर्द्धक अथवा स्वास्थ्य सम्बन्धी। स्वच्छ। Promoting or pertaining to health, clean.

Sanitary napkin (सेनीटरी नेप्किन) मासिक धर्म के रक्त का अवशोषण करने के काम आने वाला सेनीटरी पैड। Sanitary pad used for absorbing menstrual blood.

Sanitation (सेनीटेशन) स्वास्थ्यरक्षा, स्वच्छता। The establishment of conditions favorable to health, cleanliness.

Sanitizer (सेनीटाइजर) स्वच्छ करने वाला। That which makes clean.

Sanity (सेनिटी) मस्तिष्क की स्वस्थ्यता, स्वस्थचित्रता। Soundness of mind.

Sap (सैप) किसी प्राणी का जीवित रहने के लिये आवश्यक प्राकृतिक रस। Natural juice of an organism essential for vitality.

Saphena (सैफेना) जघनशिरा, नस की दो बड़ी शिराओं के लिये प्रयुक्त नाम। A name given to two large veins of the leg.

Saphenous nerve (सैफेनस नर्व) अरू तंत्रिका की एक शाखा जो पैर, टखने तथा पाँव के मध्यवर्ती पार्श्व की आपूर्ति करती है। A branch of femoral-nerve supplying the medical side of the leg, ankle and foot.

Saphenous veins (सैफेनस वेन्स) टाँग की दो उपास्थि, लघु एवं वृहत जघन शिरायें। Two superficial, small and great saphenous veins of the leg.

Saponification (सेपोनीफिकेशन) किसी तेल अथवा वसा को किसी साबुन में परिवर्तित करना, साबुनीकरण। Conversion of an oil or fat into a soap.

Saporific (सेपोरीफिक) किसी स्वाद अथवा सुगन्ध को प्रदान करने वाला, सुस्वाद। Imparting a taste or flavor.

Saprogen (सेप्रोजन) मवाद बनाने वाला अथवा मवाद पड़ जाने से उत्पन्न कोई भी सूक्ष्मजीव। Any microorganism causing or produced by putrefaction.

Saprophyte (सेप्रोफाइट) सड़ते हुए अथवा मृत कार्बनिक पदार्थ पर जीवित रहने वाला कोई भी जीव, मृतजीवी। Any organism living upon decaying or dead organic matter.

Sarcoblast (सार्कोब्लास्ट) पेशीमांसप्रसू। Myoblast, embryonic cell that develops into a muscle cell.

Sarcocarcinoma (सार्कोकार्सिनोमा) सार्कोमा एवं कार्सिनोमा प्रकृति का एक दुर्दम अबुर्द। A malignant tumor of sarcomatous and carcinomatous nature.

Sarcocele (सार्कोसील) शुक्रग्रन्थि का मांसल शोथ अथवा अबुर्द, वृशणमांसार्बुद। Fleshy swelling or tumor of the testis.

Sarcoid (सार्कोयड) मांस के समान, सार्कायडोसिस की गुलिकाभ विक्षति। Resembling flesh, tuberculoid lesion of sarcoidosis.

Sarcoidosis (सार्कायडोसिस) एक ऐसा रोग जिसके कारण का पता नहीं होता जिसमें कणिकागुल्मीय विक्षतियाँ उत्पन्न होती है जो शरीर के किसी भी अंग या ऊतक को प्रभावित कर सकती है। A disease of unknown cause characterized by granulomatous lesions that may affect any organ or tissue of the body.

Sarcolemma (सार्कोलेम्मा) प्रत्येक रेखित पेशी तन्तु को आच्छादित करने वाली एक झिल्ली। A membrane covering each striated muscle fiber.

Sarcolemmal (सार्कोलेमल) सार्कोलम्मा से सम्बन्धित। Pertaining to the sarcolemma.

Sarcolysis (सार्कोलाइसिस) शरीर के कोमल ऊतको अथवा माँस का विघटन होना। Decomposition of the soft tissues or flesh of the body.

Sarcoma (सार्कोमा) संजोजी ऊतक जैसे पेशी अथवा अस्थि का एक अबुर्द या कैन्सर जो हड्डियों, मूत्राशय, वृक्कों, यकृत, प्लीहा तथा फेफड़ों आदि को प्रभावित

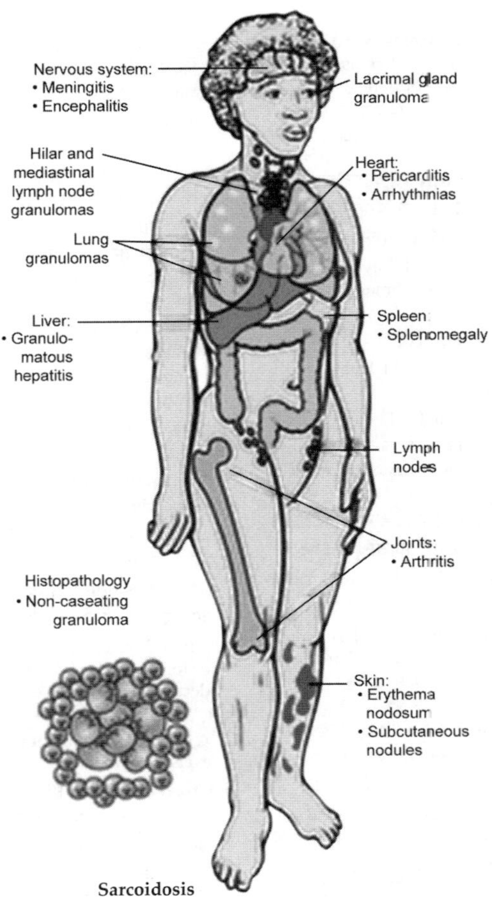

Sarcoidosis

कर सकता है, सार्काबुर्द। A malignant tumor or cancer of the connective tissue such as muscle or bone, which may affect the bones, bladder kidneys liver, spleen and lung, etc.

Sarcomatosis (सार्कोमेटोसिस) बहुत से स्थानों पर बहुत से सार्कोमाओं का बनना, सार्कोरूग्णता। Development of many sarcomas at various sites.

Sarcophagy (सार्कोफेजी) माँस खाने की आदत। Habit of eating flesh.

Sarcoplasm (सार्कोप्लाज्म) पेशी कोशिकाओं का कोशिका द्रव्य। The cytoplasm of the muscles cells.

Sarcoptes (सार्कोप्टीस) कुटियों का एक वंश जिसमें सार्कोप्टीस स्केबाई का समावेश होता है जिससे मनुष्य में स्कैबीज या पामा रोग उत्पन्न होता है। A genus of mites, including sarcoptes scabiei, which causes scabies in man.

Sarcoptic (सार्कोप्टिक) सार्कोप्टीस वंश की कुटियों का, उनसे सम्बन्धी अथवा उनके द्वारा उत्पन्न। Of, pertaining to or caused by mites of the genus sarcoptes.

Sarcostosis (सार्कोस्टोसिस) मांसल अथवा पेशीय ऊतक में अस्थिभवन या अस्थिकरण होना। Ossification of fleshy or muscular tissue.

Satellite (सेटेलिटी) धमनी के साथ–साथ चलती हुई शिरा, धमनीसहचराशिरा। A vein accompanying an artery.

Satiety (सेटाइटी) पूर्णतया विशेषकर भोजन से तृप्ति, परिपूर्णता। Full satisfaction, especially with food.

Saturation (सेचुरेशन) संतृप्ति, संतृप्तिकरण। The state of being saturated or the act of saturating.

Satyriasis (सेटीरिएसिस) पुरूष में अत्यधिक बढ़ी हुई कामेच्छा, पुरूष-अतिकामुकता। Excessive sexual desire in the male.

Saucerization (सौसेराइजेशन) किसी ऊतक में शल्यक्रिया द्वारा गड्ढा बनाना अथवा चोट लग जाने पर गड्ढा बन जाना। Surgical formation or formation by trauma of depression in a tissue.

Saw (सा) क्रकच, आरी। A surgical instrument for the excision of a bone.

Saxifragant (सैक्सीफ्रेगेन्ट) पथरियों को विशेषकर मूत्राशय में घोलने अथवा तोड़ने वाला। Dissolving or breaking the calculi, especially in the bladder.

Scab (स्कैब) किसी त्वचीय अथवा उपरिस्थ (ऊपरी) व्रण की पपड़ी जो स्राव के सूख जाने से बन जाती है। Crust of a cutaneous or superficial wound formed by drying up to the discharge.

Scabicidal (स्कैबीसाइडल) पामा कुटकी के लिए विनाशकारी। Destructive to scabies mite.

Scabicide (स्कैबीसाइड) पामा या स्कैबीज़ को उत्पन्न करने वाली कुटकी को मारने वाला, पामानाशी। Killing the mite sacroptes scabiei, causing scabies.

Scabies (स्कैबीज़) कण्डू (खुजली) कुटकी सार्कोप्टीस स्कैबियाड द्वारा उत्पन्न एक अति सांसर्गिक त्वचा रोग। A highly contagious skin disease caused by the itch mite, sarcoptes scabiei.

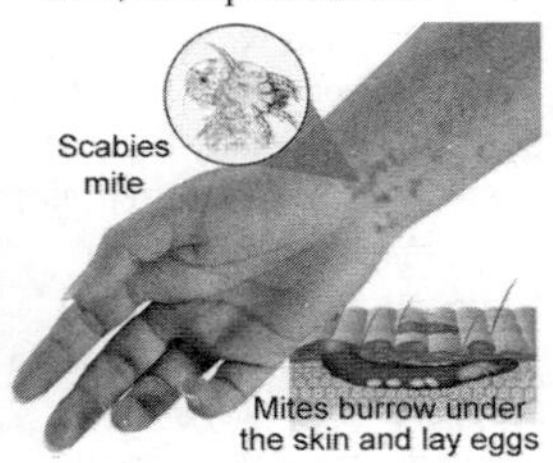

Scabrities (स्कैबराइटिस) नाखूनों का अस्वाभाविक मोटापन, नखस्थूलता। Abnormal thickening of the finger nails.

Scala (स्केला) कोई आशयनुमा अंग, अधःकुल्य।
A bladder-like organ; the cochlear canal.

Scald (स्केल्ड) भाप या गर्म पानी से जल कर बनने वाला घाव, तप्तद्रवदाह।
Any injury caused by moist heat.

Scalding (स्केल्डिंग) मूत्र त्याग करने पर जलन के साथ दर्द होना। A burning pain on urinating.

Scale (स्केल) पर्पटी, शल्क, पपड़ी, खुरण्ड, माप, पपड़ी उतरना या उतारना। A thin crust covering the skin, measurements to desquamate.

Scaler (स्केलर) दांतों से पथरी को निकालने वाला एक दन्त-यन्त्र।
A dental instrument for removal of calculus from the teeth.

Scaling (स्केलिंग) दाँतों से दन्तमल (टार्टर) अथवा पथरी को अलग करने की क्रिया। Removal of tartar or calculus from the teeth.

Scalp (स्कैल्प) कपाल का आवरण जिसमें बालों सहित त्वचा तथा अवत्वक ऊतक आदि होते है, शिरोवल्क।
Covering of the cranium, which includes skin with hair

- The scalp is a multilayered structure with layers that can be defined by the word itself:

S-skin
C-connective tissue (dense)
A-aponeurotic layer (galea aponeurotica)
L-loose connective tissue
P-pericranium

Scalp

and subcutaneous tissue, etc.

Scalpel (स्कैल्पल) एक छोटा, सीधा शल्यक्रिया सम्बन्धी चाकू जिसका एक किनारा उन्नतोदार होता है, छुरी। A small straight surgical knife with a convex edge.

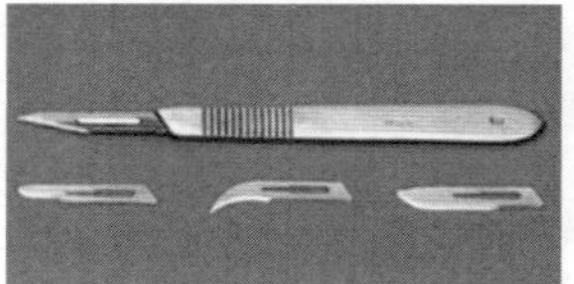

Scalpriform (स्कैलप्रीफोर्म) छेनी के आकार का। Shaped like a chisel.

Scalprum (स्कैप्रम) हड्डियों के टुकड़ों को निकालने के लिये एक दांतेदार यंत्र। A toothed instrument for removing the bone pieces.

Scanner (स्कैनर) स्कैनिंग के लिए प्रयोग में लाया जाने वाला एक उपकरण। An apparatus used for scanning.

Scaphocephalic (स्कैफोसिफैलिक) नाव के आकार के सिर वाला। Having boat-shaped head.

Scaphohydrocephaly (स्कैफोहाइड्रोसिफैली) जलशीर्षता एवं नौकाकार-करोटि संयुक्त रूप में। Hydrocephaly and scaphocephaly combined.

Scaphoid (स्कैफॉयड) नौकाकार, नाव के आकार का, मणिबन्ध (कलाई) अथवा पदकूर्च की समीपस्थ नौकाकार हड्डी। Boat-shaped, a proximal boat-shaped bone of the carpus or tarsus.

Scaphoiditis (स्कैफॉयडाइटिस) नौकाभ अस्थि का शोथ। Inflammation of the scaphoid bone.

Scapula (स्कैपुला) कन्धे के पश्च भाग को बनाने वाली एक बड़ी, चपटी, तकोनी हड्डी, असफलक, स्कन्धफलक। Shoulder blade. The large flat, triangular bone forming the posterior part of the shoulder.

Scapulalgia (स्कैपुलेल्जिया) स्कन्धाफलक में दर्द होना। Pain in the shoulder blade.

Scapulectomy (स्कैपुलेक्टॉमी) शल्यक्रिया द्वारा सम्पूर्ण स्कैपुला हड्डी को अथवा उसके किसी भाग को काट कर निकाल देना। Surgical excision or resection of the scapula bone.

Scapulodynia (स्कैपुलोडाइनिया) कन्धे में दर्द होना। Pain occurring in the shoulder.

Scapulopexy (स्कैपुलोपैक्सी) स्कैपुला हड्डी का पसलियों के साथ स्थिरीकरण करना। Fixation of the scapula bone to the ribs.

Scar (स्कार) क्राचिन्ह, क्षतचिन्ह, घाव का निशान। Cicatrix. A mark left after healing of a wound or injury.

Scarificator (स्कैरीफिकेटर) त्वचा में छोटे-छोटे चीरे लगाने वाला एक यंत्र, प्रच्छानक। An instrument for making small incisions in the skin.

Scarlatina (स्कार्लटिन) स्कार्लेट-ज्वर, रक्त-ज्वर। Scarlet fever.

Scarlatiniform (स्कार्लेटीनिफोर्म) आरक्तज्वर जैसा,आरक्तज्वर-रूप। Resembling scarlatina; scarlatinoid.

Scarlet fever (स्कार्लेट फीवर) एक तीव्र सांसर्गिक रोग जिसमें गला खराब हो जाता है, ज्वर हो जाता है तथा नाड़ी की गति तेज हो जाती है जिसके पश्चात् दाने निकल आते है। An acute contagious disease characterized by sore throat, fever with rapid pulse, followed by rash.

Scatologic (स्केटोलॉजिक) मल पदार्थ से सम्बन्धित। Concerning fecal matter.

Scatophagy (स्केटोफेजी) मलभक्षण। Eating of excrements.

Scatoscopy (स्केटोस्कॉपी) नैदानिक उद्देश्यों से मल का परीक्षण करना। Examination of the feces for diagnostic purpose.

Schick test (शिक टैस्ट) तनु डिफ्थीरिया टॉक्सिन का 0.1 मिलीलीटर का एक अन्तस्त्वचीय इन्जैक्शन लगाकर डिफ्थीरिया के

प्रति रोगक्षमता के अंश को निर्धारित करने वाला एक परीक्षण। यदि 3 से 4 दिन पश्चात् इन्जैक्शन के स्थान पर एक लाल सूजन उत्पन्न होती है, तो परीक्षण का परिणाम धनात्मक होता है, यदि थोड़ी या बिल्कुल ही कोई प्रतिक्रिया नहीं होती है तो परीक्षण का परिणाम कुछ ही धनात्मक या बिल्कुल ही ऋणात्मक होता है। A Test for determining the degree of immunity to diphtheria, by giving an intradermal injection of 0.1 ml of dilute diphtheria toxin. If after 3 to 4 days a red inflamed area is developed at the point of injection the test result is positive. If there is little or no reaction, the test result is slightly positive or entirely negative.

Schiffner's dots (शफनर्ज डाट्स) लाल रक्त कोशिकाओं के मलेरिया परजीवी प्लाज्मोडियम वाइवैक्स से संक्रमित होने पर उनमें पाये जाने वाले कण। Granules present in the red blood cells when they are infected by malarial parasite, *Plasmodium vivax*.

Schiller's test (शिलर्स टैस्ट) उपरिस्थ कैन्सर, विशेषकर गर्भाशय ग्रीवा के कैन्सर के लिए एक परीक्षण। गर्भाशयग्रीवा को आयोडीन घोल से पेन्ट कर दिया जाता है। कैन्सर कोशिकाओं में ग्लाइकोजन नहीं होने के कारण वे आयोडीन घोल से अभिरंजित नहीं होती जिससे उनकी विद्यमानता का पता लगाया जा सकता है। A test for superficial cancer, especially of the cervix of uterus. The cervix is painted with iodine solution. Cancer cells due to absence of glycogen do not stain with iodine solution, by which their presence can be detected.

Schistocormia (स्किस्टोकोर्मिया) ऐसा भ्रूण जिसके धड़ में विदर या फटन होती है। A fetus with a cleft trunk.

Schistocyts (सिस्टोसाइट) रक्तसंलायी रक्ताल्पता में रक्त में पाया जाने वाला लाल रक्त कोशिका का एक टुकड़ा, विखण्डित लोहित कोशिका। A fragment of a red blood cell seen in the blood in hemolytic anemia.

Schistoprosopia (शिस्टोप्रोसोपिया) चेहरे की जन्मजात फटन। Congenital fissure of the face.

Schistosoma (शिस्टोसोमा) वर्ग ट्रेमेटोडा के कुल शिस्टोसोमेटीडी के रक्तपर्ण-कृमियों का एक वंश। A genus of blood- flukes belonging to the family schistosomatidae, class trematoda.

Schistosomiasis (शिस्टोसोमिएसिस) रक्त पर्णकृमि शिस्टोसोमा द्वारा उत्पन्न एक परजीवी रोग। A parasitic disease caused by blood fluke schistosoma.

Schistosomicide (शिस्टोसोमीसाइड) शिस्टोसोमों को नष्ट करने वाला। Destroying schistosomes.

Schizogony (शाइज़ोगोनी) शरीर में स्पोरोजुआइट का बहु विखण्डन द्वारा अलैंगिक जनन जिससे मीरोजुआइट उत्पन्न होते हैं। The asexual reproduction of a sporozoite by multiple fission within the body of the host, giving rise to merozoites, especially in the life cycle of malarial parasites.

Schizoid (शाइजॉयड) विखण्डित मानसिकता या शाइजोफ्रेनिया के समान अथवा उससे ग्रस्त। Resembling or affected with schizophrenia.

Schizont (शाइजोन्ट) विखण्डीजनन द्वारा बढ़ता हुआ कोई बीजाणु, खण्डप्रसू। Any adult sporozoan which is multiplied by schizogony.

Schizonychia (शाइजोनीकिया) नाखूनों का फटना। Splitting of the nails.

Schizophrenia (शाइजोफ्रेनिया) एक मानसिक विकार जिसमें मानसिक क्रियाशीलता का ह्रास हो जाता है। A mental disorder characterized by deterioration of mental activity.

(*i*) **Catatonic Schizophrenia** (केटाटोनिक शाइजोफ्रेनिया) एक प्रकार का शाइजोफ्रेनिया जिसमें रोगी बिल्कुल निष्क्रिय रहता है अथवा बहुत उत्तेजित हो जाता है, कभी-कभी हिंसात्मक भी हो जाता है। A form of schizophrenia in which the patient remains quits inactive or becomes very excited, sometimes even violent. (*ii*) **Reactive Schizophrenia** (रिएक्टिव शाइजोफ्रेनिया) वातावरणीय दशाओं से उत्पन्न होने वाला शाइजोफ्रेनिया। Schizophrenia caused by environmental conditions.

Schizotrichia (शाइज़ोट्राइकिया) बालों का किनारों पर फट जाना। Splitting of hair at the ends.

Schwann cell (श्वॉन सैल) परिसरीय तन्त्रिका-तंत्र की एक कोशिका जिससे परिसरीय तंत्रिका तन्तुओं के माइलिन आवरण एवं तंत्रिकाच्छद का निर्माण होता है। A cell of the peripheral nervous system that form the myelin sheath and neurilemma of the peripheral nerve fibers.

Sciatic (शियाटिक) शियाटिक तंत्रिका अथवा इस्कियम से सम्बन्धित। Pertaining to the sciatic nerve of ischium.

Scirrhus (सिरह्स) तन्तुमय ऊतक की अतिवृद्धि के कारण कठोर कैंसरीय अबुर्द। Hard cancerous tumor due to overgrowth of fibrous tissue.

Scission (सीशन) विखण्डन, विगलन, विभाजन। A splitting, separation or division.

Scissura (सीशुरा) विदर, दराद अथवा फटन। A cleft or fissure.

Sclera (स्क्लेरा) नेत्रगोलक की सफेद व ठोस कला (झिल्ली), श्वेतपटल। The white, tough membrane of the eyeball, sclerotica.

Sclerectasia (स्क्लेरेक्टेसिया) श्वेतपटल का बाहर को निकल आना। Protrusion of the sclera.

Scleritis (स्क्लेराइटिस) श्वेतपटल का प्रदाह, श्वेतपटलशोथ। Inflammation of the sclera.

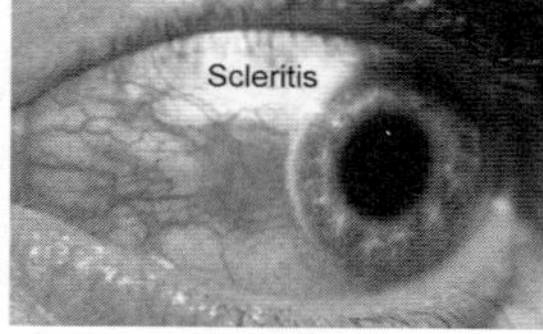

Sclerochoroiditis (स्क्लेरोकोरॉयडाइटिस) श्वेतपटल एवं रंजितपटल का शोथ। Inflammation of the sclera and choroid.

Sclerodactyly (स्क्लेरोडेक्टीली) उँगली की चमड़ी की कठोरता। Digital sclerodermas; sclerodactylia.

Scleroderma (स्क्लेरोडर्मा) त्वचा एवं शरीर के किसी भाग की कठोरता एवं सिकुड़न, त्वचा-कठिनता। Chronic hardening and shrinkage of the skin and any part of the body.

Sclerogenous (स्क्लेरोजीनस) ऊतक का कठिन्य अथवा उसकी कठोरता उत्पन्न करने वाला। Producing sclerosis or hardening of the tissue.

Sclerokeratitis (स्क्लेरोकेराटाइटिस) श्वेतपटल या स्क्लेरा एवं कार्निया का शोथ। Inflammation of the sclera and cornea.

Scleromalacia (स्क्लेरोमैलेशिया) श्वेतपटल या स्क्लेरा का कोमल हो जाना। Softening of the sclera.

Scleronyxis (स्क्लेरोनिक्सिस) श्वेतपटल का शल्यक्रिया द्वारा वेधन। Surgical puncture of the sclera.

Scleroplasty (स्क्लेरोप्लास्टी) श्वेतपटल या स्क्लेरा की प्लास्टिक सर्जरी करना। Plastic surgery of the sclera.

Sclerosis (स्क्लेरोसिस) शोथ, ह्रास अथवा तन्तुमय ऊतक के बनने से किसी अंग या ऊतक की कठोरता अथवा दृढ़ता, काठिन्य। A hardening or induration of an organ or tissue, due to inflammation, degeneration of fibrous tissue formation.

Sclerostenosis (स्क्लेरोस्टेनोसिस) ऊतकों की कठोरता एवं इनका संकुचन दोनों संयुक्त। Hardening combined with contraction of the tissue.

Sclerothrix (स्क्लेरोथ्रिक्स) बालों की भंगुरता (भुरभुरापन) हो जाना। Brittleness of the hair.

Sclerotome (स्क्लेरोटोम) श्वेतपटल या स्क्लेरा में चीरा लगाने के काम आने वाला एक चाकू। A knife used in the incision of sclera.

Scobinate (स्कोबिनेट) खुरदरी, विषम अथवा पर्विल सतह से युक्त। Having a rough, uneven or nodular surface.

Scolecoid (स्कोलीकॉयड) कीड़े से मिलता-जुलता। Resembling a worm.

Scolex (स्कोलेक्स) फीताकृमि का सिर जिसमें हुक या चूशक लगे होते हैं जिनसे यह अपने को आँत की दीवार से चिपका लेता है। The head of the tapeworm containing hooks or suckers by which it attaches itself to the wall of the intestine.

Scoliorachitic (स्कोलियोरेकिटिक) रिकेट के द्वारा उत्पन्न मेरू-दण्ड की वक्रता से सम्बन्धित अथवा उससे ग्रस्त। Pertaining to or afflicted with curvature of the spinal column caused by rickets.

Scoliosis (स्कोलियोसिस) कशेरूका-दण्ड की पार्श्वक वक्रता। Lateral curvature of the vertebral column.

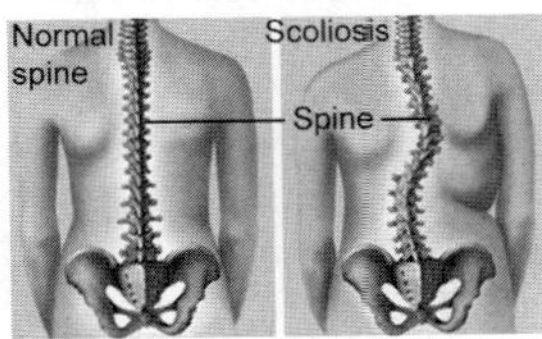

Scoop (स्कूप) चम्मच के आकार का शल्यचिकित्सीय यंत्र। Spoon-shaped surgical instrument.

Scorbutic (स्कार्ब्यूटिक) स्कर्वी से सम्बन्धित अथवा उससे ग्रस्त, स्कर्वीग्रस्त। Pertaining to or affected with scurvy.

Score (स्कोर) गणना जिसकी किसी प्रमाणिक गणना से तुलना

की जाती है। Reckoning as compared to a standard one.

Scoto (स्कोटो) अंधेरे के साथ होने वाले संबंध का संकेत देने वाला उपसर्ग। A prefix indicating relationship to darkness.

Scotoma (स्कोटोमा) दृष्टि-क्षेत्र में स्थित एक अल्प-दृष्टि का स्थान जो चारों ओर कम घटी अथवा सामान्य दृष्टि से घिरा होता है। An area of depressed vision in the visual field surrounded by an area of less depressed or normal vision.

Scotometry (स्कोटोमीट्री) अन्धक्षेत्रों का पता लगाना एवं उनकी माप लेना। The detection and measurement of scotomata.

Scotopic vision (स्कोटोपीक वीजन) धुंधले प्रकाश में भली-भाँति दिखाई देना। The ability to see well in poor light; scotopia.

Scratch test (स्क्रैच टेस्ट) परीक्षण पदार्थ जिसका एक एलर्जेन होने का संदेह होता है, के उचित हल्के घोल की कुछ बूँदों को खरोंची गई त्वचा के ऊपर रखना। यदि पदार्थ कोई एलेर्जेन है तो 15 मिनट के भीतर एक स्फोट बन जायेगा।
To place a few drops on a scratched area of the skin, of appropriately diluted solution of the test material, suspected of being an allergen. If the material is an allergen, a wheal will be developed within 15 minutes.

Screen (स्क्रीन) 1. एक समतल स्थान जिस पर चलचित्रों अथवा स्लाइडों को देखा जाता है या एक्स-रे चित्रों को दिखाया जाता है। 2. प्रतिदीप्तिदर्शी परीक्षण करना। 3. परदे के समान एक रचना। 1. A flat area upon which moving pictures or slides are viewed or X-ray picture are visualized.
2. To make a fluoroscopic examination. 3. A structure or substance resembling a curtain.

Scrofula (स्क्रोफुला) यक्ष्मज ग्रैव लसीकापर्व-शोथ, कण्ठमाला। Tuberculous cervical lymphadenitis.

Scrotal (स्क्रोटल) वृशण सम्बन्धी, अण्डकोशीय। Pertaining to the scrotum.

Scrotitis (स्क्रोटाइटिस) वृशणशोथ, अण्डकोशशोथ। Inflammation of the scrotum.

Scrotum (स्क्रोटम) वृषणकोश, अणुकोश। Bag holding the testes.

Scrubbing (स्क्रबिंग) कस कर रगड़ कर साफ करना। Cleaning by rubbing hardly.

Scum (स्कम) किसी सम्वर्धन की सतह पर तैरने वाली जीवाणुओं अथवा मैल की छोटी पतली परत, फेन। A small thin layer of bacteria or impurities floating on the surface of a culture.

Scurvy (स्कर्वी) एस्कॉर्बिक एसिड विटामीन सी की कमी से होने वाला एक रोग जिसमें रक्ताल्पता हो जाती है, मसूड़े स्पंज के समान पोले हो जाते है जिनसे रक्तस्राव होने लगता है। A disease due to deficiency of ascorbic acid 'vitamin-c' characterized by anemia, spongy gums with a tendency of bleeding.

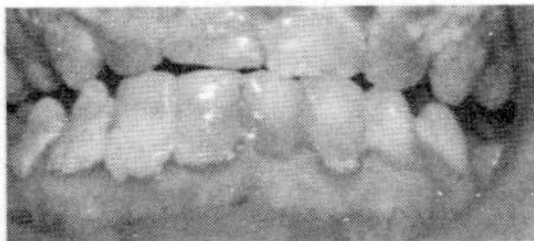

It includes gum disease and loss of teeth

Scutiform (स्क्यूटीफॉर्म) कवच या ढाल के आकार का। Shield shaped.

Scybala (स्काइबेला) कठोर मल, मलगांठ। Hard masses of fecal matter.

Scyphoid (स्काइफॉयड) प्याले के आकार जैसा। Cup-shaped.

Seasickness (सीसिकनैस) पानी के जहाज से यात्रा करने से उत्पन्न गति-रूग्णता, समुद्री-रूग्णता। Motion sickness caused by travelling in the ship.

Sebaceous (सीबेसियस) त्वग्वसा से सम्बन्धित, उसे धारण करने वाला अथवा उसे स्रावित करने वाला, त्वग्वसीय। Pertaining to, containing, or secreting sebum.

Sebaceous cyst (सीबेसियस सिस्ट) पुटी जिसमें सीबम या त्वग्वसा भरा होता है। त्वग्सीय पुटी। A cyst filled with sebum.

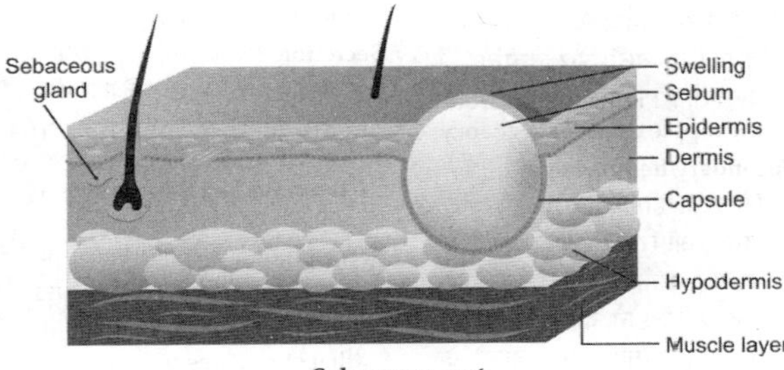

Sebaceous cyst

Sebaceous glands (सीबेसियस ग्लैण्ड्स) त्वचा की त्वग्वसा या सीबम स्रावित करने वाली ग्रन्थियाँ जो रोमकूपों में खुलती है। The glands of the skin secreting sebum, which open into the hair fallicles.

Seborrhea (सीबोरीह्या) त्वग्वसीय ग्रन्थियों से अत्यधिक स्राव निकलना, त्वग्वसास्त्रव। Excessive secretion of the sebaceous glands.

Sebum (सीबम) त्वचा की त्वग्वसीय ग्रन्थियों का तैलीय स्राव, त्वग्वसा। The oily secretion of the sebaceous gland of the skin.

Second intention (सेकण्ड इन्टैंशन) दो कणांकुर युक्त सतहों का आवलेश (चिपकाव) द्वारा विरोहण (भरना)। Healing by adhesion of two granulated surfaces.

Secondary areola (सैकण्ड्री एरियोला) गर्भावस्था के दौरान चूचुकों के चारों ओर उत्पन्न वर्णकता। Pigmentation around the nipple during pregnancy.

Secondary hemorrhage (सेकण्ड्री हीमोरेह्ज) किसी चोट लगने, ऑपरेशन अथवा प्रसव के पश्चात् गर्भाशय से 24 घण्टों के बाद प्रकट होने वाला रक्तस्राव जो पूतिता (मवाद पड़ जाना) के कारण होता है। Hemorrhage appearing more than 24 hours after an injury or operation or from the uterus after delivery that is due to sepsis.

Secreta (सीक्रिटा) स्राव के उत्पाद, उत्सृष्ट पदार्थ। The products of secretion.

Secretagogue (सिक्रीटोगौग) स्रावर्धक, स्राव बढ़ाने वाला। A substence which promotes secretion.

Secretin (सेक्रेटिन) अम्ल काइम के आँत में प्रवेश करने पर ह्योडिनम एवं जेजुनम की श्लेष्मिक कला से स्रावित होने वाला एक हार्मोन। यह अग्न्याशयी तथा पित्त या बाइल एवं आंत्तीय स्राव को उत्तेजित करता है। A hormone secreted by the mucous membrane of duodenum and jejunum when acid chyme enters the intestine. It stimulates the secretion of pancreatic juice and bile and intestinal secretion.

Secretion (सिक्रीशन) वह क्रिया जिसके द्वारा कोई ग्रन्थिल अंग किसी पदार्थ को उत्पन्न करता है। The process by which a glandular organ produces a substance.

Secretomotor (सिक्रीटोमोटर) वह विशेषकर कोई तंत्रिका जो स्राव को उत्तेजित करती है। Agent that stimulates secretion.

Sectile (सैक्टाइल) कट जाने योग्य। Capable of being cut.

Sector (सैक्टर) किसी वृत्त के दो अर्द्धव्यासों एवं एक चाप के बीच का स्थान। The area of a circle between two radii and an arc.

Secundiparity (सेकण्डीपैरिटी) दूसरी बार गर्भवती होने की अवस्था। The condition of being secundipara.

Sedate (सिडेट) शान्त करना। To calm.

Sedative (सिडेटिव) उत्तेजना को शान्त करने वाला, शामक। Soothing, calming. Allaying excitement.

Sedentary (सिडेन्ट्री) ऐसे व्यवसाय से सम्बन्धित जिसमें शारीरिक श्रम की न्यूनतम आवश्यकता होती है। Pertaining to an occupation requiring minimal physical exercise.

Sediment (सैडीमेन्ट) तलछट। वह पदार्थ जो किसी द्रव की तली में बैठ जाता है। Precipitate. The substance that settles down at the bottom of a liquid.

Sediment Rate (सैडिमेन्ट रेट) अवसादन दर। Laboratory test of speed at which erythrocytes settle.

Segment (सैग्मैन्ट) खण्ड, खण्डांश, एक छोटा-सा टुकड़ा। A part or section of an organ or body, lobe, a small piece.

Segmentation (सैग्मैन्टेशन) एक से भागों में विभाजित, खण्डीभवन, खण्डांशी भवन। Cleavage, division into similar parts.

Segregation (सैग्रीगेशन) पृथक्करण। Separation.

Seisesthesia (सीसेस्थीसिया) संघटन या आघात का बोध होना। Perception of concussion.

Seizure (सीज़र) दर्द अथवा किसी रोग जैसे अपस्मार (मिर्गी) का अचानक आक्रमण हो जाना अथवा दौरा पड़ जाना, ग्रह। A sudden attack of pain, or of a disease such as epilepsy.

Selene (सैलीन) नाखूनों पर सफेद धब्बे पड़ना। White spots on the nails.

Self-conscious (सैल्फ-कॉन्शस) अपने अस्तित्व को जानने वाला। Conscious of one's self.

Self-limited (सैल्फ-लिमिटेड) ऐसे रोग को बताने वाला जो चिकित्सा के बिना एक निश्चित काल के पश्चात् समाप्त हो जाने वाला होता है जैसे इन्फ्लुएन्जा। Denoting a disease that without treatment tends to cease after a definite period, e.g. influenza.

Sella turcica (शेला टर्सिका) स्फैनॉयड हड्डी की ऊपरी सतह पर स्थित एक गड्ढा जिसमें

पीयूष ग्रन्थि स्थित रहती है, पर्याणिका। A depression on the upper surface of the sphenoid bone, in which the pituitary gland is situated.

Semeiosis (सेमियोसिस) लक्षणों के द्वारा किसी रोग का अध्ययन करना। Study of the disease by symptoms.

Semen (सीमेन) वीर्य पुरूष में स्खलन में मूत्रमार्ग से निकलने वाला एक गाढ़ा, दूधिया पदार्थ जैसा, चिपचिपा स्राव। A thick, opalescent, viscid secretion discharge at ejaculation from urethra of the male.

Semenarche (सीमेनार्की) यौवनारम्भ के दौरान वीर्य उत्पादन का आरम्भ होना। The beginning of the production of the semen during puberty.

Semi (सेमी) एक उपसर्ग जिसका अर्थ आधा होता है। A prefix meaning half.

Semicircular (सेमीसर्कुलर) अर्द्धवृत्ताकार। In the form of a half circle.

Semicoma (सेमीकॉमा) अर्धमूर्च्छा, अर्धसन्यास। Partial impairment of the consciousness from which the patient may be aroused.

Semilunar (सेमील्यूनर) अर्द्धचन्द्राकार। Shaped like a crescent or half-moon.

Semimembranous (सेमीमेम्ब्रेनस) जिसका कुछ भाग किसी झिल्ली का बना होता है। Composed partly of a membrane.

Seminal (सेमीनल) वीर्य सम्बन्धी। Pertaining to semen.

Seminal emission (सेमीनल एमिसन) वीर्य का निकलना। Discharge of semen.

Seminoma (सेमीनोमा) शुक्रग्रन्थि का दुर्दम अबुर्द। A malignant tumor of the testis.

Semirecumbent (सेमीरिकम्बैन्ट) आधा लेटा हुआ। Half lying down.

Semitendinous (सेमीटैण्डीनस) आंशिका रूप से कण्डरा का होना। Being partially tendinous.

Senescence (सेनेस्सेन्स) वृद्ध होना, जरा। The process of growing old.

Senility (सैनीलिटी) वृद्धावस्था के साथ होने वाली शारीरिक एवं मानसिक दुर्बलता, जरा-दोर्बल्य। The physical and mental weakness associated with the old age.

Senna (सैन्ना) मार्कण्डी, स्वर्णपत्री, सनाय, एक रेचक पौधे की पत्तियाँ और फलियाँ। Leaves and pods of a purgative plant from Egypt and India.

Sensation (सैन्सेशन) किसी उत्तेजित अभिवाही तंत्रिका द्वारा मस्तिष्क में संवेदना क्षेत्र को ले जाये गये आवेगों के द्वारा उत्पन्न प्रभाव, संवेदना, अनुभूति। The effect produced by impulses conveyed by a stimulated afferent nerve to the sensorium.

Sense (सैन्स) मानसिक शक्ति जिसके द्वारा शरीर के भीतर या बाहर वस्तुओं की दशाओं अथवा गुणों का बोध होता है। The faculty by which the conditions or properties of the things outside or inside the body are perceived.

(*i*) **Muscular sense** (मस्कुलर सैन्स) संवेद जिसके द्वारा पेशीय गतियों का ज्ञान होता है। The sense by which muscular movements are perceived.

(*ii*) **Tactile sense** (टैक्टाइल सैन्स) स्पर्श का संवेद। Sense of touch. (*iii*) **Time Sense** (टाइम सैन्स) जिसके द्वारा समयावकाशों की भिन्नताओं का पता चलता है। The sense by which difference in time intervals is detected.

Sensible (सैन्सीबल) संवदेनशील। Perceptible to the sense.

Sensitive (सैन्सीटिव) उद्दीपनों का प्रत्युत्तर देने के सक्षम अथवा किसी पदार्थ जैसे औषधि या बाह्य प्रोटीन के प्रति असामान्य रूप से ग्रहणशील, सुग्राही। Able to respond to stimuli or abnormally susceptible to a substance, as a drug or foreign protein.

Sensitivity (सैन्सीटिविटी) सुग्राहिता अथवा सूक्ष्न ग्रहिता। The condition or quality of being sensitive.

Sensitization (सैन्सीटाइजेशन) सुग्रहीकरण, सुग्राहीभवन, संवेदनशील करना। Rendering sensitive.

Sensitizer (सैन्सीटाइजर) वह पदार्थ जो ग्रहणशील व्यक्ति को उसी अथवा अन्य क्षोभकों के प्रति प्रतिक्रिया करने योग्य बनाती है। The substance which makes the susceptible person react to the some or other irritants.

Sensorial (सैन्सोरियल) मस्तिष्क में स्थित संवेदना क्षेत्र से सम्बन्धित। Pertaining to the sensorium, the area of sensation in the brain.

Sensorimotor (सैन्सरीमोटर) जो संवेदी एवं प्रेरक दोनो हो, संवेदीप्रेरक। Sensorimotor, both, sensory and motor.

Sensorium (सैन्सीरियम) प्रमस्तिष्कीय प्रान्तस्था का वह भाग जो संवेदनाओं के केन्द्र की भांति कार्य करता है। The portion of the cerebral cortex that acts as a center of sensations.

Sensory area (सैन्सरी एरिया) प्रमस्तिष्कीय प्रान्तस्था का कोई भी स्थान जहाँ पर संवेदनाएँ ग्रहण की जाती है। Any area of the cerebral cortex in which sensations are perceived.

Sensualism (सैन्सुआलिज्म) ऐसी दशा जिसमें किसी व्यक्ति के कार्यो पर भावावेगों की प्रधानता होती है। The condition in which one's actions are dominated by emotions.

Sensuous (सैन्सुअस) संवेदों से सम्बन्धित अथवा उन्हें प्रभावित करने वाला। Pertaining to or affecting the senses.

Sentiment (सैन्टीमैन्ट) भावावेग, अनुभूति। Emotion, feeling.

Separator (सेप्रेटर) पृथक्कारी, करोटि से करोटिआवरण को अलग करने का यंत्र। An instrument for separating pericranium from the skull separatory.

Sepsis (सेप्सिस) पूति, रक्तपूतिता, रक्त-विषणता, पूतिजीवरक्तता। Putrefaction, septicemia, blood poisoning.

Septa (सेप्ता) पट, पटल, दीवार। Partition.

Septan (सेप्टान) प्रत्येक सातवें दिन पुनः उत्पन्न होने वाला। Recurring every seventh day.

Septate (सेप्टेट) किसी पट द्वारा विभाजित। Divided by a septum.

Septic (सेप्टिक) रोगजनक जीवधारियों अथवा उनके जीव-विषाक्त पदार्थों से सम्बन्धित। Pertaining to pathogenic organism or their toxins.

Septicemia (सेप्टीसीमिया) रक्त विशाक्तता, जीवाणुरक्तता। रक्त से विकृतिजनक या रोगोत्पादक जीवाणुओं का पाया जाना। Blood poisoning. Bacterium presence of pathogenic bacteria in the blood.

Septicophlebitis (सेप्टीकोफ्लेबाइटिस) शिरा का पूतिज शोथ। Septic inflammation of a vein.

Septigravida (सेप्टीग्रेविडा) सातवीं बार गर्भवती होने वाली स्त्री। A woman pregnant for the seventh time.

Septoplasty (सेप्टोप्लास्टी) नासा-पट की प्लास्टिक सर्जरी करना। Plastic surgery of the nasal septum.

Septostomy (सेप्टोस्टॉमी) किसी पट में शल्यक्रिया द्वारा एक छिद्र बनाना।
Surgical formation of an opening in a septum.

Septum (सेप्टम) दो गुहाओं में पैदा होने वाले 7 बच्चों में से

एक। One of seven children produced at one birth.

Sequela (सीक्यूला) किसी रोग के पश्चात् अथवा उसके परिणामस्वरूप उत्पन्न होने वाली विकृत दशा, अनुगम। A morbid condition following resulting from a disease.

Sequester (सीक्वैस्टर) सम्पूर्ण शरीर से किसी छोटे से टुकड़े को अलग करना। To separate a small portion from the whole body.

Sequestration (सीक्वैस्ट्रेशन) विविक्त का बनना, किसी रोगी को अलग रखना। The formation of requestrum, isolation of a patient.

Sequestrum (सीक्वैस्ट्रम) चारों ओर के ऊतक से अलग हुआ परिगलित हड्डी का एक टुकड़ा, विविक्त, विविक्तांश। A piece of necrosed bone separated from the surrounding tissue.

Seralbumin (सीराल्ब्युमिन) रक्त एल्ब्युमिन। Albumin of the blood.

Serious (सीरियस) गम्भीर। Grave.

Seroconversion (सीरोकनवर्जन) किसी संक्रामक रोग अथवा रोगक्षमीकरण की अनुक्रिया में सीरम में विशिष्ट एण्टीबॉडियों का विकसित हो जाना। Development of the specific antibodies in the serum in response to an infections disease or immunization.

Seroculture (सीरोकल्चर) रक्त में सीरम में जीवाणु सम्वर्धन। A bacterial culture in blood serum.

Serodiagnosis (सीरोडायग्नोसिस) रक्त सीरम की प्रतिक्रियाओं को देख कर रोग निदान करना। Diagnosis of disease made by observing the reactions of blood serum.

Serofibrous (सीरोफाइब्रस) सीरमी एवं तन्तुमय सतह से सम्बन्धित। Pertaining to serous and fibrous surface.

Serology (सीरोलॉजी) सीरम का वैज्ञानिक अध्ययन, सीरमविज्ञान। The scientific study of serum.

Seromucoid (सीरोम्यूकॉयड) सीरम एवं श्लेष्मा जैसा, सीरमश्लेष्माभ। Resembling the serum and mucus.

Seronegative (सीरोनिगेटिव) सीरमी परीक्षणों में ऋणात्मक प्रतिक्रिया उत्पन्न करने वाला। Producing a negative reaction to serological tests.

Seroprophylaxis (सीरोप्रोफाइलैक्सिस) सीरम देकर किसी रोग की रोकथाम करना। Sero-prevention. Prevention of a disease by the administration of serum.

Serosa (सीरोसा) कोई भी सीरमी झिल्ली जैसे पेरीओनियम, सीरमी कला। Any serous membrane such as peritoneum.

Serosanguineous (सीरोसैंग्वीनियस) सीरम एवं रक्त से बना हुआ अथवा उन दोनों की प्रकृति वाला। Composed of or of the nature of serum and blood.

Serositis (सीरोसाइटिस) किसी सिरमी झिल्ली का शोथ। Inflammation of a serous membrane.

Serosynovial (सीरोसाइनोवियल) सीरमी तथा श्लेषक-पदार्थ से सम्बन्धित। Pertaining to serous and synovial material.

Serotherapy (सीरोथिरैपी) रक्तोद-प्रयोग द्वारा की जाने वाली रोगों की चिकित्सा, सीरम-चिकित्सा। Treatment of disease by the use of blood serum, serum therapy.

Serotonin (सीरोटोनिन) रक्त प्लेटलेटों, जठरान्त्र-श्लेष्म कला, पीनियल काय, मास्ट कोशिकाओं तथा केन्द्रीय तंत्रिका तंत्र में पाया जाने वाला एसक हार्मोन 5-हाइड्रोक्सीट्रिप्टाइमाइन (5-एच टी) जो आमाशयिक स्राव को कम करता है। A hormone 5-hydroxytryptamine (5HT), present in blood platelets, gastrointestinal mucosa, pineal body, mast cells, and central nervous system, which inhibits gastric secretion.

Serotype (सीरोटाइप) किसी सूक्ष्म जीवधारी की वह किस्म जिसे उसके घटक एण्टिजनों के द्वारा सुनिश्चित किया जाता है। The type of a microorganism determined by its constituent antigens.

Serpiginous (सर्पीजीनस) रेंगने वाला, सर्पी। Creeping.

Serrate (सिरेट) दन्तुर, दान्तेदार, दन्तुरित। Notched like a saw, dentate, serrated.

Serrefine (सेरेफाइन) रक्तस्रावी वाहिनियों को दबाने वाली एक प्रकार की चीमटी। A type of forceps for compressing bleeding vessels.

Serum (सीरम) रक्त के जमने के पश्चात् रक्त का जलीय भाग सीरम कहलाता है जो फाइब्रिनोजन से रक्षित प्लाज्मा होता है। After clotting, the watery portion of blood is called as serum which is plasma excluding fibrinogen.

Serum sickness (सीरम सिकनैस) किसी प्रतिसीरम के देने अथवा किसी औषधि चिकित्सा से कुछ दिन पश्चात् उत्पन्न होने वाली एक अतिसुग्राहिता प्रतिक्रिया

जिसमें त्वचा पर दाने निकल आते है, लसीका पर्व बढ़ जाते है, ज्वर हो जाता है तथा जोड़ों में दर्द होता है। A hypersensitivity reaction occurring several days after administration of an antiserum or certain drug therapy characterized by skin rash, enlarged lymph nodes, fever and pain in the joints.

Sesquihora (सैसक्वीहॉरा) प्रत्येक ड़ेढ घण्टें पर। Every one and half hour.

Setting (सैटिंग) कठोर होना जैसे एमल्गम का कठोर होना। Hardening, as of amalgam.

Sex (सैक्स) एक विशेष लक्षण जो अधिकतर जन्तुओं एवं पौधों में नर तथा मादाओं को भिन्न करता है। A distinctive character that differentiate males and females in most animals and plants.

Sex chromosomes (सैक्स क्रोमोसोम्स) लिंग निर्धारण से सम्बन्धित गुणसूत्र जो मानव में एक्स (स्त्री) तथा वाई (पुरूष) है। सामान्य स्त्री में दो एक्स गुणसूत्र तथा सामान्य पुरूष में एक एक्स एवं एक वाई गुणसूत्र होता है। Chromosomes concerned with the determination of sex, which in humans are X (female) and Y (Male). The normal female has two X chromosome and the normal male has one X and one Y chromosome.

Sex drive (सैक्स ड्राइव) लैंगिक आनन्द के लिए अभिप्रेरण। Motivation for sexual pleasure.

Sex chromatin (सैक्स क्रोमैटिन) सैक्स क्रोमैटिन सामान्य स्त्री कायिक कोशिकाओं के केन्द्रकों के भीतर दिखाई देने वाला पिण्ड होता है। स्त्री की प्रत्येक कायिक या दैहिक कोशिका में दो एक्स गूणसूत्रों में से एक जीनी रूप से निष्क्रिय हो जाता है। सैक्स अथवा लिंग क्रोमैटिन निष्क्रिय हुए एक्स गुणसूत्र को प्रदर्शित करता है। Sex chromatine is the mass seen within nuclei of the normal female somatic cells one of the two X chromosomes in each somatic cell of the female is genetically inactivated. The sex chromatin represents the inactivated X chromosome.

Sex-linked (सैक्स लिंक्ड) लिंग गुणसूत्र पर स्थापित किसी जीन के द्वारा नियंत्रित। Controlled by a gene located on the sex chromosome.

Sextan (सैक्सटान) प्रत्येक छठे दिन उत्पन्न होने वाला, षट्दिवसीय। Occurring every sixth day.

Sextuplet (सैक्सटुप्लेट) एक ही गर्भावस्था से पैदा होने वाले छः बच्चों में से एक, शटक। One of six children born of a single pregnancy.

Sexual abuse (सैक्सुअल एब्यूज) लैंगिक छेड़छाड़ या उत्पीड़न अथवा बलात्कार। Sexual molestation or rape.

Sexual reflex (सैक्सुअल रिफ्लैक्स) जननानांगों की प्रत्यक्ष उत्तेजना से अथवा प्रत्यक्ष रूप से सोते समय या जागृत अवस्था में भावावेग में उत्तेजित होने के फलस्वरूप लिंगोंत्थान एवं वीर्य स्खलन होना। Erection of the penis and ejaculation resulting from direct stimulation of the genital organs or indirectly from emotion during sleeping or awaking.

Shakes (शेक्स) कंपकंपी, पुराने शराबियों के शरीर में होने वाली थरथराहट, (कम्पन) Shivering or tremulousness.

Shaking shallow (शेकिंग शैलो) हल्लन, कम्पन, कम्प, संक्षोभ उथला या छिछला। Shivering, having little depth.

Sheath (शीथ) एक ढक्कन वाली विशेषकर किसी लम्बे भाग को ढकने वाली रचना, आच्छद, आवरण। A covering structure, usually of an elongated part.

Shedding (शैडिंग) बाह्यत्वचा की बाह्य परत का कैंचुली के रूप में झड़ना। Casting off surface layer of epidermis.

Sheet (शीट) पलंग की चादर। A rectangular piece of cotton or cloth for bed covering.

Shield (शील्ड) कोई भी रक्षक संरचना अथवा उपकरण, कवच जैसे चूचुक कवच। Any protective structure or device as nipple shield.

Shigella (शाइगेला) एण्ट्रोबैक्टीरियेसी कुल के अगतिशील, ग्राम-ऋणात्मक, दण्डाकार जीवाणुओं का एक वंश जिससे हल्के दस्त आने से लेकर गम्भीर तथा प्राणघातक तथा पेचिश उत्पन्न हो जाती है। A genus of nonmotile, Gram-negative, rod-shaped bacteria, belonging to the family enterobacteriaceae which causes digestive trouble ranging from mild diarrhea to severe and fatal dysentery.

Shigellosis (शाइगेलोसिस) शाइगेला का संक्रमण जिससे खूनी पेचिश हो जाती है। Infection with shigella causing bacillary dysentery.

Shin (शिन) टिबिया हड्डी का अगला किनारा अथवा पैर का घुटने से टखने तक का भाग,

प्रजंघिका। Shank, the anterior edge of the tibia or the portion of leg from knee to the ankle.

Shiver (शिविर) एक मृदु कम्पन्न जैसे ठण्ड अथवा भय से होता है। A slight temor, as from cold or fear.

Shock (शॉक) रक्तस्राव, निर्जलीकरण, औषधि प्रतिक्रिया, आघात संक्रमण, विशक्तता एवं हृदपेशी-रोधगलन आदि के द्वारा उत्पन्न तीव्र परिसरीय परिसंचरणपात के कारण सामान्य कार्य करने के लिए हृदय में अपर्याप्त रक्त की वापसी होना इसमें तापमान एवं रक्त-चाप का कम हो जाना, शीघ्रगामी तथा क्षीण नाड़ी का पाया जाना और त्वचा का पीलापन विशिष्टताएँ होती है, स्तब्धता।

Insufficient return of blood to the heart for normal function, due to severe peripheral circulatory failure caused by hemorrhage, dehydration, drug reaction, trauma, infection, poisoning and myocardial infarction, etc. It is characterized by low temperature and low blood pressure, rapid and thready pulse and paleness of the skin. (*i*) **Hemorrhagic-Shock** (हीमोरैह्जिक-शॉक) तीव्र रक्त-स्राव होने के परिणामस्वरूप उत्पन्न स्तब्धता। Shock resulting from acute hemorrhage. (*ii*) **Protein shock** (प्रोटीन शॉक) किसी प्रोटीन का इन्जैक्शन लगाने के बाद होने वाली स्तब्धता। Shock occurring after administration of an injection of a protein.

Shooting (शूटिंग) तेज (तीव्र) या गम्भीर। Acute or severe.

Shortsightedness (शॉर्टसाइटेडनैस) निकट दृष्टिता। Myopia, Nearsightedness.

Shot (शॉट) इंजेक्शन, अन्तःक्षेपण, स्वापक। A vermicular term for an injection, used also to denote a dose of narcotic.

Shoulder (शोल्डर) क्लैविकल एवं स्कैपुला का संगम जहां पर बाँह धड़ से जुड़ती है, कन्धा, स्कन्ध। The junction of the clavicle and scapula where the arm joins the trunk.

Shoulder blade (शोल्डर ब्लेड) स्कन्धफलक, स्कैपुला हड्डी। Scapula bone.

Show (शो) प्रसव अथवा मासिक धर्म से ठीक पहले योनि से दिखाई देने वाला रक्त, प्रसवसूचकस्राव। Appearance of blood through vagina just prior to labor or menstruations.

Shrapnell's membrane (श्रापनील्समेम्ब्रेन) श्लथ-कला, कर्णपट का त्रिकोणक अंश, श्रैपनेल कला। Membrane flaccida, the triangular portion of the tympanic membrane.

Shreds (श्रैड्स) हाल में उत्सर्जित मूत्र में दिखाई देने वाली श्लेष्मा की बारीक-बारीक धागे के समान रचनाऐं जो मूत्र-पथ अथवा सम्बद्ध अंगों में सूजन होने का संकेत देती है। Fine threadlike structures of mucus seen in recently excreted urine, that indicates the inflammation of urinary tract or associated organs.

Shudder (शडर) भय से काँपना। Trembling with fear.

Shunt (शन्ट) दो प्राकृतिक नलिकाओं विशेषकर रक्त वाहिनियों के बीच एक शरीर-वृत्रिक मार्ग। A physiological passage between two natural channels, especially between blood vessels.

Sialadenitis (सियालेडीनाइटिस) किसी लार-ग्रन्थि का शोथ। Inflammation of a salivary gland.

Sialagogue (सियालेगौग) लार का स्राव बढ़ाने वाला, लारवर्धक। Sialogogue, increasing flow of saliva.

Siale angiectasis (सियालोएन्जियक्टेसिस) किसी लार-ग्रन्थि वाहिनी का चौड़ा हो जाना। Dilatation of salivary gland duct.

Sialoadenectomy (सियालोएडीनेक्टॉमी) किसी लार-ग्रन्थि को शल्यक्रिया द्वारा काट कर अलग कर देना। Excision of a salivary gland.

Sialogenous (सियालोजीनस) थूक बनाने वाला। Forming saliva.

Sialography (सियालोग्राफी) किसी रेडियो अपारदर्शक पदार्थ का इन्जैक्शन लगाकर लार-ग्रन्थियों एवं उनकी वाहिनियों का एक्स-रे परीक्षण करना, लालावाहिनाचित्रण। Sialoangiography, X-ray examination of the salivary glands and their ducts after injection of a radiopaque substance.

Sialolithiasis (सियालोलिथिएसिस) लार-ग्रन्थियों में पथरियों का बनना, लालास्मरता। The formation of calculi in the salivary glands.

Sialoporia (सियालोपोरिया) लार का अल्प स्राव होना। Deficient secretion of saliva.

Sib (सिब) 1. भाई अथवा बहिन। 2. एक खून का रिश्तेदार,

सहोदर। 1. Sibling, a brother or sister. 2. A blood relative.

Sibilant (सिबिलैन्ट) सीटी की जैसी आवाज उत्पन्न करने अथवा फुफकारें वाला। Whistling or hissing.

Sibilismus (सिबिलिस्मस) फुफकार की आवाज। A hissing sound.

Sibling (सिबलिंग) एक भाई अथवा बहिन। A brother or sister.

Siccus (सिक्कस) शुष्क, सूखा हुआ। Dry.

Sick (सिक) रोगी, किसी रोग से पीड़ित व्यक्ति, बीमार। Patient, suffering from a disease.

Sickling (सिकलिंग) रक्त में लाल रक्त कोशिकाओं का दात्रलोहितकोशिकाओं में विकसित होना। Development of red blood cells into sickle cells in the blood.

Sickness (सिक्नैस) रोग, व्याधि, बीमारी, अस्वस्थता। Illness, disease, state of being unwell.

Sicolabile (सिक्कोलेबाइल) सुखाने से परिवर्तित होने अथवा नष्ट होने वाला। Altered or destroyed by drying.

Side-effect (साइड-इफैक्ट) अनुषंगी-प्रभाव। The effect of a drug other than desired.

Siderocyte (साइड्रोसाइट) एक लाल रक्त कोशिका जिसमें हिमोग्लोबिन रहित लोहा होता है। A red blood cell containing non-hemoglobin iron.

Sideropenia (साइड्रोपीनिया) रक्त में लोहे की कमी हो जाना। Deficiency of iron in the blood.

Siderophil (साइडेरोफिल) ऐसी कोशिका जिसका लोहे से लगाव होता है। A cell having affinity for iron.

Siderosis (साइडेरोसिस) लोहे के कणों के साँस के साथ खींच कर अन्दर पहुँचने से उत्पन्न एक प्रकार की फुफ्फुसधूलिमयता। A form of pneumoconiosis due to inhalation of iron particles.

Sieve (सीव) चलनी। A mesh with uniform sized pores.

Sigh (साइ) गहरी साँस लेकर साँस निकालना जिसमें हल्की-सी आवाज, सुनाई देती है, आह भरना। A deep inspiration followed by expiration during which a slow sound is heard.

Sight (साइट) दृष्टि या नजर। Vision, power of seeing.

Sigmoid (सिग्मॉयड) कोलन के अवग्राहान्त्र वंक से सम्बन्धित, अवग्रहान्त्र। Pertaining to the sigmoid flexure of the colon.

Sigmoid flexure (सिग्मॉयड फ्लेक्सर) अवग्रहांत्र आनमन। S-shaped portion of the colon above the rectum.

Sigmoiditis (सिग्मॉयडाइटिस) सिग्मॉयड कोलन का शोथ। Inflammation of the sigmoid colon.

Sigmoidoproctostomy (सिग्मॉयडोप्रोक्टोस्टॉमी) अवग्रहांत्रमलांत्रसिम्मिलन। Artificial communication of sigmoid flexure with colon.

Sigmoidoscope (सिग्मॉयडोस्कोप) सिग्मॉयड कोलन का दृष्टि परीक्षण करने के लिए एक गुहान्तदर्शी, अवग्रहान्त्रदर्शी। An endoscope for visual examination of the sigmoid colon.

Sigmoidoscopy (सिग्मॉयडोस्कोपी) अवग्रहान्त्रदर्शी का प्रयोग करके सिग्मॉयड कोलन का निरीक्षण करना, अवग्रहान्त्रदर्शन। Inspection of the sigmoid colon by use of sigmoidoscope.

Sigmoidosigmoidostomy (सिग्मॉयडोसिग्मॉयडोस्टॉमी) सिग्मॉयड कोलन के दो खण्डों के बीच शल्यक्रिया द्वारा सम्बन्ध स्थापित करना। Surgical creation of connection between two segments of the sigmoid colon.

Sigmoidotomy (सिग्मॉयडोटॉमी) सिग्मॉयड कोलन में चीरा लगाना। To make an incision into the sigmoid colon.

Sign (साइन) 1. किसी वस्तु का अस्तित्व होने का संकेत। 2. स्वानुभूत प्रमाणों (लक्षणों) के विपरीत जिनका रोगी को पता चलता हैं, चिन्ह, निशान। 1. An indication of the existence of something. 2. Any objective evidence of a disease.

Signal (सिग्नल) वह जिससे कोई कार्य होता है, संकेत, इशारा। Something that causes an action.

Silicosis (सिलिकोसिस) सिलिका की धूल के साँस के साथ खिंचकर अन्दर जाने से उत्पन्न एक प्रकार की फुफ्फुस-धूलिमयता जिसमें अलग-अलग छोटे-छोटे पर्व बन जाते है। A type of pneumoconiosis due to inhalation of the dust of silica, characterized by the formation of small discrete nodules.

Silver (सील्वर) रजत, चाँदी। Argentum, a metal of white lustrous color.

Silver fork deformity (सिल्वर फोर्क डिफोर्मिटी) कलाई तथा हाथ के कालेस फ्रैक्चर में विद्यमान एक विकृत जो काँटे की पीठ की वक्रता के समान प्रतीत होती है। A deformity in the Colles' fracture of the wrist and hand resembling the curvature of the back of a table fork.

Simian crease (साइमियन क्रीज) हथेली की कोई क्रीज या सिकुड़न। A crease on the plam of the hand.

Similimum (साइमिलीमम) रोगी के लक्षणों से समानता रखने वाली औषधि। The remedy that corresponds most nearly to the existing symptoms of the patient.

Simmond's disease (साइमण्ड्स डिजीज) ऐसा रोग जिसमें पीयूष ग्रन्थि के पूर्ण अपक्षय से थाइरॉयड ग्रन्थि एड्रीनल ग्रन्थियाँ तथा जनन ग्रन्थियाँ कार्य नहीं करती है जननांगों का अपक्षय एवं द्वितीयक लिंग विशिष्टताओं का अभाव हो जाता है, कालपूर्व वृद्धावस्था आ जाती है तथा कृशता उत्पन्न हो जाती है। The condition in which complete atrophy of the pituitary gland causes loss of function of the thyroid gland, adrenal glands and gonads covariance and testes, with atrophy of the genital organs and loss of secondary sex characteristics, premature senility and emaciation.

Simple Inflammation (सिम्पल इन्फ्लेमेशन) शोथ जिसमें पस नहीं बनता। Inflammation without formation of pus.

Simulation (साइमुलेशन) एक रोग के लक्षणों का दूसरे रोग के द्वारा अनुकरण करना। Imitation of symptoms of one disease by another.

Simulator (साइमुलेटर) एक उपकरण जो वांछित अवस्था के समान अवस्था बनाता है।
An apparatus which creates a condition, similar.

Sinciput (सिन्सीपुट) सिर का ऊपरी एवं आगे का भाग, अग्रोपरिशीर्ष। The upper and front part of the head.

Sinew (साइनीव) कण्डरा, अस्थिमांसपेशी। A tendon or ligament.

Singer's node (सिंगरस नॉड) कण्ड-पर्व, गले की गिल्टी। A small ovoid nodule on the edge of the vocal cord in singers.

Singulation (सिंगुलेशन) हिचकी लेना। Hiccupping.

Sinister (सिनिस्टर) बायाँ, बायीं ओर। Left, on the left side.

Sinistrality (सिनिस्ट्रलिटी) बायें हाथ से कार्य करने का गुण, वाहहस्तता। Left-handedness.

Sinistraural (सिनिस्ट्रॉरल) बायें कान से अच्छी तरह से सुनने वाला। Hearing better with the left ear.

Sinistrocular (सिनिस्ट्रोकुलर) बाई आँख से जिसे अच्छा दिखाई देता हो, वामनेत्री।
Seeing better with the left eye.

Sinistromanual (सिनिस्ट्रोमैनुअल) बॉयें हाथ से कार्य करने वाला। Left-handed.

Sinistrous (सिनिस्ट्रस) भद्दा, अकुशल। Awkward, unskilled.

Sinogram (साइनोग्राम) किसी विवर में एक्स-रे अभेध्य पदार्थ का इन्जैक्शन लगाकर उसकी ली गई एक्स-रे फिल्म। X-ray film of a sinus after injecting a rodiopaque substance into it.

Sinography (साइनोग्राफी) विवरों का एक्स-रे चित्रण करना। Radiography of the sinuses.

Sinuous (साइनुअस) ऐंठा हुआ, सर्पिल, पेंचदार।
Twisted.

Sinus (साइनस) किसी हड्डी में स्थित एक गुहा जैसे परानासिक विवर जो खोपड़ी की हड्डियों में स्थित वायु से युक्त गुहायें होती हैं और नासा-गुहाओं।
A cavity within a bone, e.g. paranasal sinuses which are air containing cavities in the bones of the skull continuous with the nasal cavities.

Sinus arrhythmia (साइनस अरीहदमिया) सांस लेते समय हृदय गति का बढ़ जाना तथा सांस निकालते समय घट जाना। An increase in heart rate during inspiration and decrease on expiration.

Sinus rhythm (साइनस रिह्दम) शिरा-अलिन्द पर्व से उत्पन्न होने वाला सामान्य हृदय-ताल। The normal cardiac rhythm commencing at the sinoatrial node.

Sinusitis (साइनुसाइटिस) किसी विवर विशेषकर किसी परानासिक विवर का शोथ। Inflammation of a sinus, especially a para-nasal sinus.

Sinusoid (साइनुसॉयड) शिरानालाभ। Resembling a sinus.

Siphon (साइफन) एक मुड़ी हुई नली जिसकी असमान लम्बाई की दो भुजाऐं होती हैं। जो विभिन्न ऊँचाइयों पर रखे दो पात्रों से संलग्न रहती है तथा वायुमण्डलीय दाब द्वारा ऊँचाई पर रखे पात्र से नीचे रखे पात्र में तरलों को स्थानान्तरित करने के लिए प्रयुक्त होती है।
A bent tube with two arms of unequal length, attached to two containers placed at different levels and used to transfer liquids from the container of higher level to that of lower level, by atmospheric pressure.

Sismotherapy (सिस्मोथिरैपी) कम्पनशील मालिश द्वारा रोग की चिकित्सा करना। Seismotherapy, treatment of disease by vibratory massage.

Site (साइट) स्थल, स्थान, स्थिति। Location, place, position.

Sitophobia (साइटोफोबिया) भोजन का रोगोत्पादक भय, आहारभीति। Morbid fear of food.

Sitotoxin (साइटोटॉक्सिन) भोजन में उत्पन्न कोई भी विष। Any poison developed in food.

Situs (साइटस) स्थिति अथवा स्थान। A position or site.

Sitz bath (सिट्ज बाथ) कटि-स्नान, नितम्ब-स्नान। Immersion of patient's buttocks and perineal region in hot water.

Skatole (स्केटोल) मल में पाया जाने वाला एक बदबूदार, रवेदार पदार्थ बीटामिथाइल इन्डोल जो आँत में प्रोटीन के विघटन से बनता है। A malodorous, crystalline substance betamethyl indole found in the feces, formed by protein decomposition in the intestine.

Skeletal muscle (स्केलेटल मसल) कंकाल के किसी भाग से संलग्न पेशी जो शरीर के भागों में गति उत्पन्न करती है। A muscle attached to bone and involved in body movements.

Skeletogenous (स्केलेटोजीनस) कंकाल बनाने वाला। Forming skeleton.

Skeleton (स्केलेटन) शरीर के हड्डियों का ढाँचा जिसमें 206 हड्डियाँ होती हैं, 80 धड़ की तथा 126 भुजाओं की होती है, कंकाल, अस्थिपंजर। The bony framework of the body consisting of 206 bones, 80 of the trunks and 126 of the limbs.

Skene's glands (स्कीनीज़ ग्लैण्ड्स) स्त्री में दो छोटी-छोटी ग्रन्थियाँ जिनमें से एक अपनी वाहिनी द्वारा मूत्र-मार्ग के पिछले भाग के भूतल के प्रत्येक पार्श्व में खुलती है, स्कीन ग्रन्थियाँ। Paraurethral glands, two small glands one by its duct opening on each side of the floor of posterior portion of urethra in female.

Skew (स्कीव) एक ओर को घूमा हुआ, असम रूप, बेडौल। Turned to one side, asymmetrical.

Skiascopy (स्कायास्कोपी) दृष्टिपटलदर्शन, प्रतिदीप्तिदर्शन। Retinoscopy, fluoroscopy.

Skin (स्किन) चर्म, त्वक, त्वचा, चमड़ी, खाल। External covering of the body; cutis. (*i*) **Elastic skin** (इलास्टिक स्किन) त्वचा जिसमें

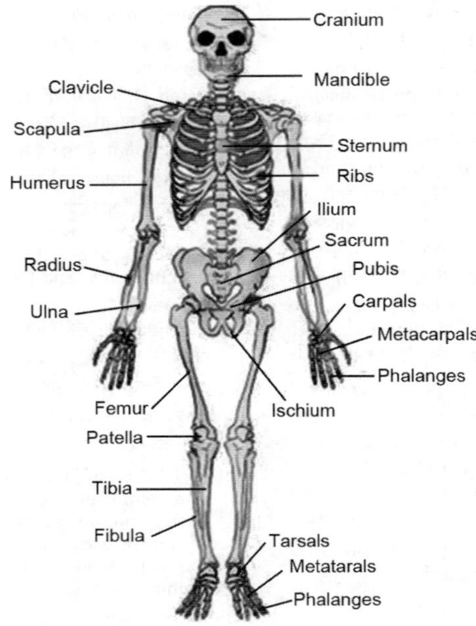

Skeleton

अत्यधिक लचीलापन होता है। Skin with the property of great elasticity.

(*ii*) **Glassy skin** (ग्लॉसी स्किन) चिकनी एवं चमकीली त्वचा। Smooth and shining skin.

(*iii*) **Parchment skin** (पार्चमैंट स्किन) त्वचा का शोष जिसके साथ वह फैल जाती है। Atrophy of the skin with stretching.

(*iv*) **Photodamaged skin** (फोटोडैमेज्ड-स्किन) जीर्ण सूर्य अनावरण के कारण क्षतिग्रस्त त्वचा। Damaged skin due to chronic sun exposure.

(*v*) **True skin** (ट्रू स्किन) अन्तस्त्वचा (यथार्थ त्वचा)

अथवा त्वचा की आन्तरिक परत, वास्तविक त्वचा। Corium (dermis) or the inner layer of the skin.

Skull (स्कल) सिर की हड्डियों का ढाँचा जो 8 कपाल की तथा 14 चेहरे की हड्डियों एवं दाँतों से मिल कर बनता है, खोपड़ी, करोटि। The bony framework of the head, composed of 8 cranial and 14 facial bones and the teeth.

Sleep (स्लीप) शरीर एवं मस्तिष्क के लिए एक विश्राम काल जिसमें शरीर के क्रियात्मक कार्य कम होते हैं तथा चेतना घट जाती है और शरीर के एच्छिक कार्य नहीं होते। सुप्ति, निद्रा, नींद। A period of rest for the body and mind in which physiological functions of the body and consciousness are diminished and voluntary body function is absent.

Sleep apnea (स्लीप एप्निया) नींद के दौरान श्वसन में नियतकालिक अवरोध होना। Periodic cessation of respiration during sleep.

Sleep disease (स्लीप डिज़ीज) निद्रारोग। Sleeping sickness.

Slide (स्लाइड) काँच अथवा अन्य किसी पारदर्शक पदार्थ की एक पतली प्लेट जिस पर सूक्ष्मदर्शी द्वारा परीक्षित होने वाले पदार्थ को रखा जाता है। A thin plate of glass or other transparent substance on which the material to be examined under the microscope is placed.

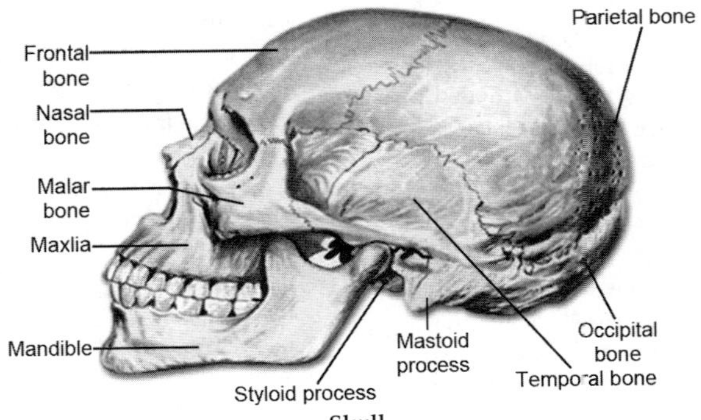

Skull

Slime (स्लाइम) चिपचिपा पदार्थ Viscous substance.

Sling (स्लिंग) गोफन, लटकन। A suspensory bandage for supporting a part of the body.

Slit (स्लिट) तंग छेद, रेखा छिद्र। A narrow opening.

Slit lamp (स्लिट लैम्प) नेत्ररोगविज्ञान में, आयताकार प्रकाश स्त्रोत के साथ संयुक्त सूक्ष्मदर्शी का बना एक यंत्र जिसमें प्रकाश को एक रेखा-छिद्र के रूप में संकीर्ण किया जा सकता है। In ophthalmology, an instrument consisting of a microscope combined with a rectangular light source that can be narrowed into a slit.

Slough (स्लफ) जीवित ऊतक अथवा किसी जख्म से अलग हुआ मृत या परिगलित ऊतक, मृत्तोतक। Dead or necrosed tissue separated from the living tissue or a wound.

Sludge (स्लज) शहर, कारखानों तथा व्यापारिक क्षेत्रों का कूड़ा-करकट अथवा कचरा, अवमल, अवर्पक। Waste material of the city, industries and commercial areas.

Sluggish (स्लगिश) मन्दगतिक, सुस्त। Slow moving, inactive.

Smallpox (स्मालपॉक्स) मसूरिका, शीतला, चेचक, बड़ी माता। A serious and highly contagious virus disease.

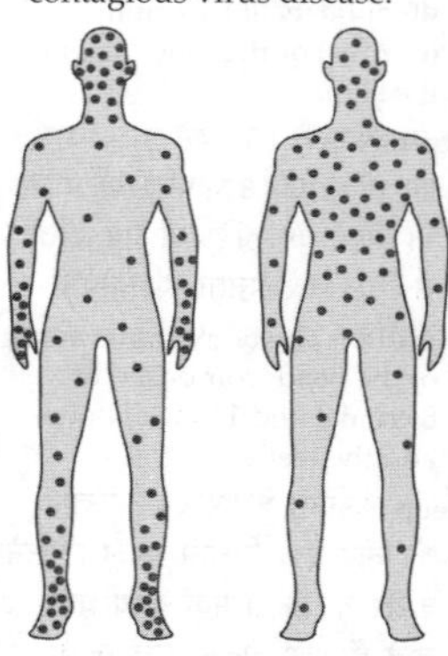

Small pox **Chicken pox**

Smear (स्मीयर) लेपन, आलेप, लेप। A film of material spread out on a glass slide for microscopic examination.

Smegma (स्मैग्मा) त्वग्वसीय ग्रन्थियों का गाढ़ा पनीर जैसा स्राव जिससे बदबू आती है और जो स्त्री में अगशिश्निका (क्लाइटोरिस) के आस–पास लघु भगोष्ठों के नीचे तथा पुरूष में शिश्न के शिश्नमुण्डच्छद के नीचे पाया जाता है, शिश्नमल, भगोष्ठमल। Thick cheesy secretion of the sebaceous glands emitting foul smell, found under labia minora about the clitoris in female and under the prepuce of penis in male.

Smegmalith (स्मैग्मालिथ) शिश्नमल या भगोष्ठमल में स्थित पथरी। A calcareous concretion in the smegma.

Smelling salt (स्मैलिंग साल्ट) अमोनियम कार्बोनेट। Ammonium carbonate.

Smith-Petersen nail (स्मिथ-पीटरसन नेल) फीमर हड्डी की गर्दन के अस्थिभंग में दृढता प्रदान करने के लिए प्रयोग में लाई जाने वाली तीन उठे हुए किनारों वाली एक विशिष्ट कील। A special nail possessing 3 flanges, for stabilizing fractures of the neck of femur bone.

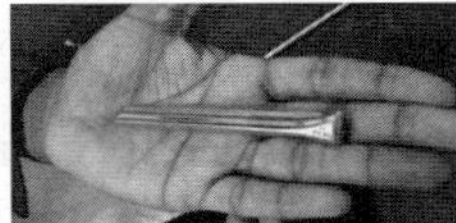

Smith-Petersen nail for trochanteric

Smog (स्मॉग) कुहरा एवं धुआँ दोनों मिले हुए। Fog and smoke combined.

Snap (स्नेप) स्फुटन A short sharp sound.

Snare (स्नेयर) पाशः नाक के पॉलिप को हटाने के लिए प्रयुक्त किया जाने वाला एक शल्य-यंत्र। A surgical instrument with a wire loop at the end, used for removal of polyp.

Sneeze (स्नीज़) नासिका की श्लेष्मिक कला के क्षोभण से निःश्वसन की पेशियों के ऐंठनयुक्त संकुचन द्वारा नाक तथा मुँह से बलपूर्वक वायु को बाहर निकालना, छींक। To expel air forcibly through the nose and mouth by spasmodic contraction of muscles of expiration due to irritation of the nasal mucous membrane.

Snellen's chart (स्नेलेन्स चार्ट) दृष्टि-तीक्ष्णता के परीक्षण के लिए पढ़ा जाने वाला चार्ट जिसमें नीचे तली पर सबसे छोटे अक्षरों से धीरे-धीरे बढ़ते परिमाण में

E	1	20/200
F P	2	20/100
T O Z	3	20/70
L P E D	4	20/50
P E C F D	5	20/40
E D F C Z P	6	20/30
F E L O P Z D	7	20/25
D E F P O T E C	8	20/20
L E F O D P C T	9	
F D P L T C E O	10	
P E Z O L C F T D	11	

शिखर पर सबसे बड़े काले अक्षर छपे होते है। Reading chart for testing visual acuity, on which block letters gradually increasing in size from smallest on the bottom to largest on the top are printed.

Snore (स्नोर) निद्राघूर्णन, खर्राटे लेना। To produce such sounds during sleep.

Snuff (स्नफ) नाक से साँस के साथ अन्दर खींचा जाने वाला औषधीय पाऊडर, नस्य, सुंघनी। A medicinal powder inhaled through the nose.

Soap (सोप) एक सफाई करने वाला रासायनिक यौगिक जो वसीय अम्ल जैसे सोडियम स्टिएरेट पर किसी क्षार की क्रिया से बनता है, साबुन। A cleaning chemical compound formed by an alkali acting on fatty acid, such as sodium stearate.

Social phobia (सोशल फोबिया) सामाजिक होने का विकृत भय। Fear of being social.

Sociology (सोशियोलॉजी) मनुष्य के सामाजिक व्यवहार समाज के नियम तथा रीतिरिवाजों एवं समाज के कार्यों का। The study of human social behavior, laws and customs and functions of the society.

Sociomedical (सोशियोमेडिकल) समाजशास्त्र एवं चिकित्साशास्त्र से सम्बन्धित। Pertaining to sociology and medicine.

Sociopathy (सोशियोपैथी) समाज विरोधी होना। The condition of being antisocial.

Socket (सॉकेट) शरीर में स्थित एक गड्ढा जिसमें कोई तुल्य अंग फिट होता है। A hollow in the body into which a corresponding organ is fitted.

Soda (सोडा) साधारण सोडा, सामान्य सोडियम बाइकार्बोनेट या खाने का सोडा। The common sodium bicarbonate; soda-ash.

Sodium (सोडियम) यह एक कोमल धात्विक तत्व है यह शीघ्र ही वायु अथवा जल में ऑक्सीकृत हो जाता है। इसके लवण शरीर में पाये जाते है और उनका चिकित्सा में व्यापक रूप से प्रयोग किया जाता है। सोडियम आयन शरीर में बहिर्कोशिकीय तरलों का मुख्य घटक होता है। It is a soft metalic element. It is readily oxidized in the air or water, its salts are found in the body and are extensively used in medicine, sodium ions is the chief constituent of extracellular fluids in the body.

Sodomy (सोडोमी) गुदामैथुन जो अधिकतर पुरूषों के बीच होता है। Anal intercourse, usually between males.

Soft palate (सॉफ्ट पैलेट) मृदु तालु, कोमल तालु। The rear portion of the roof of the mouth.

Soft sore (सॉफ्ट सोर) मृदुव्रव, मृदुक्षत, कोमल घाव। The primary ulcer of genitalia, occurring in the venereal disease, chancroid.

Solac (सोलेक) कोई वस्तु अथवा व्यक्ति जो दर्द अथवा मानसिक परेशानियों में आराम पहुँचाता है। An object or a person that gives relief in pain or mental disturbance.

Solar (सौलर) सौर, सूर्य अथवा धूप या सूर्य की रोशनी सम्बन्धी। Relating to the sun or sunlight.

Soleus (सोलियस) पैर की पिण्डली की एक चपटी, चौड़ी पेशी, पिण्डिका। A flat, broad muscle of the calf of the leg.

Solidify (सॉलिडिफाइ) ठोस बनाना या होना। To make or become solid.

Solitary (सॉलिटरी) अकेला अथवा अलग-अलग स्थित रहने वाला, एकाकी। Single or existing separately.

Solubility (सॉल्युबिलिटी) विलेयता, घुलन-शीलता। The quality of being dissolved.

Solum (सोलम) तली (पेंदी) अथवा सबसे निचला भाग। Bottom or the lowest part.

Solute (सॉल्यूट) विलयन बनाने के लिए किसी विलायक में घुला हुआ पदार्थ, विलेय। The substance dissolved in a solvent to form a solution.

Solution (सॉल्यूशन) अपने अन्दर घुले हुए पदार्थो से युक्त द्रव, विलयन, घोल। Liquid containing dissolved substances.

(*i*) **Aqueous solution** (एक्विस सॉल्यूशन) ऐसा घोल जिसमें जल विलायक या घोलक के रूप में होता है। A solution containing water as the solvent.

(*ii*) **Isotonic solution** (आइसोटॉनिक सॉल्यूशन) वह विलयन जिसका परासरणी दाब कोशिकाओं अथवा शरीर के तरलों के परासरणी दाब के समान होता है। A solution that has same osmotic pressure as that of the cells or body fluids.

Solvent (सॉल्वेन्ट) विलायक, घोलक अथवा घोल बनाने वाला। Dissolving or forming a solution.

Soma (सोमा) मस्तिष्क से पृथक शरीर, देह। The body as distinguished from the mind.

Somatalgia (सोमेटैल्जिया) शारीरिक वेदना। Bodily pain.

Somatesthesia (सोमेटोस्थीसिया) शरीर की चेतना अथवा उसका बोध होना, कायिक अभिज्ञा। Consciousness or awareness of the body.

Somatic (सोमेटिक) शरीर सम्बन्धी, दैहिक, कायिक। Pertaining to the body.

Somatization (सोमेटाइज़ेशन) मानसिक विकारों का शारीरिक लक्षणों में परिवर्तित होना। The conversion of mental disorders into bodily symptoms.

Somatopagus (सोमेटोपेगस) दो भ्रूण जो धड़ पर आपस में जुड़े होते है। Two fetuses fused together at the trunk.

Somatopathy (सोमेटोपैथी) शारीरिक रोग। Disease of the body.

Somatopsychosis (सोमेटोसाइकोसिस) कोई भी मानसिक रोग जो किसी शारीरिक रोग के लक्षण के रूप में होता है। Any mental disease that is a symptom of a bodily disease.

Somatostatin (सोमेटोस्टेटिन) हाइपोथैलेमस का एक हार्मोन जो सोमेटोट्रॉपिन हार्मोन के मुक्त होने तथा इन्सुलिन एवं गैस्ट्रिन के स्राव को रोकता है। A hormone of hypothalamus that inhibits the release of somatotropin hormone and the secretion of insulin and gastrin.

Somatotomy (सोमेटोटॉमी) मानवशरीर-रचना। The anatomy of the human body.

Somatotropin (सोमेटोट्रॉपिन) वृद्धि-उद्दीपक हार्मोन। Growth-stimulating hormone.

Somite (सोमाइट) भ्रूणकायखण्ड, भ्रूणकाय, भ्रूणदेह। A mesoblastic segment.

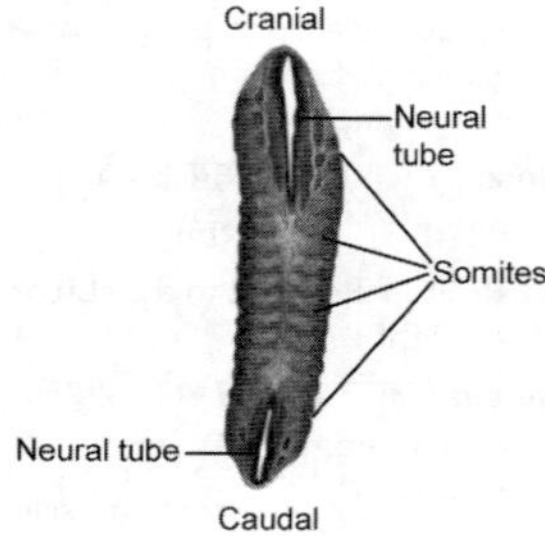

Somnambulism (सोमनेम्बुलिज्म) नींद में चलना, निन्द्राचलन, निद्राभ्रमण। Sleep walking.

Somniferous (सोमनीफेरस) नींद लाने वाला। Producing sleep.

Somniloquism (सोमनीलोक्विज्म) किसी का सोते समय बात करना। Talking in one's sleep.

Somnolence (सोमनोलैन्स) निद्रा लेने की इच्छा। Sleepiness.

Somnolism (सोमेनोलिज्म) कृत्रिम निद्रा में होने की अवस्था। Condition of being in hypnotic state.

Sonification (सोनीफिकेशन) ध्वनि अथवा ध्वनि तरंगों का उत्पन्न होना। The production of sound, or of sound waves.

Sonogram (सोनोग्राम) पराश्रव्यचित्रण में, अल्ट्रासाउण्ड तंरगों को पीछे अपने स्त्रोत को परिवर्तित न करने अर्थात् प्रतिध्वनियाँ न उत्पन्न करने वाला। In ultrasonography, not reflecting the ultrasound waves back to their source, e.g. not producing the echoes.

Sonorous (सोनोरस) अनुनादी, शोर करने वाला, ध्वनिक। Resonant, making noise.

Soporific (सोपोरीफिक) गहरी नींद लाने वाला अथवा स्वापक या मादक, निद्रापक। Producing deep sleep, or narcotic.

Sorbitol (सोर्बिटॉल) मधसार, सुरासार। A crystalline alcohol used as sweetening agent.

Sordes (सोर्ड्स) साधारणतया हल्के बुखार में दाँतों पर तथा होठों के आस-पास पाई जाने वाली कत्थइरंग की बदबूदार पपड़ियाँ, दन्तमल, मुखमल। Foul brown crusts on the teeth and about the lips, usually found in low grade pyrexia.

Sore (सोर) स्पर्शसह्य या दाबवेदनायुक्त अथवा वेदनायुक्त। Tender or painful.

Sorption (जार्प्शन) अवशोषित होना। The condition of being absorbed.

Souffle (सूफिल) परिश्रवण में सुनाई देने वाली कोमल सीटी जैसी ध्वनि अथवा परिश्रवणीय मर्मर, ब्रुईत या विरूत। A soft blowing sound heard on auscultation, or auscultatory murmur, a bruit.

Sound (साउण्ड) वायु अथवा अन्य माध्यम के कम्पनों के द्वारा कान में उत्पन्न संवेदना अथवा अनुभूति, शोर। Sensation produced in the ear by vibrations of the air or other medium, a noise.

(*i*) **Breath sounds** (ब्रेद साउण्ड्स) परिश्रवण करने पर सुनाई देने वाली श्वसन-ध्वनियाँ। Respiratory sounds heard on auscultation.

(*ii*) **Fetal heart sound** (फीटल हर्ट साउण्ड्स) भ्रूण के हृदय द्वारा उत्पन्न ध्वनि। Sound produced by the heart of the fetus. (*iii*) **Percussion sound** (पर्कसन साउण्ड्स) परिताड़न करने से उत्पन्न कोई भी

ध्वनि। A sound made by percussion.

Soup (सूप) सूप अथवा शोरबा। A liquid food prepared from vegetables or meat.

Space medicine (स्पेस मेडीसिन) हवाई यात्रा करने वाले व्यक्तियों की स्वास्थ्य समस्याओं से सम्बन्धित चिकित्सा-शास्त्र की शाखा। The branch of medical science concerned with the health problems of the person travelling in air.

Span (स्पान) विस्तार अथवा अवधि जैसे जीवन की अवधि। Full extent as the full extent of life.

Spargosis (स्पार्गोसिस) दूध से स्त्री स्तनों का फूल जाना, त्वचा का मोटा हो जाना। Distention of the female breasts with milk, elephantiasis thickening of the skin.

Spasm (स्पाज्म) पेशियों में अचानक होने वाला अनियंत्रित, ऐंठन, आकश्मिक। A sudden involuntary contraction of the muscles. (*i*) **Clonic Spasm** (क्लोनिक स्पाज्म) पेशियों का बारी-बारी से संकुचित एवं शिथिलन होना। Alternate contraction and relaxation of the muscles. (*ii*) **Tonic spasm** (टॉनिक स्पाज्म) अधिक समय तक रहने वाले अनियंत्रित पेशिय संकुचन। Involuntary muscular contraction continued for a long time.

Spasmogenic (स्पाज्मोज़ेनिक) ऐंठन उत्पन्न करने वाला, आकर्षजन। Causing spasms.

Spasmophila (स्पाज्मोफीलिया) ऐंठन अथवा आपेक्ष की असामान्य प्रवृत्ति। Abnormal tendency to spasm or convulsion.

Spasticity (स्पास्टीसिटी) पेशियों की तान अथवा उनके संकुचनों का बढ़ जाना जिससे कठोरता उत्पन्न हो जाती है एवं मद्दी गतिया होती है, संस्तम्भता। A condition of increased tone or contractions of muscles causing stiffness and awkward movements.

Spatial (स्पेसियल) स्थान या अवकाश सम्बन्धी, अवकाशीय। Pertaining to space.

Spatula (स्पैचुला) एक चपटा, पतला कुछ लचीला चाकू के आकार का यंत्र, चमस, लेपनी। A flat, thin, somewhat flexible knife-shaped instrument.

Species (स्पेसीजी) जाति, वर्ण, नस्ल। A subdivision of a genus.

Specific gravity (स्पेसीफिक ग्रेविटी) विशिष्ट गुरूत्व। The weight of a substance compared with that of water of equal volume.

Spectral (स्पैक्ट्रल) दृश्यभासी, प्रतिबिम्ब सम्बन्धी, चमक रेखा सम्बन्धी। Pertaining to the spectrum.

Spectrometer (स्पैक्ट्रोमीटर) किसी स्पैक्ट्रोस्कोप या स्पैक्ट्रमदर्शी द्वारा उत्पन्न प्रकाश की तरंगदैर्ध्य का पता लगाने वाला एक यंत्र। An instrument used for determining the wavelength of light produced by a spectroscope.

Spectrophotometry (स्पैक्ट्रोफोटोमीट्री) स्पैक्ट्रोफोटोमीटर या स्पैक्ट्रम प्रकाशमापी द्वारा किसी विलयन में रंग की मात्रा का पता लगाना। Determination of the quantity of color in a solution by the use of a spectrophotometer.

Spectroscope (स्पैक्ट्रोस्कोप) प्रतिबिम्बदर्शी, स्पैक्ट्रमदर्शी। An instrument for observing spectra of light.

Spectrum (स्पैक्ट्रम) श्वेत प्रकाश के काँच की त्रिभुजाकृति (प्रिज्म) से होकर गुजरने से बनी सात रंगों की एक पट्टी। प्रतिबिम्ब, चमकरेखा, दृश्याभास। A bond of seven colors formed by passage of the white light through a glass prism.

Speculum (स्पैकुलम) दृष्टि-परीक्षण के लिए शरीर के किसी छिद्र, नलिका अथवा गुहा को खोलने या फैलाने के लिए एक यंत्र, वीक्षक। An instrument for opening or distending an orifice, canal or cavity of the body for visual examination.

Speech (स्पीच) बोले गये शब्दों द्वारा विचारों की अभिव्यक्ति। Expression of thoughts by spoken words.

Sperm (स्पर्म) शुक्राणु। Semen containing protozoa, spermatozoon.

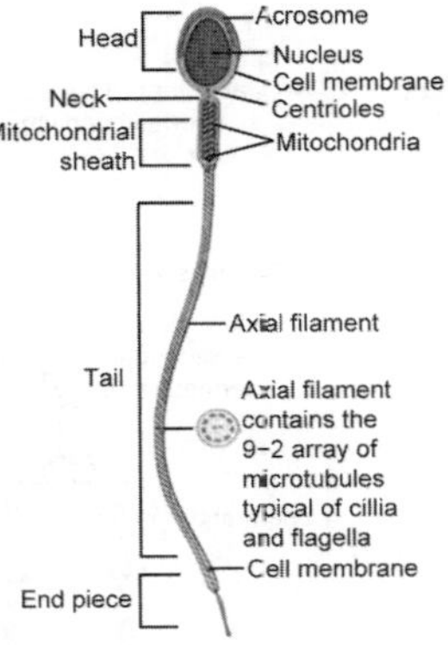

Spermatemphraxis (स्पर्मेटेमफ्रेक्सिस) वीर्य के निकलने में अवरोध उत्पन्न हो जाना। Obstruction in the ejection of semen.

Spermatic cord (स्पर्मेटिक कॉर्ड) वृषण-रज्जु। The suspensory cord of the testes.

Spermaticidal (स्पर्मेटीसाइडल) शुक्राणुओं के लिए विनाशकारी अथवा उन्हें मारने वाला, शुक्राणुनाशक। Destructive to killing spermatozoa.

Spermatid (स्पर्मेटिड) प्राक्शुक्राणु, शुक्राणुप्रसू। A cell produced by fission of a secondary spermatocyte.

Spermatin (स्पर्मेटिन) वीर्य में स्थित एक लेसदार पदार्थ। A mucilaginous substance in the semen.

Spermatitis (स्पर्मेटाइटिस) वृषण-रज्जु अथवा शुक्र वाहिनी का शोथ। Inflammation of the spermatic cord or of the ductus deferens.

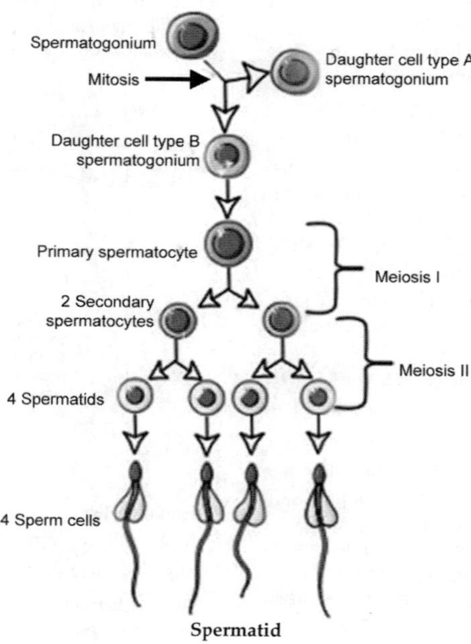

Spermatid

Spermatocele (स्पर्मेटोसील) अधिवृषण या एपिडिडीमिस का पुटीय अबुर्द जिसमें शुक्राणु होते हैं। A cystic tumor of the epididymis containing spermatozoa.

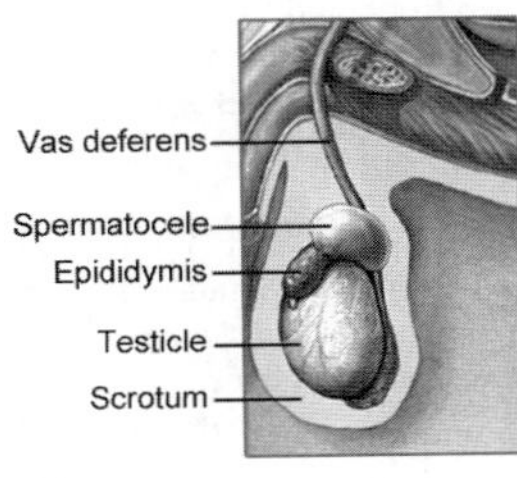

Spermatocyst (स्पर्मेटोसिस्ट) शुक्राशय, शुक्रपुटी। A seminal vesicle, spermatocele.

Spermatocystitis (स्पर्मेटोसिस्टाइटिस) किसी शुक्राशय का शोथ। Inflammation of a seminal vesicle.

Spermatocyte (स्पर्मेटोसाइट) शुक्राणुकोशिका। Germinal cell of a spermatozoon.

Spermatogenesis (स्पर्मेटोजेनेसिस) शुक्राणुओं के बनने की क्रिया, शुक्राणुजनन। The process of formation of spermatozoa.

Spermatolysin (स्पर्मेटोलाइसिन) शुक्राणुओं को नष्ट करने वाला लाइसिन। A lysin destroying spermatozoa.

Spermatopathia (स्पर्मेटोपैथिया) वीर्य का कोई भी रोग। Any disease of the semen.

Spermatorrhea (स्पर्मेटोरिह्या) लैंगिक उत्तेजना के बिना बार-बार वीर्य की अनियन्त्रित निकासी होना, शुक्रमेह, वीर्य-स्खलन। Frequent involuntary escape of the semen without sexual excitement.

Spermatozoon (स्पर्मेटोजून) शुक्राणु, पुरूषों में एक परिपक्व प्रजनन-कोशिका। A mature, male reproductive cell; sperm.

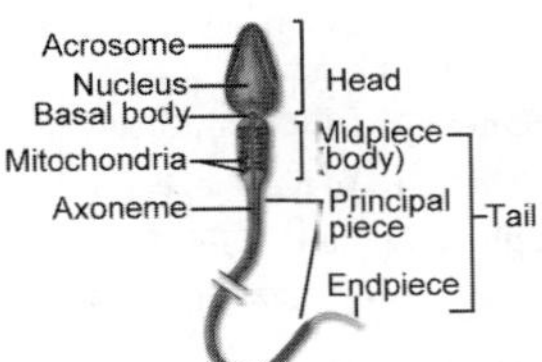

Spermaturia (स्पर्मेचूरिया) मूत्र में वीर्य का पाया जाना, शुक्रमेह। Presence of semen in the urine, seminuria.

Spermicide (स्पर्मीसाइड) शुक्राणुओं को मारने वाला, शुक्राणुनाशक। Killing spermatozoa.

Spermolith (स्पर्मोलिथ) शुक्रनली की पथरी, शुक्रवाहिकाश्मरी।

A stone in the spermatic duct. (*i*) **Aphonic speech** (एफोनिक स्पीच) कानाफूसी करना। Whispering. (*ii*) **Slurring speech** (स्लरिंग स्पीच) अस्पष्ट उच्चारण, सरवलिय उच्चारण। Indistinct pronunciation

Spermoplasm (स्पर्मोप्लाज्म) शुक्रनली का जीवद्रव्य। The protoplasm of the spermatozoon.

Sphacelate (स्फेसीलेट) कोथयुक्त अथवा परिगलित होना। To become gangrenous or necrotic.

Sphenocephalus (स्फैनोसिफैलस) ऐसा भ्रूण जिसका सिर कीलाकार होता है। A fetus with wedge-shaped head.

Sphenoid (स्फैनॉयड) कीलाकार, जतूक। Wedge-shaped.

Sphenoid bone (स्फैनॉयड बोन) सामने पश्चकपालीय एवं झर्झरिका अस्थियों तथा पार्श्व में पार्श्वकास्थि एवं शंखास्थि के बीच स्थित खोपड़ी के आधा की बड़ी हड्डी। The large bone at the base of the skull between the occipital and ethmoid bones in front, and the parietal and temporal bones at the side.

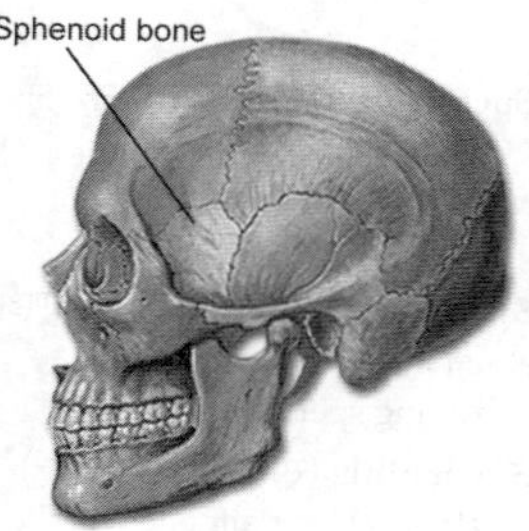

Sphenoiditis (स्फैनॉयडाइटिस) स्फैनॉयड के विवर का शोथ अथवा स्फैनॉयड हड्डी का परिगलन। Inflammation of the sphenoidal sinus or necrosis of the sphenoid bone.

Sphenoidotomy (स्फैनॉयडोटॉमी) स्फैनॉयड हड्डी में चीरा लगाना। To make an incision into the sphenoid bone.

Sphenorbital (स्फैनोर्बिटल) स्फैनॉयड हड्डी एवं नेत्र गुहाओं से सम्बन्धित। Pertaining to the sphenoid bone, and the orbits.

Sphere (स्फेरी) गोल, कोई गोलाकार पिण्ड। A ball or a globular body.

Spherocyte (स्फेरोसाइट) गोलाकार लाल रक्त कोशिका, गोलक-कोशिका। A spherical red blood cell.

Spherocytosis (स्फेरोसाइटोसिस) रक्त में गोलक-कोशिका का पाया जाना, गोलक-कोशिकता। Presence of spherocytes in blood.

Spherodial (स्फेरॉयडल) गोले से मिलता-जुलता, गोलाभ। Resembling a sphere.

Sphincter (स्फिक्चर) किसी प्रकृति द्वार अथवा मार्ग को बन्द करने वाली एक वृत्ताकार पेशी। A circular muscle closing a natural orifice or passage.

Sphincteralgia (स्फिंक्ट्रैल्जिया) मलद्वार की पीड़ा, गुदार्ति। Pain about the anus.

Sphincterismus (स्फिंक्चरिसमस) गुदा अवरोधिनी पेशियों में ऐंठन हो जाना। Spasm of anal sphincter muscles.

Sphincterotome (स्फिंक्चिरोटोम) किसी संवरणी या अवरोधिनी को काटने वाला एक यंत्र। An instrument for cutting a sphincter.

Sphygmo (स्फाइग्मो) नाड़ी या नब्ज का संकेत देने वाला एक उपसर्ग। A prefix indicating pulse.

Sphygmograph (स्फाइग्मोग्राफ) स्पन्दनलेखी। Polygraph.

Sphygmomanometer (स्फाइग्मोमैनोमीटर) धमनीय रक्त-चाप मापने का एक यंत्र यह एनेरॉयड तथा मर्करी दो प्रकार का होता है। An instrument for measuring the arterial blood pressure. It is of two types aneroid and mercury.

Sphygmophone (स्फ इग्मोफोन) नाड़ी स्पन्द को सुनने वाला एक यंत्र। An instrument for hearing the pulse beat.

Spica (स्पाइका) अंग्रेजो के आठ के अंक के समान पट्टी घुमाव एक दूसरे को पार कर जाते है, स्वभाविक पट्टिका। A figure of 8 bandage, with turns crossing each other.

Spicule (स्पाइक्यूल) एक छोटी, तेज सुई के आकार की रचना, कंटिका। A small, sharp needle-shaped structure.

Spider nevus (स्पाइडर नीवस) त्वचा की एक वृद्धि जिसमें एक केन्द्रीय लाल बिन्दु से विस्फारित कोशिकायें फैलती है जो मकड़ी के समान प्रतीत होती है। Nevus araneus. A growth of the skin in which dilated capillaries radiate from a central red point resembling a spider.

Spill (स्पिल) अति प्रवाह, अत्यधिक बहाव। An overflow.

Spina (स्पाइना) मेरूदण्ड, रीढ़, कंटक। The spine.

Spinal anesthesia (स्पाइनल एनीस्थीज़िया) मेरू-नलिका में किसी संज्ञाहारी का इन्जैक्शन लगाने से उत्पन्न संज्ञाहरण। Necrosis. Anesthesia produced by an anesthesic injected into the spinal canal.

Spinal canal (स्पाइनल कैनाल) कशेरूका-दण्ड का नाल जिसमें सुषुम्ना स्थित रहती है। Canal of the vertebral column containing the spinal cord.

Spinal column (स्पाइनल कालम) मेरू-दण्ड, पृष्ठवंश, रीढ़ की हड्डी। The backbone.

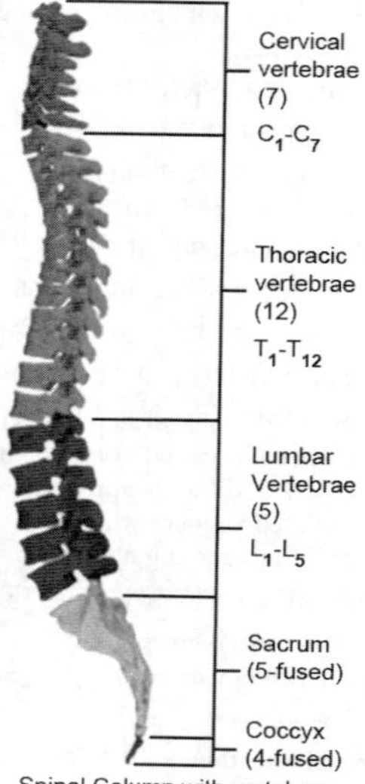

Spinal Column with vertebrae

Spinal cord (स्पाइनल कॉर्ड) सुषुम्ना, मेरू-रज्जु। The nerve structure running within the spinal cord of the spinal column.

Spinal fluid (स्पाइनल फ्लूड) मेरू-द्रव। Cerebrospinal fluid.

Spinalgia (स्पाइनैल्जिया) कषेरूका-दण्ड के क्षेत्र में दर्द होना। Pain in the region of the vertebral column.

Spinal nerves (स्पाइनल नर्वज) मेरू-रज्जु से निकलने वाली तंत्रिकाओं के 31 जोड़े जिनमें से 8 ग्रैव, 12 वक्षीय, 5 कटिपरक, 5 त्रिकास्थिज या सैक्रल तथा 1 अनुत्रकीय होता है। ये जोड़े मेरू-कषेरूकाओं के अनुरूप होते है। 31 pairs of nerves arising from the spinal cord consisting of 8 cervical, 12 thoracic, 5 lumber, 5 sacral and 1 coccygeal corresponding with the spinal vertebrae.

Spinal stenosis (स्पाइनल स्टेनोसिस) मेरू-नलिका का तंग होना। Narrowing of the spinal canal.

Spindle (स्पिन्डल) तकुवे के आकार का अथवा दोनों किनारों पर धीरे-धीरे पलता हो जाने वाला, तर्कु। A fusiform or tapering on both ends.

Spine (स्पाइन) हड्डी का काँटे के समान तेज प्रवर्ध। A sharp thorn-like processed projection of vertebrae.

Spinocerebellar (स्पाइनोसेरीबेलर) सुशुम्ना-रज्जु एवं अनुमस्तिष्क से

सम्बन्धित। Concerning spinal cord and cerebellum

Spinothalamic (स्पाइनोथैलेमिक) मेरू-रज्जु एवं चेतक सम्बन्धी। Pertaining to the spinal cord and thalamus.

Spiral (स्पाइरल) चक्करदार, ऐंठा हुआ, पेंचदार या सर्पिल। Coiled, twisted, and winding like a screw.

Spirituous (स्प्रिचुअस) एल्कोहॉल से सम्बन्धित। Pertaining to alcohol.

Spirochaeta (स्पाइरोकीटा) सर्पकीट, चक्रकीट। A bacterium having a spiral shape.

Spirochetolysis (स्पाइरोकीटोलाइसिस) अपघटन द्वारा स्पाइरोकीटों का नष्ट होना। Destruction of spirochetes by lysis.

Spirochetosis (स्पाइरोकीटोसिस) स्पाइरोकीटों का कोई भी संक्रमण। Any infection with spirochetes.

Spirogram (स्पाइरोग्राम) श्वसनलेख, श्वास लेख। The tracing made by the spirograph.

Spirograph (स्पाइरोग्राफ) श्वासलेखयंत्र। An instrument for recording respiration.

Spirometer (स्पाइरोमीटर) श्वसनमापी। An instrument for measuring respiration.

Spissated (स्पाइसेटेड) घनीभूत, सघन, गाढ़ा। Thickened, inspissated.

Spit (स्पिट) थूकना। To expectorate saliva.

Splanchnectopia (स्प्लैंक्नेक्टोपिया) एक अंतरांग अथवा अन्तरांगों का विस्थापन। Displacement of viscus or the viscera.

Splanchnic (स्प्लैंक्निक) अंतरांगों अथवा आन्तरिक अंगों से सम्बन्धित, आशयिक। Pertaining to the viscera or internal organs.

Splanchnicotomy (स्प्लैंक्नीकोटॉमी) किसी आशयिक तंत्रिका का पारपरिच्छेदन करना। Transection of a splanchnic nerve.

Splanchnodynia (स्प्लैंक्नोडाइनिया) उदरीय क्षेत्र में दर्द होना। Pain accruing in the abdominal region.

Splanchnomicria (स्प्लैंक्नोमाइक्रिया) छोटे अंतरांगों का होना। The condition of having small viscera.

Splanchnosclerosis (स्प्लैंक्नोस्क्लेरोसिस) अन्तरांगों का कठोर होना। Hardening of the viscera.

Splanchnotomy (स्प्लैंक्नोटॉमी) अंतरांगों का व्यवच्छेदन (चीर-फाड़) करना, आशय

उच्छेदन। Dissection of the viscera.

Spleen (स्प्लीन) उदर-गुहा में ऊपरी बाँये भाग में आमाशय के हृदय-अन्त के पार्श्व में स्थित एक बड़ी, गहरे लाल रंग की तथा स्पंज के समान ग्रन्थि। प्लीहा, तिल्ली। A large, dark red and spongy gland situated in the upper left part of the abdominal cavity lateral to the cardiac end of the stomach.

Splenalgia (स्प्लीनैल्जिया) प्लीहा या तिल्ली में दर्द होना। Splenodynia pain in the spleen.

Splenectomy (स्प्लीनेक्टॉमी) शल्यक्रिया द्वारा प्लीहा को काट कर निकाल देना, प्लीहाच्छेदन। Excision of spleen.

Splenemia (स्प्लीनीमिया) प्लीहा का रक्ताधिक्य हो जाना। Congestion of spleen with blood.

Splenitis (स्प्लीनाइटिस) प्लीहाशोथ। Inflammation of the spleen

Splenocolic (स्प्लीनोकोलिक) प्लीहा एवं कोलन से सम्बन्धित। Pertaining to the spleen and colon.

Splenoid (स्प्लीनॉयड) प्लीहा के समान, प्लीहाभ। Like spleen.

Splenolysin (स्प्लीनोलाइसिन) प्लीहा-ऊतक को नष्ट करने वाला लाइसिन। A lysin which destroys the splenic tissue.

Splenomalacia (स्प्लीनोमैलेशिया) प्लीहा का कोमल हो जाना, प्लीहामृदुता। Softening of the spleen.

Splenomegaly (स्प्लेनोमेगाली) प्लीहा का बढ़ जाना। Enlargement of the spleen.

Splenonephroptosis (स्प्लीनोनेफ्रोप्टोसिस) प्लीहा एवं वृक्क का नीचे की ओर विस्थापन। Downward placement of the spleen and kidney.

Splenopathy (स्प्लीनोपैथी) प्लीहा का कोई भी रोग, प्लीहाविकृति। Any disease of spleen.

Splenoportogram (स्प्लीनोपोर्टोग्राम) प्लीहाप्रति-हारचित्र। Radiographic picture of the spleen and portal vein after injection of radio-opaque medium.

Splenoptosis (स्प्लीनोप्टोसिस) प्लीहा का नीचे की ओर विस्थापन। Downward displacement of spleen.

Splenorrhagia (स्प्लीनोरैह्जिया) प्लीहा से रक्तस्राव होना। Hemorrhage from the spleen

Splenorrhaphy (स्प्लीनोरैह्फी) प्लीहा के जख्म की सिलाई करना। Suture of wound of the spleen.

Splint (स्प्लिन्ट) शरीर के विस्थापित गतिशील अथवा क्षतिग्रस्त अंगों के स्थिरीकरण अथवा उनकी रक्षा हेतु प्रयोग में लाया जाने वाला लकड़ी या धातु का बना एक उपकरण। An appliance made of wood or metal used for the fixation or protection of displaced, movable or injured parts of the body.

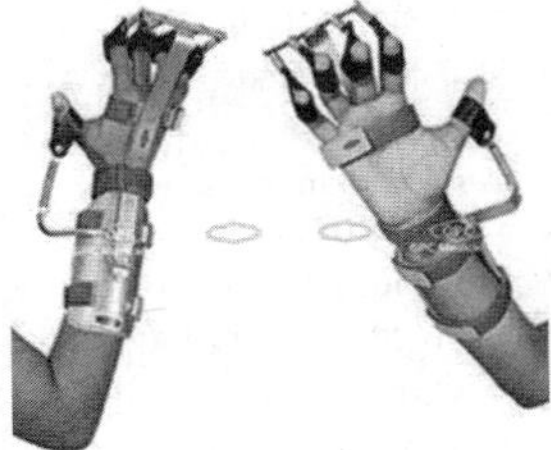

Splinting (स्प्लिन्टिंग) स्प्लिन्ट से किसी सन्धिच्युति अथवा अस्थिभंग को स्थिर करना, स्थिरीकरण, कुषानुप्रयोग। Fixation of dislocation or fracture with a splint.

Split (स्प्लिट) एक लम्बी फटन। A longitudinal fissure.

Split tongue (स्प्लिट टंग) विदीर्ण अथवा द्विषाखित जिह्वा। Cleft or bifid tongue.

Spondylalgia (स्पॉण्डीलैल्जिया) कषेरूकाओं में दर्द होना। Pain occurring in the spine or vertebrae.

Spondylexarthrosis (स्पॉण्डीलेक्सारथ्रोसिस) किसी कषेरूका का विस्थापन। Dislocation of the vertebra.

Spondylitis (स्पॉण्डीलाइटिस) एक या अधिक कषेरूकाओं का शोथ। Inflammation of cne or more vertebrae.

Spondylolisthesis (स्पॉण्डीलोलिस्थेसिस) किसी निचली कटि-कषेरूका का आगे का सैक्रम के ऊपर विस्थापित हो जाना, कषेरूकाग्रसर्पण। Forward displacement of a lower lumbar vertebra over the sacrum.

Spondylolysis (स्पॉण्डीलोलाइसिस) किसी कषेरूका का टूटना। The breaking down of vertebrae.

Spondylomalacia (स्पॉण्डीलोमैलेशिया) कषेरूकाओं का कोमल हो जाना। Softening of the vertebrae.

Spondylosis (स्पॉण्डीलोसिस) कषेरूका सन्धिग्रह। Vertebral ankylosis.

Spondylotherapy (स्पॉण्डीलोथिरैपी) रोगी की चिकित्सा में मेरूदण्ड को हाथ से घुमाना-फिराना। Manipulation of the spinal column in the treatment of disease.

Spondylotomy (स्पॉण्डीलोटॉमी) कषेरूकासंधि-उच्छेदन। Section of a vertebra.

Sponge (स्पन्ज) एक छिद्रिल, अवशोषक पिण्ड जैसे गॉज की गद्दी या गॉज से चारों ओर से लिपटी हुई रूई अथवा कुछ समुद्री जानवरों का इलास्टिक तन्तुमय कंकाल। A porous, absorbent mass as a pad of gauze or cotton surrounded by gauze, or the elastic fibrous skeleton of certain marine animals.

Spongiform (स्पन्जीफॉर्म) स्पन्ज के समान। Like sponge.

Spongiocyte (स्पॉन्जियोसाइट) तंत्रिकाबन्ध-कोशिका। A neuroglial cell.

Spontaneous-fracture (स्पान्टेनियस फ्रैक्चर) विखनिजीकृत अस्थि में जैसे अस्थि सुशिरता में स्वतः अस्थि भंग हो जाना जिसमें दर्द नहीं होता। Fracture of a demineralized bone as in osteoporosis, which is painless.

Spoon-nail (स्पून-नैल) चमसनख, चम्मच जैसा गड्ढेदार नाखुन। A nail with a concave outer surface.

Sporadic (स्पोरेडिक) कभी-कभी उत्पन्न होने वाला। Occurring occasionally.

Spore (स्पोर) छोटे-छोटे जीवधारियों जैसे एककोशिकीय जन्तु, कवक तथा शैल या काई आदि की एक लैंगिक अथवा अलैंगिक जनन कोशिका बीजाणु। Sexual or asexual reproductive cell of the lower animals, such as protozoa fungi and algae, etc.

Sporocyst (स्पोरोसिस्ट) बीजाणु पुटी, बीज पुटी। एक कोश या थैली जिसमें बीजाणु अथवा जनन कोशिकाऐं होती है। A sac containing spores or reproductive cells.

Sporogenous (स्पोरोजींनस) बीजाणुओं के उत्पादन से सम्बन्धित। Concerning sporogenesis.

Sporogony (स्पोरोगोनी) स्पोरोजुआ, विशेषकर मच्छर में मलेरिया-परजीवी के स्पोरोजुआ का लैंगिक जीवन-चक्र। The sexual life-cycle of sporozoa, especially that of the malarial parasite in the mosquito.

Sporotrichosis (स्पोरोट्राइकोसिस) स्पोरोट्राइकम कवक द्वारा उत्पन्न त्वचा एवं उपस्थित लसीका ग्रन्थियों का जीर्ण कवक रोग जिसमें फोड़े, गाँठें तथा जख्म बन जाते है। Chronic fungal disease of the skin and superficial lymph nodes, caused by the fungus sporotrichum, characterized by the formation of abscesses, nodes and ulcers.

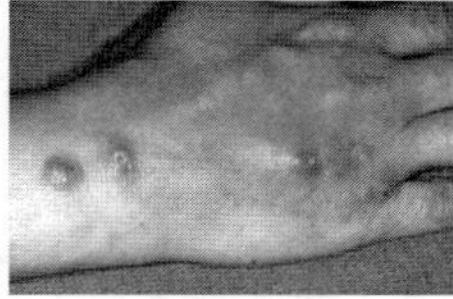

Sporozoite (स्पोरोज्वाइट) मलेरिया-परजीवी के जीवनचक्र में युग्मकपुटी के भीतर स्पोरोब्लास्ट से उत्पन्न होने वाली एक लम्बी हंसिऐं के आकार की कोशिका। An elongated sickle-shaped cell developing from the sporoblast within the oocyst in the life cycle of malarial parasite.

Sporulation (स्पोरूलेशन) बीजाणुओं का उत्पन्न होना, बीजाणुजनन। Production of spores.

Spot (स्पॉट) बिन्दु, चित्ती, धब्बा। A macule; macula.

Spotted fever (स्पॉटेड फीवर) कुर्बर ज्वर, मस्तिष्क मेरू-ज्वर, चित्तीदार बुखार। Cerebrospinal fever.

Spotting (स्पॉटिंग) साधारणतया मासिक धर्मों के बीच अथवा प्रसव के प्रारम्भ में योनि से प्रकट होने वाला हल्के से रक्त के साथ मिश्रित स्राव। Appearance of bloodtinged discharge from the vagina, usually between menstrual periods or at the onset of labor.

Sprain (स्प्रेन) मोच जो अधिकतर पाँव अथवा टखने के जोड़े में होती है। Wrenching of a joint with partial rupture of its ligaments, which generally occurs in foot or ankle joint.

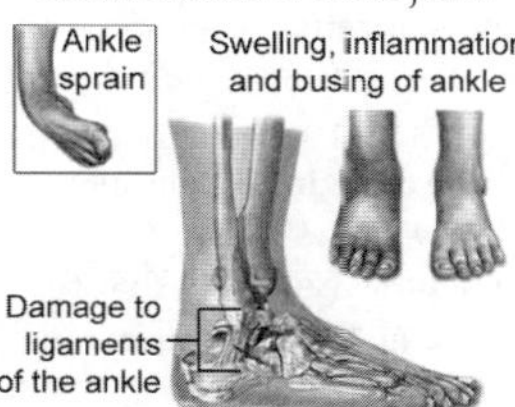

Spray (स्प्रे) सूक्ष्म उड़नशील कणों में परिवर्तित कोई औषधियुक्त द्रव, फुहार, बौछार। A medicated liquid converted into minute flying particles.

Sprue (स्प्रू) प्रसर, नख, लांगूलिका, उपांगुष्ठ। A projecting portion.

Spud (स्पड) किसी बाह्य पदार्थ को हटाने के लिए एक छोटा फावड़े के समान ब्लेड। A small spadelike blade to dislodge a foreign substance.

Spur (स्पर) एक तेज, नुकीली, बाह्यवृद्धि। A sharp, pointed bony outgrowth.

Spurious (स्युरियस) मिथ्या, जो वास्तविक न हो, मिलावट से अशुद्ध किया हुआ। False; not genuine; adulterated.

Sputum (स्प्यूटम) खाँस कर मुख से निकाला गया पदार्थ जो फेंफडों से आता है। बलगम, कफ। Matter expelled from the mouth by coughing which comes from the lungs.

Squamatization (स्क्वेमेटाइजेशन) कोशिकाओं का पट्टकी कोशिकाओं में परिवर्तित होना। The changing of cells into squamous cells.

Squamosa (स्क्वेमोसा) शंखास्थि की पट्टकी भाग। The squamous part of temporal bone.

Squamous (स्क्वेमस) पपड़ी अथवा पतली प्लेट के समान रचना, पट्टकी, शल्कीय। Scale like on thin plate like structure.

Squamous bone (स्क्वेमस बोन) शंखास्थि का ऊपरी अगला भाग। Upper anterior portion of temporal bone.

Squamous cells (स्क्वेमस सैल्स) उपकला की चपटी, पपड़ीदार कोशिकाएँ। Flat, scaly cells of the epithelium.

Squamous-occipital (स्क्वेमस-ऑक्सीपिटल) पश्चकपालीय हड्डी के पट्टिका भाग से सम्बन्धित। Pertaining to the squamous portion of the occipital bone.

Squint (स्क्विट) तिर्यकदृष्टि, तिरछी नजर, बहंगापन। Strabismus.

Stab (स्टेब) छुरा भोंकना, वेधना। To pierce with a knife.

Stagnant (स्टेग्नैन्ट) प्रवाहहीन, निश्चल। Not flowing

Stain (स्टेन) अभिरंजक, दाग, धब्बा। A dye, a discoloration

Stalagmometer (स्टेलेग्मोमीटर) किसी तरल की दी इुई मात्रा में बूंदों की संख्या का पता लगाने वाला एक यंत्र। An instrument for determining the number of drops in a given amount of fluid.

Stamina (स्टेमिना) शक्ति, सहनशीलता, ओजस्विता, दम। Strength, patience.

Stammering (स्टेमरिंग) एक वाणी दोष जिसमें कोई व्यक्ति हकलाते हुए बोलता है, हकलाना। A speech defect in which one speaks with hesitation and repetition.

Stand-still (स्टेण्ड-स्टील) विराम, अपरिवर्तित। Arrest, cessation of activity, unchanged.

Stapedectomy (स्टेपीडेक्टॉमी) श्रवण में सुधार करने हेतु कान की स्टेपीस हड्डी को शल्यक्रिया द्वारा काट कर निकाल देना, रकाब-उच्छेदन। Excision of the stapes bone in the ear in order to improving hearing.

Stapes (स्टेपीस) मध्य कर्ण में स्थित एक अस्थिका जो इन्कस से जुड़कर जोड़ बनाती है, रकाब। An ossicle in the middle ear that articulates with the incus.

Staphyle (स्टेफाइल) काकलन। Uvula.

Staphylitis (स्टेफाइलाइटिस) काकलकशोथ। Inflammation of the uvula.

Staphylococcus (स्टैफिलोकॉकस) स्टैफिलोकॉकस वंश का एक ग्राम धनात्मक जीवाणु जो त्वचा पर तथा ऊर्ध्व श्वसन पथ में रहता है जिससे फोड़ा बनता है तथा ऊर्ध्व श्वसन-पथ का संक्रमण उत्पन्न होता है, स्तवकगोलाणु। A Gram-positive bacteria of the genus staphylococcus present on the skin and in the upper respiratory tract, which causes abscess formation and upper respiratory infection.

Staphyloma (स्टेफिलोमा) आँख के कॉर्निया या स्क्लेरा का बाहर को निकल आना, अजका। Protrusion of the cornea or sclera of the eye.

Staphyloplasty (स्टेफाइलोप्लास्टी) कॉकलक अथवा कोमल तालु की प्लास्टिक सर्जरी करना। Plastic surgery of the uvula of soft plate.

Staphyloschisis (स्टेफाइलोस्चाइसिस) कॉकलक एवं कोमल तालु की फटन होना। Fissure of the uvula and soft palate.

Stapling (स्टेपलिंग) शल्यचिकित्सा में ऊतकों के अनुकूल विशेष स्टेपलों का प्रयोग करके दो ऊतकों को जैसे आँत के दो किनारों को आपस में जोड़ने की प्रक्रिया। In surgery, the process of uniting two tissues together, such as the two ends of the intestine, by using special staples compatible with the tissue.

Starch (स्टार्च) पौधों में कार्बोहाइड्रेटों का मुख्य भण्डार। The chief storage of carbohydrates in plant.

Starvation (स्टावेशन) आहारहीनता, भुखमरी। Long continued deprival of food; death from hunger.

Stasis (स्टेसिस) तरलों के जैसे रक्त तथा मूत्र आदि के बहाव में रूकावट पैदा हो जाना, स्थैतिकता। Stoppage of flow of fluids as of the blood and urine, etc.

State (स्टेट) अवस्था, दशा अथवा स्थिति। Condition or situation.

Static (स्टेटिक) विश्राम अवस्था में, जो गतिशील न हो, साम्यावस्था

में अथवा सन्तुलित, स्थैतिक। At rest, not in motion; in equilibrium.

Statistics (स्टेटिस्टिक्स) सांख्यिकी। A numeric collection of facts.

Statoconia (स्टेटोकोनिया) कर्णाष्मरियाँ। Otoliths.

Statokinetic (स्टेटोकाइनेटिक) गति होने से उत्पन्न शरीर की प्रतिक्रिया से सम्बन्धित। Pertaining to reactions of the body caused by movement.

Status (स्टेटस) दशा या अवस्था, सतत अवस्था। Condition or state.

Staunch (स्टॉन्च) किसी जख्म से खून के बहाव को रोकना। To stop the flow of blood from a wound.

Steal (स्टील) रक्त प्रवाह का अपने सामान्य मार्ग से विचलित हो जाना। The deviation of blood flow from its normal passage.

Steariform (स्टीयरीफार्म) वसा के समान, वसारूप। Resembling fat.

Steatocele (स्टीयेटोसील) अण्डकोश के भीतर वसीय अबुर्द। Fatty tumor within the scrotum.

Steatomatous (स्टीयेटोमेटस) बहुत सी त्वग्वसीय पुटियों से चिन्हित। Marked with numerous sebaceous cysts.

Steatorrhea (स्टीयेटोरिह्या) मल में अत्यधिक वसा का पाया जाना, वसापुरीश। Presence of excess of fat in the feces.

Stellate (स्टीलेट) ताराकार, इस प्रकार व्यवस्थित कि भाग कर केन्द्र से फैले हुए होते है। Star-shaped; arranged in such a way that the parts rediate from a center.

Stem (स्टैम) डण्ठल के समान सहारा देने वाली कोई भी रचना, तना, स्तम्भ। Any stalk like supporting structure.

Stenocephaly (स्टेनोसिफैली) कपाल अथवा सिर का तंग हो जाना, संकीर्णकपालीयता। Narrowness of the cranium or head.

Stenosis (स्टेनोसिस) शरीर के किसी छिद्र अथवा मार्ग का संकीर्ण या तंग हो जाना, संकीर्णता। Stricture. Constriction or narrowing of an opening or passage of the body.

Stenostomia (स्टेनोस्टोमिया) मुख का तंग हो जाना। Narrowing of the mouth.

Stensen's duct (स्टेनसेन्स डक्ट) कर्णपूर्व ग्रन्थि की उत्सर्गी नली जो मुख-गुहा में खुलती है। The excretory duct of the parotid gland which open into the oral cavity.

Stent (स्टेन्ट) किसी ऊतक को जगह पर थामे रखने अथवा किसी त्वचा निरोप या सम्मिलित नलिकाकार रचनाओं को सहारा देने के लिए एक उपकरण अथवा किसी उचित पदार्थ का सांचा। A device or mold of a suitable substance used to hold a tissue in place or to support a skin graft or the tubular structures that are being anastomosed.

Stentorophonic (स्टेन्टोरोफोनिक) तेज बोलने वाला अथवा तेज आवाज पैदा करने वाला। Speaking loudly or producing loud sound.

Stercobilin (स्टर्कोबिलिन) बाइल या पित्त से उत्पन्न एक भूरा वर्णक जो मल को उसका विशिष्ट रंग प्रदान करता है। A brown pigment derived from bile which gives the characteristic color to feces.

Stercolith (स्टर्कोलिथ) मलाश्मरी। A fecal calculus.

Stercus (स्टर्क्स) बिष्ठा, मल, गोबर। Feces, dung, excrement.

Stereognosis (स्टीरीयोग्नोसिस) स्पर्श द्वारा ठोस वस्तु की आकृति पहचानने में समर्थता। Ability to recognize form of the solid things by touch.

Stereoisomerism (स्टीरीयोआइसोमेरिज्म) ऐसी दशा जिसमें दो अथवा अधिक पदार्थों का एक ही एमप्रीकल फार्मूला होता है परन्तु स्ट्रक्चल फार्मूला भिन्न होता है, त्रिविमसमायवता। The condition in which two or more substances have the same empirical formula but different structural formulas.

Stereology (स्टीरीयोलॉजी) वस्तुओं के लम्बाई, चौड़ाई एवं ऊँचाई तीनों पहलुओं का अध्ययन करना। Study of three-dimensional aspects of objects.

Stereophotography (स्टीरीयोफोटोग्राफी) ऐसी फोटोग्राफी जो चित्त में ठोसपन अथवा गहराई के प्रभाव को उत्पन्न करती है। Photography that produces effect of solidity or depth in the picture.

Stereoscope (स्टीरीयोस्कोप) ऐसा यंत्र जो किसी वस्तु के दो चित्त के प्रतिबिम्ब को मिलाकर देखने पर उस वस्तु की घनता (ठोसपन) अथवा गहराई को दर्शाता है। An instrument showing the solidity or depth of an object seen by combining image of two pictures.

Stereotropic (स्टीरीयोट्रॉपिक) घन-वृत्ति से सम्बन्धित। Pertaining to stereotropism.

Stereotypy (स्टीरीयोटिपी) बेमतलब के शब्दों अथवा कार्यों के लगातार बार-बार दुहराना। Persistent repetition of senseless words or acts.

Sterile (स्टेराइल) अपूतित अथवा जीवित सूक्ष्मजीवों से रहित, निर्जीवाणुक। Aseptic or free from living microorganism.

Sterility (स्टेरीलिटी) जीवित सूक्ष्मजीवों से रहित रहना, निर्जीवाणुकता, विसंक्रमणता। Condition of being free from living microorganism.

(*i*) **Acquired sterility** (एक्वायर्ड स्टेरीलिटी) एक बार बच्चा पैदा करने के बाद गर्भधारण न होना। The failure of further conception after once produced a child.

(*ii*) **Female Sterility** (फीमेल स्टेरीलिटी) किसी स्त्री की गर्भधारण करने में असमर्थता। Inability of a woman to conceive.

Sterilization (स्टेरीलाइजेशन) गर्मी से, गैस तथा आयनन विकिरण के प्रति अनावृत करके किसी पदार्थ के सभी सूक्ष्म जीवों को पूर्णतया अलग करने अथवा उन्हें नष्ट करने की क्रिया, निर्जीवाणुकरण। Process of completely removing or destroying all microorganisms on a substance by heat, by exposure to gas, exposure to ionizing radiation.

Sterilizer (स्टेरीलाइज़र) सूक्ष्मजीवों को नष्ट करने वाला एक उपकरण, विसंक्रामक यंत्र जैसे वाष्पदाबी, विसंक्रामक यंत्र। An apparatus for destroying microorganisms as an autoclave.

Sternal (स्टर्नल) स्टर्नल सम्बन्धी, उरोस्थिक। Pertaining to the sternum.

Sternal Puncture (स्टर्नल पंक्चर) उरोस्थि से अस्थि मज्जा का नमूना उपलब्ध करने हेतु बड़े छिद्र वाली सूई से उरोस्थि को छेदित करना। To pierce the sternum with a large-bone needle to obtain a specimen of bone marrow from the sternum.

Sternohyoid (स्टर्नोहॉयड) स्टर्नम एवं हॉयड हड्डी से संबन्धित। Pertaining to the sternum and hyoid bone.

Sternoschisis (स्टर्नोस्काइसिस) स्टर्नम की जन्मजात फटन। Congenital fissure of the sternum.

Sternum (स्टर्नम) वक्ष या छाती में आगे मध्यम रेखा में स्थित एक लम्बी, चपटी हड्डी। An elongated flat bone in the median line of the thorax in front.

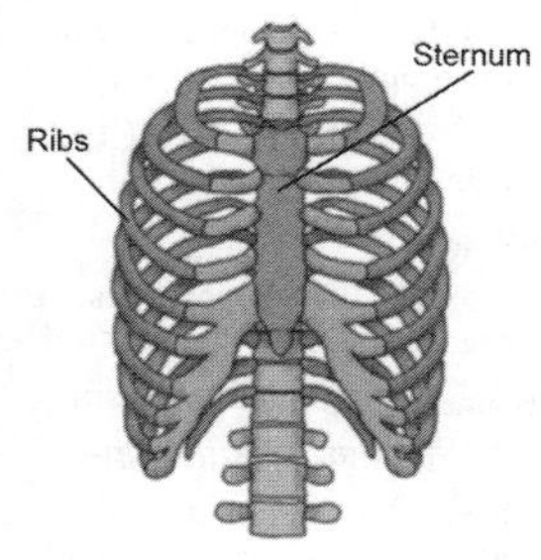

Sternum

Steroid (स्टैरॉयड) यौगिकों के किसी वर्ग में से कोई एक जिसमें लिंग हार्मोन, एड्रीनल कॉर्टेक्स के हार्मोन, पित्त अम्लों तथा कुछ कैंसरजनक पदार्थों का समावेश होता है। Any of a group of compounds which includes sex hormones and hormones of the adrenal cortex, bile acids and certain carcinogenic substances.

Steroidogenesis (स्टैरॉयडोजेनेसिस) स्टैरॉयडों की उत्पत्ति जैसे कि एड्रीनल ग्रन्थियों के द्वारा होती है। Production of steroids as by the adrenal glands.

Sterol (स्टैराल) एक स्टैरॉयड जिसमें एक ओ.एच. (एल्कॉहॉल) वर्ग होता है जैसे कोलेस्ट्रॉल एवं अरगोस्ट्रॉल। A steroid with one OH (alcohol) group, e.g. cholesterol, ergosterol.

Stertorous (स्टैरटोरस) घर्घराहटयुक्त, खर्राटेदार। With deep snoring.

Stethoscope (स्टेथोस्कोप) एक मध्यस्थित यंत्र जो परिश्रवण करने पर शरीर में उत्पन्न ध्वनियों को परीक्षक के कानों तक संचारित करता है, परिश्रवण यंत्र, परिश्रावक। An intervening instrument which transmits the sounds produced in the body to the ear of examiner. on auscultation.

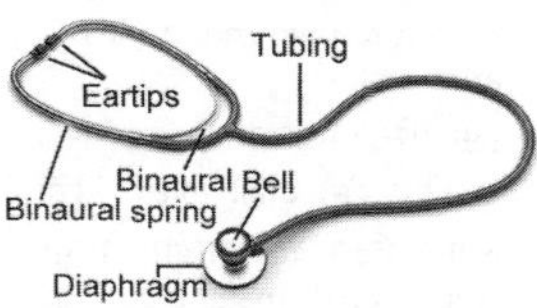

Sthenia (स्थेनिया) असाधारण शक्ति होना, बल, स्फूर्ति। A condition of unusual strength.

Stigma (स्टिग्मा) लांछन चमड़ी पर कोई लाल धब्बा। A red spot on the skin; marks of disease, or congenital abnormalities.

Stilet (स्टीलेट) एक छोटी तेज नुकीली एषणी। A small sharp-pointed probe.

Stillbirth (स्टिलबर्थ) मृत बच्चे का जन्म, मृतजन्म। Birth of a dead child.

Still's disease (स्टिलस डिजीज) किशोरावस्था में होने वाला

गठियारूप संन्धिशोथ। Juvenile rheumatoid arthritis.

Stimulant (स्टिमुलैन्ट) शरीर की क्रियात्मक सक्रियता को बढाने वाला साधन, उत्तेजक। An agent which increase the functional activity of the body.

Stimulus (स्टिमुलस) उद्दीपक, उत्तेजक, उत्तेजन, शील, उद्दीपन। Anything which excites an organ.

Sting (स्टिंग) दशानुभूति, दंश, डंक। Sharp, smarting sensation a punctured wound made by an insect.

Stitch (स्टिच) अचानक क्षण भर के लिए होने वाली काटने जैसी अथवा ऐंठन की स्थानीय वेदना। A sudden, transient, cutting or spasmodic local pain.

Stoke (स्टोक) किसी तरल की श्यानता अथवा चिपचिपेपन की एक इकाई जो .0001 वर्ग मीटर प्रति सेकण्ड होती है। A unit of viscosity of a fluid equal to .0001 square meter per second.

Stokes-Adams Syndrome (स्टीक्स-एडेम्स सिण्ड्रोम) मस्तिष्क के रक्त प्रवाह में बाधा उत्पन्न हो जाने के कारण बेहोशी हो जाना तथा दौरे पड़ना। Unconsciousness with convulsion caused by interference in blood flow of the brain.

Stoma (स्टोमा) मुख, द्वार या छिद्र। A mouth, opening or pore.

Stomach (स्टोमक) आमाशय, जठर, पेट। The chief digestive organ.

Stomachic (स्टोमेकिक) आमाशय की क्रियात्मक सक्रियता बढ़ाने वाली औषधि। A medicine that increases the functional activity of the stomach.

Stomal (स्टोमल) किसी मुख, द्वारा या छिद्र से सम्बन्धित। Pertaining to a Stoma.

Stomatitis (स्टोमेटाइटिस) मुख की श्लेष्मिक कला की सूजन, मुखपाक। Inflammation of the oral mucosa.

(*i*) **Membranous Stomatitis** (मेम्ब्रेनस स्टोमेटाइटिस) मुखपाक जिसमें कूट कला बन जाती है। Stomatitis with the formation of a false membrane.

Stomatognathic (स्टोमेटोग्नेथिक) मुख एवं जबड़ों को एक साथ प्रदर्शित करने वाला। Denoting the mouth and jaws together.

Stomatomenia (स्टोमेटोमीनिया) मासिक धर्म के समय मुँह से खून बहना। Bleeding from the mouth at the time of menstruation.

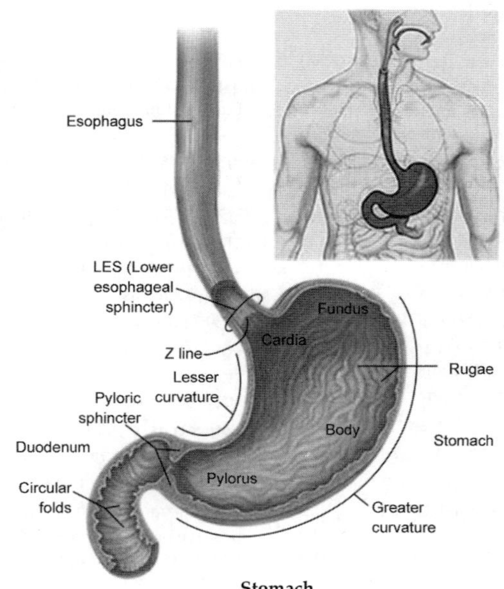

Stomach

Stomatopathy (स्टोमेटोपैथी) मुख का कोई भी रोग। Any disease of the mouth.

Stomatorrhagia (स्टोमेटोरैहजिया) मुँह से खून बहना। Bleeding from the mouth.

Stone (स्टोन) अश्मरी, पथरी। Calculus.

Strabismus (स्ट्राबिस्मस) एक दृष्टि-दोष जिसमें दोनों नेत्रों के दृष्टि-अक्ष किसी वस्तु पर एक साथ नहीं टिकते। तिर्यक दृष्टि, टेढ़ा देखना, ढेरना। A visual defect in which visual axes of both eyes are not directed towards an object simultaneously.

Strain (स्ट्रेन) मोच, तनाव, दबाव, छानना। A sprain, tension, pressure, to filter.

Strait (स्ट्रेट) एक संकीर्ण अथवा तंग मार्ग।

A constricted or narrow passage.

Straited Muscle (स्ट्रियेटेड मसल) रेखित पेशी। Stripped or voluntary muscle which is subject to control by will.

Strangle (स्ट्रेंगिल) श्वास-प्रणाल के दबाव से दम घोटना या दम घुटना। To suffocate or be suffocated from compression of the trachea.

Strangury (स्ट्रेन्गारी) दर्द के साथ बूँद-बूँद करके पेशाब होना, बिन्दूमूत्रकृच्छ। Painful drop by drop urination.

Strap (स्ट्रैप) मरहम पट्टी को स्थान पर थामें रखने अथवा किसी जख्म की सतहों को मिलाने के लिए एक बन्धन या पट्टी जैसे एडहीसिव प्लास्टर की। A band, as of adhesive plaster, used to hold dressing in place or to attach the surface of a wound.

Stratification (स्ट्रेटीफिकेशन) परतों में व्यवस्थापन। Arrangement in layers.

Stratum (स्ट्रेटम) एक परत जैसे स्ट्रेटम कॉर्निया, बाह्यत्वचा के सबसे बाहरी परत, अस्तर। A layer, e.g. stratum corium, the outermost layer of the epidermis.

Strawberry Tongue (स्ट्रॉवेरी टंग) हल्की-हल्की लाल दानेदार जीभ, कणिकाकारक्त जिह्वा। The papillated tongue of scarlet fever.

Streak (स्ट्रीक) रेखा, धारी, लकीर। Furrow, line, bend or color mark.

Streptococcemia (स्ट्रैप्टोकॉक्सीमिया) रक्त में स्ट्रैप्टोकॉकस जीवाणुओं का पाया जाना। Strepticemia. Presence of streptococci in the blood.

Streptococcicosis (स्ट्रैप्टोकॉक्सीकोसिस) स्ट्रैप्टोकॉकस का कोई भी संक्रमण। Any infection with streptococcus.

Streptococcus (स्ट्रैप्टोकॉकस) स्ट्रैप्टोकॉकस वंश तथा स्ट्रैप्टोकॉकेसी कुल का एक ग्राम-धनात्मक जीवाणु। A Gram-positive bacteria of the genus streptococcus belonging to the family streptococcaceae.

Stress (स्ट्रैस) किसी शब्द, वाक्य अथवा बात पर जोर देना। शारीरिक जोर दबाव, यांत्रिक बल, रोगजनक जीव तथा आघात, प्रयास। Emphasis, physical stress-pressure, mechanical force, pathogenic organism and injury, effort.

Stressor (स्ट्रैसर) दबाव उत्पन्न करने वाला साधन अथवा दशा। An agent or condition which produces stress.

Stretch (स्ट्रैच) फैलाना, तनाव। To extend.

Stretcher (स्ट्रेचर) बीमार, चोट खाए हुए अथवा मृत व्यक्ति को ले जाने वाली ट्रोली। A litter for carrying the sick, injured or dead person.

Stria (स्ट्रिया) रेखा, लकीर, खरोंच, धारी। A streak or line.

Striated (स्ट्रियेटेड) धारीदार, जिस पर रेखाएँ या लकीरें हों, रेखित। Striped; having striae or streaks.

Stricture (स्ट्रिक्चर) किसी नली, वाहिनी, मार्ग अथवा खोखले अंग जैसे मूत्र नली या गवीनी, मूत्र-मार्ग अथवा ग्रासनली का असामान्य रूप से तंग हो जाना, निकोचन। An abnormal narrowing of a tube, duct, passage or hollow organ, such as ureter, urethra or esophagus.

Stridor (स्ट्रीडोर) एक कर्कश या रूक्ष, ऊँची श्वसनीय ध्वनि, घर्घर। A harsh, high-pitched respiratory sound.

Strip (स्ट्रिप) छिलका उतारना या छीलना। To remove, pull or tear the covering on outer layer from something.

Stroke (स्ट्रोक) एक तेज मुक्का, आघात या प्रहार, आकस्मिक आक्रमण। A sharp blow, A sudden attack.

Stroke volume (स्ट्रोक वोल्यूम) प्रत्येक स्पन्द पर बाँयें निलय से फेंके गये रक्त की मात्रा जो आयु लिंग तथा श्रम के अनुसार बदलती रहती है। The amounts of blood ejected by the left ventricle at each beat, which varies with the age, sex.

Stroma (स्ट्रोमा) किसी अंग को संभाले रहने वाला ऊतक अथवा आधारक। The supporting tissue or matrix of an organ.

Strophocephaly (स्ट्रोफोसिफैली) सिर एवं चेहरे का जन्मजात विरूपण।
Congenital distortion of the head and face.

Struma (स्ट्रूमा) गलगण्ड, घेंघा या ग्वॉयटर, अवटुरता। Goiter.

Strumitis (स्ट्रूमाइटिस) थाइरॉयड ग्रन्थि की सूजन, अवटुशोथ। Inflammation of a thyroid gland.

Strychnine (स्ट्रिकनीन) स्टिकनस नक्स-वोमिका पौधे से उपलब्ध एक विषैला एल्केलॉयड। A poisonous alkaloid obtained from the plant strychnous nux-vomica.

Stump (स्टम्प) अंगोच्छेदन के पश्चात छूटा किसी भुजा का दूरस्थ सिरा, स्थूणक, ठूँठ। The distal end of a lumb left after amputation.

Stun (स्टन) मुक्का मार कर या चोट पहुँचा कर बेहोश कर देना। To make unconscious by a blow or injury.

Stupe (स्ट्यूप) किसी औषधि से युक्त गर्म पानी में भिगोया गया एक कपड़ा या स्पंज जिसे सिकाई के लिए प्रयुक्त किया जाता है। A cloth or sponge mode wet with hot water containing a medicine, used for formation.

Stupor (स्ट्यूपर) ऐसी दशा जिसमें रोगी से कम ही प्रत्युत्तर प्राप्त होता है। जड़िमा। A condition of reduced responsiveness.

Stuttering (स्टटरिंग) हकलाहट। Speech defect with stumbling and spasmodic repetition of same syllable.

Stye (स्टाइ) आँख की पलक की किसी त्वग्वसीय ग्रन्थि का शोथ। Inflammation of a sebaceous gland of the eye-lid.

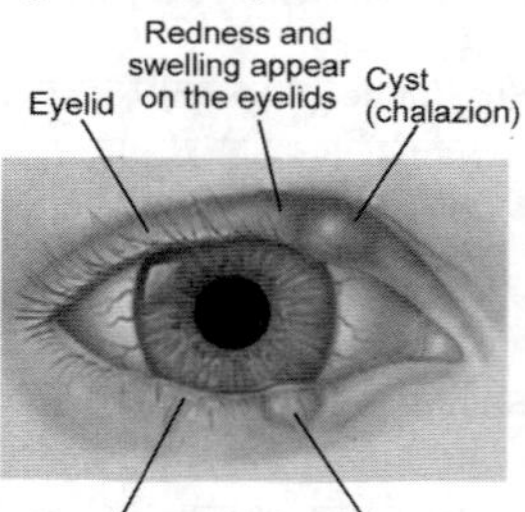

Stylet (स्टाइलेट) एक पतली एशणी। A thin probe.

Styliform (स्टाइलीफार्म) लम्बा एवं नुकीला। Long and pointed.

Styloid process (स्टीलॉयड प्रोसेस) नीचे की ओर को उभरा हुआ शंखास्थि का एक नुकीला पदार्थ। A pointed process of the temporal bone projecting downwards.

Stylus (स्टाइलस) बाह्य प्रयोग के लिये पेन्सिल के समान नुकीला औषधीय योग, शर। Pencil-like pointed medicinal preparation for external application.

Styptic (स्टिप्टिक) स्तम्भ। Astringent.

Sub (सब) एक उपसर्ग जिसका अर्थ नीचे या कम, भीतर, कम मात्रा में, सामान्य से कम तथा मामूली। A prefix which means below, beneath or under inside, in small quantity, less than normal, and moderately.

Subacidity (सबएसिडिटी) अल्प अम्लता। Deficient acidity.

Subanconeus (सबएन्कोनियस) कोहनी से नीचे। Below the elbow.

Subareolar (सबएरियोलर) परिवेश या मण्डल से नीचे। Below the areola.

Subaural (एबऔरल) कान से नीचे, अवकर्णी। Below the ear.

Subchoroidal (सबकोरॉयडल) नेत्र के रंजितपटल अस्तर के नीचे। Beneath the choroid coat of the eyes.

Subclinical (सबक्लीनिकल) किसी रोग की उसके विशिष्ट लक्षणों के प्रकट होने से पूर्व की अवस्था से सम्बन्धित। Pertaining to the stage of a disease before appearance of its typical symptoms.

Subconsciousness (सबकॉनशियसनैस) आंशिक रूप से चेतन होना। The state of being partially conscious.

Subcortex (सबकॉर्टेकस) मस्तिष्क का कार्टेक्स के नीचे स्थित श्वेत पदार्थ। White substance of the brain underlying the cortex.

Subcostal (सबकॉस्टल) पसलियों के नीचे, अवपर्षुक। Beneath the ribs.

Subcutaneous (सबक्यूटेनियस) त्वचा के नीचे, अवत्वक, अवत्वचीय। Hypodermic. Beneath the skin.

Subendothelial (सबएण्डोथीलियल) एण्डोथीलियम से नीचे अवअन्तःकलायज। Below the endothelium.

Subfamily (सबफेमिली) कुल एवं वंश के बीच का विभाजन। A division between family and genus.

Subglossitis (सबग्लोसाइटिस) जिह्वा के नीचे की सतह या ऊतकों का शोथ। Inflammation of the under surface or tissues of the tongue.

Subilium (सबइलियम) इलियम का सबसे निचला भाग। The lowest part of the ilium.

Subjective (सब्जैक्टिव) जिसका केवल रोगी को पता लगता है। परीक्षक को नहीं जैसे लक्षणों का पता लगाना। Perceived only by patient and not by examiner, as perception of the symptoms.

Subjective Symptom (सब्जैक्टिव सिम्प्टम) वह लक्षण जिसका ज्ञान केवल रोगी को होता है। Symptom that is perceptible only to the patient.

Sublatio (सबलेशियों) शरीर के किसी भाग का ऊपर को उठना अथवा अलग हो जाना। Elevation, removal or detachment of a part of the body.

Sublimate (सब्लीमेट) उत्सादन से प्राप्त अथवा तैयार किया गया एक पदार्थ। A substance obtained or prepared by sublimation.

Subluxation (सबलक्जेशन) आंशिक सन्धिच्युति या विस्थापन, अनुसन्धिच्युति। Partial dislocation.

Submaxillary (सबमैक्सिलरी) ऊर्ध्वहनु या मैक्जिला से नीचे। Below the maxilla.

Submicron (सबमाइक्रोन) एक माइक्रोन से कम की माप। A measure of less than 1 micron.

Submucosa (सबम्यूकोसा) किसी श्लेष्मिक झिल्ली के नीचे सछिद्र संयोजी ऊतक की परत, अवश्लेष्मिकलकला। The layer of areolar connective tissue beneath a mucous membrane.

Submuscular (सबमस्कुलर) पेशी के नीचे, अवपेशीय। Below the muscle.

Subneural (सबन्यूरल) किसी तंत्रिका के नीचे। Beneath a nerve.

Subnormality (सबनॉर्मलिटी) सामान्य से नीचे होना। The condition of being subnormal.

Suborder (सबआर्डर) जन्तु वर्गीकरण में, किसी गण एवं कुल के बीच।
In animal classification, between an order and a family.

Subpharyngeal (सबफेरिन्जियल) ग्रसनी या गले से नीचे। Beneath the pharynx.

Subpial (सबपायल) पाया मेटर के नीचे। Beneath the pia mater

Subpontine (सबपोन्टाइन) पोन्स से नीचे। Below the pons.

Subpulmonary (सबपल्मोनरी) फेफड़ो के नीचे। Below the lung.

Subscription (सब्सक्रिप्शन) नुस्खे का वह भाग जिसमें घटकों को मिलाने का निर्देश दिया होता है, अवनिर्देश। That part of a prescription in which direction for compounding the ingredients is given.

Subsidence (सब्सीडैन्स) किसी रोग का धीरे-धीरे लुप्त होना, लोप। Gradual disappearance of a disease.

Subsistence (सबसिस्टैन्स) जीवन के लिए अनिवार्य किसी वस्तु जैसे भोजन की न्यूनतम मात्रा। The minimum amount of something essential for life as that of food.

Subspinous (सबस्पाइनस) किसी कंटक प्रवर्ध अथवा मेरू-दण्ड के नीचे। Below a spinous process or the spinal column.

Substitude (सब्स्टीट्यूड) कोई भी वस्तु अथवा औषधि जिसका दूसरी वस्तु अथवा औषधि की एवज में प्रयोग किया जा सकता है। Anything or medicine which may be used in place of another.

Subtarsal (सबटार्सल) पदकूर्च या गुल्फ के नीचे। Below the tarsus.

Subtetanic (सबटिटेनिक) मृदु टेटनस से पीड़ित। Suffering from mild tetanus

Subtle (सब्ट्ल) तीक्ष्ण बुद्धि, अति सूक्ष्म। Mentally acute, very fine.

Subtrochlear (सबट्रॉक्लियर) चक्रक से नीचे। Below the trochlea.

Subvaginal (सबवैजाइनल) किसी नलिकाकार चादर के भीतर अथवा योनि से नीचे। Inside a tubular sheath, or below the vagina.

Succedaneum (सक्सेडेनीयम) एक स्थानापन्न एवं एवजी अर्थात् कोई औषधि या अन्य वस्तु जिसे दूसरे के स्थान पर काम मे लाया जा सकता है। A substitute, i.e. a drug or other thing that can be used in place of another.

Succenturiate (सक्सेनटियूरीएट) सहायक, अनुषंगी। Accessory.

Succus (सक्कस) जीवित ऊतकों के द्वारा स्रावित कोई भी तरल अथवा रस जैसे जठर रस या आमाशयिक रस जो आमाशय की दिवारों का स्राव होता है, रस। Any fluid or juice secreted by the living tissue as gastric juice which is the secretion of stomach walls.

Succussion (सक्कुसन) जल से पूर्ण होने पर उत्पन्न होने वाली छपछप की ध्वनि को सुनकर शरीर की गुहा विशेषकर वक्ष में तरल एवं वायु की विद्यमानता का पता लगाने के लिये शरीर को हिलाना, हल्लन। Shaking of the body to detect the presence of fluid and air in the body cavity, especially in the thorax, by listening the splashing sound.

Suck (सक) चूशण जैसे स्तन से दूध का चूशण करना, चूसना। To draw a fluid into the mouth as milk from the breast.

Suckle (सक्ल) स्तनपान कराना, दूध पिलाना। To feed at the breast.

Sucrose (सुक्रोज) ईख की चीनी। Cane—sugar.

Suction (सक्शन) किस तरल या गैस के ऊपर वायु दाब कम करके चूशित्त या एस्पिरेटर द्वारा उसे खींचना। Withdrawing of a fluid or gas by reduction of air pressure over it, with an aspirator.

Sudomotor (सुडोमोटर) स्वेद ग्रन्थि के स्राव को उत्तेजित करने वाला। Stimulating the secretion of sweat gland.

Sudor (सुडोर) पसीना, स्वेद। Sweat; perspiration.

Sudoriferous (सुडोरीफेरस) स्वेद को उत्पन्न करने अथवा इसका वहन करने वाला।

Producing or conveying sweat.

Suffocation (सफोकेशन) दम घुटना, घुटन, श्वासावरोध। Impairment of respiration.

Sufusion (सफ्यूजन) शरीर के किसी तरल का चारों ओर के ऊतकों में फैल जाना, परिप्लावन। Extraversions. Spreading of a body fluid into the surrounding tissues.

Sugar (शुगर) एक मीठा कार्बोहाइड्रेट जिसके दो मुख्य वर्ग डाइसैकेराइड एवं मोनोसैकेराइड होते है। A sweet carbohydrate, the two principal groups of which are disaccharides and monosaccharides.

Suggestion (सजेस्शन) प्रस्ताव, संसूचन, सुझाव। Presentation of an idea to the mind.

Suicide (सुसाइड) आत्महत्या, आत्मघात। The act of killing one-self; self-murder.

Sulcate (सल्केट) खातिकायुक्त या खांचेदार। Furrowed or grooved.

Sulcus (सल्कस) एक खातिका, खाँचा या हल्का-सा गड्ढा, परिखा जो विशेषकर मस्तिष्क की सतह पर स्थित होती है। A furrow, groove or slight depression, especially on the surface of the brain.

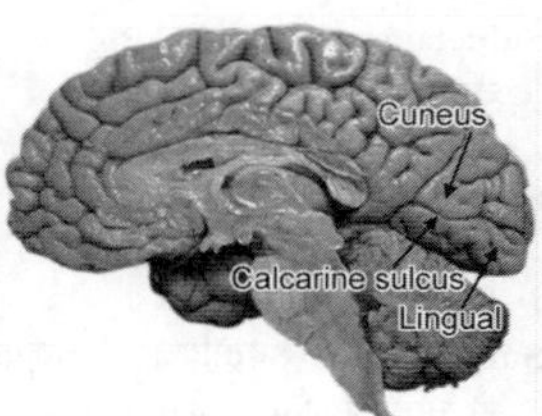

Sunburn (सनबर्न) सूर्यप्रकाश में अत्यधिक रहने उत्पन्न त्वक्शोथ, आतपदाह। Dermatitis due to excessive exposure to sunlight.

Sunscreen (सनस्क्रीन) मरहम अथवा क्रीम के रूप में कोई पदार्थ जो सूर्य किरणों से त्वचा की रक्षा करने के लिए प्रयोग में लाया जाता है। Any substance in the form of an ointment or cream, used to protect the skin from sun rays.

Sunstroke (सनस्ट्रोक) आतपघात, सूर्यघात, घामाघात, लू लगना। Heat-stroke from direct rays of the Sun.

Superabduction (सुपरएब्डक्शन) अत्यधिक दूर को खींच ले जाना। To draw away extremely.

Superciliary (सुपरसिलियरी) आँख की भौंह से सम्बन्धित अथवा उसके क्षेत्र में स्थित। Pertaining to or situated in the region of an eyebrow.

Superego (सुपरइगो) अहम बढ़ जाना। Overgrowth of ego.

Superextension (सुपरएक्सटेन्शन) अत्यधिक खिंचाव होना। Extreme extension.

Superfecundation (सुपरफिकण्डेशन) दो अलग-अलग लैंगिक ससंर्गो द्वारा एक ही आवर्त चक्र में दो या अधिक डिम्बों का गर्भाधान होना, अधिसंफलन, अतिप्रजनन। Fertilization of two or more ova during the same menstrual cycle, by two separate sexual intercourse.

Superfetation (सुपरफिटेशन) दो भिन्न मासिकधर्म-काल में दो डिम्बाणुओं का निषेचन होने के कारण गर्भाशय में भिन्न आयु के दो भ्रूणों का पाया जाना। The presence of two fetuses of different ages in the uterus, due to fertilization of two at different menstrual periods.

Superior (सुपिरीयर) ऊर्ध्व, उत्कृष्ट, प्रवर, वरिष्ठ। The upper of the two or more parts, more vital.

Superiority complex (सुपीरियरिटी कॉमप्लैक्स) अपनी हीनभावना की क्षतिपूर्ति करने के लिए किसी का अपनी श्रेष्ठता का अत्यधिक किया जाने वाला प्रदर्शन। An over exhibition of one's own superiority in order to compensate for one's feeling of inferiority.

Supernatant (सुपरनेटेन्ट) अवक्षेपित अघुलनशील पदार्थ की परत के ऊपर रहने वाला साफ द्रव। The clear liquid lying above a layer of precipitated insoluble.

Supernumerary (सुपरन्यूमेरेरी) सामान्य संख्या से अधिक। More than the normal number.

Superparasite (सुपरपैरासाइट) ऐसा परजीवी जो दूसरे परजीवी होता है। A parasite that is parasitic on another parasite.

Superscription (सुपरक्रिप्शन) किसी नुस्खे का शीर्ष जिसमें आर.एक्स (Rx) चिन्ह होता है जिसका लेटिन भाषा में अभिप्राय रिसीपी होता है जिसका अर्थ 'लो' है, अधिनिर्देश। The heading of prescription containing the symbol Rx, signifying (Latin) recipe which means 'take'.

Superstructure (सुपरस्ट्रक्चर) अधिसंरचना। A structure above the surface.

Supervirulent (सुपरवाइरूलैन्ट) सामान्य से अधिक विषाक्त। More virulent than usual.

Supination (सुपिनेशन) उत्तान करने की क्रिया, उत्तानन। The act of supplanting.

Supinator (सुपिनेटर) वह पेशी जो अग्रबाहु का उत्तान करती है। A muscle which causes supination of the forearm.

Suppository (सपोज़ीटरी) शरीर के किसी छिद्र जैसे मलाशय, योनि, अथवा मूत्र-मार्ग में निवेशित करने के लिए औषधियुक्त बेलनाकार या शंक्वाकार एक पिण्ड जो वहाँ पर जाकर घुल जाता है तथा इसकी औषधि अवशोषित हो जाती है, वर्तिका। A medicated cylindrical or conical mass to be introduced into a body orifice, as the rectum, vagina or urethra where it dissolves and its medicine is absorbed.

Suppress (सप्रेस) दबाना, दमन करना, उपशमन करना। To conceal: to retain.

Suppurate (सपुरेट) पस या मवाद बनाना। To form pus.

Suppuration (सपुरेशन) पस का बनना, पूयता, पूयीभवन। Pyogenesis; Formation of pus.

Supra (सुप्रा) एक उपसर्ग जिसका अर्थ ऊपर या अधिक होता है। A prefix which means above.

Supracerebellar (सुप्रासेरीबेलर) अनुमस्तिष्क की ऊपरी सतह से ऊपर। Above the upper surface of the cerebellum.

Supraclavicular (सुप्राक्लैविकुलर) क्लैविकल के ऊपर, अधिजत्रुकीय। Above the clavicle.

Supragingival (सुप्राजिन्जाइवल) मसूड़े के ऊपर। Above the gingiva.

Supraintestinal (सुप्राइन्टैस्टाइनल) आँत के ऊपर पड़ा हुआ। Lying over the intestine.

Supramammary (सुप्रामैमरी) किसी स्तन के ऊपर। Above a breast.

Suprameatal (सुप्रामीयेटल) किसी कुहर या द्वार विशेषकर बाह्य कर्ण कुहर के ऊपर। Above a meatus, especially the external auditory meatus.

Suprarenal (सुप्रारीनल) गुर्दे के ऊपर, अधिजछनिक। Above the kidney.

Sura (सुरा) पैर की पिण्डली। Calf of the leg.

Surfactant (सर्फेक्टैन्ट) वह जो सतह तनाव को कम करता है जैसे तेल। That which lowers the surface tension, e.g. oils.

Surgery (सर्जरी) शल्यचिकित्सा, शल्यक्रिया, शल्यविज्ञान, शल्यकर्म। The branch of medicine which treats disease by operative procedure.

(*i*) **Ablative Surgery** (एब्लेटिव सर्जरी) एक ऐसा ऑपरेशन जिसमें किसी भाग को निकाल दिया जाता है। An operation in which a part is removed.

(*ii*) **Aural Surgery** (औरल सर्जरी) कान की शल्यक्रिया। Surgery of the ear.

(*iii*) **Exploratory Surgery** (एक्सप्लोरेट्री सर्जरी)

नैदानिक उद्देश्यों के लिए किया जाने वाला ऑपरेशन। An operation performed for diagnostic purposes.

Surgical neck (सर्जिकल नैक) गण्डकों के नीचे ह्यूमेरस हड्डी के काण्ड का संकुचित भाग जहाँ पर अधिकतर अस्थिभंग होता है। Constrictive part of the shaft of humerus bone below the tuberosities where fracture commonly occurs.

Surrogate (सरोगेट) प्रतिस्थापक, एक वस्तु अथवा व्यक्ति जो दूसरी वस्तु या व्यक्ति को पुनः स्थापित करता है। A substitute; a thing or person that replaces another.

Sursumversion (सर्समवर्जन) दोनों आँखों का एक साथ ऊपर को घूम जाना। The turning upward of both the eyes simultaneously.

Susceptible (ससेप्टिबल) सुग्राह्म, सुग्राही, संवेदनशील। Sensitive to an influence, liable to become affected with a disease.

Suspiration (सस्पिरेशन) आह भरना। The act of sighing.

Sustentaculum (सस्टैन्टाकुलम) एक सहारा अथवा सहारा देने वाली रचना। A support or supporting structure.

Suturation (स्यूचुरेशन) टाँके लगाना या सिलाई करना, सीवन। Application of sutures of stitching.

Suture (स्यूचर) 1. किसी अचल संधि में हड्डियों के जुड़ने की रेखा जैसे खोपड़ी की हड्डियों के बीच की रेखाएँ। 2. टाँके लगा कर किसी जख्म के किनारों को जोड़ना। 1. Line of union of bones in an immovable joint, as those between the skull bones. 2. To unite the margins of a wound by stitching.

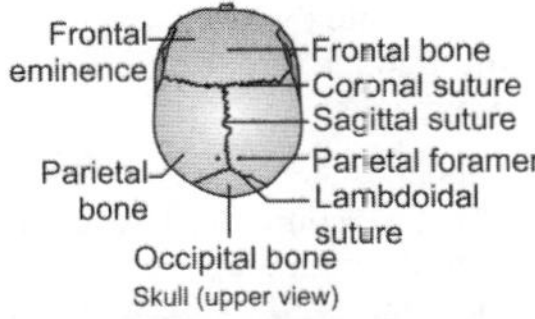

Skull (upper view)

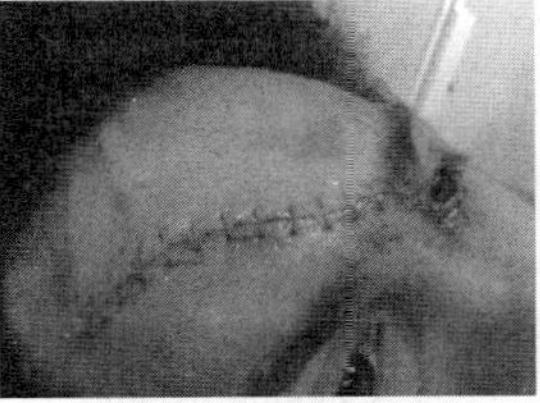

Swab (स्वाब) किसी तार या छड़ी के किनारे से संलग्न रूई, गॉज अथवा अन्य अवशोष पदार्थ की एक गद्दी जिसे गुहाओं को साफ करने, औषधि लगाने अथवा

जीवाणु विज्ञान सम्बन्धी परीक्षण के लिए ऊतक के एक टुकड़े या स्राव को प्राप्त करने हेतु प्रयोग में लाया जाता है। A pad of cotton or gauze or other absorbable material attached to the end of a wire or stick, used for clearing the cavities, applying medicines or for obtaining a piece of tissue or secretions for bacteriological examination.

Swallowing (स्वॉलोइंग) निगलने की क्रिया। The process of passing something from mouth into the stomach, through the throat, esophagus.

Sweat (स्वेट) पसीना, स्वेद, पसीना लाना। Perspiration. To excrete fluid through the pores of the skin.

Swelling (स्वैलिंग) शरीर के किसी अंग अथवा किसी हिस्से की असामान्य अल्पकालीन वृद्धि, सूजन, उत्सेघ। An abnormal transient enlargement of an organ or part of the body.

Swoom (स्वूम) मूर्च्छा, मूर्च्छित होना। A fainting, to faint.

Sycosis (साइकोसिस) जीर्ण रोमकूपशोथ, विशेषकर दाढ़ी का (साइकोसिस बार्बी)। Chronic inflammation of the hair follicles, especially of the beard.

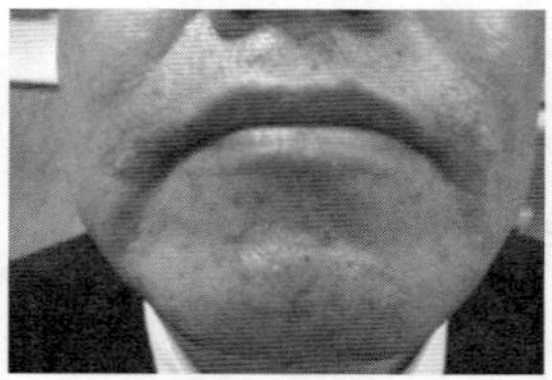

Symbiosis (सिम्बियोसिस) संहजीविता, सहजीवन। Mutualism, commensalism.

Symblepharon (सिम्बलेफेरान) आँख की पलक की नेत्रश्लेष्मा का नेत्र गोलक से चिपक जाना। Adhesion of the conjunctiva of eyelid to the eyeball.

Symbrachydactyly (सिम्ब्रेकीडैक्टाइली) हाथ की अंगुलियों का जाल युक्त होना असामान्य रूप से छोटी होती है। Webbing of the fingers that are abnormally short.

Symelus (साइमीलस) ऐसा भ्रूण जिसकी टांगे जुड़ी होती है। A fetus with fused legs.

Sympathectomy (सम्पिैथेक्टॉमी) स्वसंचालित तंत्रिका-तन्त्र के अनुकम्पी विभाजन के किसी भाग का पारपरिच्छेदन करना या उसका उच्छेदन करना अर्थात काट कर बाहर निकाल देना। Transection, resection or excision of a part of the sympathetic division of the autonomic nervous system.

Sympathetic (सिम्पैथेटिक) 1. अनुकम्पी तन्त्रिका-तंत्र से सम्बन्धित। 2. सहानुभूति से सम्बन्धित अथवा उससे उत्पन्न, संवेदी। 1. Pertaining to the sympathetic nervous system. 2. Pertaining to or caused by sympathy.

Sympatheticoparalytic (सिम्पैथेटिकोपैरालाइटिक) अनुकम्पी तन्त्रिका-तन्त्र के पक्षाघात के कारण उत्पन्न होने वाला। Occurring due to paralysis of the sympathetic nervous system.

Sympathetic plexus (सिम्पैथेटिक प्लक्सस) अनुकम्पी तन्त्रिकाओं एवं गण्डिकाओं से बनी एक जालिका। A plexus formed by the sympathetic nervous and ganglia.

Sympathiconeuritis (सिम्पैथिकोन्यूराइटिस) अनुकम्पी तंत्रिकाओं का शोथ। Inflammation of the sympathetic nerves.

Sympathicotonic (सिम्पैथिकोटॉनिक) सिम्पैथिकोटोनिया से सम्बन्धित अथवा उससे ग्रस्त। Pertaining to or characterized by sympathicotonia.

Sympathist (सिम्पैथिस्ट) वह व्यक्ति जो शीघ्र ही दूसरे व्यक्ति के प्रस्ताव अथवा राय स्वीकार कर लेता है तथा उनका प्रत्युत्तर देता है। The person who accepts and responds readily to suggestion or opinions of another.

Sympathomimetic (सिम्पैथोमाइमेटिक) अनुकम्पी तन्त्रिका-तन्त्र के उद्दीपन से उत्पन्न होने वाले प्रभावों जैसे इपिनफ्रीन के इन्जैक्शन के पश्चात् होने वाले प्रभाव, के समान प्रभाव उत्पन्न करने वाला। Adrenergic. Producing effects resembling those produced from stimulations of the sympathetic nervous system, as the effects resulting from injection of epinephrine.

Symphyseal (सिम्फाइज़ियल) किसी गंधक से सम्बन्धित। Symphysial. Pertaining to a symphysis.

Symphysiorrhaphy (सिम्फाइज़ियोरैह्फी) विभाजित संधानक में टाँकें लगाना। Suture of a divided symphysis.

Symphysiotomy (सिम्फाइज़ियोटॉमी) श्रोणि-बहिर्गम को बड़ा करके प्रसव को आसान बनाने के लिए जघन संधानक को विभाजित करना। To divide the pubic symphysis to facilitate delivery, by enlarging the pelvic outlet.

Symphysis (सिम्फाइसिस) जो हड्डियों की संयोजन रेखा जैसे

जघनास्थियों का सामने मध्य रेखा पर संगम, संधानक। The line of fusion of two bones, e.g. the junction of pubic bones on midline in front.

Symptom (सिम्पटम) शरीर में अथवा इसके कार्य में कोई परिवर्तन होना जिसका व्यक्ति को पता चल जाता है, जिससे शरीर में किसी रोग के होने का संकेत मिलता है, लक्षण। Any change in the body or its functions recognized by the person that indicates the presence of a disease in the body.

(*i*) **Delayed Symptom** (डिलेड सिम्पटम) देर से प्रकट होने वाला लक्षण। Symptom appearing late. (*ii*) **Local Symptom** (लोकल सिम्पटम) स्थानिक लक्षण। Symptom occurring locally.

Symptomatic (सिम्पटोमेटिक) लाक्षणिक, लक्षण सम्बन्धी। Pertaining to a symptom.

Sympus (सिम्पस) ऐसा भ्रूण जिसकी टांगे जुड़ी होती है। A fetus with fused legs.

Synactosis (साइनेक्टोसिस) शरीर के भागों के असामान्य संयोजन के परिणामस्वरूप होने वाली कुरचना। Malformation resulting from abnormal fusion of parts of the body.

Synapse (साइनेप्स) दो तंत्रिकाकोशिकाओं के प्रवर्धो के बीच अथवा एक तंत्रिका कोशिका एवं एक प्रेरक अंग के बीच का संगम जहाँ पर तंत्रिका-आवेगों का संचारण होता है। The junction between the processes of two neurons or between a neuron and an effector organ where neural impulses are transmitted.

Synarthrophysis (साइनार्थ्रोफाइसिस) जोड़ों में धीरे-धीरे बढ़ने वाला सन्धिग्रह। Pro-gressive ankylosis in the joints.

Synarthrosis (साइनारथ्रोसिस) अचल संधि। Immovable joint.

Synchilia (सिन्काइलिया) होठों का जन्म से चिपका होना। Congenital adhesion of the lips.

Synchondrosis (सिन्कॉण्ड्रोसिस) उपास्थिसंधि, उपास्थि का जोड़। Union by intervening cartilage.

Synchronous (सिन्क्रोनस) एक ही समय में उत्पन्न होने वाला, समकालीन। Occurring at the same time.

Syncope (सिन्कोप) मूर्च्छा, सम्मूर्च्छा, बेहोशी। Fainting or swooning.

Syncytium (सिनसाइटियम) कोशिका भित्तियों के घुल जाने से उत्पन्न जीवद्रव्य का एक

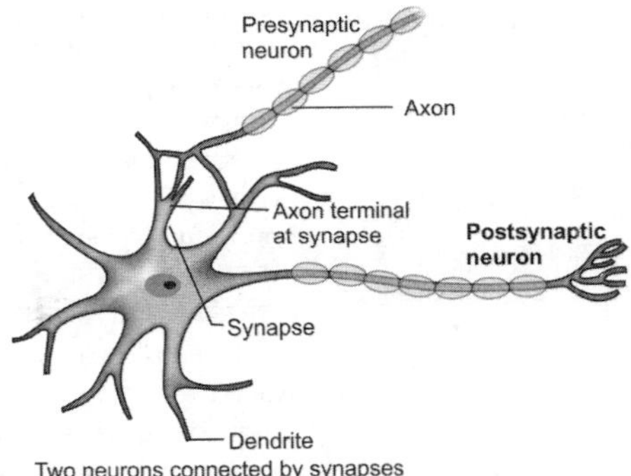

Two neurons connected by synapses

Synapse

बहुकेन्द्रिय ढेर जैसे कोई रेखित पेशी तन्तु। A multinucleated mass or protoplasm produced by dissolution of the cell walls, e.g. a striated muscles fiber.

Syndesmitis (सिण्डेस्माइटिस) तन्तुसंधि शोथ। Inflammation of ligament.

Syndesmology (सिण्डेस्मोलॉजी) स्नायु, सन्धियों, उनकी गतियों तथा उनके रोगों का अध्ययन, सन्धि प्रकरण। Study of the ligaments, joints, their movements, and their diseases.

Syndesmosis (सिण्डेस्मोसिस) ऐसा जोड़ जिसमें हड्डियों लिगामैन्टो से बन्धी होती है। A joint in which the bones are bounded by ligaments.

Syndrome (सिण्ड्रोम) संलक्षण। A commonly observed combination of symptoms.

Synechia (साइनीकिया) शरीर के भागों का चिपक जाना विशेषकर आइरिस का कार्निया या लैन्स से चिपक जाना, संसक्ति। Adhesion of parts of the body, especially adhesion of iris to the cornea or lens.

Synechotomy (साइनीकोटॉमी) किसी चिपकाव को तोड़ देना। The breaking up of an adhesion.

Synergism (सिनर्जिस्म) दो या अधिक पदार्थों जैसे औषधियों की संयुक्त क्रिया जिससे ऐसा प्रभाव उत्पन्न होता है जो प्रत्येक औषधि से अलग-अलग उत्पन्न प्रभावों के कुल योग से बड़ा होता है,

योगवाहिता। Combined action of two or more agents such as drugs producing an effect that is greater than the total effects produced by each drug separately.

Synergist (सिनर्जिस्ट) योगवाहिता सम्बन्धी, साथ-साथ कार्य करने वाला। Pertaining to synergy, acting together.

Synergy (सिनर्जी) दो या अधिक रचनाओं अथवा औषधियों की परस्पर सम्बन्धित क्रिया या सहकारिता, योगवाहिता। Correlated action or cooperation of two or more structures or drugs.

Synezesis (साइनेज़ेसिस) पुतली का बन्द होना। Closure of the pupil.

Syngamy (सिनगैमी) गर्भधान में युग्मनज को बनाने के लिए दो युग्मकों का मिलन। The union of two gametes to form a zygote in fertilization.

Synkinesis (सीनकाइनेसिस) किसी ऐच्छिक गति के साथ एक अनैच्छिक गति का होना। An involuntary movement accompanying a voluntary movement.

Synopsia (साइनोप्सिया) नेत्रों का जन्मजात संयोजन। Congenital fusion of the eyes.

Synopsis (साइनोप्सिस) झांकी, झलक। Abstract of matter so arranged as to exhibit a general view of the whole.

Synosteography (साइनोस्टियोग्राफी) सन्धियों का विवरण। A description of the joints.

Synovectomy (सइनोवेक्टॉमी) किसी श्लेषक कला को शल्यक्रिया द्वारा काट कर निकाल देना। Excision of a synovial.

Synovia (सइनोविया) श्लेषक कला द्वारा स्रावित संधि गुहाओं, श्लेषपुटियों तथा कण्डरा आच्छदों में पाया जाने वाला एक रंगहीन, पारदर्शक, चिपचिपा तरल, श्लेषक। Synovial fluid, a colorless, transparent, viscid fluid found in the joint cavities, bursae and tendon sheaths, secreted by the synovial membrane.

Synovial cyst (सइनोवियल सिस्ट) श्लेषक कला की पुटी जिसमें श्लेषक तरल भरा होता है। A cyst of the synovial membrane containing synovial fluid.

Synovioma (सइनोवीओमा) श्लेषककलार्बुद, स्नेहक झिल्ली की रसौली। A tumor of the synovial membrane.

Syntaxis (सिन्टेक्सिस) सन्धि, जोड़। Articulation.

Synthesis (सिन्थेसिस) किसी यौगिक को बनाने वाले तत्वों

को जोड़कर कृत्रिम रूप से उस यौगिक को बनाना अथवा उसका प्राकृतिक रूप से बनना। Production of a compound artificially or naturally, by union of elements composing it.

Synulosis (साइनुलोसिस) वर्णचिन्ह ऊतक का बनना। Formation of scar tissue.

Syphilis (सिफिलिस) एक स्पाइरोकीट ट्रेपोनेमा पैल्डिम द्वारा उत्पन्न एक संक्रामक, जीर्ण, रजित रोग जिसमें बहुत सी त्वचा विक्षतियां उत्पन्न हो जाती है परन्तु शरीर का कोई भी अंग अथवा ऊतक ग्रस्त हो सकता है। An infection, chronic, venereal disease caused by a spirochete treponema pallidum producing many skin lesions but any organ or tissue of the body may be involved.

Syphilitic (सिफिलिटिक) सिफिलिस से सम्बन्धित, उससे उत्पन्न या ग्रस्त, उपदंशग्रस्त। Pertaining to caused by or affected with syphilis.

Syphiloma (सिफिलोमा) सिफिलिस से उत्पन्न एक अबुर्द अथवा गम्मा। A tumor orginated from syphilis or gumma.

Syphilotherapy (सिफिलोथिरैपी) सिफिलिस रोग की चिकित्सा। Treatment of syphilis.

Syringe (सिरिंज) किसी तरल का शरीर, गुहा में सूचिका भरण करने के लिये एक यंत्र तथा किसी गुहा की धुलाई करना। Instrument for injection a fluid into the body, cavity or wash out a cavity.

Syringities (सिरिंजाइटिस) कम्बुकर्णी नली या यूस्टेशियन ट्यूब का शोथ। Inflammation of the Eustachian tube.

Syringomyelia (सिरिंगोमायलिया) सुषुम्ना रज्जु के पदार्थ में तरल से भी गुहाओं का पाया जाना। Presence of fluid filled cavities in the substance of spinal cord.

Syringopontia (सिरिंगोपोन्टिया) जान्स में गुहाओं का पाया जाना Presence of cavities in the pons.

Syrinx (सिरिंक्स) नालव्रल, कम्बुकर्णी नली या यूस्टेशियन नली। Fistula Eustachian tube.

Syrup (सीरप) शुगर का जल में एक गाढ़ा घोल। A concentrated solution of sugar in water.

System (सिस्टम) आपस मे सम्बन्धित रचनाओं अथवा अंगों का एक समूह जो एक ही उद्देष्य के लिये अथवा परिणाम उत्पन्न करने के लिये जो अकेले एक की क्रिया से सम्भव नहीं होता,

एकसाथ कार्य करते हैं; संस्थान, तंत्र। A group of interconnected structures or organs that act together for a common purpose or to produce the result which is not possible by action of one alone.

Systematization (सिस्टेमेटाइज़ेशन) किसी योजना के अनुसार संगठित करना। The process of organizing according to a plan.

Systemic circulation (सिस्टेमिक सर्कुलेशन) फेफड़ों के अतिरिक्त सम्पूर्ण शरीर से होने वाला परिसंचरण। Circulation through the whole body except lungs.

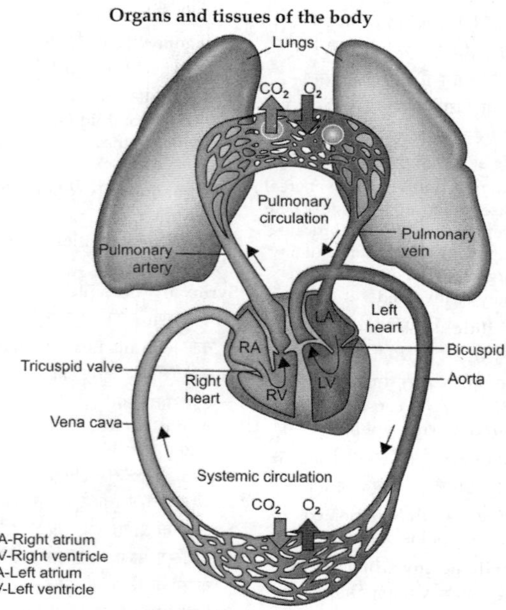

Systemic circulation

Systole (सिस्टोल) हृदय चक्र का वह भाग जिसमें हृदय संकुचित रहता है जो हृदय की प्रथम एवं द्वितीय ध्वनि के बीच के समयावकाश में होता है; प्रकुंचन। The part of the cardiac cycle in which the heart is in contraction which occurs in the interval between first and second heart sound.

Systolic (सिस्टोलिक) प्रकुंचन सम्बन्धी, प्रकुंचीय Pertaining to the systole.

Systremma (सिस्ट्रेमा) टांग की पिण्डली की पेशियों में ऐंठन हो जाना, पेशियों की एक कठोर गाँठ बन जाती है। बॉयटा आना। Cramp in the calf muscles of the leg, the muscles forming a hard knot.

T

Tabes (टेबीज) शरीर अथवा शरीर के किसी भाग का किसी जीर्ण रोग के कारण धीरे-धीरे क्षीण होते जाना, क्षय। A progressive wasting of the body or part of it due to a chronic disease.

Tabetic crisis (टेबीटिक क्राइसिस) सिफिलिस के कारण उत्पन्न होने वाला तीव्र उदर शूल। Acute abdominal pain causing due to Syphilis.

Tabocism (टेबोसिज्म) जीर्ण तम्बाकू विषाक्ता। Tabocaris chronic tobacco.

Tabocosis (टेबोकोसिस) तम्बाकू से उत्पन्न होने वाली विषाक्त अवस्था। Poisoning by tobacco.

Taboo (टेबू) प्रतिबन्धित या निषिद्ध अथवा जो धार्मिक उद्देश्यों के लिए अलग कर दिया गया हो। Restricted or prohibited or set apart for religious purposes.

Tache (टैश) एक रंगीन धब्बा या चकत्ता (चित्ती)। A colored spot or macule.

Tachyarrhythmia (टेकीएरीहद्मिया) सामान्य हृदय गति ताल में किसी प्रकार की अनियमितता हो जाने पर उत्पन्न तीव्र हृदय गति। Rapid heart rate associated with an irregularity in the normal heart rhythm.

Tachycardia (टेकीकार्डिया) हृदय गति का असामान्य रूप से तेज हो जाना, हद्क्षिप्रता, दिल की धड़कन बढ़ जाना। Abnormal rapidity of the heart rate.

Tachylalia (टेकीलेलिया) बोलने में शीघ्रता। Rapidity of speech.

Tachyphrasia (टेकीफ्रेज़िया) बहुत बोलना अथवा जल्दी-जल्दी बोलना। Tachyphasia. Excessive speech or rapid speech.

Tachypnea (टेकीप्निया) अति तीव्र श्वसन, श्वासक्षिप्रता, क्षिप्रश्वसन। Very rapid respiration.

Tactile (टैक्टाइल) स्पर्श सम्बन्धी, स्पर्श द्वारा जिसका ज्ञान होता है। Pertaining to touch perceptible to touch.

Tactometer (टेक्टोमीटर) स्पर्श-संवेदनशीलता को मापने वाला एक यंत्र, स्पर्श ज्ञानमापी। An instrument for measuring sensibility of touch.

Taenia (टीनिया) फीताकृमि, कोई भी पट्टे के समान रचना। Tapeworm, any band like structure.

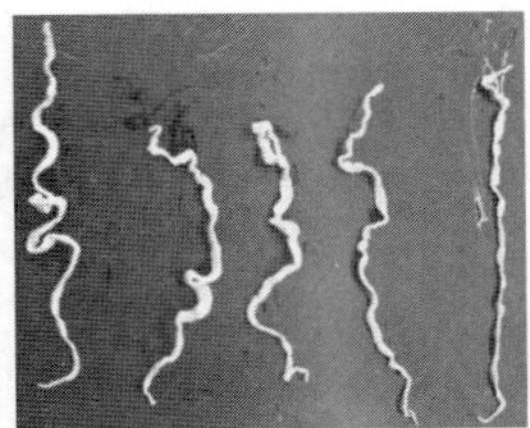

Tag (टैग) एक छोटा पुर्वंगक (पॉलिप) या छोटी वृद्धि। A small polyp or growth.

Talalgia (टैलेल्जिया) टखने या ऐड़ी में दर्द होना। Pain in the heel or ankle.

Talc (टैल्क) साबुन बनाने के लिये प्रयुक्त किए जाने वाले पत्थर का चूर्ण। Powdered Soapstone.

Talipes (टेलीपीज) मुद्गरपाद, पाद की एक जन्मजात विकृति जिसमें पाद अपनी सामान्य स्थिति से विचलित हो जाता है। Clubfoot, a congenital deformity of the foot in which the foot is deviated out of its normal position.

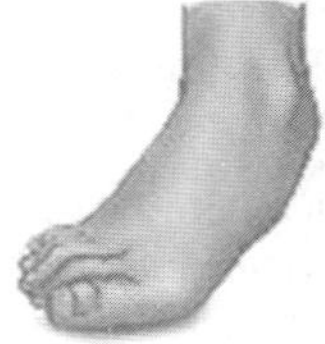

Talipes equinovalgus

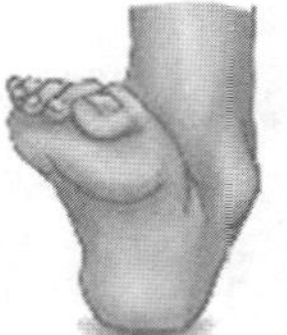

Talipes calcanecvalgus

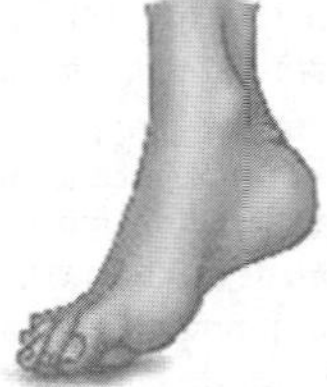

Talipes equinovarus

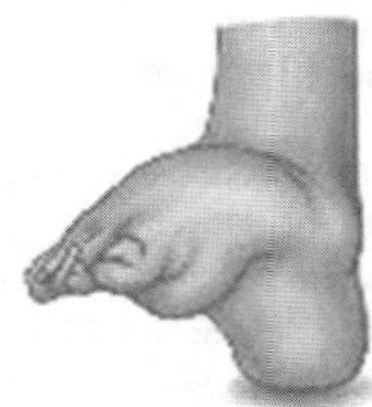

Talipes calcaneocavus

Talocrural (टेलोक्रूरल, टेलस एवं पैर की हड्डी से सम्बन्धित। Pertaining to the talus and leg bones.

Talus (टेलस) टखने की हड्डी, घुटिकास्थि। The second largest bone of the ankle; the astragalus.

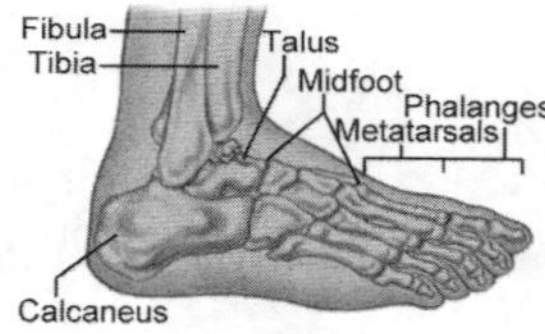

Talus

Tampon (टेम्पन) रक्तस्राव को रोकने के लिये किसी मुलायम कपड़े या रूई की डाट, पिचु। A plug of lint or cotton used for plugging a bleeding orifice.

Tamponade (टेम्पोनेड) शरीर के किसी अंग या हिस्से का विकृतिजन्य स्पीडन, तीव्र स्पीडन। Pathologic compression of an organ or part.

Tantrum (टेनट्रम) आवेश। A fit of bad temper.

Tap (टैप) वेध, वेधन, रेपन। To perform paracentesis.

Tapeworm (टेपवर्म) वर्ग केस्टोडा, संघ प्लेटीहैल्मिन्थीज का एक लम्बा, चपटा, फीते के आकार का आंत्रिक परजीवी जिसमें एक स्कोलेक्स होता है जिस पर आन्त्रीय भित्ति से चिपकने के लिए हुक एवं चूशक लगे होते है तथा खण्डों की एक श्रृंखला होती है, फीताकृमि। A long, flattened, tape-shaped intestinal parasite belonging to the class cestoda phylum platyhelminthes which consist of a scolex with hooks and suckers for attachment to the intestinal wall, and a series of segments.

Taphephobia (टेफीफोबिया) जीवित जमीन मे दफन किए जाने का विकृत भय। Abnormal fear of being buried alive.

Tapinocephaly (टेपिनोसिफैली) खोपड़ी के शिखर का चपटा होना। Flatness of top of the skull.

Tapping (टैपिंग) द्रवनिष्कासन शोफ में पानी बाहर निकालने के लिए किया जाने वाला ऑपरेशन। The operation for drawing off the effused fluid or water in dropsy.

Tar (टैर) तारकोल, अलकतरा, बिरोजा। A viscous mass obtained from the distillation of pine wood.

Target cell (टार्गेट सैल) एक लाल रक्त कोशिका जिसमें एक गोल गाढ़ा केन्द्रीय क्षेत्र होता है जो चारों ओर से एक हल्के छल्ले से घिरा होता है। A red blood cell with a rounded dense central area surrounded by a light ring.

Tarsal (टार्सल) नेत्रच्छदपट्टिका या टखने से सम्बन्धित। Pertaining to the tarsus of eyelid or to the ankle.

Tarsitis (टार्साइटिस) 1. नेत्रच्छदपट्टिका का शोथ, वर्त्मान्तशोथ। 2. पदकूर्च या गुल्फ

का शोथ। 1. Inflammation of the tarsal border of an eyelid. 2. Inflammation of the tarsus of the foot.

Tarsomalacia (टॉर्सोमैलेशिया) किसी नेत्रच्छदपट्टिका का कोमल हो जाना। Softening of the tarsus of an eyelid.

Tarsometatarsal (टार्सोमेटाटार्सल) गुल्फ एवं प्रपदिका से सम्बन्धित, पदकूर्चप्रपदिक। Pertaining to the tarsus and metatarsus.

Tarsorrhaphy (टार्सोरैह्फी) नेत्रच्छद-विदर को कम करने अथवा इसे पूर्णतया बन्द करने के लिए आँख की ऊपरी एवं निचली पलकों के किनारों को सीना, वर्त्मसीवन। Suture of the margins of upper and lower eyelids together to reduce or entirely close the palpebral fissure.

Tarsus (टार्सस) पदकूर्च, गुल्फ, नेत्रच्छदपट्टिका, वर्त्मपट्टिका, वर्त्मगुल्फ, पलकों की उपास्थि। Instep, cartilages of the eyelid.

Taste (टेस्ट) स्वाद। The peculiar sensation caused by contact of substances with the tongue.

Taste buds (टेस्ट बड्स) जिह्वा की सतह, कोमल तालु, कण्डच्छद तथा ग्रसनी के कुछ भाग में स्थित अण्डाकार रचनाएँ–स्वाद कलिकाएँ जिनमें संवेदी एवं स्वाद कोशिकाएँ होती है। उद्दीप्त होने पर ये स्वाद के संवेदी को उत्पन्न करती है। Oval structures situated on the surface of the tongue, soft palate, epiglottis and some portion of the pharynx containing sensory and taste cells. On stimulation they give rise to sense of taste.

Taxis (टैक्सिस) किसी जीव की किसी उद्दीपन के प्रति अनुक्रिया, उसकी उद्दीपक की ओर गति करना अथवा उद्दीपन से दूर जाना अनुक्रिया होती है, अनुचालन। The response of an organism to a stimuli, moving towards or away from the stimulus.

Taxonomy (टैक्सोनॉमी) जीवधारियों के वर्गीकरण से सम्बन्धित विज्ञान, वर्गिकी, वर्गीकरण। The branch of science dealing with the classification of organisms.

T-cells (टी-सैल्स) लसीका कोशिकायें जो थाइमस ग्रन्थि में परिपक्व होती है, टी कोशिकायें कहलाती है। जब ये रक्त परिसंचरण में प्रवेश कर जाती हैं तो एण्टीबॉडी बनाने वाली कोशिकाओं के उत्पादन को बढ़ा कर विलम्ब से रोगक्षमता उत्पन्न करती है। Lymphocytes which mature in the thymus gland are called T cells. When they enter the blood circulation they produce delayed immunity by enhancing the production of antibody forming cells.

Tears (टीयर्स) अश्रु, आँसू। The drops of fluid secreted by the lacrimal glands.

Teaspoon (टीस्पून) आयतन की एक घरेलू इकाई जो लगभग 5 मिलीलीटर के बराबर होती है। A household unit of volume which is equal to approximately 5 milliliters.

Teat (टीट) स्तन-ग्रन्थि का चूचुक अथवा चुचूक के समान कोई कोई भी उभार। Nipple of the mammary gland or any protuberance resembling a nipple.

Technology (टैक्नोलॉजी) तकनीकी-विज्ञान, प्रौद्योगिकी। The science of techniques.

Tectorium (टैक्टोरियम) आवरण, छद। An overlaying structure.

Tectum (टैक्टम) 1. छत के समान कोई भी संरचना। 2. मध्यमस्तिष्क का पृष्ठीय भाग। 1. Any roof like structure. 2. The dorsal portion of the midbrain.

Teeth (टीथ) प्रत्येक जबड़े से निकलने वाले चबाने का कार्य करने वाले अंग, दाँत, दन्त। Organs of mastication projecting from each other.

(*i*) **Desiduous Teeth** (डेसीड्यूयस टीथ) अस्थायी दाँत, दूध के दाँत। Temporary teeth milk-teeth.

(*ii*) **Incisor Teeth** (इन्सीज़र टीथ) कृन्तक दन्त। Having knife like edge for biting food.

(*iii*) **Wisdom Teeth** (विस्डम टीथ) कृन्तक दन्त। Having knife-like edge for biting food.

Tegmen (टेग्मेन) शरीर के किसी भाग को ढकने वाली रचना अथवा छत छद। A structure that covers a part of the body, or roof.

Tegmentum (टेग्मेन्टम) मध्य-मस्तिष्क का पृष्ठीय भाग। Dorsal portion of the midbrain.

Tegument (टेगुमेन्ट) त्वचा या शरीर का आवरण। The skin or the covering of the body.

Tela (टेला) जाली के समान कोई भी ऊतक अथवा रचना। Any weblike tissue or structure.

Telangiectasia (टीलैन्जियेक्टेसिया) रक्त कोशिकाओं अथवा सूक्ष्म रक्त वाहिनियों के एक समूह का विस्फारण, वाहिकास्फीति। Dilatation of a group of blood capillaries or small blood vessels.

Teleangitis (टीलैन्जाइटिस) केशिकाओं का शोथ। Inflammation of the capillaries.

Telecardiography (टेलीकार्डियोग्राफी) टेलीकार्डियोग्राम लेने की क्रिया। Process of taking telecardiogram.

Telediagnosis (टेलीडायग्नोसिस) इलैक्ट्रोनिक विधि से चिकित्सक को संचारित होने वाली आंकड़ों के आधार पर रोगी से दूर किसी स्थान पर रह कर उसके रोग का निदान करना। To make the diagnosis of a disease at a place distant from the patient, on the basis of data transmitted electronically to the physician.

Telekinesis (टेलीकाइनेसिस) बिना स्पर्श किये किसी वस्तु को इच्छानुसार चला देना, अस्पर्श। To move an object according to the will without touching.

Telemetry (टेलीमीट्री) अपने से दूर स्थित किसी वस्तु की माप लेना जिसके आँकड़े इलैक्ट्रॉनिक विधि से संचारित हो जाते है। The making of measurements of a distant object, the data being transmitted electronically.

Telencephalon (टेलीन्सिफेलॉन) भ्रूणीय अन्तमस्तिष्क, उन्ममस्तिष्क। The embryonic endbrain.

Teleopsia (टेलीऑप्सिया) एक दृष्टि-दोष जिसमें वस्तुये वास्तव में जितनी दूरी पर होती है, उससे दूर नजर आती है। A visual defect in which object appears to be farther away than they actually are.

Telepathy (टेलीपैथी) संवेदी अंगों अथवा भौतिक साधनों का प्रयोग किए बिना एक व्यक्ति के विचारों का दूर स्थित दूसरे व्यक्ति के मस्तिष्क में पहुँच जाना। The transmission of thoughts of one person to the mind of another person at a distance without use of sensory organs or physical agents.

Telescope (टेलीस्कोप) दूर-दर्शक यंत्र। An optical instrument for viewing distant objects.

Telophase (टीलोफेज) सूत्री विभाजन की अन्तिम प्रावस्था, सूत्री विभाजन अन्तावस्था। The last phase of mitosis.

Temper (टैम्पर) किसी व्यक्ति की चित्तवृत्ति की दशा। State of one's mood.

Temperament (टेम्पर मेंट) प्रकृति, स्वभाव अथवा मिजाज। Nature, disposition or mental state.

Temperate (टेम्पेरट) मामूली, संयमी, शांत। Moderate, self restrained, calm.

Temperature (टैम्प्रेचर) ऊष्णता का अंश, तापमान। Degree of hotness. (*i*) **Ambient Temperature** (एम्बिएन्ट टैम्प्रेचर) वातावरण अथवा किसी स्थान का तापमान। Temperature of the environment or of a place. (*ii*) **Normal Temperature** (नॉर्मल टैम्प्रेचर) एक स्वस्थ्य मनुष्य के शरीर का मुख से लिया गया तापमान जो 98.6°फे. (37°से) होता है। Temperature of the body of a healthy person taken orally which is 98.6°F (37°C). (*iii*) **Rectal Temperature** (रैक्टल टैम्प्रेचर) थर्मामीटर को गुदीय नली में घुसा कर लिया गया तापमान। Temperature taken by inserting a thermometer into the anal canal.

Temple (टैम्पल) सिर के प्रत्येक ओर कान के समान तथा गण्डास्थिक चाप के ऊपर का क्षेत्र, कर्णपटी, शंख। The region of the head on each side in front of the ear and over the zygomatic arch.

Temporal (टैम्पोरल) समय से सम्बन्धित अथवा समय में सीमित। Related to or limited in time.

Temporomaxillary (टेम्पोरोमैक्जिलरी) टैम्पोरल एवं मैक्टिला हड्डी से सम्बन्धित। Pertaining to the temporal and maxillary bones.

Temporoparietal (टैम्पोरोपैराइटल) टेम्पोरल एवं पैराइटल हड्डी से सम्बन्धित। Pertaining to the temporal and the parietal bones.

Tenacious (टिनेशियस) चिपचिपा, आष्लेशी, तन्य। Adhesive.

Tenacity (टिनेसिटी) चिपचिपाहट, तन्यता। Adhesiveness.

Tenaculum (टेनाकुलम) किसी भाग जैसे किसी धमनी को पकड़ने एवं थामें रखने के लिए हुक के समान, नुकीला शल्यक्रिया सम्बन्धी यंत्र। Hook like, pointed surgical instrument for grasping and holding a part, as an artery.

Tenderness (टैन्डरनैस) स्पर्श अथवा दाब के प्रति संवेदनशीलता स्पर्शसहता, दाब-वेदना। Sensitiveness to touch or pressure.

Tendinitis (टैन्डीनाइटिस) कण्डाराशोथ, कण्डरा-प्रदाह। Inflammation of the tendon; tendonitis.

Tendon (टैण्डन) कण्डरा। तन्तुमय संयोजी ऊतक की एक रज्जु जो पेशी में विलीन हो जाती है तथा उसे किसी हड्डी या अन्य भागों से संलग्न करती है। A cord of fibrous connective tissue continuous with the muscle and attaching it to a bone or other parts.

Tendon reflex (टैण्डन रिफ्लैक्स) किसी पेशी के कण्डरा का परिताड़न करने पर पेशी का संकुचित होना। Contraction of a muscle on percussion of its tendon.

Tenesmus (टिनेस्मस) मलद्वारा अथवा मूत्राशयी संवरणी का ऐंठन युक्त संकुचन जिसमें दर्द होता है तथा मल-त्याग या मूत्रण के लिए जोर लगाना पड़ता है जिसका कोई असर नहीं होता, स्पीडन कुंथन। Spasmodic contraction of anal or vesical sphincter with pain and ineffectual straining at defecation or urination.

Tenifuge (टेनीफ्यूज) फीताकृमियों को बाहर निकालने वाला। That which expels tapeworms.

Tennis elbow (टेनिस एल्बो) सामान्यतया टेनिस खेलने में जोर पड़ने पर उत्पन्न एक रोग जिसमें ह्मेरस हड्डी के पार्श्वीय अधिस्थूलक पर दर्द होता है जो बाहु तथा अग्रबाहु के बाहर की ओर फैल जाता है एक कलाई के अभिपृष्ठ-आंकुचन और उत्तानन (सीधा करने) से बढ़ जाती है तथा वस्तुओं को पकड़ने में कठिनाई होती है। A condition usually coused by strain in playing tennis, characterized by pain over lateral epicondyle of the humerus bone radiating to outer side of the arm and forearm and aggravated by dorsiflexion and supination of the wrist. There is weakness of the wrist and difficulty in grasping object.

Tenodynia (टीनोडाइनिया) किसी कण्डरा में दर्द होना, कण्डरार्ति। Tenalgia. Pain in a tendon.

Tenomyotomy (टीनोनायोटॉमी) किसी कण्डरा एवं पेशी के किसी भाग को काट कर निकाल देना। Excision of a portion of a tendon and muscle.

Tenon's Capsule (टेनन्स कैप्सूल) नेत्रश्लेष्मा के पीछे नेत्रगोलक का एक पतला संयोजी ऊतक का आवरण। A thin connective tissue covering of the eyeball behind the conjunctive.

Tenorrhaphy (टीनोरैड्फी) किसी कण्डरा को सीना, कण्डरासीवन। Suture of a tendon.

Tenosynovectomy (टीनोसाइनोवेक्टॉमी) किसी कण्डरा-आच्छद को शल्यक्रिया द्वारा काट कर अलग कर देना। Excision of a tendon sheath.

Tenosynovities (टीनोसाइनोवाइटिस) किसी कण्डरा आच्छद की सूजन, कण्डराशोथ। Inflammation of a tendon sheath.

Tenotome (टीनोटोम) किसी कण्डरा को आर-पार काटने के लिए एक यंत्र। An instrument for making across section of a tendon.

Tenotomy (टीनोटॉमी) शल्यक्रिया द्वारा कण्डरा को काटना कण्डराच्छेदन। Surgical section of a tendon.

Tension (टैन्शन) खींचने की क्रिया अथवा खिंचा होना। मानसिक दाब, तनाव। The act of stretching or the condition of being stretched. Mental stress.

Tensor (टेन्सर) कोई भी पेशी जो किसी भाग को तनावयुक्त बनाती है, तानिका। Any muscle that makes a part tense.

Tentacle (टेन्टाकल) भोजन ग्रहण करने, परिग्रहण अथवा चलने-फिरने के लिए अपवृष्टवंशियों में पाया जाने वाला एक लम्बा तथा पलता प्रवध। A slender process in invertebrates for feeding, prehension or locomotion.

Tentorium cerebella (टेन्टोरियम-सेरीबेला) प्रमस्तिष्क एवं अनुमस्तिष्क के बीच पश्चकपालीय खण्ड़ों को सहारा देने वाला दृढ़तानिका का प्रवर्ध, अनुमस्तिष्क छदि। The process of dura mater between the cerebrum and cerebellum supporting the occipital lobes.

Tepid (टेपिड) हल्का गर्म, गुनगुना। Slightly warm; lukewarm.

Teras (टेरास) विकृत भ्रूण, दैत्य। Deformed fetus, a monster.

Teratoblastoma (टेराटोब्लास्टोमा) एक अबुर्द जिसमें भ्रूणीय पदार्थ होता है जो तीनों जनन स्तरों को प्रस्तुत नहीं करता। A tumor containing embryonic material that does not represent all three germinal layers.

Teratocarcinoma (टेराटोकार्सिनोमा) अपरूपार्बुद या टेराटोमा की उपकला-कोशिकाओं से उत्पन्न होने वाला कैन्सर। A carcinoma developing from the epithelial cells of a teratoma.

Teratogen (टेराटोजन) अपरूपजनन उत्पन्न करने वाली कोई भी वस्तु, अपरूपजनन। Anything that causes teratogenesis.

Teratogenicity (टेराटोजेनिसिटी) कुरचना उत्पन्न करने का गुण अथवा ऐसा करने की क्षमता। The property or capability of producing malformation.

Teratology (टेराटोलॉजी) अपरूपविज्ञान, विरूपविज्ञान। Scientific study of teratogens and their mode of action.

Teratoma (टेराटोमा) कोई संकर अथवा जन्मजात अबुर्द, अपारूपार्बुद। A complex or congenital tumor, teratoblastoma.

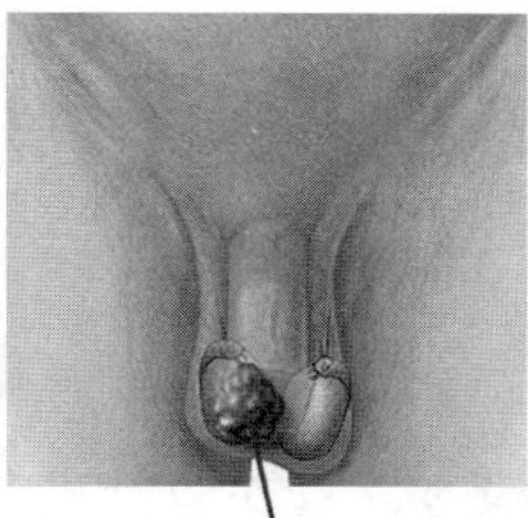

Malignant teratoma

Teratosis (टेराटोसिस) विकृत भ्रूण का होना। The condition of being a deformed fetus.

Teres (टेरिस) बेलनाकार, सिलिंड्राकार। Round and long; cylindrical.

Tergal (टर्गल) पीठ अथवा पृष्ठीय सतह से सम्बन्धित। Pertaining to the back or dorsal surface.

Terminal (टर्मिनल) अन्त्य, अन्तस्थ, सीमान्त, अन्तिम। Towards the extremity or terminus; endings final.

Terminal illness (टर्मिनल इलनैस) ऐसी बीमारी जिससे रोगी की मृत्यु हो जाती है। An illness which causes the patient to die.

Terminology (टर्मिनोलॉजी) नामवाली। Nomenclature.

Tertiary (टर्शियरी) क्रम अथवा अवस्था में तीसरा जैसे तृतीयक सिफिलिस। Third in order or stage as tertiary syphilis.

Tertion (टर्षियन) प्रत्येक तीसरे दिन होने वाला, ऐसा सामान्यतया मलेरिया ज्वर के लिए कहा जाता है, तृतीयक।
Accruing every third day usually said of malaria fever.

Test (टैस्ट) परीक्षण, जांच। An examination or trial.

Testa (टैस्टा) छिलका। A shell.

Testis (टेस्टिस) वृषण या अण्डकोश के भीतर स्थित पुरूष की दो जनन ग्रन्थियों में से एक जिसमें वीर्य एवं पुरूष लिंग हार्मोन–टेस्टोस्टरोन उत्पन्न होता है, शुक्रग्रन्थि। One of the two reproductive glands of male contained in the scrotum that produces semen and male sex hormones—testosterone.

Test meal (टैस्ट मील) आमाशय की सामग्रियों के रासायनिक विश्लेषण या आमाशय के रोगों के एक्स-रे निदान के लिए रोगी को दिया जाने वाला एक थोड़ा तथा निश्चित मात्रा एवं संघटन का आहार, परीक्षणाहार।
A small meal of definite quantity and composition given to the patient for chemical analysis of the stomach contents or X-ray diagnosis of the stomach diseases.

Testosterone (टेस्टोस्टेरोन) शुक्रग्रन्थियों से उत्पन्न एक

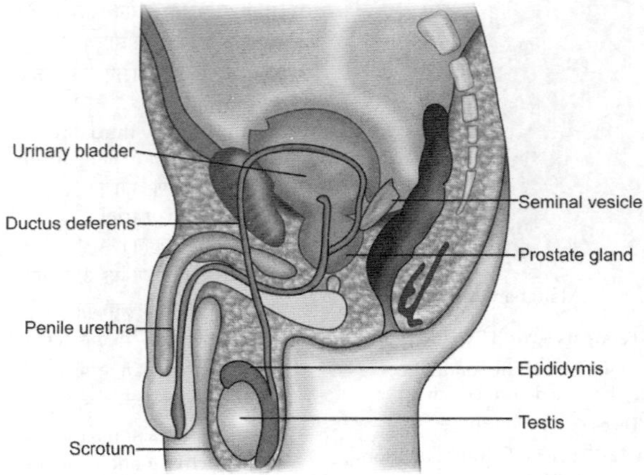

Testis

पुरूष लिंग हार्मोन। A male sex hormone produced by the testes.

Test tube baby (टैस्ट ट्यूब बेबी) ऐसी माँ से पैदा होने वाला बच्चा जिसके डिम्ब को अलग कर किसी टैस्ट ट्यूब (परीक्षण नली) में गर्भित किया जाता है तथा फिर इसे उसके गर्भाशय में आरोपित कर दिया जाता है। A baby born to a mother whose ovum was removed, fertilized in test tube, and then implanted in her uterus.

Tetanic (टिटेनिक) टिटेनस से सम्बन्धित अथवा उसे उत्पन्न करने वाला, धनुस्तम्भी। Pertaining to or producing tetanus.

Tetanospasmin (टिटेनोस्पाजमिन) टिटेनस को उत्पन्न करने वाले बेसीलस क्लॉस्ट्रीडियम टिटेनाइ के द्वारा उत्पन्न जीवविष का तन्त्रिका विषाक्त घटक जिससे टिटेनस में आपेक्ष आते है। The neurotoxin component of the toxin produced by clostridium tetani, the causative bacillus of tetanus which causes convulsions in tetanus.

Tetanus (टिटेनस) किसी जख्म से शरीर में प्रवेश करने वाले टिटेनस बेसीलस कलास्ट्रीडियम टिटेनाइ के तंत्रिकाप्रेरक जीवविष द्वारा उत्पन्न एक तीव्र संक्रामक रोग जो अधिकतर प्राणघातक होता है। An acute infectious disease, often fatal caused by neurotoxin of tetanus bacillus clostridium tetani, entering the body through a wound.

(*i*) **Anticus tetanus** (एन्टीकस टिटेनस) टिटेनस जिसमें शरीर पीछे को मुड़ जाता है। Tetanus in which the body is bent backward.

(*ii*) **Local tetanus** (लोकल टिटेनस) टिटेनस जिसमें जख्म के पास कुछ पेशियों में ऐंठन हो जाती है। Tetanus characterized by spasm of certain muscles near the wound. (*iii*) **Puerperal tetanus** (प्यूरपीरल टिटेनस) बच्चा पैदा होने के पश्चात् होने वाली टिटेनस। Tetanus occurring following childbirth.

Tetanus antitoxin (टिटेनस एण्टिटॉक्सिन) टिटेनस बेसीलस क्लॉस्ट्रीडियम टिटेनाइ के संक्रमण के परिणामस्वरूप अथवा टिटेनस टॉक्सिन या टॉक्सॉयड के संरोपण (टीका लगाने) से रक्त में उत्पन्न होने वाली एक एण्टीबॉडी। An antibody that develops in the blood as a result of infection by the tetanus bacillus. Clostridium tetani or inoculation with tetanus toxin or toxoid.

Tetanus toxoid (टिटेनस टाक्सॉयड) यह टिटेनस टॉक्सिन होता है जिसे रूपान्तरित कर देया जाता है जिससे इसकी विषाक्तता बहुत कम हो जाती है परन्तु इसकी सक्रिय रोगक्षमता उत्पन्न करने की क्षमता नहीं बदलती। It is tetanus toxin which is modified so that its toxicity is greatly reduced but its capacity to produce anti-immunity is not changed.

Tetany (टेटेनी), माँसपेशियों की अत्यधिक उत्तेजित अवस्था, अपतानिका, माँसपेशियों की अकडन। Condition of muscular hyper excitability in which mild stimuli produce cramps and spasms.

Tetrabrachius (टैट्राब्रेकियस) विकृत भ्रूण जिसके चार बाहें होती है। A deformed fetus having four arms.

Tetrad (टैट्रॉड) चार वस्तुओं का एक समूह, चतुष्क। A group of four things.

Tetradactyly (टैट्राडैक्टाइली) किसी हाथ अथवा पॉव में चार अंगुलियों का पाया जाना। The presence of four digits on a hand or foot.

Tetralogy (टैट्रालोगी) चार लक्षणों अथवा तत्वों का संयोजन, चतुष्क। The combination of four symptoms or elements.

Tetramastous (टैट्रामैस्टस) चार स्तनों से युक्त। Having four breasts.

Tetraplegia (टैट्राप्लीजिया) चतुरांगधात। Quadriplegia.

Tetrascelus (टेट्रास्केलस) ऐसा विकृत भ्रूण जिसके चार टाँगे होती है।
A deformed fetus with four legs.

Textiform (टैक्सटीफोर्म) जाल के समान बना हुआ। Formed like a network.

Thalamocele (थैलेमोसील) मस्तिष्क का तीसरा निलय।
The third ventricle of the brain.

Thalamotomy (थैलेमोटॉमी) चेतक के किसी भाग को शल्य कर्म द्वारा नष्ट करना। Surgical destruction of a portion of thalamus.

Thalamus (थैलेमस) अधश्चेतक एवं अधिचेतक बीच आन्तर अग्रमस्तिष्क का सबसे बड़ा भाग जो मस्तिष्क के तीसरे निलय की पार्श्वीय प्राचीर के एक भाग को बनता है। गन्ध, दृष्टि तथा श्रवण। Largest part of diencephalon, lying between hypothalamus and epithalamium, forming a portion of the lateral wall of 3rd ventricle of the brain. All sensory impulses except olfactory, visual and auditory impulses are received by the thalamus and relayed to the cerebral cortex.

Thalassemia (थैलासीमिया) एक आनुवांशिक रक्तसंलायी।
A hereditary hemolytic anemia.

Thalassotherapy (थैलासोथिरैपी) समुद्री जल द्वारा रोगों की चिकित्सा करना।
Treatment of the disease by sea-water.

Thanatology (थैनेटोलॉजी) मृत्यु विज्ञान।
The science of death.

Thanatophobia (थैनेटोफोबिया) मृत्युभिति, मौत का डर।
Fear of death.

Theca (थीका) एक आच्छद, आवरण या खोल जैसे हृदय को ढकने वाला हृदयावरण या पैरीकार्डियम, पिधान। A sheath or case, as pericardium covering the heart.

Thecitis (थीकाइटिस) किसी कण्डरा के आवरण का शोथ।

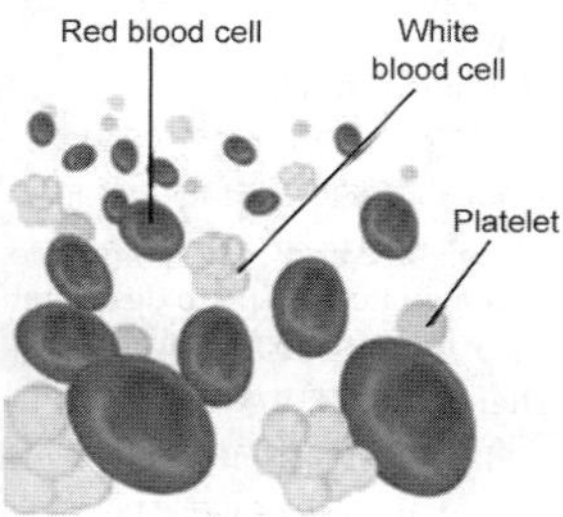

Normal

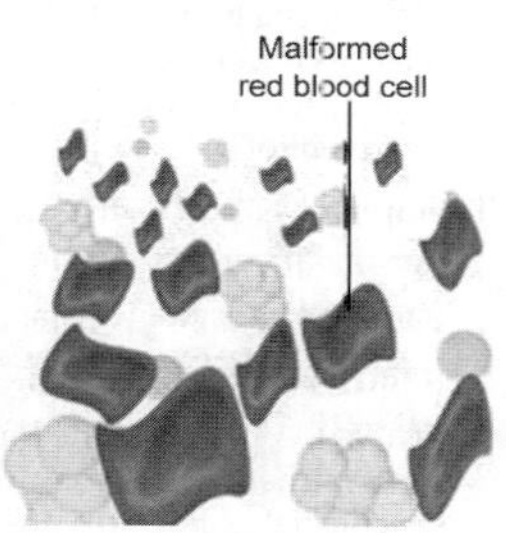

Thalassemia

Inflammation of the sheath of a tendon.

Thecoma (थीकोमा) डिम्बग्रन्थि का अबुर्द। A tumor of the ovary.

Thelalgia (थीलैल्जिया) चूचुकों में दर्द होना, चूचुकवेदना। Pain in the nipples.

Thelarche (थीलार्के) यौवनारम्भ पर स्तनों के विकास का आरम्भ होना। The beginning of development of breasts at puberty.

Theloncus (थीलोन्कस) चूचुक का अबुर्द। A tumor of a nipple.

Thelygenic (थीलाइजेनिक) केवल स्त्री सन्तान उत्पन्न करने वाली। Producing only female offspring.

Thenar (थीनर) 1. हाथ की हथेली अथवा पैर का तलवा। 2. अंगूठे के आधार पर हाथ का मांसल भाग। 1. Palm of the hand or sole of the foot. 2. Rounded fleshy part of the base of the thumb.

Theomania (थियोमैनिया) धार्मिक उन्माद। Religious mania.

Theory (थियोरी) एक कल्पना अथवा अनुमान जो सार्वजनिक रूप से स्वीकृत हो जाने पर सिद्धान्त बन जाता है। A supposition or assumption which becomes principle when generally accepted.

Therapeutic (थिराप्यूटिक) रोग निवारक। A curative.

Therapeutics (थिराप्यूटिक्स) चिकित्सा-विज्ञान की वह शाखा जिसका सम्बन्ध औषधियों अथवा उपायों का प्रयोग करने तथा रोगों की चिकित्सा से है, उपचार-

विज्ञान। The branch of medical science concerned with the application of remedies and treatment of disease.

Therapist (थिरापिस्ट) स्वास्थ्य रक्षा के विशिष्ट क्षेत्र में रोगों की चिकित्सा करने में कुशल व्यक्ति जैसे भौतिक चिकित्सा-विशेषज्ञ। A person skilled in the treatment of diseases in a specific field of health care, as physiotherapist.

Therapy (थिरैपी) किसी रोग अथवा विकृतिजनक अवस्था की चिकित्सा। Treatment of a disease or pathological condition.

Thermalgesia (थर्मेल्जैसिया) गर्मी से होने वाला दर्द, तापवेदना। Pain caused by heat.

Thermic (थर्मिक) ऊष्मा सम्बन्धी, तापीय। Pertaining to heat.

Thermoanesthesia (थर्मोएनीस्थीजिया) गर्मी एवं ठण्ड को पहचानने में असमर्थता, तापसंवेदनाभाव। Thermanesthesia, inability to recognize heat and cold.

Thermobiotic (थर्मोबायोटिक) उच्च तापमान पर जीवित रहने के सक्षम। Able to exist at high temperature.

Thermocautery (थर्मोकॉटरी) गर्म किये गए तार से दहन करना। Cauterization by a heated wire.

Thermocoagulation (थर्मोकोगुलेशन) ऊतक को नष्ट करने के लिए उच्च-बारम्बारता वाली धाराओं से इसे जमाना। To coagulate a tissue to destroy it by high-frequency currents.

Thermode (थर्मोड) शरीर के किसी भाग को गर्म अथवा ठण्डा करने वाला एक उपकरण। An apparatus for heating or cooling a part of the body.

Thermoelectric (थर्मोइलैक्ट्रिक) ऊष्मा द्वारा उत्पन्न विद्युत। Electricity generated by heat.

Thermogenesis (थर्मोजेनेसिस) ऊष्मा की उत्पत्ति, विशेषकर शरीर में, तापजनन। The production of heat, especially in the body.

Thermography (थर्मोग्राफी) शरीर के तापमान परिवर्तनों का तापलेखी द्वारा रेखाचित्र–अभिलेखन करना, तापलेखन। The graphic recording of temperature variations of the body by thermograph.

Thermolabile (थर्मोलेबाइल) जो गर्मी से आसानी से परिवर्तित अथवा नष्ट हो जाता हो, तापपरिवर्ती। Changed or destroyed easily by heat.

Thermometer (थर्मामीटर) तापमान का पता लगाने वाला एक यंत्र,

तापमापी। An instrument for determining the temperature.

Thermometry (थर्मामीटरी) तापमान को मापना। Measurement of temperatures.

Thermophilic (थर्मोफिलीक) तापरागी। Requiring great heat for growth.

Thermophobia (थर्मोफोबिया) गर्मी का विकृत भय। Morbid fear of heat.

Thermoplegia (थर्मोप्लीजिया) तापघात। Heat-stroke.

Thermoregulation (थर्मोरेगुलेषन) ऊष्मा-नियमन, तापनियमन। Heat regulation.

Thermostat (थर्मोस्टेट) स्वतः तापमान को नियमित करने वाला उपकरण, ताप-नियंत्रक। An apparatus regulating the temperature automatically.

Thermotaxis (थर्मोटैक्सिस) तापानुचलन। Regulation of the temperature of the body.

Thermotoxin (थर्मोटॉक्सिन) अत्यधिक गर्मी से ऊतकों में उत्पन्न होने वाला एक विष। A poison formed in the tissue due to excessive heat.

Thiersch's Graft (थीरषेज़ ग्राफ्ट) त्वचा निरोपण की एक विधि जिसमें बाह्यत्वचा को एवं अन्तस्त्वचा के एक भाग को प्रयोग में लाया जाता है। A method of skin grafting in which the epidermis and portion of dermis is used.

Thigmesthesia (थिग्मेस्थीजिया) स्पर्श के प्रति सूक्ष्मग्रहिता या संवेदनशीलता। Sensitivity to touch.

Thinking (थिंकिंग) सोचना, विचारना। To consider.

Thirst (थर्स्ट) प्यास। A desire for drink.

Thomas Splint (थोमास स्पलिन्ट) कूल्हे पर एक छल्ले से आरम्भ होकर पाँव के तार तक फैली एक कमची या कुशा जिससे टूटी हुई टांग के लम्ब अक्ष में उस पर खिंचाव उत्पन्न होता है। A splint extending from a ring at the hip to beyond the foot, allowing traction on a fractured leg, in its long axis.

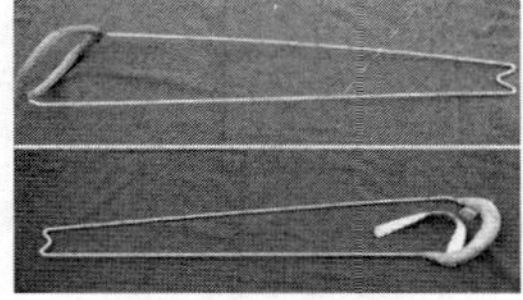

Thomson's disease (थॉमसन डिज़ीज) पेशीतानता, थामसन रोग। Congenital myotonia.

Thoracentesis (थोरेसेन्टेसिस) वक्षवेधन। Puncture of chest wall to drain out pleural fluids.

Thoracic cage (थोरैसिक केज) वक्ष को चारों ओर से घेरने वाली अस्थिल रचना। The bony structure surrounding the thorax.

Thoracocentesis (थोरैकोसेन्टेसिस) सुई का प्रयोग करके वक्ष-गुहा से तरल का चूषण करने के लिए शल्यक्रिया द्वारा वक्ष भित्ति का छेदन करना, वक्षवेधन। Surgical puncture of the chest wall for aspiration of fluid from the thoracic cavity, by using a needle.

Thoracolumbar (थोरैकोलम्बर) वक्ष एवं कटि-कशेरूकाओं से सम्बन्धित। Pertaining to the thorax and the lumbar vertebrae.

Thoracomyodynia (थोरैकोमायोडाइनिया) छाती की पेशियों में दर्द होना। Pain in the muscles of the chest.

Thoracoplasty (थौरैकोप्लास्टी) पसलियों के भागों को शल्यक्रिया द्वारा काट कर निकाल देना जिससे वक्ष की प्राचीर रोगग्रस्त फेफड़े को पिचका सके, वक्षसंधान। Surgical removal of portions of the ribs, so that the chest wall may collapse a diseased lung.

Thoracoscopy (थोरैकोस्कोपी) वक्षदर्शी द्वारा फुफ्फुसावरणी गुहा का निरीक्षण करना, वक्षदर्शन। Inspection of the pleural cavity with a thoracoscope.

Thoracostomy (थोरैकॉस्टॉमी) वक्ष भित्ति में चीरा लगाना जिसमें छिद्र को निकासी के लिए कायम रखा जाता है। To make an incision in the chest wall, with maintenance of the opening for drainage.

Thorax (थोरैक्स) शरीर में गर्दन के आधार एवं मध्यपट या डायफ्राम के बीच का भाग जो पसलियों से घिरा होता है, वक्ष, उर। Chest part of the body between base of the neck and the diaphragm, surrounded by ribs.

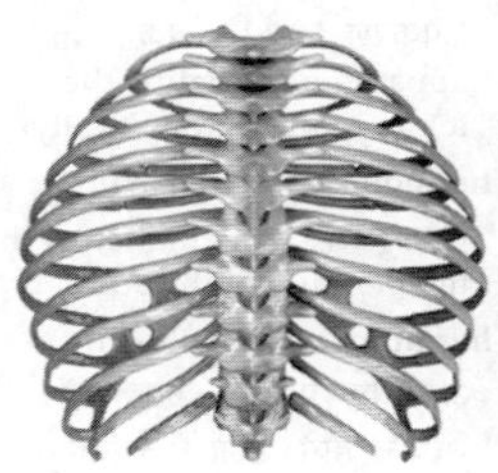

Threadworm (थ्रेडवर्म) धागे के समान, लम्बा एवं पतला आँत में रहने वाला कीड़ा, सूत्रकृमि। Enterobius vermicularis, pinworm. A threadlike, long and thin intestinal worm.

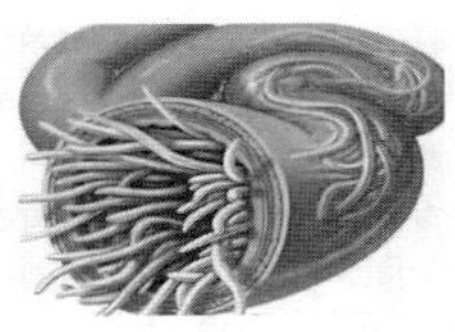

Threadworm

Threshold (थ्रीशोल्ड) प्रभावसीमा। वह बिन्दु जिस पर कोई प्रभाव उत्पन्न होना शुरू होता है। The point at which an effect begins to be produced.

Threshold dose (थ्रीशोल्ड डोज़) न्यूनतम मात्रा जिससे रोगी पर कोई प्रभाव होता है। Minimum dose that will produce an effect on the patient.

Thrill (थ्रिल) परिस्पर्शन द्वारा अनुभव किया जाने वाला कम्पन्न। Fremitus, a vibration felt on palpation.

Thrix (थ्रिक्स) बाल, केश, रोम। Hair.

Throat (थ्रोट) ग्रसनी एवं गलतोरणिका, कण्ठ। The pharynx and the fauces.

Throbbing (थ्रॉबिंग) धड़कने वाला, प्रस्पन्द। Pulsating or beating.

Thrombectomy (थ्रोम्बेक्टॉमी) किसी रक्त वाहिनी से शल्यक्रिया द्वारा थक्के को बाहर निकाल देना, घनास्त्रनिष्कासन। Surgical removal of a clot from a blood vessel.

Thrombin (थ्रॉम्बिन) थ्रॉम्बिन रक्त प्लाज्मा में विद्यमान एक पदार्थ होता है। An enzyme derived from prothrombin by action of thromboplastin.

Thromboangitis (थ्रोम्बोएन्जाइटिस) किसी रक्त वाहिनी के भीतरी स्तर की सूजन जिसके साथ रक्त का थक्का बन जाता है। Inflammation of the inner coat of a blood vessels with the formation of blood clot.

Thrombocyst (थ्रॉम्बोसिस्ट) किसी घनास्त्र या थ्रॉम्बस के चारों ओर बनने वाला झिल्लीनुमा कोश (थैली)। A membranous sac formed around a thrombus.

Thrombocythemia (थ्रोम्बोसाइथीमिया) रक्त में प्लेटलेटों की संख्या बढ़ जाना, बिम्बाणु–बहुलता। An increase in number of platelets in the blood.

Thrombocytopenia (थ्रोम्बोसाइटोपीनिया) बिम्बाणुओं की कमी। Decrease below normal in number or platelets.

Thrombocytosis (थ्रोम्बोसाइटोसिस) बिम्बाणुओं की बहुलता। An increase in the number of platelets in the blood.

Thromboembolectomy (थ्रोम्बोएम्बोलैक्टॉमी) शल्यक्रिया

द्वारा किसी अन्तःशल्यीय घनास्त्र को निकाल देना। Excision of an embolic thrombus.

Thromboembolism (थ्रोम्बोएम्बोलिज्म) किसी रक्त वाहिनी का किसी ऐसे घनास्त्र या थ्रॉम्बस के द्वारा बन्द हो जाना जो अपने बनने के स्थान से अलग हो चुका होता है तथा रक्त के द्वारा उस रक्त वाहिनी तक पहुँचा है। The blocking of a blood vessels by a thrombus that has been detached from the site of its formation and carried by blood to this blood vessel.

Thrombogenesis (थ्रॉम्बोजेनेसिस) रक्त थक्के का बनना, घनास्त्र जनक। The formation of a blood clot.

Thrombokinase (थ्रॉम्बोकाइनेस) रक्त स्कन्दन कारण 10। Blood coagulation factor X.

Thrombolysis (थ्रोम्बोलाइसिस) किसी थ्रॉम्बस का टूटना। The breaking up of a thrombus.

Thrombophlebitis (थ्रोम्बोफ्लेबाइटिस) थ्रॉम्बस बनने के साथ किसी शिरा की सूजन हो जाना, घनास्त्र-शिराशोथ। Inflammation of a vein associated with thrombus formation.

Thromboplastin (थ्रोम्बोप्लास्टिन) तीसरा रक्त स्कन्दन कारक, रक्त एवं ऊतकों में पाया जाने वाला एक पदार्थ जो कैल्सियम ऑयनों की विद्यमानता में प्रोथ्रॉम्बिन के थ्रॉम्बिन में परिवर्तित होने में सहायता पहुँचाता है। The third blood coagulation factor, a substance in the blood and tissues which in the presence of calcium ions, aids in the conversion of prothrombin to thrombin.

Thrombosis (थ्रोम्बोसिस) किसी रक्त वाहिनी में रक्त थक्के का बनना अथवा उसका पाया जाना, घनास्त्रता। The formation or presence of a blood clot within a blood vessel.

Thrombus (थ्रॉम्बस) रक्तवाहिनियों में थक्का विद्यमान रहना, घनास्र। The presence of a clot in the blood vessels.

Thrush (थ्रश) मुखव्रण, छाले। Apathies, small white ulcers of the mouth.

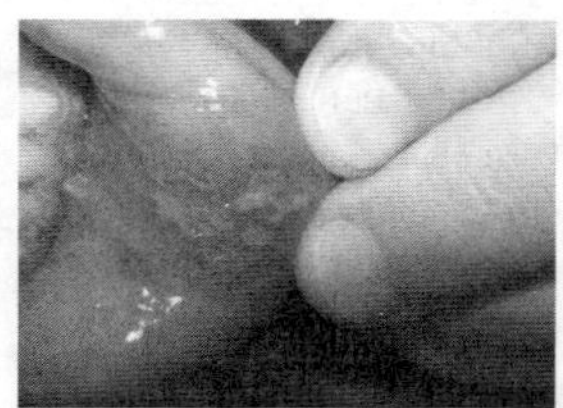

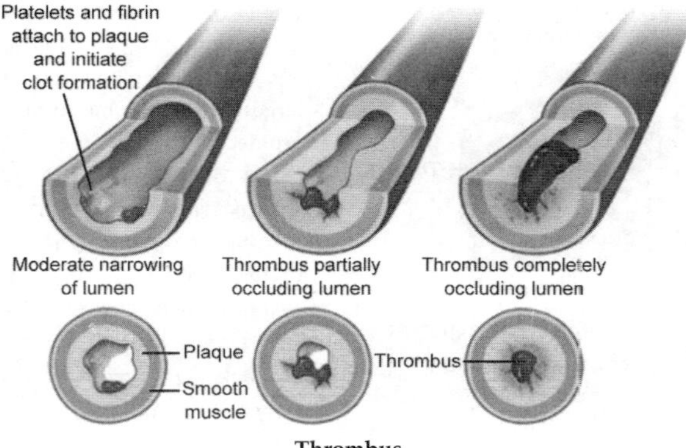

Thrombus

Thumb (थम्ब) हाथ की रेडियल हड्डी के ओर की पहली, छोटी तथा मोटी अंगूली जिसमें दो अंगुथ्ल्यस्थियाँ होती है। Pollex, the first short and thick digit on the radial side of the hand having two phalanges.

Thymectomy (थाइमैक्टॉमी) थाइमस ग्रन्थि का शल्यक्रिया द्वारा उच्छेदन। Excision of the thymus gland.

Thymocyte (थाइमोसाइट) थाइमस ग्रन्थि से उत्पन्न होने वाली एक लसीकाकोशिका। A lymphocyte derived from the thymus gland.

Thymokesis (थाइमोकेसिस) थाइमस ग्रन्थि की असामान्य वृद्धि। Abnormal enlargement of the thymus gland.

Thymolytic (थाइमोलाइटिक) थाइमस ग्रन्थि ऊतक के लिए विनाशकारी। Destructive to thymus gland tissue.

Thymoma (थाइमोमा) बाल्यग्रन्थि में बनने वाली कोई रसौली। A tumor arising in the thymus.

Thymus (थाइमस) मध्यस्थानिक-गुहा में हृदय के आगे एवं ऊपर स्थित एक लसीकाभ ग्रन्थि जो लगभग यौवनारम्भ पर अपने अधिकतम भार को ग्रहण कर लेता है और फिर इसका प्रत्यावर्तन होने लगता है। A lymphoid gland situated in the mediastinal cavity anterior to gland above the heart, which reaches its maximum weight at about puberty and then undergoes involution.

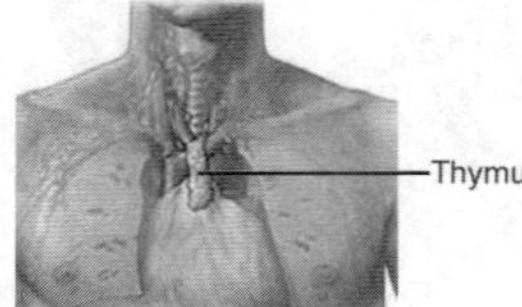

Thymus

Thyroadenitis (थाइरोएडीनाइटिस) थाइरॉयड ग्रन्थि का शोथ। Inflammation of the thyroid gland.

Thyrocardiac (थाइरोकार्डियक) थाइरॉयड ग्रन्थि एवं हृदय से सम्बन्धित। Pertaining to the thyroid gland and heart.

Thyroglobulin (थाइरोग्लोबुलिन) थॉइरॉयड ग्रन्थि द्वारा स्त्रावित तथा इसके कोलॉइड पदार्थ में संचित एक आयोडीनयुक्त ग्लाइकोप्रोटीन। An iodine-containing glycoprotein secreted by the thyroid gland and stored in its colloid substance.

Thyroglossal duct (थाइरोग्लौसल डक्ट) अण्टुजिह्वा नली अवटुग्रन्थि एवं जिह्वा के मध्य स्थित एक भ्रूण नली। A fetal passage between the thyroid gland and the tongue.

Thyroid cartilage (थाइरॉयड कार्टिलेज) अवटु-उपास्थि, स्वरयंत्र की सबसे बड़ी उपास्थि। The largest cartilage of the larynx.

Thyroidectomize (थाइरॉयडेक्टामोइज) थायरॉड ग्रन्थि को शल्यक्रिया द्वारा काट कर निकलना। To excise the thyroid gland.

Thyroidectomy (थाइरॉयडेक्टॉमी) थाइरॉड ग्रन्थि को शर्ल्य क्रर्म द्वारा काट कर निकाल देना, अवटु-अच्छेदन। Excision of the thyroid gland.

Thyroid gland (थाइरॉयड ग्लैण्ड) गर्दन के आधार पर, स्वरयंत्र के निचले भाग तथा श्वासप्रणाल के ऊपरी भाग के दोनों ओर स्थित एक अन्तःस्त्रावी ग्रन्थि, अवटु ग्रन्थि। An endocrine gland situated at base of the neck, on both sides of lower part of the larynx and upper part of the trachea.

Thyroiditis (थाइरॉयडाइटिस) थाइरॉयड ग्रन्थि का शोथ, अवटुशोथ। Inflammation of the thyroid gland.

Thyroid-stimulating hormone (थाइरॉयड स्टिमुलेटिंग हार्मोन) अग्रज पीयूष ग्रन्थि से स्रावित होने वाला एक हार्मोन जो थाइरॉयड को अपने दो हार्मोन थाइरॉक्सिन

एवं ट्राइआयडोथाइरोनीन को स्रावित करने के लिए उसे उद्दीप्त करता है। A hormone secreted by the anterior pituitary gland that stimulates the thyroid to secrete its two hormones—thyroxine and triiodothyronine.

Thyroid storm (थाइरॉयड स्टॉर्म) अवटु-विषाक्तता का एक उपद्रव जिसमें अचानक ज्वर हो जाता है, पसीना आता है, दिल की धड़कन बढ़ जाती है, फुफ्फुसीय शोथ या रक्तसंकुल हृदपात हो जाता है, कँपकपी एवं बेचैनी होती है।

A complication of thyrotoxicosis in which there is sudden onset of fever, sweating tachycardia, pulmonary edema or congestive heart failure, tremulousness and restlessness.

Thyromegaly (थाइरोमेगैली) थाइरॉयड ग्रन्थि का बढ़ जाना। Enlargement of the thyroid gland.

Thyroptosis (थाइरोप्टोसिस) थाइरॉयड ग्रन्थि का नीचे की ओर वक्ष में विस्थापित हो जाना। Downward displacement of the thyroid gland into the thorax.

Thyrotoxic (थाइरोटॉक्सिक) थाइरॉयड ग्रन्थि की विषैली क्रियाशीलता से सम्बन्धित अथवा उससे ग्रस्त, अवटुविषज। Pertaining to or affected with toxic activity of the thyroid gland.

Thyrotoxicosis

(थाइरोटॉक्सिकोसिस) अवटुविषाक्तता, एक स्वक्षम अवटु रोग। One of the autoimmune thyroid diseases.

Thyrotropic (थाइरोट्रॉपिक) थाइरॉयड ग्रन्थि के प्रति लगाव रखने अथवा उसे उत्तेजित करने वाला, अवटुप्रेरक। Having affinity for, or stimulating the thyroid gland.

Thyrotropism (थाइरोट्रॉपिज्म) थाइरॉयड ग्रन्थि के प्रति लगाव। Affinity for the thyroid gland.

Thyroxin (थाइरॉक्सिन) थाइरॉयड ग्रन्थि का एक आयोडीन-युक्त हार्मोन जो कोशिका की चयापचय दर को बढ़ाता है। यह अवटुअल्पक्रियता की चिकित्सा में प्रयोग में लाया जाता है। An iodine-containing hormone of the thyroid gland which increases the rate of cell metabolism. It is used in the treatment of hypothyroidism.

Tibia (टिबिया) टांग की अन्दरूनी व सबसे लम्बी हड्डी, अन्तर्जंघिका। The inner and large bone of the leg.

Tibialgia (टिबिएल्जिया) टिबिया हड्डी में दर्द होना। Pain in the tibia bone.

Tibiofemoral (टिबियोफिमोरल) टिबिया एवं फीमर हड्डियों से सम्बन्धित। Pertaining to the tibia and femur bones.

Tic (टिक) एक ऐंठनयुक्त, अनैच्छिक बारम्बार होने वाला पेशीय संकुचन जिसमें चेहरे, गर्दन अथवा कन्धे की पेशियाँ सबसे अधिक प्रभावित होती है, स्वभावाकर्ष। A spasmodic, involuntary, repetitive muscular contraction most commonly affecting the face neck or shoulder muscles.

Tick (टिक) एक रक्त-चूषक परजीवी। A blood sucking parasite.

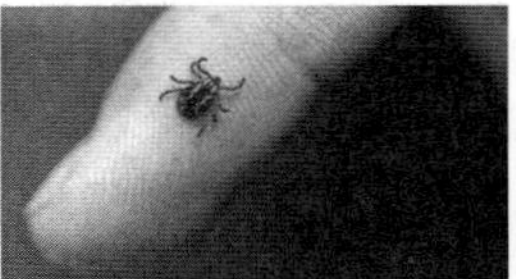

Tickling (टिक्लिंग) गुदगुदी, त्वक्-तंत्रिका की उत्तेजना के कारण होने वाली एक विशेष प्रकार की संवेदना। A peculiar sensation resulting from excitation of the cutaneous nerve, titilation.

Tidal (टाइडल) नियत अवधि पर उठने एवं गिरने या बढ़ने तथा घटने वाला। Periodically rising and falling or increasing and decreasing.

Tinctorial (टिंक्टोरियल) अभिरंजन या रंग से सम्बन्धित। Pertaining to staining or color.

Tincture (टिंक्चर) किसी जन्तु अथवा वनस्पति औषधि या रासायनिक पदार्थ का एक एल्कोहॉलयुक्त घोल जैसे टिंक्चर आयोडीन। An alcoholic solution prepared from an animal or vegetable drug or a chemical substance, e.g. tincture of iodine.

Tinea (टीनिया) त्वचा का कवक संक्रमण, दाद। Fungus infection.

Tinea capitis (टीनिया केपीटिस) शिरोवल्क का कवक संक्रमण। Fungus infection of the scalp.

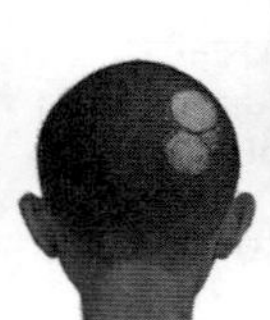

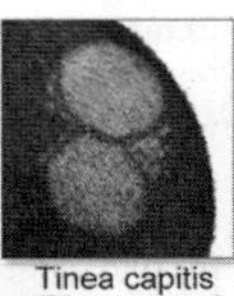

Tinea capitis (Ringworm of the scalp)

Tinea corporis (टीनिया कॉर्पोरिस) काय-दद्रु, बहुचक्री दद्रु। Ringworm of the body.

Tinea nigra (टीनिया नाइग्रा) हथेली की त्वचा का कवक संक्रमण।

Pityriasis, fungus infection of the skin of the palm.

Tinea pedis (टीनिया पेडिस) पाँव की त्वचा का जीर्ण कवक संक्रमण, पाद-दद्रु। Athlete's foot, chronic fungal infection of skin of the foot.

Tingle (टिंगल) नुकीली वस्तु के चुभने अथवा डंक लगने जैसी संवेदना। A prickling or stinging sensation.

Tinnitus (टिनाइटस) रोगी द्वारा कान में सुनाई देने वाली घंटी के बजने जैसी, भिनभिनाहट अथवा ध्वनियाँ। Ringing, buzzing or other sounds heard in the ear by the patient.

Tintometry (टिन्टोमीट्री) रंगों के पैमाने से तुलना करके रंग का पता लगाना। Determination of color by comparison with a scale of colors.

Tiqueur (टिक्व्यूअर) पेशीस्फुरण से पीड़ित व्यक्ति। The person afflicted with a tic.

Tissue (टिशू) एक-सी कोशिकाओं का एक समूह जो मिलकर किसी विशेष कार्य को करती है, ऊतक। A group of similar cells which together perform a particular function. (*i*) **Bony tissue** (बोनी टिशू) हड्डी, अस्थि। Bone.

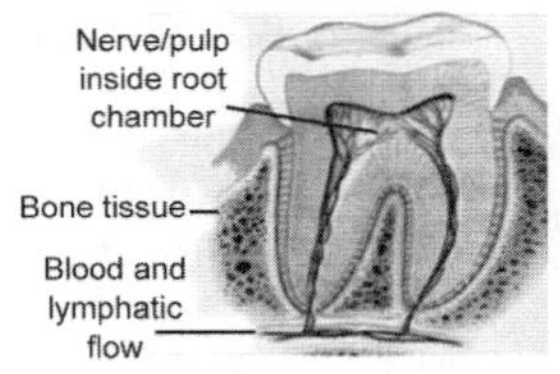

(*ii*) **Cartilaginous tissue** (कार्टिलेजिनस टिशू) उपास्थि का पदार्थ। The substance of cartilage.

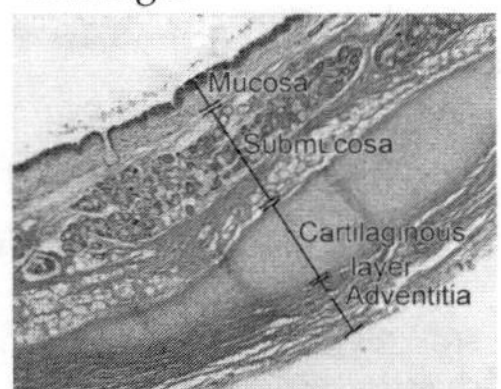

(*iii*) **Fatty tissue** (फैटी टिशू) शरीर की वसा से बनने वाला ऊतक। Tissue consisting of body fat. (*iv*) **Muscular tissue** (मस्कुलर टिशू) पेशी का पदार्थ, पेशी ऊतक। The substance of the muscle.

(*v*) **Osseous tissue** (ओसियस टिशू) हड्डी को बनाने वाला विशिष्ट ऊतक। The specialized tissue forming the bone.

Tissular titillation (टिशूलर टाइटीलेशन) जीवित ऊतकों से

सम्बन्धित। Pertaining to living tissues.

Titillation (टाइटीलेशन) गुदगुदाहट। A pleasant feeling.

Titration (टाइट्रेशन) सीरम में एण्टीबॉडी की मात्रा का अनुमापन करना, अनुमापन। Determination of quantity of antibody in the serum.

Titubation (टाइट्यूबेशन) प्रस्खलन, लड़खड़ाना, बेचैनी, घबराहट। The staggering gait of the diseased.

Toadskin (टोडास्किन) एक ऐसा रोग जिसमें त्वचा अत्यधिक शुष्क हो जाती है, उसमें झुर्रिया पड़ जाती है तथा परतों के रूप में झड़ने लगती है। A condition characterized by excessive dryness, wrinkling and scaling of the skin.

Tobacco (टोबैको) तम्बाकु। The dried leaves of *Nicotina tabocum*.

Tocology (टोकोलॉजी) प्रसूतिविज्ञान, धातृविज्ञान। Midwifery.

Tocolysis (टोकोलाइसिस) गर्भाशयी संकुचनों में अवरोध उत्पन्न हो जाना। Inhibition of uterine contractions.

Toe (टो) पैर की एक अंगुली, पादांगुली। A digit of the foot.

Toilet training (टॉयलेट ट्रेनिंग) बच्चे को मल एंव मूत्र के विसर्जन पर नियंत्रण रखना सिखलाना जब तक वह टॉयलेट पर नहीं बैठा दिया जाता। To train the child to control urination and defecation until he/she is placed on a toilet.

Tolerance (टोलेरैन्स) बिना विपरीत प्रभाव के उत्पन्न हुए सहन करने की क्षमता, सहनशक्ति। The ability to endure without any adverse effect.

Tolerogenesis (टोलेरोजेनेसिस) रोगक्षमता सम्बन्धी सह्मता का उत्पन्न होना। Production of immunologic tolerance.

Tomography (टोमोग्राफी) टोमोग्राफ द्वारा किसी ऊतक खण्ड या किसी ऊतक अथवा अंग की किसी खास गहराई का एक्स-रे चित्र लेना। Obtaining of the X-ray picture by tomo-graph of a tissue section or of particular depth of a tissue or of an organ.

Tone (टोन) किसी पेशी या वाहिनी का तनाव अथवा उसे बढ़ाने या खींचने के प्रति प्रतिरोध, तान। The tension or resistance of a muscles or vessel against an elongation or stretch.

Tongue (टंग) जिह्वा, जीभ। The organ of the taste and speech.

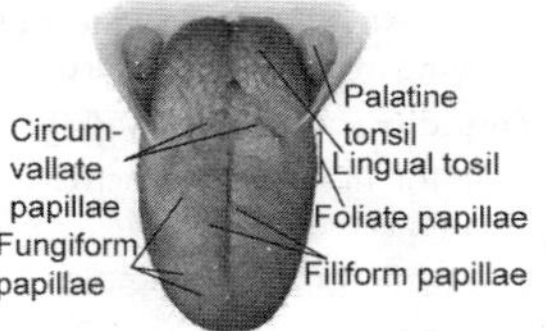

Tongue-tie (टंग-टाइ) जिह्वा-बद्धता। Ankylogossia.

Tonicity (टॉनिसिटी) तान विशेषकर पेशीय तान से युक्त होने का गुण, तानता। Property of possessing tone, especially muscular tone.

Tonoclonic (टोनोक्लोनिक) जो तानिक एवं अवमोटनीय दोनों हो, ऐसा पेशीय ऐंठनों के लिए कहा जाता है। Both tonic and colonic said of muscular spasms.

Tonofilament (टोनोफिलामैंट) टोनोफाइब्रिल का एक सूत्र। A filament of a tonofibril.

Tonography (टोनोग्राफी) अन्तरिक्ष-दाब (आँख के भीतर के दाब) में होने वाले परिवर्तनों का अभिलेखन करना, तनावअभिलेखन। The recording of changes in intraocular pressure.

Tonometer (टोनोमीटर) तनावमापी, तनाव मापने का यंत्र। An instrument to measure tension.

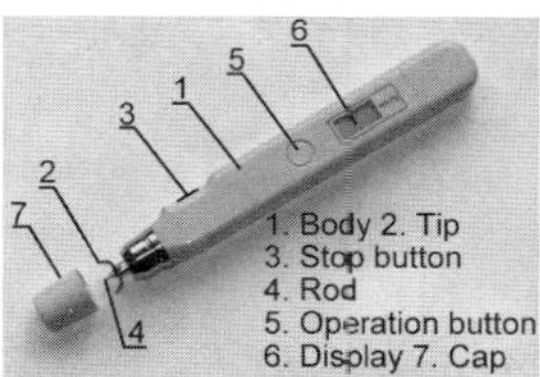

Tonometry (टोनोमीट्री) तनावमिति, तनावमापन। Measuring the tension.

Tonsil (टॉन्सिल) लसीकाभ ऊतक का एक पिण्ड गलततुण्डिका। A mass of lymphcid tissue.

Tonsillectomy (टॉन्सिलेक्टॉमी) शल्यक्रिया द्वारा किसी टॉन्सिल को काट कर निकाल देना। Surgical removal of a tonsil.

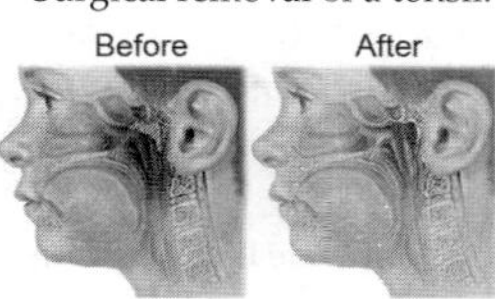

Tonsillitis (टॉन्सिलाइटिस) किसी टॉन्सिल या गलतुण्डिका विशेषकर तालु-गलतुण्डिका का शोथ। Inflammation of a tonsil, especially the palatine tonsil.

Tonsilloscopy (टॉन्सिलोस्कोपी) टॉन्सिलो का निरीक्षण करना। Inspection of the tonsils.

Tooth (टूथ) दन्त, दान्त, दांत। Singular form of teeth.

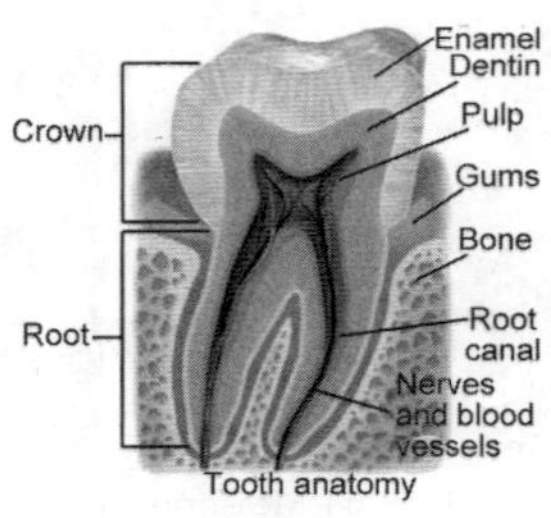

Tooth

Topagnosis (टीपेग्नोसिस) स्पर्श संवेदना के स्थान को निर्धारित करने में असमर्थता। Inability to localize the site of sensation of touch.

Tophaceous (टोफेसियस) टोफस से सम्बन्धित। Related to tophus.

Tophus (टोफस) गाऊट में कान की उपास्थि में अथवा सन्धियों के आस-पास के ऊतकों में सोडियम यूरेट का जमाव। A deposit of sodium urate in the cartilage of ear or in the tissue about the joints in gout.

Topical (टोपिकल) किसी स्थान विशेष से सम्बन्धित। Pertaining to a particular area, local.

Topography (टोपोग्राफी) शरीर के किसी भाग का विवरण देना, अंगरेखांकन। Description of a part of the body.

Topophobia (टोपोफोबिया) किसी क्षेत्र विशेष में होने का विकृत भय, स्थलभीति। Morbid fear of being in a particular place.

Torpidity (टोर्पीडिटी) निष्क्रियता, मन्दता या धीमापन। Inactivity, sluggishness.

Torr (टोर्र) सामान्य वायुमण्डलीय तापमान एवं दाब में 1 मि.मी. पारे का दाब। A pressure of 1 mm of mercury under normal atmospheric temperature and pressure.

Torsion (टार्शन) अपने अक्ष पर ऐंठ जाने की क्रिया अथवा ऐंठ जाना, मरोड़। Act of twisting or condition of being twisted at its axis.

Torso (टॉर्सो) धड़। Trunk.

Torticollar (टॉर्टीकॉलर) मन्यास्तम्य से सम्बन्धित। Pertaining to torticollis.

Torticollis (टॉर्टीकॉलिस) गर्दन की पेशियों के ऐंठनयुक्त संकुचन से अकड़ी हुई एवं ऐंठी हुई गर्दन, गीवास्तम्भ, मन्यास्तम्भ। Wryneck. Stiff neck with torsion caused by spasmodic contraction of the neck muscles.

Tortuous (टार्चुअस) ऐंठा हुआ, कुटिल, बहुत-सी ऐंठनों अथवा घुमावों वाला। Twisted, having many twists or turns.

Torture (टॉर्चर) मानसिक अथवा शारीरिक कष्ट पहुँचाना, उत्पीड़ित

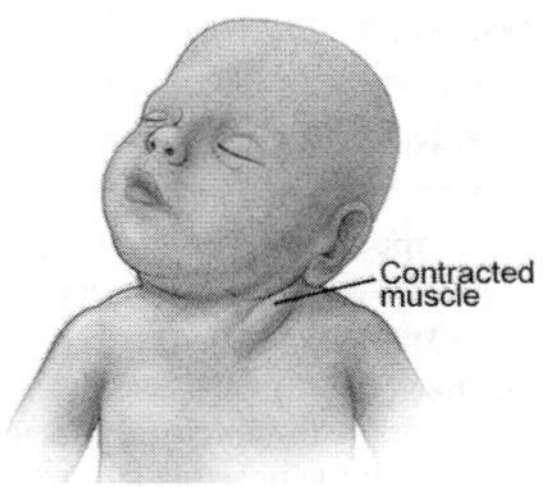

Torticollis

करना। To inflict mental or physical trouble.

Totipotent (टोटीपोटेन्ट) पूर्णशक्तिमान, पूर्णविभवी। Relating to totipotency.

Touch (टच) स्पर्श, परिस्पर्शन। The sense by which contact of an object with the skin is recognized.

Tourniquet (टोर्नीकुयट) अस्थायी रूप से दूरस्थ स्थान में परिसंचरण को रोकने, रक्त स्राव को रोकने अथवा अन्तःशिराभ इन्जैक्शन या शिरावेध को आसान बनाने के लिए भुजा के चारों ओर कस कर बांधा जाने वाला पट्टा। A band to be bound tightly around a limb to arrest the circulation temporarily in distal area, to stop bleeding injection or venipuncture.

Toxemia (टॉक्सीमिया) रक्त धारा द्वारा जीवाणुज जीवविषों के सम्पूर्ण शरीर में फैले जाने से उत्पन्न दशा, जीवविषरक्तता। The condition caused from the spread of bacterial toxins throughout the body by blood-stream.

Toxic (टॉक्सिक) जीवाणुओं की क्रिया द्वारा उत्पत्ति विषान्नसर, जीवविष, विष। A poisonous albumin produced by the action of bacteria.

Toxicoderma (टॉक्सिकोडर्मा) किसी विष के परिणामरूप उत्पन्न कोई भी त्वचा रोग। Any skin disease resulting from a poison.

Toxicology (टॉक्सिकोलॉजी) विषविज्ञान, जीवविषविज्ञान, अगदन्त्र। The branch of science concerned with the nature, effects, and detection of poisons.

Toxicosis (टॉक्सिकोसिस) विष से उत्पन्न कोई भी रोगावस्था, विषाक्तता, विषण्णता। Any diseased condition resulting from poisoning.

Toxiferous (टॉक्सीफेरस) विषवाहक। Carrying poison.

Toxigenic (टॉक्सिजेनिक) जीवविषों अथवा विषों को उत्पन्न करने वाला, जीवविषजनक। Producing toxins or poisons.

Toxigenicity (टॉक्सिजेनीसिटी) जीवविषों को उत्पन्न करने का

गुण, जीवविषजनकता। The property of production toxins.

Toxinosis (टॉक्सिनोसिस) किसी जीवविष द्वारा उत्पन्न कोई भी रोग। Any disease caused by a toxin.

Toxoid (टाक्सॉयड) रोगक्षम-क्रिया को उत्तेजित करने वाला विष पदार्थ, जीवविषाभ। A toxin that has been deprived by power to injure but which still stimulates immunity formation.

Toxophil (टॉक्सोफिल) जीवविषों के प्रति विशेष रूप से आकर्षित होने वाला। Specially attracted towards toxins.

Toxophorous (टॉक्सोफोरस) किसी टॉक्सोफोर से सम्बन्धित। Pertaining to a toxophore.

Trabecula (ट्रेबीकुला) किसी अंग की भित्ति अथवा कैप्सुल से बढ़कर उसके पदार्थ में पहुँचने वाला संयोजी ऊतक का एक तन्तुमय पट्‌टा, रज्जु, बन्धक। A fibrous band of connective tissue extending from the wall or capsule of an organ into its substance.

Trabecularism (ट्रेबीकुलेरिज्म) बन्धक या रज्जु धारण करना। Condition of having a trabecula.

Trace (ट्रेस) बहुत ही थोड़ी मात्रा। A very small quantity.

Tracer (ट्रेसर) किसी वस्तु की बाह्य रूपरेखा अथवा गतियों का रेखा चित्रण द्वारा अभिलेखन करने वाला एक उपकरण। An apparatus for recording graphically the outline or movements of an object.

Trachea (ट्रेकिया) श्वासप्रवाल। Windpipe in which air passes through the nose via larynx.

Tracheitis (ट्रेकाइटिस) श्वास-प्रणालशोथ। Inflammation of the trachea.

Trachelitis (ट्रेकीलाइटिस) ग्रर्भाशयग्रीवाशोथ। Inflammation of the mucos membrane of cervix uteri.

Trachelology (ट्रेकिलोलॉजी) गर्दन एवं इसके रोगों का वैज्ञानिक अध्ययन। Scientific study of the neck and its diseases.

Trachelorrhaphy (ट्रेकिलोरैह्फी) फटी हुई गर्भाशयग्रीवा में टांके लगाना, गर्भाशयग्रीवा-सीवन। Suturing of a torn cervix uteri.

Tracheobronchomegaly (ट्रेकियोब्रोन्कोमेगैली) सामान्यतः जन्मजात श्वास-प्रणाल एवं प्रमुख श्वासनलियों का चौड़ा होना। Widening of the trachea and main bronchi, usually congenitally.

Tracheocele (ट्रेकियोसील) श्वास-प्रणाल की श्लेष्मिक कला का बहिःसरण, श्वास-प्रणाल,

हर्निया। Herniation of the mucous membrane of the trachea.

Tracheomalacia (ट्रेकियोमैलेशिया) श्वास-प्रणाल की उपस्थियों का कोमल हो जाना। Softening of the cartilages of trachea.

Tracheoscope (ट्रेकियोस्कोप) श्वासप्रणाल-दर्शन में प्रयुक्त एक यंत्र। An instrument used in tracheoscopy.

Tracheostenosis (ट्रेकियोस्टेनोसिस) श्वासप्रणाल की सिकुड़न। A narrowing of the trachea.

Tracheostomy (ट्रेकियोस्टॉमी) गर्दन से होकर श्वास-प्रणाल में छेद करना, श्वासप्रणाल-छिद्रीकरण। To make an opening into the trachea through the neck.

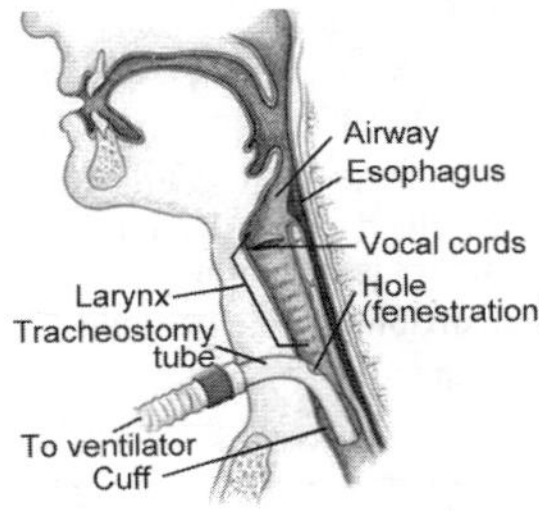

Traching (ट्रेसिंग) किसी सक्रियता जैसे श्वसनीय गतियों, हृदय स्पन्द अथवा मस्तिष्क की वैधुत सक्रियता का रेखाचित्र-अभिलेखन, अनुरेखण। A graphic record of some activity such as respiratory movement, heartbeat on electrical activity of the brain.

Trachoma (ट्रेकोमा) क्लेमाइडिया ट्रेकोमेटिस के किसी उपभेद द्वारा उत्पन्न एक प्रकार का जीर्ण सांसर्गिक नेत्रश्लेष्मलाशोथ। A form of chronic contagious conjunctivitis, caused by a stain of *Chlamydia trachomatis.*

Trachomatous (ट्रेकोमेटस) रोहे से सम्बन्धित अथवा रोहयुक्त। Pertaing to or having trachoma.

Trachopyosis (ट्रेकियोपायोसिस) श्वास-प्रणाल का शोथ जिसमें पस बन जाता है। Tracheitis with pus formation.

Tract (ट्रेक्ट) मार्ग या नली, एक-सा कार्य करने वाले ऊतकों अथवा अंगों का लम्बान में एक संग्रह। A pathway, a longitudinal assemblage of tissue or organs having the same function.

Traction (ट्रेक्शन) कर्षण, खिंचाव। The act of drawing or pulling

(*i*) **Axis traction** (एक्सिस ट्रैक्शन) लम्ब अक्ष की रेखा में जैसे श्रोणि को लम्ब अक्ष की रेखा में खींचना जिसके द्वारा भ्रूण को बाहर को खींचा जाता है, अक्ष कर्षण। Traction in line with the long axis, as of the pelvis through which a fetus is to be drawn. (*ii*) **Elastic traction** (इलास्टिक ट्रेक्शन) इलास्टिक साधनों जैसे रबर की पट्टियों द्वारा लगाया जाने वाला खिंचाव। Traction exerted by elastic agents such as rubber bands.

Tractor (ट्रेक्टर) खिंचाव पैदा करने के लिए एक उपकरण। An apparatus for applying traction.

Tractotomy (ट्रेक्टोटोमी) पथछेदन, स्नायुपथ छेदन। Incision of a nerve tract in the brainstem and spinal cord.

Tragescent (ट्रागेसेंट) फूला हुआ। Distended.

Tragus (ट्रेगस) कान के बाह्य छिद्र के सामने स्थित उपास्थि का प्रक्षेपण, तुंगिका। A small pointed eminence of the external ear in front of and partly closing the passage to the organs of hearing.

Trait (ट्रेट) विशेषक। Any characteristic peculiar to an individual.

Trance (ट्रांस) उपसमाधि। An alter state of consciousness.

Tranquilizer (ट्रेन्क्वीलाइजर) एक औषधि जो मानसिक तनाव एवं चिन्ता को कम करने का कार्य करती है। A drug that acts to reduce mental tension and anxiety.

Transatrial (ट्रान्सएट्रियल) अलिन्द से गुजार कर किया गया। Performed through the atrium.

Transcortical (ट्रान्सकॉर्टिकल) प्रमस्तिष्कीय प्रान्तस्था के दो भागों को जोड़ने वाला। Joining two parts of the cerebral cortex.

Transducer (ट्रान्सड्यूसर) एक प्रकार की शक्ति को दूसरे प्रकार की शक्ति में परिवर्तित करने वाला एक उपकरण जैसे दाब या तापमान को वैधुत आवेग में परिवर्तित करने वाला। An apparatus for converting one form of energy to another.

Transection (ट्रान्सैक्शन) किसी लम्ब अक्ष के आर-पार काटना, पारपरिच्छेदन। The cutting across a long axis.

Transferrin (ट्रान्सफेरिन) रक्त सीरम में विद्यमान एक ग्लोबुलिन जो लोहे को बान्धता एवं उसका वहन करता है। A globulin in the blood serum that binds and transports iron.

Transfixion (ट्रान्सफिक्शन) भीतर से बाहर की ओर आर-पार काटना जैसे किसी अंगोच्छेदन या विच्छेदन में किया जाता है। A cutting across from within outward as in amputation.

Transforation (ट्रान्सफोरेशन) भ्रूण की खोपड़ी के आधार पर छेद करना। Perforation of the fetal.

Transfusion (ट्रान्सफ्यूजन) रक्त, रक्त के किसी घटक, सैलाइन अथवा अन्य घोल को किसी शिरा द्वारा रक्त धारा में प्रविष्ट करना, आधान। Introduction of blood, a blood component, saline or other solution, into the blood stream through a vein.

Transillumination (ट्रान्सइलुमिनेशन) किसी गुहा अथवा अंग की दूसरी ओर से इसकी प्राचीर से तेज रोशनी गुजार कर इसका निरीक्षण करना, पार-प्रदीपन। Inspection of a cavity or organ by passing strong light through its wall from the opposite side.

Translocation (ट्रान्सलोकेशन) स्थानांतरण, स्थलान्तरण। The displacement of part or whole of chromosome to another.

Translucent (ट्रान्सलुसैन्ट) अर्द्धपारदर्शक। Semi-transparent.

Transmigration (ट्रान्समाइग्रेशन) आर-पार या से होकर भ्रमण करना विशेषकर श्वेत रक्त कोशिकाओं का कोशिकाओं की भित्तियों से होकर ऊतकों में पहुँचना। The wandering across or through, especially the passage of white blood cells.

Transmission (ट्रान्समिशन) स्थानांतरण, संचरण, संचारण, प्रेषण। Transfer, as of a disease.

Transmural (ट्रान्स्म्यूरल) किसी अंग अथवा गुहा की भित्ति की सम्पूर्ण मोटाई से होकर फैलने अथवा उसे ग्रस्त करने वाला। Spreading or involving the entire thickness of the wall of an organ or cavity.

Transnasal (ट्रान्सनेज़ल) पारनासी, नाक में अथवा नाक द्वारा। Through the nose.

Transparent (ट्रान्सपैरेन्ट) पारदर्शक। Admitting the passage of the rays of light.

Transparietal (ट्रान्सपैराइटल) प्राचीर से होकर। Through the wall.

Transplant (ट्रान्सप्लान्ट) प्रतिरोपण करना। To transfer from one part to another.

Transplantation (ट्रान्सप्लान्टेशन) शरीर के किसी एक भाग से जीवित ऊतक अथवा अंग को लेकर उसे दूसरे भाग पर अथवा दूसरे व्यक्ति में निरोपित करना, प्रतिरोपण। The grafting of living tissue or organ taken from one part of the body to another part, or to another person.

Transpleural (ट्रान्सप्लूरल) फुफ्फुसावरणों से होकर। Through the pleurae.

Transposition (ट्रान्सपोजिशन) स्थिति-अन्तरण। An interchange of position.

Transsexual (ट्रान्ससैक्सुअल) विपरीत लिंग का होने की तीव्र इच्छा रखने वाला व्यक्ति। The person possessing intense desire to be of the opposite sex.

Transthermia (ट्रान्सथर्मिया) विद्युतधारा द्वारा गहरे ऊतकों में ऊष्मा उत्पन्न करना। Production of heat in the deep tissues by electric current.

Transthoracic (ट्रान्सथोरैसिक) वक्ष या छाती के पार, पारवक्षीय। Across the thorax.

Transudate (ट्रान्सूडेट) किसी झिल्ली विशेषकर कोशिकाओं की भित्तियों से निकलने वाला एक तरल पदार्थ, पारस्राव, रिसाव। Fluid substance that has passed through a membrane.

Transudation (ट्रान्सुडेशन) किसी झिल्ली से किसी तरल का विशेषकर सीरम का कोशिकाओं की भित्तियों से होकर रिसना, पारस्रवण। Oozing of a fluid through a membrane.

Transurethral (ट्रान्सयूरेथ्रल मूत्र-मार्ग से गुजार कर किया गया। Performed through the urethra.

Transvenous (ट्रान्सवेनस) किसी शिरा से होकर। Through a vein.

Transversectomy (ट्रान्सवर्सेक्टॉमी) किसी कशेरूका के अनुप्रस्थ प्रवर्ध को शल्यक्रिया द्वारा काट कर निकाल देना। Excision of a transverse process of a vertebra.

Trapeziform (ट्रेपीजीफॉर्म) यमलम्बाभ आकृति का। Trapezoid-shaped.

Trapezium (ट्रेपीज़ियम) कलाई की हड्डियों की दूरस्थ पंक्ति की रेडियम हड्डी की ओर की प्रथम हड्डी जो अँगूठे की करभास्थि से मिलकर जोड़ बनाती है, समलम्बक अस्थि। The first bone on radial side of the distal row of bone of the wrist, which articulates with the metacarpal bone of the thumb.

Trauma (ट्रॉमा) शारीरिक अथवा मानसिक आघात, चोट, अभिघात। Physical or psychological injury.

Traumatize (ट्रॉमेटाइज़) चोट पहुँचाना। To cause trauma.

Traumatology (ट्रॉमेटोलॉजी) शल्यचिकित्सा की वह शाखा जिसका सम्बन्ध चोटों एवं जख्मों से होता है, अभिघातविज्ञान। The branch of surgery dealing with the injuries and wounds.

Traumatopyra (ट्रॉमेटोपाइरा) किसी चोट लगने के फलस्वरूप उत्पन्न ज्वर। Fever resulting from a trauma.

Treatment (ट्रीटमैन्ट) किसी रोग अथवा विकार की काट करना, चिकित्सा, उपचार, इलाज। The combating of a disease or disorder (*i*) **Dental Treatment** (डैन्टल ट्रीटमैन्ट) दन्त-रोगों की चिकित्सा। Treatment of the dental disease (*ii*) **Domiciliary Treatment** (डोमीसिलियरी ट्रीटमैन्ट) गृह-चिकित्सा। Treatment given at home. (*iii*) **Empiric Treatment** (एम्पीरिक ट्रीटमैन्ट) निरीक्षण एवं अनुभवों के आधार पर की जाने वाली रोगों की चिकित्सा, किसी वैज्ञानिक आधार पर नहीं। Treatment of the disease based on observation and experience and not on a scientific basis. (*iv*) **Expectant Treatment** (एक्सपैक्टेन्ट) लक्षणों के उत्पन्न होने पर उनमें आराम पहुँचाने के लिए की जाने वाली चिकित्सा, रोगमुक्ति के प्रकृति पर छोड़ दिया जाता है। Treatment for relief of symptoms as they arise, leaving cure of the disease to nature. (*v*) **Palliative Treatment** (पैलिएटिव ट्रीटमैन्ट) रोग से मुक्ति दिलाने की अपेक्षा लक्षणों में आराम पहुँचाने के लिए की जाने वाली चिकित्सा। Treatment for relief of symptoms rather than curing the disease. (*vi*) **Rational Treatment** (रेशनल ट्रीटमैन्ट) वैज्ञानिक आधार पर की जाने वाली चिकित्सा। Treatment instituted on scientific basis.

Trematoda (ट्रेमेटोडा) संघ प्लेटीहैल्मिन्थीज़ (चपटे क्रमियों) का एक वर्ग। A class of the phylum platy helminthes (the flat worms).

Tremble (ट्रेम्ब्ल) काँपना। To shiver.

Tremograph (ट्रेमोग्राफ) कम्पनों का अभिलेखन करने वाला एक उपकरण। An apparatus for recording tremors.

Tremolous (ट्रेमुलस) काँपता हुआ अथवा हिलता हुआ, कम्पायमान। Trembling or shaking.

Tremor (ट्रेमर) कम्प, कम्पन। An involuntary trembling. (*i*) **Coarse tremor** (कोर्स ट्रेमर) धीमी गति से होने वाला कम्पन्न। Slow tremor. (*ii*) **Fine tremor** (फाइन ट्रेमर) जल्दी-जल्दी होने वाला कम्पन्न। A rapid tremor. (*iii*) **Pastural tremor** (पोस्चुरल ट्रेमर) भुजाओं या धड़ को कुछ स्थितियों में रखने पर होने वाला

कम्पन्न। Tremor that accrue when the limbs or tremor are kept in certain positions.

(*iv*) **Senile tremor** (सैनाइल ट्रेमर) वृद्धावस्था में होने वाला कम्पन्न। A tremor accruing in old age.

Trench fever (ट्रेंच फिवर) खाई-ज्वर, खात-ज्वर। Fever with a sudden onset with dizziness, headache pain in lumbar region and legs, especially shins.

Trench foot (ट्रेंच फूट) हिमदाह के समान एक रोग जो ठण्डे पानी में बहुत समय तक खड़े रहने वाले सैनिकों के पैरों को ग्रस्त करता है। A condition resembling frostbite involving the feet of soldiers who stand in cold water for long period of time.

Trench mouth (ट्रेंच माउथ) तीव्र परिगलनकारी व्रणयुक्त मसूड़ाशोथ। Acute necrotizing ulcerative gingivitis.

Trephine (ट्रेफाइन) खोपड़ी से हड्डी का वृत्ताकार टुकड़ा अलग करने के लिए एक बेलनाकार आरी। Trepan, cylindrical saw for removing circular piece of bone from the skull.

Trepidation (ट्रेपीडेशन) काँपना, भय, चिन्ता। A trembling, fear, anxiety.

Treponema (ट्रेपोनीमा) ट्रेपोनीमेटेसी कुल का मनुष्य में परजीवी के रूप में रहने वाला स्पाइरोकीटों का एक वंश। ट्रेपोनीमा पैलीडम सिफिलिस रोग उत्पन्न करने वाला जीव होता है। A genus of Spirochetes, parasite in man that belongs to the family spirochaetaceae, *Treponema pallidum* is the causative organism of syphilis.

Treponemiasis (ट्रेपोनीमिएसिस) ट्रेपोनीमा से पीड़ित रोग। Infestation with treponema.

Triad (ट्रॉयड) तीन सम्बद्ध वस्तुओं का एक वर्ग, त्रिक। A group of three associated things.

Triangle (ट्रॉयन्गल) त्रिभुज, त्रिकोण। A space bounded by three lines or sides.

Tribadism (ट्रॉइबेडिस्म) परस्परस्त्री-मैथुन, औरतों द्वारा आपस में मैथुन करना। Unnatural intercourse between women.

Tribrachius (ट्राइब्रेकियस) तीन बाहों वाला भ्रूण। A fetus with three arms.

Triceps (ट्राइसेप्स) तीन सिर वाला जैसे ट्राइसेप्स पेशी होती है, त्रिशीर्षपेशी। Three-headed, as a triceps muscle.

Trichiasis (ट्राइकिएसिस) आँखों की पलकों के बालों का अन्दर की ओर वृद्धि करना जिससे

वे कॉर्निया को रगड़ कर चिड़चिड़ाहट पैदा करते है, पक्ष्मावर्तन। In growing of the eyelashes so that they rub against the cornea, causing irritation.

Trichoanesthesia (ट्राइकोएनिस्थीज़िया) केश संवेदनशीलता का अभाव होना। Loss of sensibility of hair.

Trichobezoar (ट्राइकोबेज़ोर) आमाशय अथवा आँत में विद्यमान बालों की एक गेंद। A hair ball in the stomach or intestine.

Trichocryptosis (ट्राइकोक्रिप्टोसिस) रोमकूपों का कोई भी रोग। Any disease of the hair follicles.

Trichogen (ट्राइकोजन) बालों की वृद्धि को उत्तेजित करने वाला साधन।
An agent stimulating the growth of hair.

Trichology (ट्राइकोलॉजी) केश, इसके रोगों एवं उनकी चिकित्सा का अध्ययन, रोम-विज्ञान। Study of the hair, its disease and treatment.

Trichomatic (ट्राइकोमैटिक) सामान्य वर्णदृष्टि, त्रिवर्णदृष्टि। Able to differentiate three primary colors, which means normal color vision.

Trichomatosis (ट्राइकोमेटोसिस) शिरोवल्क के कवक रोग एवं सफाई के अभाव में फंसे हुए उलझे हुए बालों का पाया जाना। Entangled matted hair due to fungus disease of the scalp and lack of cleanliness.

Trichomonas (ट्राइकोनोनास) कशाभी परजीवीय एककोशिकीय जन्तुओं का एक वंश। A genus of flagellated parasitic unicellular protozoa species.

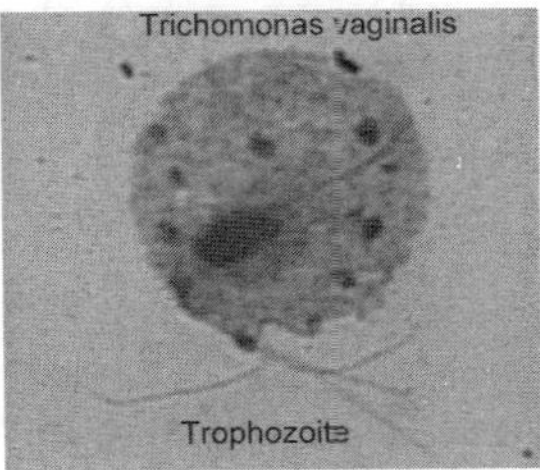

Trichomycosis (ट्राइकोमाइकोसिस) किसी कवक द्वारा उत्पन्न बालों का कोई भी रोग। Any disease of the hair caused by fungus.

Trichophagia (ट्राइकोफेजिया) बालों को खाने की आदत। The habit of eating hair.

Trichophytobezoar (ट्राइकोफाइटो-बेजोआर) आमाशय अथवा आँत में पाई जाने वाली बालों की गेंद। A hairball found in the stomach or intestine.

Trichophyton (ट्राइकोफाइटोन) परजीवीय कवकों का एक वंश जो त्वचा, बालों तथा नाखूनों में वास

करते है एवं बहुत से त्वचाकवकता और दद्रु संक्रमण उत्पन्न करते है। A genus of parasitic fungi that live in the skin, hair and nails and cause various dermatomycosis and ringworm infection.

Trichorrhexomania (ट्राइकोरैह्क्सोमैनिया) हाथ के नाखूनों से बालों को तोड़ने का उन्माद। Mania for breaking off the hair with fingernails.

Trichotillomania (ट्राइकोटिलोमैनिया) बालों को नोचने की सनक, लोमकर्षणोन्माद। Mania for pulling out hair.

Trichuriasis (ट्राइक्यूरिएसिस) आँत में ट्राइक्यूरिस वंश के कृमियों का पाया जाना, कशाकृमिरूग्णता। Presence of worms of genus trichuris in the intestine.

Tricipital (ट्राइसिपिटल) तीन सिर वाला। Three-headed.

Tricrotic (ट्राइक्रोटिक) एक नाड़ी स्पन्द के स्पन्दनलेखी अनुरेखण पर तीन खाँचों से युक्त। Having three notches on a sphygmographic tracing from one beat of the pulse.

Tricuspid (ट्राइकस्पिड) तीन नोकों अथवा कपर्दिकाओं वाला जैसे हृदय का कोई कपाट, त्रिकपर्दी। Having three points or cusps, as a valve of the heart.

Tricuspid atresia (ट्राइकस्पिड एट्रैसिया) त्रिकपर्दी कपाट की संकीर्णता। Stenosis of the Tricuspid valve.

Tricuspid Value (ट्राइकस्पिड वाल्व) दायाँ अलिन्द-निलय-कपाट। Right atrioventricular valve.

Trident (ट्राइडैन्ट) तीन दाँतों वाला। Having three-pronged spear.

Trifurcation (ट्राइफर्केशन) तीन शाखाओं में विभाजन। Division into three branches.

Trigeminal nerve (ट्राइजेमिनल नर्व) पाँचवीं कपालीय तंत्रिका, त्रिधारातन्त्रिका। Fifth cranial nerve.

Trigeminal neuralgia (ट्राइजेमिनल न्यूरैल्जिया) आनन-तन्त्रिकाशूल, त्रिधारातन्त्रिका की प्रगति के साथ-साथ होने वाला तीव्र शूल। Facial neuralgia, sharp pain along the course of trigeminal nerve.

Trigger (ट्रीगर) उद्दीपक या उद्दीपन, यकायक आरम्भ हो जाना। Stimulus, to start suddenly.

Trigger finger (ट्रीगर फिंगर) ऐसी दशा जिसमें हाथ या पैर की किसी अंगुली का आंकुचन अथवा प्रसार अस्थायी रूप से रूक जाता है परन्तु एक झटके के साथ अंगुली अपनी सामान्य

अवस्था में वापिस आ जाती है। The condition in which flexion or extension of a digit is arrested temporarily but the digit returns to its normal with a jerk.

Triglycerides (ट्राइग्लाइसेराइड्स) रक्त में ग्लिसरॉल का पाँच विभिन्न वसीय अम्लों में से तीन के साथ संयोजन। Combination of glycerol with three of five different fatty oxide in the blood.

Trigone (ट्राइगोन) एक त्रिभुजाकार स्थान, विशेषकर मूत्राशय के आधार पर मूत्रनलियों के दो छिद्रों एवं मूत्रमार्ग के बीच का त्रिभुजाकार स्थान, त्रिकोण। Trigonum: A triangular area, especially at the base of the urinary bladder between the two openings of the urethra.

Trigonitis (ट्राइगोनाइटिस) मूत्राशय के त्रिकोण का शोथ। Inflammation of the trigone of the bladder.

Tri-iodothyronine (ट्राइ-आयडोथाइरोनीन) थाइरॉयड ग्रन्थि का एक हार्मोन। A harmone of the thyroid gland.

Trilaminar (ट्राइलेमिनर) तीन परतों वाला। Three-layered.

Trilobate (ट्राइलोबेट) तीन खण्डों वाला। Having three lobes.

Trilocular (ट्राइलोकुलर) तीन अवकाशों अथवा गुहाओं से युक्त। Having three spaces or cavities.

Trimester (ट्राइमेस्टर) त्रिमास, तीन महीने की अवधि। A period of three month.

Trimmer (ट्राइमर) ऐसा यंत्र जो किसी वस्तु के किनारे-किनारे से सामग्री को काट कर उसे आकार प्रदान करता है। An instrument used to shape something by cutting of the material along its margin.

Trimorphous (ट्राइमॉर्फस) तीन विभिन्न रूपों में जीवित रहने वाला। Living in three different forms.

Triophthalmos (ट्रायोफ्थैल्मोस) एक विकृत भ्रूण जिसके तीन आँखें होती है। A deformed fetus with three eyes.

Triorchidism (ट्राइआर्किडिज्म) तीन शुक्रग्रन्थियों का पाया जाना। The presence of three testes.

Triplet (ट्रिपलेट) एक जन्म से उत्पन्न होने वाले तीन बच्चों में से एक। One of three children produced at one birth.

Triplex (ट्रिपलैक्स) त्रिगुण, तिगुना। Three-fold.

Triploidy (ट्रिप्लॉयडी) गुणसूत्रों की अगुणित संख्या के तिगुने का

पाया जाना। The presence of triple the haploid number of chromosomes.

Tripod (ट्राइपोड) तीन पदों वाला। Having three feet.

Tripsis (ट्रिप्सिस) सम्पेषण (घोटने) की क्रिया, मालिश। The process of trifurcation, massage.

Triquetrum (ट्राइक्वेट्रम) तीन कोनों वाला। Three-cornered.

Triradiate (ट्राइरेडिएट) तीन किरणों वाला, तीन दिशाओं में विकिरणशील। Having three rays; radiating in three directions.

Trismus (ट्रिज्मस) चर्वण-पेशियों की ऐंठन जिसके फलस्वरूप जबड़े भींच जाते है। हनुस्तम्भ। Spasm of the muscles of mastication resulting in lockjaw.

Trisomy (ट्राइसोमी) त्रिगुणित कोशिका में एक प्रकार के एक अतिरिक्त (तीसरा) गुणसूत्र का पाया जाना, त्रिगुणसूत्रता। The presence of an additional (3rd) chromosome of one type in a diploid cell.

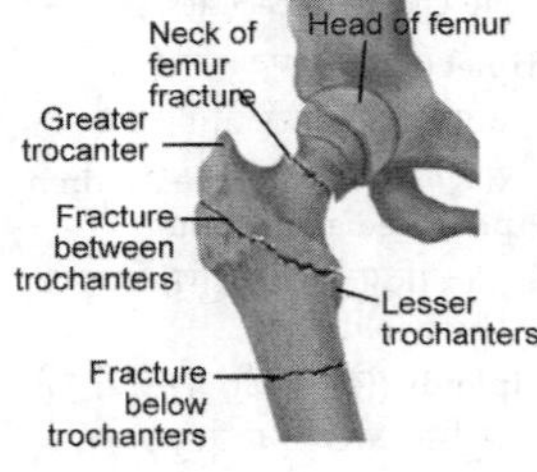

Trisulcate (ट्राइसल्केट) तीन खातिकाओं वाला। Having three furrows.

Tritanopia (ट्राइटैनोपिया) नीलकर्णान्धता, नीले रंग का दिखाई न देना। Blue blindness.

Triturate (ट्राइटुरेट) रगड़ का पाउडर बनाना। To make powder by rubbing.

Trituration (ट्राइटुरेशन) रगड़ कर या पीस कर पाउडर बनाने की क्रिया, अवपेषण, घोटना। The process of making powder by rubbing or grinding.

Trocar (ट्रोकार) धातु की एक प्रवेशिनी में बन्द एक तेज नुकीला यंत्र जो गुहा भित्ति का वेधन करने एवं तरल खींचने के लिए प्रयोग में लाया जाता है। A sharp-pointed instrument contained in a mental cannula, used to puncture a cavity wall and to withdraw fluid.

Trochanter (ट्रोकैन्टर) फीमर हड्डी की ग्रीवा के नीचे दो अस्थिल प्रवर्धों में से एक। Either of the two bony processes below the neck of the femur bone.

Trochanterplasty (ट्रोकैन्टरप्लास्टी) प्लास्टिक सर्जरी द्वारा फीमर की ग्रीवा की मरम्मत करना। Repair of the neck of the femur by plastic surgery.

Trochlea (ट्रोक्लिया) 1. किसी हड्डी की जोड़ बनाने वाली चिकनी सतह जिस पर कोई दूसरी हड्डी खिसकती है, चक्रिक। 2. घिरनी का कार्य करने वाली एक रचना। 1. The articular smooth surface of bone upon which an another bone glides. 2. A structure having thefunction of a pulley.

Trochleariform (ट्रोक्लियरीफार्म) घिरनी के आकार की। Pulley-shaped.

Trophic (ट्रॉफिक) पोषण से सम्बन्धित अथवा उस पर निर्भर रहने वाला। Pertaining to as dependent upon nutrition.

Trophoblast (ट्रोफोब्लास्ट) बीजपुटी की सबसे बाहरी परत जो गर्भित डिम्ब को गर्भाशय भित्ति से संलग्न करती है तथा अपरा बन जाती है, बीजपोशक। The outermost layer of the blastocyst, which attaches the fertilized ovum to the uterine wall and becomes placenta.

Trophology (ट्रोफोलॉजी) पोषणविज्ञान, आहारविज्ञान। The science of nutrition.

Trophozoite (ट्रोफोज्वाइट) एक बीजाणु परजीवी जो अपनी वृद्धि की अवस्था में अपने पोषद से पोषण ग्रहण करता है। Sporozoan parasite receiving nourishment forms its host during its growing stage.

Tropin (ट्रॉपिन) एक प्रत्यय जो किसी पदार्थ के उद्दीपक प्रभाव का, विशेष क्रम रूप से किसी हार्मोन के उसके लक्ष्य अंग पर प्रभाव का संकेत देता है। A suffix indicating the stimulating effect of a substance, especially a hormone, on its target organ.

Tropism (ट्रॉपिज्म) किसी जीव की किसी बाह्य उद्दीपक जैसे प्रकाश, अंधेरा, गर्मी या ठण्ड आदि की ओर अथवा उससे दूर होने वाली अनैच्छिक गति। Involuntary movement of an organism towards or away from an external stimulus such as light, darkness, heat or cold, etc.

Trousseau's sign (ट्रूसॉज साइन) गुप्त टिटेनी रोग का एक चिन्ह जिसमें ऊपरी बाहु की तंत्रिकाओं एवं वाहिनियों पर दाब लगाने के परिणामस्वरूप पेशीय ऐंठन हो जाती है। A sign of latent tetany in which spasm occurs as a result of pressure applied to nerves and vessels of the upper arm.

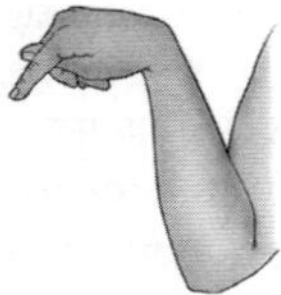

Trousseau's sign

True ribs (ट्रू रिब्स) ऊपरी सात पसलियाँ। Seven upper ribs.

Truncus (ट्रँकस) धड़, काण्ड, प्रकाण्ड, वृहत्वाहिका। A trunk, a large vessel.

Truncus arteriosus (ट्रंकस आर्टिरियोसस) धमनी कांड। The large artery of the primitive heart giving off the two aortas.

Trunk (ट्रंक) सिर एवं भुजाओं के अतिरिक्त शरीर का शेष भाग अथवा एक बड़ी रचना जैसे रक्त वाहिनी, तंत्रिका या लसीका, वाहिनी जिससे छोटी-छोटी शाखाएँ निकलती है अथवा जो इन शाखाओं के मिलने से बनती है, धड़, प्रकाण्ड, काण्ड। The part of the body excluding head and limbs or a large structure, e.g. blood vessels from which smaller branches arise, or which is formed by the union of these branches.

Truss (ट्रस) हर्निया के लिए प्रयोग में लाई जाने वाली पेटी, हर्निया-पेटी। A belt used for hernia.

Trypanosoma (ट्रिपेनोसोमा) परजीवीय, कशाभी एककोशिकीय जन्तुओं का एक वंश जो रक्त में पाया जाता है जिसकी गति टी. रोह्डेसिएन्सी टीसेट्सी मक्खी द्वारा संचारित होती है तथा पूर्वी अफ्रीका में निद्रा रोग लाती है। A genus of parasitic, flagellated protozoa found in the blood, species of T-rhodesiense is transmitted by the tsetse fly and causes sleeping sickness in East Africa.

Trypanosomic (ट्रिपेनोसोमिक) ट्रिपेनोसोमा से सम्बन्धित। Pertaining to trypanosomes.

Trypsin (ट्रिप्सिन) आँत में एन्ट्रोकाइनेस की अग्नाशय से स्रावित ट्रिप्सीनोजन पर क्रिया होने से बनने वाला एक प्रोटीन-अपघटनकारी एन्जाइम। A protecting enzyme formed in the intestine by the action of enterokinase on trypsinogen, secreted by the pancreas.

Trypsinogen (ट्रिप्सीनोजन) अग्नाशयी रस में पाया जाने वाला ट्रिप्सिन का निष्क्रिय रूप जो आँत में एन्ट्रोकाइनेस के साथ मिश्रित होकर सक्रिय हो जाता है। The inactive form of trypins found in pancreatic juice becomes activated when mixed with enterokinase in the intestine.

Tsetse fly (टीसेट्सी फ्लाइ) अफ्रीका की एक मक्खी जो निद्रा रोग उत्पन्न करती है। An African fly which causes sleeping sickness.

Tsp (टीएसपी) चाय की चम्मच। Teaspoon.

Tubal nephritis (ट्यूबल नेफ्राइटिस) वृक्क नलिकाओं का शोथ। Inflammation of the kidney tubules.

Tube (ट्यूब) एक लम्बा, खोखला, बेलनाकार अंग अथवा यंत्र, नली, नाल। A long, hollow, cylindrical organ or instrument.

Tubectomy (ट्यूबेक्टॉमी) किसी नली विशेषकर डिम्ब वाहिनी को सम्पूर्ण को अथवा उसके किसी भाग को शल्यक्रिया द्वारा काट कर अलग कर देना। Surgical removal of all or part of a tube, especially the fallopian tube.

Tuber (ट्यूबर) कन्द, गुलिका, स्थानिक सूजन। A localized swelling.

Tubercle (ट्यूबरकल) किसी हड्डी पर कण्डरा की संलग्नता के लिए स्थित अथवा त्वचा या श्लेष्मिक झिल्ली पर स्थित एक छोटी पर्विका या उत्सेघ, गुलिका। A small nodule or eminence on a bone for attachments of a tendon, or on the skin or mucous membrane.

Tuberculid (ट्यूबरकुलिड) यक्ष्मा के जीवविषों द्वारा उत्पन्न एक विटिकीय (फुन्सीदार) त्वचा विस्फोट। Tuberculoderma a popular skin eruption caused by toxins of tuberculosis.

Tuberculin (ट्यूबरकुलिन) ट्यूबरकल बेसीलस से निकाला गया एक तरल जिसे यक्ष्मा के निदान के लिए प्रयोग में लाया जाता है। A liquid extracted from tubercle bacillus, used in the diagnosis of tuberculosis.

Tuberculitis (ट्यूबरकुलाइटिस) किसी गुलिका का शोथ। Inflammation of a tubercle.

Tuberculoma (ट्यूबरकुलोमा) एक यक्ष्मज अबुर्द अथवा फोड़ा यक्ष्मिकागुल्म। A tuberculosis tumor or abscess.

Tuberculosis (ट्यूबरकुलोसिस) क्षय रोग। An infectious bacterial disease characterized by the growth of nodule (tubercles) in the tissue. (*i*) **Aerogenic tuberculosis** (एरोजेनिक ट्युबरकुलोसिस) अन्दर खींच लेने पर वायु द्वारा उत्पन्न यक्ष्मा रोग। Tuberculosis occurring through air, by inhaling infected droplets. (*ii*) **Endogenous tuberculosis** (एण्डोजीनस ट्यूबरकुलोसिस) शरीर के अन्य स्थान में स्थित गुलिका

से उत्पन्न होने वाली यक्ष्मा। Tuberculosis arising from a tubercle in another site of the body.

(*iii*) **Pulmonary tuberculosis** (पल्मोनरी ट्यूबरकुलोसिस) फुफ्फुसीय यक्ष्मा, राजयक्ष्मा। Tuberculosis of the lungs.

Tuberculotic (ट्यूबरकुलोटिक) यक्ष्मा से सम्बन्धित अथवा उससे पीड़ित, यक्ष्मज। Pertaining to or suffering from tuberculosis.

Tuberculum (ट्यूबरकुलम) गुलिका, दण्डाणु। Tubercle.

Tuberosity (ट्यूबरोसिटी) किसी हड्डी पर स्थित एक उठान जिससे कोई पेशी संलग्न होती है। An elevation on a bone to which a muscle is attached.

Tubo-ovarian (ट्यूबो-ओवेरियन) डिम्ब वाहिनी एवं डिम्बग्रन्थि से सम्बन्धित। Pertaining to the fallopian tube and the ovary.

Tubo-ovaritis (टयूबो-ओवेराइटिस) डिम्ब वाहिनी एवं डिम्बग्रन्थि का शोथ। Inflammation of the fallopian tube and ovary.

Tubotorsion (टयृबोटॉर्शन) किसी नली को ऐंठने का कार्य। The act of twisting a tube.

Tubovaginal (ट्यूबोवैजाइनल) डिम्बवाहिनी एवं योनि से सम्बन्धित। Pertaining to the fallopian tube and vagina.

Tubule (ट्यूब्यूल) एक छोटी नली अथवा नलिका जैसे वृक्कीय नलिकाएँ तथा शुक्र जनक नलिकाएँ आदि। A small tube or canal, e.g. renal tubules and seminiferous.

Tubulorrhexis (ट्यूब्यूलोरैहक्सिस) वृक्क नलिकाओं का फट जाना। Rupture of the renal tubules.

Tubulous (ट्यूब्यूलस) नलिकाओं से युक्त। Containing tubules.

Tuft (टफ्ट) एक छोटा गुच्छा या समूह अथवा चक्करदार पिण्ड। A small clump cluster or coiled mass.

Tularemia (टूलेरीमिया) फ्रान्सीसेला टुलेरेन्सिस द्वारा उत्पन्न एक तीव्र प्लेग के समान संक्रामक रोग जो किसी संक्रमित किलनी और संक्रमित कीडो व जीव जन्तुओं के सीधे सम्पर्क मे आने के कारण होता है। An acute plague-like infectious disease caused by *Francisella tularensis*, which is transmitted through the bite of an infected tick or direct contact with infected animals.

Tumescence (ट्यूमेसेन्स) सूजन या फुलाव। A swelling.

Tumor (ट्यूमर) फुलाव अथवा फैलाव, अबुर्द, गुल्म, रसौली। Swelling or enlargement.

(*i*) **Benign Tumor** (बैनाइन ट्यूमर) यह प्रगतिशील नहीं

होता, निकाल देने के पश्चात् फिर से उत्पन्न नहीं होता और स्थलान्तरण को उत्पन्न नहीं करता तथा अधिकतर एक तन्तुमय कैप्सूल से चारों ओर से घिरा होता है, सुदम अबुर्द। It is not progressive, not recurring after removal and not giving rise to metastasis and usually surrounded by a fibrous capsule.

(*ii*) **Mixed tumor** (मिक्सड ट्यूमर) दो या अधिक प्रकार के ऊतक से बना अबुर्द। A tumor composed of two or more types of tissue.

Tumoricidal (ट्यूमोरीसाइडल) अबुर्द कोशिकाओं के लिए विनाशकारी। Destructive to tumor cells.

Tumorous (ट्यूमोरस) अबुर्द के समान। Tumor-like.

Tunica (ट्यूनिका) शरीर के किसी भाग अथवा अंग को आच्छादित करने या आस्तरित करने वाली एक झिल्ली अथवा अन्य संरचना, कंचुक, आवरण। A membrane or other structure covering or lining a body part or organ.

Tunica adventitia (ट्यूनिका एडवेन्टीशिया) किसी धमनी या नलिकाकार रचना का बाह्य स्तर, बहिःकंचुक। Outer coat of an artery or an tubular structure.

Tunica intima (ट्यूनिका इन्टिमा) धमनी का भीतरी स्तर। Inner coat of an artery.

Tunica media (ट्यूनिका मीडिया) धमनी का बीच का पेशीय स्तर। Middle muscular coat of an artery.

Tunica vaginalis (ट्यूनिका वैजा. इनालिस) शुक्रग्रन्थि के सामने के भय एवं पार्श्वो को ढँकने वाली सीरमी झिल्ली, अण्डधर कंचुक। The serous membrane covering the front and sides of the testis.

Tunnel (टनल) ठोस काय में स्थित आने-जाने का एक तंग मार्ग, सुरंग। A narrow passageway through a solid body.

Turbid (टर्बिड) गंदला, जो साफ न हो, आविल। Muddy; not clear.

Turbidimeter (टर्बिडीमीटर) किसी तरल के गंदलेपन को मापने वाला एक उपकरण। An apparatus for measuring the turbidity of a fluid.

Turbidity (टर्बिडिटी) गदलापन, धुंधलापन, आविलता। Muddiness, cloudiness.

Turbinate (टर्बिनेट) उल्टे शंकु के आकार का, लट्टू-रूप। Shaped like an inverted cone.

Turbinotomy (टर्बिनोटॉमी) किसी टर्बिनेट हड्डी को चीरना, नासाशुक्तिकाछेदन। Incision of a tubinate bone.

Turgor (टर्गर) कोशिका में सामान्य तनाव। Normal tension in a cell.

Tussiculation (टसीकुलेशन) थोड़ी देर के लिये उठने वाली सूखी खांसी। A short, dry cough.

Tutamen (ट्यूटामेन) एक रक्षक आवरण अथवा संरचना जैसे आँखों के लिये पलकें तथा पलकों के बाल। A protecting covering or structure, as eyelids and eyelashes for the eyes.

Twig (ट्विग) किसी रक्त वाहिनी अथवा तंत्रिका की अन्तिम शाखा। A final branch of a blood vessel or nerve.

Twin (ट्विन) जुड़वाँ बच्चों में से एक, यमल।
One of the two children born at one birth.
(*i*) **Dizygotic twins** (डाइजाइगोटिक ट्विन्स) एक ही समय में गर्भित होने वाले दो अलग-अलग डिम्बों से विकसित होने वाले यमल, द्विडिम्बी यमल। Twins developed from two separate ova fertilized at the same time.
(*ii*) **Monozygotic twins** (मोनोजाइगोटिक ट्विन्स) एक गर्भित डिम्ब से विकसित होने वाले यमल। Twins that developed from one fertilized ovum.
(*iii*) **Parasitic twins** (पैरासाइटिक ट्विन्स) छोटे-बड़े संयुक्त यमलों में से छोटा यमल। The smaller of the unequal cojoined twins.

Twitch (ट्विच) किसी पेशी का तुरन्त होने वाला ऐंठनयुक्त संकुचन, स्फुरण।
A quick spasmodic contraction of a muscle.

Tyloma (टाइलोमा) किण, घट्टा। A callus or callosity.

Tympanectomy (टिम्पैनेक्टॉमी) मध्यकर्ण कला को शल्यक्रिया द्वारा काटकर निकाल देना। Excession of the tympanic membrane.

Tympanic membrane (टिम्पैनिक मेम्ब्रेन) मध्य कर्ण की गुहा की पार्श्व भित्ति को बनाने वाली झिल्ली, मध्यकर्णिक कला। Membrane forming the lateral wall of the cavity of the middle ear.

Tympanites (टिम्पैनाइट्स) आँतों में गैस के होने से पेट का फूल जाना, आध्मान, आफरा। Distention of abdomen due to presence of gas in the intestines.

Tympanitis (टिम्पैनाइटिस) मध्यकर्णीय झिल्ली का प्रदाह, मध्यकर्णशोथ।

Inflammation of the tympanic membrane, myringitis.

Tympanography (टिम्पैनोग्राफी) किसी भेदन माध्यम को प्रविष्ट करके यूस्टेशियन नली एवं मध्य कर्ण का एक्स-रे परीक्षण करना। X-ray examination of the Eustachian tube and middle ear after introducing a contrast medium.

Tympanomalleal (टिम्पैनोमेलियल) मध्यकर्ण-कला एवं मुदगर अस्थि से सम्बन्धित। Pertaining to the tympanic membrane and the malleus bone.

Tympanoplasty (टिम्पैनोप्लास्टी) मध्यकर्ण-कला की प्लास्टिक सर्जरी करना, मध्यकर्ण-सन्धान। Plastic surgery of the tympanic membrane.

Tympanum (टिम्पैनम) मध्यकर्ण-गुहा। Eardurm cavity of the middle ear.

Tympany (टिम्पैनी) आधमान या अफारा, अनुनाद। Tympanites, resonance.

Typhlectasis (टिफ्लेक्टेसिस) सीकम या अन्धान्त्र का फूल जाना। Distention of the cecum.

Typhlitis (टिफ्लाइटिस) सीकम या अन्धान्त्र की सूजन, अन्धान्त्रशोथ। Inflammation of the cecum.

Typhlomegaly (टिफ्लोमेगैली) सीकम या अन्धान्त्र का असामान्य रूप से बढ़ जाना। An abnormal enlargement of the cecum.

Typhlopexy (टिफ्लोपैक्सी) गतिशील सीकम को उदरीय भित्ति के साथ सीना। Suturing of the movable cecum to the abdominal wall.

Typhlospasm (टिफ्लोस्पाज्म) सीकम का ऐंठ जाना। Spasm of the cecum.

Typhlostomy (टिफ्लोस्टॉमी) एक स्थायी अन्धान्त्र नालव्रण स्थापित करना। To establish a permanent cecal fistula.

Typhoid (टाइफॉयड) टाइफस के समान। Resembling typhus.

Typhoid fever (टाइफॉयड फीवर) साल्मोनेला टाइफाइ द्वारा उत्पन्न एक तीव्र संक्रामक रोग जिसमें निरन्तर ज्वर रहता है, आंत्रिक ज्वर, मियादी बुखार। Enteric fever. An acute infectious disease characterized by *Salmonella typhi.*

Typholysin (टाइफोलाइसिन) टाइफॉयड बेसीलसों के लिए विनाशकारी लाइसिन। A lysin destructive to typhoid bacillity.

Typhopneumonia (टाइफोन्यूमोनिया) टाइफॉयड ज्वर के साथ न्यूमोनिया होना। Pneunonia occurring with typhoid fever.

Typhus (टाइफस) तीव्र संक्रामक रोगों के एक वर्ग का कोई रोग जिसमें तीव्र ज्वर होता है, तीसरे से सातवें दिन के बीच चित्रीपिटिकीय विस्फोट निकल आते हैं, सिर में तेज दर्द होता है, कमजोरी बहुत होती है तथा तन्त्रिका लक्षण उत्पन्न हो जाते हैं, टाइफस। Any of a group of acute infectious diseases with high fever, maculopapular eruption appearing from the third to seventh day severe headache, great prostration and nervous symptoms.

Tyremesis (टाइरीमेसिस) शिशुओं द्वारा दही जैसे पदार्थ की उल्टी होना। Tyrosis vomiting of curdy material by infants.

Tyroma (टाइरोमा) पनीर जैसे पदार्थ से युक्त एक अबुर्द। A tumor containing cheesy material.

Tyrosinemia (टाइरोसाइनीमिया) एक आनुवंशिक रोग जिसमें रक्त में टाइरोसीन बढ़ जाता है और यह मूत्र में आने लगता है जिसके परिणामस्वरूप यकृत का सिरहोसिस हो जाता है, वृक्कीय नलिकाएँ ग्रस्त हो जाती है तथा अल्पग्लूकोजरक्तता हो जाती है। A hereditary disease marked by excess of tyrosine in the blood, and it passes in the urine, resulting in cirrhosis of the liver, renal tubular involvement and hypoglycemia.

Tyrosinuria (टाइरोसीनूरिया) मूत्र में टाइरोसीन का पाया जाना। Presence of tyrosine in the urine.

Tysonitis (टाइसोनाइटिस) शिश्नमुण्डच्छदीय ग्रन्थियों का शोथ। Inflammation of Tyson' glands (preputial glands).

U

U (यू) 1. इकाई 2. यूरेनियम का रासायनिक प्रतीक। 1. Unit 2. Chemical symbol for Uranium.

Uberous (यूबेरस) फलदायक या उपजाऊ जननक्षय या अबंध्य। Fruitful; fertile.

Ulalgia (यूलैल्जिया) मसूड़ों में दर्द होना। Pain in the gums.

Ulcer (अल्सर) घाव, फोड़ा। A sore on any soft part of the body attended with discharge of pus.

Ulcerogangrenous (अल्सेरोगैंग्रीनस) व्रण एवं कोथ दोनों के बनने की विशिष्टता से युक्त। Characterized by the formation of both, ulcer and gangrene.

Ulcerogenic (अल्सरोजेनिक) जख्म बनने वाला। Producing ulcer.

Uliginous (यूलीजीनस) मिट्टी या कीचड़ से युक्त। Muddy.

Ulitis (यूलाइटिस) मसूड़ों का प्रदाह। Inflammation of the gums.

Ulna (अलना) अन्तःप्रकोष्ठिका। The medial and larger of the two bones of the forearms.

Uloglossitis (यूलोग्लोसाइटिस) मसूड़ों एवं जीभ की सूजन। Inflammation of the gums and tongue.

Ulorrhagia (यूलोरैह्जिया) मसूडों से रक्तस्राव होना। Bleeding from the gums.

Ulorrhea (यूलोरीह्या) मसूड़ों से स्राव निकलना। Discharge from the gums.

Ulotrichous (यूलोट्राइकस) छोटे-छोटे ऊन जैसे बालों को धारण करने वाला। Having short woolly hair.

Ultrafiltration (अल्ट्राफिल्ट्रेशन) ऐसे निस्यन्दक के द्वारा छानना जो अतिसूक्ष्मदर्शीय कणों को अलग करता है। Filtration through a filter which removes ultramicroscopic particles.

Ultrasonic (अल्ट्रॉसोनिक) पराध्वनिक, प्रतिध्वनिक। Relating to mechanical vibrations of very high frequency.

Ultrasonography (अल्ट्रॉसोनोग्राफी) अल्ट्रॉसाउण्ड का प्रयोग करके किसी अंग अथवा ऊतक का प्रतिबिम्ब या चित्र प्राप्त करना। To obtain image or photograph of an organ or tissue by using ultrasound.

Ultrasound (अल्ट्रॉसाउण्ड) सुनाई न देने वाली ध्वनि जिसकी बारम्बारता 20,000 से 10,000,000,000 चक्र प्रति सेकण्ड होती है। Inaudible sound with the frequency of 20,000 to 10,000,000,000 cycles per second.

Ultrastructure (अल्ट्रॉस्ट्रक्चर) बहुत सूक्ष्म संरचना जिसे केवल अतिसूक्ष्मदर्शी द्वारा ही देखा जा सकता है। A very minute structure visible only under the ultramicroscope.

Ultraviolet rays (अल्ट्रॉवायेलेट रेज) पराबैंगनी किरणें। Invisible actinic rays of the spectrum which are beyond the visible violet end, violet rays.

Umbilical cord (अम्बिलाइकल कॉर्ड) नाभि-रज्जु। The navel string.

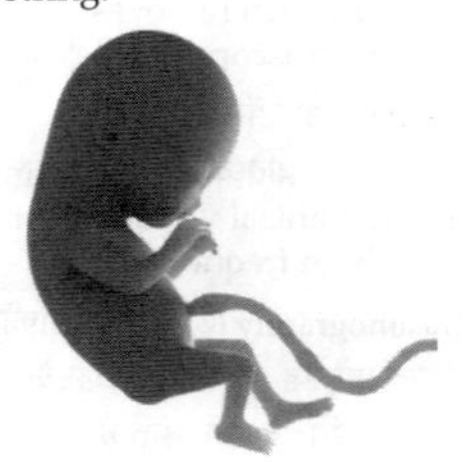

Umbilical souffle (अम्बिलाइकल सूफ्ल) नाभि-रज्जु से उत्पन्न होने वाली सी-सी करने की आवाज। A hissing sound arising from the umbilical cord.

Umbilication (अम्बिलाइकेशन) 1. एक गड्ढा जो नाभि के समान होता है। 2. किसी फोड़े अथवा जलस्फोट के शिखर पर एक गड्ढे का बनना। 1. A depression resembling the umbilicus. 2. Formation of a depression on the top of an abscess or vesicle.

Umbilicus (अम्बिलाइकस) नाभि। Navel.

Umbo (अम्बो) ककुद। A boss; any central convex eminence.

Uncinate (अनसाइनेट) हुक के आकार का, हुक से युक्त। Hook-shaped; hooked.

Unconditioned-reflex (अनकण्डीशन्ड-रिफ्लैक्स) उत्पन्न प्रतिवर्त क्रिया, उपार्जित नहीं। Reflex action, not acquired.

Unconscious (अनकॉनशस) बेहोश। Senseless.

Uncus (अन्कस) अंकुश। A hook.

Underweight (अण्डरवेट) ऐसी दशा जिसमें किसी व्यक्ति के शरीर का भार उसके सामान्य भार से कम से कम 10% कम होता है। A condition in which the body weight of a person is at least 10% less than what is normal for that person.

Undine (अन्डाइन) आँखों की धुलाई करने के लिये एक छोटा काँच

का फ्लास्क। A small glass flask for washing eyes.

Undulation (अनडुलेशन) उर्मिलता, लहरदार गति या धड़कन तरंगण। A wavelike motion or pulsation.

Ungual (अॅग्वल) नाखूनों से सम्बन्धित अथवा उनसे मिलता-जुलता। Pertaining to or resembling the nails.

Unguentum (अंग्वैन्टम) मरहम। Ointment.

Unicorn (यूनीकॉर्न) केवल एक सींग धारण करने वाला। Having a single cornu or horn.

Unicuspid (यूनीकस्पिड) केवल एक कपर्दिका धारण करने वाला। Having a single cusp.

Uniforate (यूनीफोरेट) केवल एक छिद्र वाला। Having only one opening.

Unilateral (यूनीलेट्रल) एकपार्श्विक, केवल एक पार्श्व को प्रभावित करने वाला। Affected, or confined to, but on one side.

Uninuclear (यूनीन्यूक्लियर) केवल एक केन्द्रक वाला। Having only one nucleus.

Union (यूनीयन) जोड़, विरोहण प्रक्रिया। Joining; the process of healing.

Uniparous (यूनीपेरस) एक समय में केवल एक बच्चे को जन्म देने वाली। Producing one child at a birth.

Unipolar (यूनीपोलर) केवल एक ध्रुव वाली कोशिका। A cell with one pole.

Unit (यूनिट) कोई अकेली चीज। A single entity.

Univalent (यूनीवैलेन्ट) एक की वैलेन्सी वाला। Having a valence of one.

Universal-antidote (यूनीवर्सल एन्टिडोट) विषाक्तता में प्रयुक्त एक प्रतिकारक जब विशिष्ट प्रतिकारक का पता नहीं होता अथवा वह उपलब्ध नहीं होता। An antidote used in poisoning where the specific antidote is unknown or not available.

Universal donor (यूनीवर्सल डोनर) O रक्त वर्ग का व्यक्ति जिसके रक्त को बिना खतरे के A, B, O रक्त वर्गों में से किसी भी रक्त वर्ग के व्यक्ति में चढ़ाया जा सकता है। A person of blood group O whose blood may be transfused to a person of the other A,B,O blood group, without danger.

Unmyelinated (अनमाइलीनेटेड) माइलिन आच्छद से रहित। Without a myelin sheath.

Unsaturated (अनसेचुरेटेड) असंतृप्त। Not saturated.

Uptake (अपटेक) अवशोषण। The absorption by a tissue of same substance.

Uracrasia (यूरेक्रेसिया) 1. मूत्र की विकृत अवस्था। 2. मूत्र को रोकने में असमर्थता।
1. Disordered state of the urine. 2. Inability to retain the urine.

Uranium (यूरेनियम) यूरेनियम। A feebly radioactive metallic element.

Urapostema (यूरेपोस्टीमा) एक फोड़ा जिसमें मूत्र भरा होता है। An abscess filled with urine.

Uratemia (यूरेटीमिया) रक्त में यूरेट विशेषकर सोडियम यूरेट में पाया जाना। Presence of urates, especially sodium urate in the blood.

Uratosis (यूरेटोसिस) ऊतकों में यूरेटों का जमाव। The deposit of urates in the tissues.

Urea (यूरिया) मूत्र का मुख्य नाइट्रोजनी घटक तथा प्रोटीन चयापचय का मुख्य नाइट्रोजनी अंतिम उत्पाद जो अमीनों-अम्ल एवं अमोनिया यौगिकों से यकृत में बनता है। मिहेय। The chief solid constituent of urine and principal nitrogenous product of tissue catabolism, which is formed in the liver from amino acids and ammonia compounds.

Urea frost (यूरिया फ्रोस्ट) बढ़े हुए यूरीमिया के रोगियों की त्वचा पर दिखाई देने वाले यूरिया के श्वेत परतदार जमाव। White flaky deposits of urea seen on the skin of patients with advanced uremia.

Urelcosis (यूरेल्कोसिस) मूत्र-पथ में जख्म बनना। Ulceration of the urinary tract.

Ureter (यूरेटर) मूत्रनली, गवीनी। Tube carrying urine from the renal pelvis of the kidney to the bladder.

Ureterocele (यूरेटेरोसील) मूत्रनली का मूत्राशय में खुलने वाले स्थान के पास पुटी के समान विस्फारण। Cyst-like dilatation of the ureter near its opening into the bladder.

Ureterostomy (यूरेटेरोस्टोमी) गवीनीछिद्रीकरण। The formation of a urethral fistula.

Urethra (यूरेथ्रा) मूत्रमार्ग, मूत्रपथ। The excretory canal of the bladder.

Urethritis (यूरेथ्राइटिस) मूत्रमार्ग का प्रदाह। Inflammation of the urethra.

Urethropexy (यूरेथ्रोपैक्सी) मूत्रमार्ग का शल्य क्रिया द्वारा स्थिरीकरण। Surgical fixation of the urethra.

Urethrophraxis (यूरेथ्रोफ्रेक्सिस) मूत्रमार्ग में अवरोध उत्पन्न हो

जाना। Obstruction of the urethra.

Urethroplasty (यूरेथ्रोप्लास्टी) मूत्रमार्ग की प्लास्टिक सर्जरी करना। Plastic surgery of the urethra.

Urethrorrhea (यूरेथ्रोरिह्या) मूत्रमार्ग से असामान्य स्राव निकलना। Abnormal discharge from the urethra.

Urethroscope (यूरेथ्रोस्कोप) मूत्रमार्गदर्शी। An instrument for visual examination of the interior of the urethra.

Uretic (यूरेटिक) मूत्र का बहाव बढ़ाने वाला पदार्थ। An agent promoting the flow of urine.

Urging (यूरगिंग) इच्छा, रूचि। Desire.

Urinary calculus (यूरिनरी कैल्कुलस) मूत्रीय पथ में बनने वाली पथरी। A calculus formed in the urinary tract.

Urination (यूरिनेशन) मूत्र-त्याग की क्रिया। The act of passing urine from the bladder.

Urine (यूरिन) मूत्र, पेशाब। Water excreted from the bladder.

Urinoma (यूरिनोमा) एक पुटी जिसमें मूत्र होता है। A cyst containing urine.

Urinometer (यूरिनोमीटर) मूत्र के विशिष्ट गुरूत्व का पता लगाने वाला उपकरण। An apparatus for determining the specific gravity of urine.

Urobilin (यूरोबिलिन) यूरोबिलिनोजन के ऑक्सीकरण से बना एक भूरा वर्णक। A brown pigment formed by oxidation of urobilinogen.

Urobilinogen (यूरोबिलिनोजन) आंत्रीय जीवाणुओं की बिलिरूबिन के ऊपर होने वाली क्रिया से आँत में बनने वाला एक रंगहीन यौगिक। A colorless compound formed in the intestine by the action of intestinal bacteria on bilirubin.

Urobilinuria (यूरोबिलिन्यूरिया) मूत्र में यूरोबिलिन की अधिकता। Excess of urobilin in the urine.

Urocele (यूरोसील) वृषणकोश के अंदर पेशाब का जमाव होना। An effusion of urine in the scrotum.

Urochrome (यूरोक्रोम) मूत्रवर्णक। A yellow urinary pigment.

Urocyanosis (यूरोसायनोसिस) मूत्र की नील विवर्णता। Blue discoloration of the urine.

Urography (यूरोग्राफी) मूत्रपथचित्रण। Radiographic description of the urinary tracts or X-ray examination.

Urolithiasis (यूरोलिथिएसिस) मूत्रपथरी बनना। The formation of urinary calculus in the urinary system.

Urology (यूरोलॉजी) मूत्र-प्रणाली के रोगों से सम्बन्धित विशिष्ट चिकित्सा, मूत्रविज्ञान। The branch of medicine and physiology concerned with the function and disorders of the urinary system.

Uroplania (यूरोप्लेनिया) मूत्रीय पथ के अतिरिक्त अन्य अंगों से मूत्र का निकलना। Discharge of urine from the organs other than the urinary tract.

Uropoiesis (यूरोपॉयसिस) यूरिया की उत्पत्ति होना। Production of urea.

Uropyoureter (यूरोपायोयूरेटर) मूत्रनली में मूत्र एवं पस का इकट्ठा होना। Accumulation of urine and pus in the ureter.

Uroschesis (यूरोस्केसिस) मूत्र का दमन अथवा अवधारण। Suppression or retention of urine.

Urosis (यूरोसिस) मूत्रांगों का कोई भी रोग। Any disease of the urinary organs.

Urticaria (अर्टिकेरिया) शीतपित्त, जुलपित्ति, छपकि। Hives (nettle-rash) shingles.

Uteroplasty (यूटेरोप्लास्टी) प्लास्टिक सर्जरी द्वारा गर्भाशय की मरम्मत करना। Repair of the uterus by plastic surgery.

Uterus (यूट्रस) बच्चेदानी, गर्भाशय। The female organ of gestation; the womb.

Utricle (यूट्रीकल) लघुकोश, क्षुद्रकोश। A little sac or pocket.

Uvea (यूवीया) रंजिटपटल, अस्तिपटल। The pigmented layer of the eyeball; Uveal tract; choroid.

Uveitis (यूवाइटिस) रंजितपटल का प्रदाह। Inflammation of uvea.

Uveoparotitis (यूवीयोपैरोटाइटिस) कर्णपूर्वग्रंथि शोथ एवं असित-पटलशोथ। Inflammation of the parotid gland and uveitis.

Uviofast (यूवियोफास्ट) अल्ट्रॉवायोलेट विकिरण से अप्रभावित। Unaffected by ultraviolet radiation.

Uviolize (यूवियोलाइज) रोगों की चिकित्सा में अल्ट्रॉवायोलेट किरणों का प्रयोग करना। To use ultraviolet rays in the treatment of disease.

Uviometer (यूवियोमीटर) अल्ट्रॉवायेलेट प्रकाश की तीव्रता मापने वाला एक यंत्र। An instrument for measuring the intensity of ultraviolet light.

Uviosensitive (यूवियोसेन्सीटिव) अल्ट्रॉवायलेट किरणों के प्रभावों के प्रति संवेदनशील। Sensitive to the effects of ultraviolet rays.

Uvula (यूव्यूला) एक लटकता हुआ छोटा मांसल पिण्ड विशेषकर तालु का काकलक। A hanging small fleshy mass, especially the palatine uvula.

Uvulatomy (यूव्यूलेटामी) काकलक को चीरना। To incise the uvula.

Uvulitis (यूव्यूलाइटिस) काकलक शोथ। Inflammation of the uvula.

Uvuloptosis (यूव्यूलोप्टेसिस) काकलक का शिथिल हो जाना एवं लटक जाना। Relaxation and hanging of the uvula.

Uvulotome (यूव्यूलोटोम्) काकलक को काट कर निकाल देने वाला एक यंत्र। An instrument for removal of the uvula.

V

V (वी) 1. वाइब्रियो, दृष्टि 2. वेनिडियम का रासायनिक प्रतीक। 1. Vibrio; Vision 2. Chemical symbol for Vanadium.

Vaccinable (वैक्सीनेबल) टीका लगवाने के सक्षम। Capable of being vaccinated.

Vaccination (वैक्सीनेशन) रोगक्षमता उत्पन्न करने के लिये टीका लगाने की क्रिया। Inoculation of a vaccine to produce immunity.

Vaccinator (वैक्सोनेटर) टीका लगाने वाला व्यक्ति। The person who vaccinates.

Vaccine (वैक्सीन) टीका। A preparation of living, weakend or killed microorganism or viruses, used in prevention of disease through immunizing of persons likely to be exposed; a genus of cowpox.

Vaccinia (वैक्सीनिया) गोशीतला, छोटी माता। Cowpox; a contagious disease amongst cattle.

Vaccinogenous (वैक्सीनोजीनस) वैक्सीन उत्पन्न करने वाला। Producing vaccine.

Vaccinostyle (वैक्सीनोस्टाइल) टीका लगाने के काम आने वाला एक नुकीला सिरा। A pointed stylus used in vaccination.

Vaccum (वैक्यूम) निर्वात। An empty space exhausted of air or gas.

Vaccum aspiration (वैक्यूम एस्पिरेशन) गर्भाशय में कैथीटर से संलग्न चूषण उपकरण द्वारा निर्मित या शून्य स्थान उत्पन्न करके उसकी सामग्रियों को निकालना। Removal of the uterine contents by creating vaccum in the uterus by a suction apparatus attached to a catheter.

Vaccum extractor (वैक्यूम एक्सट्रेक्टर) प्रसव के दौरान भ्रूण पर खिंचाव डालने के लिए भ्रूण के सिर पर लगाया जाने वाला एक चूषण कप। A suction cup attached to the fetal head for applying traction to the fetus during delivery.

Vacuole (वैक्योल) रिक्तिका। A clear space in a cell filled with air or fluid.

Vagabond's disease (वैगाबोन्ड'स डिजीज) यूकाजनिक तवग्विवर्णता।

Discoloration of the skin from lice.

Vagina (वैजाइना) 1. योनि, प्रजनन-नलिका। 2. आवरण। 1. The female genital canal extending from uterus to vulva.
2. A sheath or any sheath-like structure.

Vaginismus (वैजाइनिस्मस) योनि की दर्दनाक ऐंठन। Painful spasm of the vagina.

Vaginitis (वैजीनाइटिस) योनि-प्रदाह। Inflammation of the vagina.

Vaginoperineotomy (वैजाइनोपैरीनियोटॉमी) योनि एवं मूलाधार दोनों में एक चीरा लगाना। To make an incision into the vagina and perineum.

Vaginosis (वैजाइनोसिस) योनि का रोग। Disease of the vagina.

Vagitis (वैगाइटिस) वेगम तंत्रिका का शोथ। Inflammation of the vagus.

Vagitus (वेजीटस) शिशु का चिल्लाना। The cry of an infant.

Vagolysis (वेगोलाइसिस) शल्यक्रिया द्वारा वेगस तंत्रिका को नष्ट करना। Surgical destruction of the vagus nerve.

Vagotomy (वेगोटॉमी) शल्यक्रिया द्वारा वेगस तंत्रिका को आर-पार काट देना।
Surgical transection of the vagus nerve.

Valence, Valency (वैलेन्स, वैलेन्सी) संयोजकता। The combining power of an atom as compared with an atom of hydrogen.

Valgus (वैल्गस) शरीर का वह भाग जो बाहर की ओर शरीर की मध्य रेखा से दूर को घूमा होता है जैसे–बहिर्नत। The part of the body bent outward, away from the midline of the body, as talipes valgus.

Vallate (वैलेट) किसी गड्ढे के चारों ओर किनारे से युक्त, परिवृत्त। Having an edge around a depression, cupped.

Vallum-Unguis (वेलम-अन्विवस) नाखून को ढकने वाली त्वचा की तह, अभिनख। Fold of skin overlaping the nail.

Valve (वाल्व) कपाट, कपाटिका। A device permitting control of an opening so as to allow free passage one-way, but not the other; valva.

Valvoplasty (वाल्वोप्लास्टी) किसी कपाट में चीरा लगाना। Plastic surgery of a valve.

Valvotomy (वाल्वोटॉमी) किसी कपाट में चीरा लगाना। To make an incision into a valve.

Van den Bergh's test (वान डेन बर्ग्स टैस्ट) रक्त सीरम अथवा प्लाज्मा में बिलिरूबिन की

विद्यमानता का पता लगाने के लिए किया जाने वाला एक परीक्षण। A test to detect the presence of bilirubin in blood serum or plasma.

Vapor (वेपर) वाष्प, भाप। A gaseous form assumed by a solid or liquid substance when sufficiently heated.

Vaporize (वेपोराइज) किसी ठोस अथवा तरल पदार्थ को भाप में बदलना। To convert a solid or liquid into a vapor.

Vapotherapy (वेपोथिरेपी) वाष्प द्वारा रोगों की चिकित्सा करना। Treatment of the disease by vapor.

Variant (वेरियेन्ट) रूपान्तर, परिवर्तन। Having tendency to alter or change.

Varicella (वेरीसेला) छोटी माता। Chickenpox.

Varicocele (वेरिकोसील) अण्डकोश की रक्त वाहिनियों का बढ़ना। Abnormal enlargement of blood vessels of the spermatic cord.

Varicose (वेरिकोस) किसी शिरा का फैला हुआ भाग। The dilated portion of a vein.

Varicose vein (वेरिकोस वेन) अपस्फीत शिरा। A varix.

Varicosity (वेरिकोसिटी) 1. अपस्फीत होना। 2. एक अपस्फीत शिरां 1. The condition of being varicose. 2. Varix, a varicose vein.

Variola (वेरियोला) बड़ी माता, चेचक। Smallpox.

Varix (वेरिक्स) किसी शिरा का फूलना या बढ़ना। A venous dilation of an enlarged and tortuous vein.

Varus (वेरस) शरीर का मध्यरेखा की ओर झुकना। Displacement or angulation towards the midline of the body.

Vas (वास) वाहिका, नली। A vessel; duct.

Vasa (वासा) वास का बहुवचन। Plural of vas.

Vasalgia (वासेल्जिया) किसी वाहिनी में दर्द होना। Pain in a vessel.

Vascularization (वैस्कुलैराइजेशन) ऊतकों में नई रक्त वाहिनियों का बनना। The formation of new blood vessels in tissues.

Vasculature (वैस्कुलेचर) 1. शरीर अथवा इसके किसी भाग में रक्त वाहिनियों की व्यवस्था। 2. किसी विशिष्ट क्षेत्र को रक्त वाहिनियों की आपूर्ति। 1. The arrangement of blood vessels in the body or any part of it. 2. The supply of blood vessels to a specific region.

Vasculitis (वैस्कुलाइटिस) किसी रक्तवाहिका का प्रदाह। Inflammation of a blood vessel.

Vasculopathy (वैस्कुलोपैथी) रक्त वाहिनियों का कोई भी रोग। Any disease of the blood vessels.

Vasectomy (वासेक्टॉमी) शुक्रवाहिनी को काट कर हटाना। Excision of the vas deferens.

Vasitis (वासाइटिस) शुक्रवहानली का प्रदाह। Inflammation of ductus deferens.

Vasoconstriction (वासोकन्सट्रिक्शन) रक्त वाहिनियों के अन्तर्व्यास का घट जाना। Lose in the caliber of blood vessels.

Vasodepression (वासोडिप्रेसन) रक्त वाहिनियों का प्रतिरोध कम हो जाना जिससे रक्तचाप कम हो जाता है। Decrease in the resistance of blood vessels which causes low blood pressure.

Vasodilator (वासोडाइलेटर) रक्त वाहिकाओं के तनाव को नियमित करने वाला। Regulating the tension of the blood vessels.

Vasopressor (वासोप्रेसर) रक्तवाहिकाओं की सिकुड़न एवं रक्तचाप बढ़ाने वाला। Producing vasoconstriction and a rise in blood pressure.

Vasospasm (वासोस्पाज्म) किसी रक्त वाहिनी का ऐंठ जाना, वाहिकाकर्ष। Angiospasm, spasm of a blood vessel.

Vasotonia (वासोटोनिया) रक्त वाहिनियों की तान अथवा तनाव। The tone or tension of blood vessels.

Vasovasostomy (वासोवासोस्टॉमी) शुक्र-वाहिका के पूर्व में काटे गये सिरों को फिर से जोड़ना। Rejoining of the previously cut ends of vas deferens.

Vastus (वास्टस) बड़ा, यह पेशियों के लिए कहा जाता है। Great, said of muscle.

VCG (वी.सी.जी.) सदिशहृद् लेखन। Vectorcardiography, analysis of the direction and magnitude of the electrical forces of the heart's action.

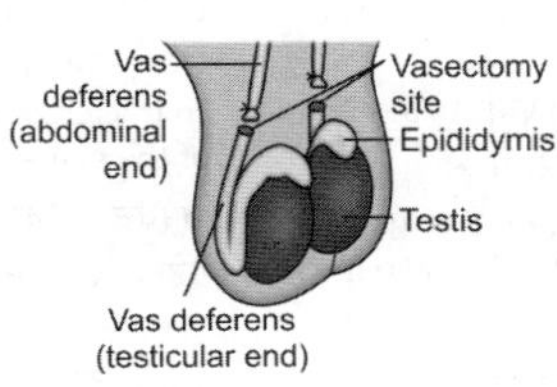

Vasectomy

Vector (वेक्टर) रोगवाहक। An inveterate animal capable of transmitting an infectious agent among vertebrates.

Vegetation (वेजीटेशन) कोई भी वृक्ष के समान कवकरूप वृद्धि। Any plant-like fungoid growth.

Vegetative (वेजीटेटिव) वर्धी, वर्धन-शक्ति से सम्पन्न। Having the power of growth.

Vehicle (वेहीक्ल) अनुपान, वाहन। Excipient.

Veil (वेल) आवरण, परदा। Cover with something, mask, shell.

Vein (वेन) शिरा, वह रक्तवाहिका जो धमनियों से रक्त लेकर हृदय को वापस करती है। Vessel that receives blood from the arteries and returns it to the heart.

Velamentous (वेलामेन्टस) आवरण रचना के समान। Like a veil.

Velamentum (वेलामेन्टम) एक कलामय आवरण। A membranous covering.

Venene (वेनेन) सांप का जहर। The snake-poison.

Venereal (वेनेरीयल) संभोग के कारण होने वाले रोगों से सम्बन्धित। Concerned with diseases contacted by sexual intercourse.

Venereal-diseases (वेनेरीयल डिज़ीज़) रतिज रोग, संभोग के कारण होने वाली बीमारी। Any disease due to venery; VD.

Venereology (वेनेरीयोलॉजी) रतिज रोगों का अध्ययन एवं उसकी चिकित्सा करना। The study and treatment of venereal diseases.

Venipuncture (वेनीपंक्चर) किसी शिरा को सुई द्वारा छेदना। Needling of a vein.

Venogram (वेनोग्राम) शिरालेख, शिराचित्र। A radiograph of venous system after an opaque media injection.

Venom (वीनम) विष, जहर। The poisonous substances injected in bites by snakes, certain spiders, bees, wasps, etc.

Venomous (वीनोमस) 1. विषैला 2. विष निकालने वाला। 1. Poisonous 2. Secreting poison.

Veno-occlusive (वेनो-ऑक्लुजिव) शिराओं में अवरोध उत्पनन हो जाने से सम्बन्धित अथवा उससे युक्त। Pertaining to or characterized by obstruction of the veins.

Vent (वेन्ट) निकास जैसे–मलद्वार, गुहा। An outlet, e.g. the anal opening.

Venter (वेन्टर) उदर, पेट। Belly or a belly-shaped part.

Ventilation (वेन्टीलेशन) संवातन, ताजी हवा का संभरण होना। The suppling of fresh air.

Ventilator (वेन्टीलेटर) फेफड़ों के कृत्रिम श्वसन के लिये एक उपकरण। An apparatus for artifical respiration of the lungs.

Ventral (वेन्ट्रल) उदर अथवा शरीर के अगले तल से सम्बन्धित, अग्र। Pertaining to the abdomen or the anterior surface of the body; anterior.

Ventricle (वेन्ट्रीक्ल) मस्तिष्क अथवा हृदय के अंदर स्थित गुहा, निलय।
A normal cavity in the brain or heart.

Ventriculitis (वेन्ट्रीकुलाइटिस) किसी निलय का शोथ।
Inflammation of a ventricle.

Ventriculocisternostomy (वेन्ट्रीकुलोसिसटर्नोस्टोमी) मस्तिष्क निलय कुंड सम्मिलन।
Artificial communication between cerebral ventricles and subarachnoid space.

Ventriculography (वेन्ट्रीकुलोग्राफी) मस्तिष्क निलय चित्रण।
The localization of tumors by radiographs of the ventricles of the brain after replacing their fluid contents.

Ventrosity (वेन्ट्रोसिटी) बढ़े हुए पेट का होना, मोटापा। The condition of having an enlarged abdomen; obesity.

Ventrosuspension (वेन्ट्रोसस्पेन्शन) गर्भाशय-अग्रनिलम्बन।
The fixation of the displaced uterus at the abdominal wall.

Verbigeration (वरबिजरेशन) अर्थहीन शब्दों की पुनरावृत्ति।
Repetition of words that are either meaningless or have no significance.

Verbomania (वर्बोमैनिया) अत्यधिक बात करने का उन्माद। Mania for excessive talking.

Verge (वर्ज) धारा, किनारा, हशिया। An edge or margin.

Vermicidal (वर्मीसाइडल) आँत के कीड़ों को मारने वाला। Killing the intestinal worms.

Vermicular (वर्मीकुलर) कृमि से मिलता-जुलता। Worm-like.

Vermiform (वर्मीफोर्म) कृमि आकार का। Worm-shaped.

Vermiform-appendix (वर्मीफोर्म-एपैण्डिक्स) उपांत्र, उण्डुकपुच्छ। A worm-shaped tube opening into the cecum.

Vermifugal (वर्मीफ्यूगल) कीड़े बाहर निकालने वाली दवा। Medicine of expelling worms.

Vermifuge (वर्मीफयूग) आंत्र कृमियों को बाहर निकालने वाला कीड़ा, पीड़क जन्तु।
An agent expelling intestinal worms.

Vermin (वर्मिन) फसलों को नष्ट करने वाला कीड़ा, पीड़क जन्तु। A noxious or parasitic insect, or the one, destructive to crops, etc.

Vermination (वर्मीनेशन) कृमियों के कारण होने वाली बीमार अवस्था। The condition of one with worms.

Vermiphobia (वर्मीफोबिया) कृमियों से पीड़ित होने का विकृत डर। Morbid fear of being infected with worms.

Vernacular (वर्नेकुलर) देशी, स्वदेशी। Indigenous.

Vernix caseosa (वर्निक्स केसेओसा) भ्रूण-स्नेह। The waxy or cheese-like white substance found coating the skin of newborn human babies.

Verruca (वरूका) मस्सा, अधिमांस। A wart; a flesh-colored growth characterized by circumscribed hypertrophy of the papillae of the corium.

Verrucosis (वेरूकोसिस) बहुत से अधिमांसों का उत्पन्न होना। The development of multiple warts.

Versicolor (वर्सीकलर) बहुत से रंगों को धारण अथवा परिवर्तित होने वाला। Having, or changeable in many colors.

Version (वर्जन) गर्भाशय का मुड़ जाना। Turning of the womb or the fetus in utero.

Vertebra (वर्टीब्रा) मेरूदण्ड का अस्थिखण्ड। One of the bony segments of the spinal column.

Vertebral canal (वर्टिब्रल कैनाल) कशेरूकाओं से रंध्रों के जुड़ने से बना लम्बा, खोखला स्थान जिसमें सुषुम्ना रज्जु होती है। The long, hollow space formed by union of vertebral foramina, which contains the spinal cord.

Vertebral column (वर्टीब्रल कॉलम) मेरूदण्ड, रीढ़ की हड्डीयाँ। The spinal column; Backbones, the series of backbones that makes vertebral column.

Vertebrate (वर्टीब्रेट) कषेरूका-दण्ड धारण करने वाला, पृष्ठवंशी। Having a vertebral column.

Vertebrectomy (वर्टीब्रेक्टॉमी) किसी कषेरूका अथवा इसके भाग को काटकर निकाल देना। Excision of a vertebra or of its part.

Vertex (वर्टेक्स) कपालशीर्ष, शीर्ष। The crown of the head.

Vertical (वर्टिकल) लम्बरूप। Perpendicular.

Vertiginous (वर्टिजिनस) चक्कर आने से सम्बन्धित या उससे पीड़ित, भ्रमिग्रस्त। Pertaining to or afflicted vertigo.

Vertigo (वर्टिगो) चक्कर आना, सिर चकराना। Giddiness or swimming of the head; dizziness.

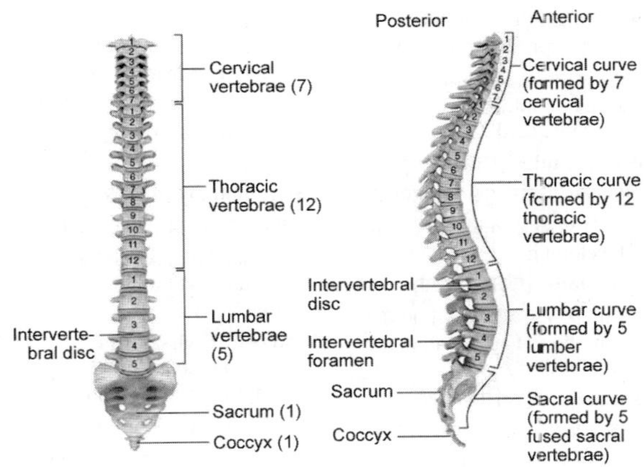

(a) Anterior view showing regions of the vertebral column.

(b) Right lateral view showing four normal curves.

Vertebral column

Vesania (वेसेनिया) पागलपन, मनोविक्षिप्त। Unsoundness of mind.

Vesica (वेसिका) मूत्राशय, आशय। The bladder; vesical.

Vesical (वेसिकल) मूत्राशय संबंधी। Pertaining to the bladder.

Vesical reflex (वैसाइकल-रिफ्लैक्स) मूत्राशय के मूत्र से भर जाने पर फूल जाने पर मूत्र-त्याग की प्रवृत्ति होना। The inclination to urinate caused by moderately distended urinary bladder with urine.

Vesicant (वेसीकैन्ट) छाले या फफोले उत्पन्न करने वाला, जलस्फोटक Blistering; producing blisters.

Vesication (वेसिकेशन) फफोले पैदा होना। The formation of blister.

Vesicle (वेसीक्ल) जलस्फोट, फफोला। A little bladder of water formed under the skin; blister.

Vesicofixation (वेसिकोफिक्सेशन) मूत्राशय को उदर-भित्ति के साथ संलग्न करना। Attachment of the urinary bladder to the abdominal wall.

Vesicoprostatic (वेसिकोप्रोस्टेटिक) मूत्राशय एवं प्रोस्टेट ग्रंथि से सम्बन्धित। Pertaining to the urinary bladder and the prostate gland.

Vesicopustule (वेसिकोपसच्यूल) फफोला जिसमें पस बन रहा होता है। A vesicle in which pus is developing.

Vesicostomy (वेसिकोस्टॉमी) मूत्राशय में एक छेद बनना। The formation of an opening into the bladder.

Vesicovaginal (वेसिकोवैजाइनल) मूत्राशय एवं योनि से सम्बन्धित। Pertaining to the urinary bladder and the vagina.

Vesiculectomy (वेसिक्यूलेक्टॉमी) शुक्राशय-उच्छेदन। Resection of a portion or all of each of the seminal vesicle.

Vesiculitis (वेसिक्युलाइटिस) शुक्राशय का प्रदाह। Inflammation of the seminal vesicles.

Vesiculogram (वेसीकुलोग्राम) शुक्राषय का एक्स-रे चित्र। An X-ray picture of the seminal vesicles.

Vessel (वेसिल) शरीर के द्रव्यों को इधर-उधर ले जाने वाली नली, वाहिका, वाहिनी। Vas, a duct, tube or canal, conveying the fluids of the body.

Vestibule (वेस्टीब्यूल) प्रघाण। A porch or threshold.

Vestibulocochlear nerve (वेस्टीबुलोकॉक्लियर नर्व) आठवीं कपालीय तंत्रिका। 8th cranial nerve.

Vestibulotomy (वेस्टीबुलोटॉमी) अन्तःकर्ण के प्रघाण में चीरा लगाना। To make an incision into the vestibule of the internal ear.

Vestige (वैस्टिज) अवशेष। A remnant of something formerly present; vestigium.

Veterinarian (वेटेरीनेरियन) पशु-चिकित्सक। A doctor of veterinary medicine.

Veterinary (वेटेरीनरी) 1. घेरलू जानवरों, उसके रोगों तथा चिकित्सा से सम्बन्धी। 2. पशु-चिकित्सक। 1. Pertaining to the domestic animals, their diseases and treatment. 2. Veterinarian.

Viability (वायाबिलिटी) जीवनक्षमता, जन्म के पश्चात् जीवित रहने की क्षमता। Ability to live after birth.

Vial (वॉयल) छोटी शीशी। A small glass bottle.

Vibrator (वाइब्रेटर) कम्पित्र, कम्पक। An apparatus for use in vibratory.

Vibrio (विब्रियो) सूक्ष्माणु। A genus of microorganism.

Vibrissa (विब्रिसा) नथुनों के अंदर रहने वाले बाल। One of the stiff hair within the nostrils.

Vicarious (विकेरीयस) दूसरे की एवज में कार्य करने वाला, असामान्य स्थिति में उत्पन्न होने वाला। Acting as a substitute; accruing in an abnormal situation.

Vicarious-menstruation (विकेरीयस-मैन्सचुएशन) मासिक धर्म के समय योनि के अतिरिक्त अन्य स्थान जैसे–नाक एवं स्तनों आदि से रक्तास्राव होना। Bleeding during menstruation from the site other than vagina, as from the nose, breasts.

Vigil (विजिल) नींद न आना। Insomnia; wakefulness.

Vigor (विगोर) शारीरिक अथवा मानसिक शक्ति। Active force or strength of body or mind.

Villiferous (विलीफेरस) अंकुरों से युक्त। Having villi.

Villositis (विलोसाइटिस) अपरा के अंकुरों की सूजन हो जाना। Inflammation of the villi of placent.

Villus (विलस) अंकुर। A tuft.

Vinculum (विनकुलम) बंध या पट्टी। A ligament; a band.

Vinous (विनस) शराब जैसा। Having the nature of wine.

Vinum (विनम) शराब। Wine; the fermented juice of grapes.

Violence (वायोलेन्स) हिंसा। Injury or physical discomfort.

Viremia (वाइरीमिया) विषाणुओं का खून में पाया जाना। Presence of viruses in the blood.

Virgin (वर्जिन) कुँवारी, वह स्त्री जिसने संभोग न किया हो। A woman who has had no sexual intercourse.

Virile (विराइल) पुल्लिंग। Masculine.

Virilism (विरीलिज्म) स्त्रियों में पुरूषों जैसी विषेशताऐं होना। The appearance of secondary male characteristic in the female.

Virillia (विरीलिया) पुरूष लैंगिक अंग। The male sexual organs.

Virology (वाइरालॉजी) विषाणुओं तथा उनके द्वारा उत्पन्न रोगों का अध्ययन। The study of viruses and the diseases caused by them.

Virucide (वाइरूसाइड) विषाणु नष्ट करने वाला पदार्थ। An agent which destroys virus.

Viruria (वाइरूरिया) विषाणुओं का मूत्र में पाया जाना। Presence of viruses in the urine.

Vis (वाइस) शक्ति, बल। Force or energy.

Visceralgia (विस्रेल्जिया) किसी भी अंतरांग में दर्द होना। Pain in any viscus.

Visceroinhibitory (विस्रोइनहीबिटरी) किसी अंतरांग की क्रिया को रोकने वाला। Inhibiting the action of a viscus.

Viscerosomatic (विस्रोसोमेटिक) अंतरांगों एवं शरीर से सम्बन्धित। Pertaining to the viscera and the body.

Viscerotopic (विस्रोटॉपिक) प्रारंभिक रूप से अन्तरांगों पर क्रिया करने वाला। Primarily acting on the viscera.

Viscid (विसिड) चिपचिपा, चिपकने वाला। Adhesive, sticky.

Viscoelasticity (विस्कोइलास्टीसिटी) चिपचिपा एवं लचीला होने का गुण। The property of being viscous and elastic.

Viscosimeter (विस्कोसीमीटर) विभिन्न द्रव्यों में व्याप्त चिपचिपेपन को मापने का यंत्र। An instrument for measuring the viscosity of various liquids.

Visibility (विजीबिलिटी) दिखाई दिये जाने का गुण। The quality of being visible.

Visible (विजिबल) 1. दृष्टि से सम्बन्धित। 2. देखी गई वस्तुओं को तुरन्त याद कर लेना। 1. Pertaining to vision. 2. Readily remembering the objects seen.

Vision (विजन) दृष्टि। Act of viewing external objects.

Visualization (विजुआलाइजेशन।) 1. दृष्टिगोचर करने की क्रिया। 2. कल्पना में किसी वस्तु को देखना। 1. The process of making visible. 2. To see an object in imagination.

Visuognosis (विजुयोग्नोसिस) जो कुछ देखा गया है उसे पहचानना एवं उसकी व्याख्या करना। The recognition and interpretation of what is seen.

Visuopsychic (विजुयोसाइकिक) जो दृष्टिपरम एवं मानसिक दोनों हो। Both visual and psychic.

Vita (वाइटा) प्राण। Life.

Vitality (वाइटालिटी) प्राणशक्ति, ताकत। The vital principle of life, strength.

Vital statistics (वाइटल स्टेटिस्टिक्स) जन्म-दर, मृत्युदर एवं अस्वस्थता दर की संख्यिकी। Statistics of birth rate, death rate and morbidity rate.

Vitamer (विटामर) एक पदार्थ अथवा यौगिक जिसमें विटामिन की सक्रियता होती है। A substance or compound which has vitamin activity.

W

Wafer (वेफर) एक चपटी योनि-वर्ति। A flat vaginal suppository.

Waist (वेस्ट) धड़ कप वक्ष एवं कूल्हों के बीच का भाग, कटि। The part of the trunk between the thorax and hips.

Wakefulness (वेकफुलनेस) अनिद्रा, जागृतावस्था, नींद का अभाव। Absence of sleep, sleeplessness.

Walk (वॉक) चलना, चाल। To move on foot, the manner of moving on foot, gait.

Walker (वाकर) बैसारवी। Crutch, a mobile device used to assist a person in walking.

Wall (वाल) प्राचीर, दीवार। An investing part enclosing a cavity, chamber, or any anatomical unit.

Walleye (वालआई) नेत्रों का बाहर की ओर घूम जाना। Turning of the eye outward.

Wandering (वाण्ड्रिंग) भ्रमणाकारी, भ्रमणशील, भ्रमी। Moving freely about.

Wandering Mind (वाण्ड्रिंग माइन्ड) अस्थिर विचलित मस्तिष्क। Fluctuated mind.

Ward (वार्ड) अस्पताल का एक बड़ा कमरा जिसमें चार से अधिक रोगियों को रखा जाता है, कक्ष। A large hosp:tal room accommodating more than 4 patients.

Wart (वार्ट) बाह्यत्वचा एवं अंकुरकों की एक स्थानीय अतिवृद्धि जो किसी विषाणु द्वारा उत्पन्न होती है अथवा यह एक सुदम अबुर्द हो सकती है, अधिमांस (मस्सा)। Verruca, a localized overgrowth of the epidermis and papillae, which is caused by a virus or it may be benign tumor. (*i*) **Plantar Wart** (प्लान्टर वार्ट) पांव के तलवे पर उत्पन्न होने वाला अधिमांस। Verruca plantaris, planter wart occurring on the sole of foot.

Warty (वार्टी) मस्सों से मिलता-जुलता या उनकी प्रकृति का, मस्साभ। Resembling or of the nature of warts.

Wassermann reaction (वासरमैन रिएक्शन) सिफिलिस के निदान के लिए सीरम पूरक बन्धन परीक्षण। Serum complement-fixation test for the diagnosis of syphilis.

Wasting (वेस्टिंग) शरीर अथवा इसके भाग के परिमाण या शक्ति को कम करने वाला, क्षयकारी। Emaciating, causing loss of size or strength of the body or of its part.

Water (वाटर) एक साफ, रंगहीन, गन्धहीन तथा स्वादहीन द्रव, H_2O, जल। A clear, colorless, odorless, tasteless liquid, H_2O.

(*i*) **Hard water** (हार्ड वाटर) ऐसा जल जिसमें मैग्नीशियम एवं कैल्सियम के लवण घुले होते हैं। कठोर जल। Water that contains salts of magnesium and calcium dissolved in it.

(*ii*) **Potable water** (पोट्बल वाटर) ऐसा जल जो संदूषण से मुक्त और पीने के लिए उपयुक्त होता है। A water free from contamination and fit for drinking.

Water bed (वाटर बैड) गर्म पानी (100 ° एफ या 37.8 °से.) से आंशिक रूप से भरा रबड़ का एक गद्दा जो शरूयाक्षत की रोकथाम तथा उसकी चिकित्सा के काम आता है। A rubber mattress partially filled with warm water (100 °F or 37.8 °C), used in preventing and treating bedsores.

Waterhouse-Friderichsen Syndrome (वाटरहाउस-फ्राइडेरीक्सेन सिण्ड्रोम) मस्तिष्कावरणशोथ द्वारा एड्रीनल ग्रन्थि में रक्तचाप होने के परिणामस्वरूप तीव्र एड्रीनल अपर्याप्तता हो जाने के कारण उत्पन्न होने वाला रोग। Acute adrenal insufficiency occurring as a result of hemorrhage into adrenal gland, caused by meningitis.

Watt (वाट) विद्युत शक्ति की एक इकाई, एक वाट एक वोल्ट के बल से बहने वाली एक एम्पियर की धारा उत्पन्न शक्ति होती है। A unit of electric power, one watt is the power produced by one ampere of current flowing with a force, of one volt.

Wave (वेव) इलैक्ट्रोकार्डियोग्राम, एन्सिफैलोग्राम के अभिलेखन में या शरीरवृतिक क्रियाशीलता के अन्य रेखाचित्र अभिलेख में दिखाई देने वाला एक दोलन या कम्पन। तरंग, लहर। An oscillation seen in the recording of an ECG, EEG or other graphic record of physiologically activity. (*i*) **Dicrotic wave** (डाइक्रोटिक वेव) द्विस्पन्दी नाड़ी में द्वितीय तंरग। Second wave in a dicrotic pulse.

(*ii*) **Excitation wave** (एक्साइटेशन वेव) उत्तेजक-

आवेग जो हृदय के शिरा-आलिन्द-पर्व से उत्पन्न होकर आलिन्द-निलय-पर्व तक पहुँचते है। The excitatory impulse that originates in the SA node of the heart and reaches the AV node.

(*iii*) **Sound wave** (साउण्ड वेव) कम्पन करते हुऐ माध्यम के कम्पन जो अन्तःकर्ण के कर्णावर्त के संवेदी ग्राहकों को उद्दीप्त करके ध्वनि की अनुभूति उत्पन्न करते हैं। Vibrations of a vibrating medium that, on stimulating sensory receptors of the cochlea in the inner ear give rise to sensations of sound.

Wavelength (वेवलैंथ) एक तंरग के शिखर से दूसरी तरंग के शिखर तक की दूरी। तरंग-दैर्ध्य। The distance from the top of one wave to the top of next one.

Wax (वैक्स) कान का मैल, मोम, मधुमक्खियों द्वारा जमा किया गया एक सुघट्य पदार्थ जिसे शुद्ध रूप से चिकित्सा में मरहम बनाने के काम में लाया जाता है। Ear wax or cerumen, Beeswax, a plastic substance deposited by honey-bees, used in medicines in pure form in making ointments.

Waxy cast (वैक्सी कॉस्ट) गम्भीर, जीर्ण वृक्कीय रोग में उत्पन्न होने वाला घना, अधिक परावर्तन (पीछे की ओर मोड़ देने योग्य) मूत्रीय निर्मोक। Dense highly refractile urinary cast, occurring in severe chronic renal disease.

Waxy degeneration (वैक्सी डीजेनेरेशन) क्षयकारी रोगों में पाया जाने वाला श्वेतसाराभ (एमीलॉयड) का ह्रास। Amyloid degeneration seen in wasting disease.

Wean (वीन) माँ के दूध की एवज में अन्य पोशक पदार्थो के उपयोग के द्वारा बच्चे को माँ का दूध पिलाना छुडा देना, स्तन-त्याग, अपस्तनता। To deprive of a child from breastfeeding by substituting other nutrient substances.

Web (वेब) आसपास की रचनाओं को सम्बन्धित करने वाला एक ऊतक या कोई झिल्ली या जाल। A tissue or membrane connecting the adjacent structure.

Webbed (वेब्ड) जालयुक्त जैसे बतख के पैर की अंगुलियाँ, जालीदार। Having a web, as the toes of a duck's feet.

Weber's test (वेबर्स टेस्ट) एकपार्श्विक अधिरता के लिए एक परीक्षण। इस परीक्षण में एक कम्पन्शील ट्यूनिंग फोर्क के

आधार को माथे के बीच में रखा जाता है एकपार्श्विक तंत्रिका जनित बधिरता से स्वस्थ कान से ध्वनि सुनाई देगी जबकि चालकता सम्बन्धी बधिरता में बहरे कान से ध्वनि सुनाई देगी। A test for unilateral deafness. In this test the base of a vibrating turning fork is placed against the middle of the forehead, in unilateral nerve-type deafness, the sound will be heard by healthy ear, whereas in a conductive type deafness, sound will be heard by the deaf ear.

Wedge shaped (वेज शेप्ड) कील के आकार का, कीलाकार। Having one end thick and the other sloping.

Weight (वेट) भारीपन की माप, भार, वजन। The measure of heaviness.

Weil's disease (वेल्स डीजीज) संक्रामी कामला, सज्वर-पीलिया। Acute febrile icterus, infective jaundice.

Wernicke's encephalopathy (वर्निक्ज एन्सिफैलोपैथी) जीर्ण मदातयय, आमाशीयक कार्सिनोमा अथवा गर्भिणी अतिवमन में विटामिन बी की कमी से उत्पन्न होने वाली मस्तिष्क-विकृति। Encephalopathy caused by vitamin B deficiency occurring in chronic alcoholism gastric carcinoma or hyperemesis gravidarum.

Wet dream (वैट ड्रीम) शक्ति में वीर्य स्खलन, स्वप्नदोष। Nocturnal seminal emission.

Wheal (व्हील) त्वचा पर उत्पन्न होने वाला एक परिसीमित उत्थान जो शीघ्र ही लुप्त हो जाता है तथा जिसमें खुजली आती है। ऐसा पित्ती, एलर्जी तथा कीट के काटने आदि में देखा जाता है, स्फोट। A circumscribed elevation on the skin disappearing quickly, and accompanied by itching. It is seen in urticaria, allergy and insect bites, etc.

Wheelchair (व्हीलचेयर) बड़े पहियों वाली एक विशेष कुर्सी जो ऐसे रोगियों को जो चल-फिर नहीं सकते, लाने-ले जाने का कार्य करती है। A special chair with large wheels for transporting the patients, who are unable to walk.

Wheeze (ह्वीज) श्वसन के दौरान सुनी जाने वाली सीटी बजाने जैसी आवाज, घरघराहट। A whistling sound heard during respiration.

Whey (व्हे) तक्र, छाछ, मट्ठा, मस्तु, पनीरजल, छैने का पानी, घोल। The milk-serum separated from the curd in coagulation.

Whipworm (व्हिपवर्म) एक गोलकृमि, कशाकृमि, प्रदोतकृमि। A roundworm which infects the intestine of man in humid tropics.

Whisky (विह्स्की) जौ से बनाई गई मदिरा। Liquor prepared from barley.

Whisper (विह्स्पर) फुसफुसाइट, बिना आवाज बोलना। Speech without phonation.

White gangrene (व्हाइट गैंग्रीन) स्थानीय रक्ताल्पता के कारण उत्पन्न कोथ। Gangrene caused by local anemia.

White leg (ह्वाइट लेग) घनास्त्रशिराशोथ। Thrombophlebitis.

Whitlow (ह्विटलो) हाथ अथवा पैर की किसी अंगुली के सिरे का फोड़ा, चिप्स या अंगुलिबेढ़ा। Felon, paronychia abscess of the end of a finger or toe.

Whoop (हूप) कूकर खाँसी (काली खाँसी) का ध्वनिक (आवाज करने वाला) तथा आक्षेपिक (कपा देने वाला) अन्तःश्वसन (साँस लेना)। The sonorous and convulsive inspiration of whooping cough.

Whooping Cough (हूपिंग कफ) बेसीलस बोर्डेटेला पर्टुसिस द्वारा उत्पन्न एक संक्रामक रोग। काली खाँसी, कूकर कास। Pertussis, an infectious disease caused by the *Bacillus bordetella* pertussis.

Whorl (व्हर्ल) चक्कदार व्यवस्थापन। Vortex, a spiral arrangement.

Widal's reaction or test (वीडाल्स रिएक्शन और टैस्ट) टायफॉयड ज्वर के लिये किया जाने वाला समूहन परीक्षण। An agglutination test for typhoid fever.

Wilms tumor (विल्मज ट्यूमर) बच्चों में उत्पन्न होने वाला वृक्क का तीव्र गति से बढने वाला अबुर्द। A rapidly developing tumor of the kidney occurring in children.

Windchill (वाइन्डचिल) अनावृत मानव त्वचा पर वायु का ठण्डा प्रभाव। The cooling effect of the wind on the exposed human skin.

Wine (वाइन) किसी भी फल का किण्वित (खमीकृत) रस, सामान्यतया अंगूरों का जिसमें 10–15 प्रतिशत एल्कोहॉल होता है। मदिरा, मद्य, शराब। Fermented juice of any fruit, usually of grapes which contains 10–15% alcohol.

Wing (विंग) पक्ष, पंख, विभाग। Ala.

Winker (विंकर) पलक मारने वाला। One who winks?

Wiring (वायरिंग) तार से हड्डी के टुकडों को जकड़ कर बाँधना।

Fastening bone fragments by wire.

Wisdom tooth (विस्डम टूथ) अन्तचर्वक दन्त, अक्ल-दाढ़। The last molar teeth on each side of the jaw.

Withdrawal syndrome (विद्ड्राल सिण्ड्रोम) शराब आदि छोड़ देने से उत्पन्न लक्षण समूह। Abstinence syndrome, a group of symptoms arising from withdrawal of alcohol, etc.

Womb (वूम) गर्भाशय। Uterus.

Wool-Fat (वूलफेट) ऊर्णवसा, लिनोलिन। A fatty substance, extracted from wool, used in ointment, waterproof coatings, etc., linolin.

Wordblindness (वर्डब्लाइण्डनैस) लिखे हुए अथवा छपे हुए शब्दों को समझने में असमर्थता, शब्दान्धता, लेखान्धता। Inability to understand the written or printed words.

Word salad (वर्ड सलड) अर्थहीन शब्दों का बोलना, निरर्थक शब्दोच्चार। The speaking of meaningless words.

Workout (वर्कआउट) हल करना। To solve.

Wound (वूण्ड) आघात या चोट के कारण त्वचा अथवा शरीर की किसी रचना का सामान्य निरन्तरता में स्थित टूटन, घाव, जख्म, व्रण अथवा क्षत। Breaking in the normal continuity of the skin or a body structure caused by injury.

(*i*) **Abraded Wound** (एब्रेडेड वूण्ड) खरोचदार घाव। Caused or resulting from abrasion.

(*ii*) **Incised Wound** (इन्साइज्ड वूण्ड) तेज काटने वाले यंत्र से बनाया गया स्पष्ट व्रण। A clear wound caused by a sharp cutting instrument.

(*iii*) **Lacerated Wound** (लेसीरेटेड वूण्ड) किसी धारहीन वस्तु अथवा डंडे या लाठी से मारने से बना फटा हुआ जख्म जिसके किनारे फटे हुये एवं ऊबड़-खाबड़ होते है। A torn wound with ragged edges (not a clean wound) caused by a blunt object or stick.

(*iv*) **Perforating wound** (पर्फोरेटिंग वूण्ड) ऐसा जख्म जिसमें जख्म बनाने वाली वस्तु शरीर में प्रवेश करती एवं बाहर निकल जाती है। Wound in which the object causing the wound enters the body and emerges out. (*v*) **Tunnel Wound** (टनल वूण्ड) ऐसा जख्म जिसके प्रवेश तथा निर्गम छिद्र बराबर व्यास के होते हैं। Wound which has the opening of entrance and exit of equal diameter.

Wrinkle (रिकल) त्वचा की झुर्री, वलय । Unevenness or fold of the skin.

Wrist Drop (रिस्ट ड्रॉप) मणिबन्धस्त्रंस, मणिबन्धघात, कलाई तथा अँगुलियों की प्रसारक पेशी का पक्षाघात। Paralysis of the extensor muscle of wrist and fingers.

Writer's Cramp (राइटर्स क्रैम्प) अधिक समय तक लिखते रहने से अंगुठे एवं पास की दो अंगुलियों की पेशियों को प्रभावित करने वाला उद्वेष्ट या ऐंठन (बॉयटा) । A cramp affecting the muscles of the thumb and two adjacent fingers after prolonged writing.

Wry Neck (री नैक) वक्र-ग्रीवास्तम्भ, अकड़ी हुई गर्दन। Torticollis.

Wuchereria (वूकेरेरीया) वर्ग नेमाटोडा के फाइलेरिया-कृमियों का एक वंश जो संसार के गर्म क्षेत्रों में पाया जाता है। A genus of filarial worms of the class nematoda, found in warm regions of the world.

X

X (एक्स) जैंथीन का प्रतीक। Symbol for Xanthine.

Xanthein (जेन्थिन) पीतरंजक, पौधे का एक पीला रंग। The yellow coloring matter of plant, xanthine.

Xanthelasma (जेन्थेलाज्मा) पीताबुर्द। Xanthoma.

Xanthine (जेन्थीन) यह प्यूरीन बेसों एडिनीन तथा ग्वानीन का एक चयापचयी उत्पाद एवं यूरिड अम्ल का एक पूर्वगामी होता है। It is a metabolic product of purine bases adenine and guanine, and a precursor of uric acid.

Xanthinuria (जेन्थीनूरिया) मूत्र में अधिक मात्रा में जेन्थीन का उत्सर्जित होना। Excretion of large amounts of xanthine in urine.

Xanthochromia (जेन्थोक्रोमिया) पीत विवर्णता जैसे त्वचा या प्रमश्तिष्कमेरू-तरल की, पीतचर्मता। Yellow discoloration, as of the skin or cerebrospindal fluid.

Xanthodont (जेन्थोडोन्ट) पीले दाँतों वाला, पीत-दन्त। Having yellow teeth.

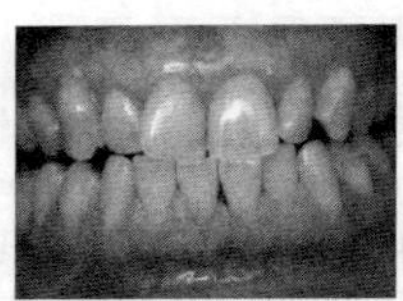

Xanthogranulomatous (जेन्थोग्रेनुलोमेटस) एक अबुर्द जिसमें कणिका गुल्म एवं पीताबुर्द दोनों के लक्षण विद्यमान रहते हैं। Pertaining to, the nature of, or affected by xanthogranuloma.

Xanthoma (जेन्थोमा) लाइपिड के जमा हो जाने के कारण त्वचा में उत्पन्न होने वाली थोड़ी उठी हुई, चपटी, कोमल पिटिका, पर्व अथवा चकता, पीताबुर्द। Slightly elevated, flat, soft papule, nodule or a palaque occurring in the skin due to deposition of lipid.

Xanthomatosis (जेन्थोमेटोसिस) बहुत से पीताबुर्दों का बनना, पीताबुर्दता। Formation of multiple xanthomas.

Xanthophyll (जेन्थोफिल) कुछ पौधों तथा अण्डे की जर्दी में पाया जाने वाला केरोटीन से उत्पन्न एक पीला वर्णक। A yellow pigment derived from carotene, present in some plants and egg yolk.

Xanthosis (जेन्थोसिस) केरोटीन वर्णक से युक्त गाजर आदि अधिक मात्रा में खाने के फलस्वरूप त्वचा का पीला हो जाना। The yellowing of the skin resulting from ingestion of excessive amount of carrots, etc. Containing the pigment carotene.

Xanthuria (जेन्थूरिया) पीतरंजकमेह। Excess of xanthine in the urine.

X Chromosome (एक्स क्रोमोसोम) वह गुणसूत्र जो स्त्री के लक्षणों को निश्चित करता है। The chromosome that determines female characteristics.

Xeno (जीनो) अजनबी अथवा बाह्य पदार्थ के अर्थ में प्रयुक्त एक उपसर्ग। A prefix meaning strange or foreign substance.

Xenomania (ज़ीनोमैनिया) विदेशमोह, विदेशी संस्कृति के प्रति मोह, प्यार या झुकाव। An inordinate attachment to foreign things.

Xenomenia (ज़ीनोमेनिया) अपथप्रवृत्तार्तव, उन्मार्गी-आर्तव, अनुकल्परज। Vicarious or supplementary menstruations.

Xenorexia (ज़ीनोरैक्सिया) क्षुधा की विकृति जिसमें कोई व्यक्ति निरन्तर बाह्य पदार्थों को खाता रहता है। An abnormality of appetite in which a person persistently eats foreign substance.

Xeransis (ज़ीरेन्सिस) ऊतकों में धीरे-धीरे नमी का अभाव होना। A gradual loss of moisture in the tissues.

Xerantic (ज़ीरेन्टिक) शुष्क बनाने वाला, शुष्ककर। Causing dryness.

Xerocheilia (ज़ीरोकीलिया) होठों की खुश्की। Dryness of lips.

Xerocytosis (ज़ीरोसाइटोसिस) रक्त में अधिक संख्या में ज़ीरोसाइटों या निर्जलीकृत लाल रक्त कोशिकाओं का पाया जाना। Presence of a large number of xerocytes or dehydrated RBC in the blood.

Xeroderma (ज़ीरोडर्मा) त्वचा की अत्यधिक शुष्कता एवं रूक्षता, मृदु मत्स्यचर्मता। Excessive dryness and roughness of the skin; milk ichthyosis.

Xeromycteria (ज़ीरोमिक्टीरिया) नासिका मार्गों का शुष्क होना। Dryness of the nasal passages.

Xerophthalmia (जीरोफ्थैल्मिया) नेत्र के किसी रोग अथवा विटामिन ए की कमी के कारण नेत्रश्लेष्मता एवं स्वच्छ मण्डल का असामान्य रूप से शुष्क एंव मोटी हो जाना। Abnormal dryness and thickening of the conjunctiva and cornea, due to some disease of the eye or to vitamin A deficiency.

Xeroradiography (जीरोरेडियोग्राफी) एक शुष्क प्रक्रिया का प्रयोग करके एक्स-रे चित्र का पुनःउत्पाद करना जिसमें पाउडर के रूप में एक पदार्थ जैसे सेलेनियम से एक प्लेट आच्छादित होती है और विद्युत से समान रूप पूरित होती है, जिसे धातु की प्लेटों के बीच में थामा जाता है। The reproduction of X-ray picture by using a dry process in which a plate covered with a powdered substance, such as selenium, electrically and evenly charged, is held between the metal plates.

Xerosis (ज़ीरोसिस) शुष्कता, रूक्षता, रूखापन। Dryness.

Xerostomia (जीरोस्टोमिया) लार या थूक के अभाव में मुँह का खुश्क हो जाना, मुख शुष्कता। Dryness of the mouth due to lack of saliva.

Xerotocia (ज़ीरोटोसिया) उल्व-तरल की कमी से प्रसव का शुष्क हो जाना। Dry labor due to diminished amount of amniotic fluid.

Xiphisternum (ज़ीफाइस्टर्नम) उरःपत्तक। Xiphoid process.

Xiphoid process (ज़ीफॉयड प्रोसेज) स्टर्नस का सबसे नीचे का तलवार के आकार का भाग, असिरूप। Ensiform, the lowest sword-shaped portion of the sternum.

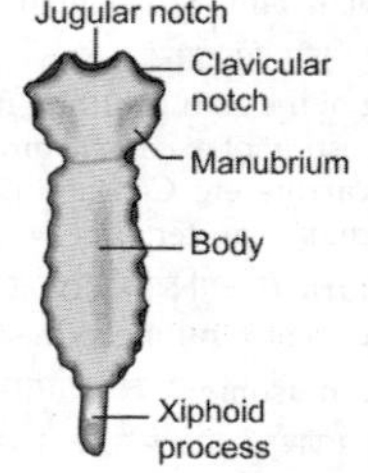

X-linked (एक्स-लिंक्ड) एक्स गुणसूत्र पर स्थित जीनों द्वारा संचारित। Sex-linked, transmitted by genes on the X chromosome.

X-Rays (एक्स-रेज़) एक उच्च-शक्ति की विद्युत चुम्बकीय तंरग जिसकी दैर्ध्य 0.05 से 100 एन्गस्ट्रॉम ईकाई होती है। एक्स-किरण। A high energy electromagnetic on the X chromosome.

Xyrospasm (ज़ाइरोस्पाज्म) अँगुलियों एवं भुजाओं का व्यावसायिक कम्पन जैसा कि नाइयों में देखा जाता है। An occupational spasm of the fingers and arms as seen in barbers.

Xyster (ज़िस्टर) निघर्षणी, खुर्चनी। An instrument used to clean the bones by scraping.

Y

Yard (यार्ड) गज, शिश्न, लिंग। A measure of three feet, the penis.

Yawn (यान) जम्हाई लेना, अंगड़ाई लेना। To gape; to open the mouth widely.

Yawning (यानिंग) जम्हाई लेने वाला। One who opens the mouth widely and takes deep inspiration.

Yaws (याज) उष्णकटिबन्धीय क्षेत्र में स्पाइरोकीट, ट्रेपोनेमा पेर्टिन्यू द्वारा अधिकतर बच्चों में उत्पन्न होने वाला एक अरतिज, दैहिक संक्रामक रोग। Frambesia, a nonvenereal, systemic infectious disease, occurring most commonly in children in the tropical region caused by spirochete, treponema pertenue.

Yeast (यीस्ट) फलों, सब्जियों, मिट्टी एंव जन्तु मल आदि में पाया जाने वाला एक कवक जो कार्बोहाइड्रेटों का किण्वन या खमीरण करने के सक्षम होता है। A fungus found in fruits, vegetables, soil and animal feces, etc. and is capable of fermenting carbohydrates.

Yellow-body (यलो बॉडी) पीत-पिण्ड। The corpus luteum.

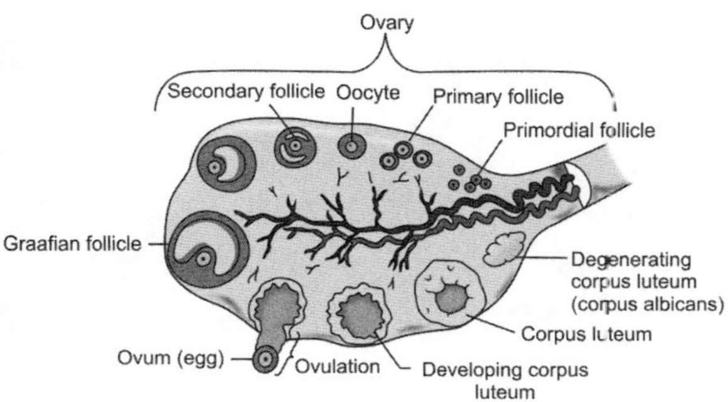

Yellow-body

Yellow fever (यलो फिवर) पीत-ज्वर। An epidemic disease with high fever, jaundice, black vomit.

Yellow spot (यलो स्पोट) प्रत्येक स्वर-रज्जु के अग्रज किनारे पर स्थित एक छोटी पीली-पीली पर्विका। Macula flava laryngis, a small yellow nodule at the anterior end of each vocal cord.

Yoga (योगा) योगा शब्द शारीरिक आसनों या स्थितियों तथा श्वसन के नियमन से सम्बद्ध होता है। This term is associated with physical postures and regulation of breathing.

Yolk (योक) डिम्ब या अण्डे मे संचित पौष्टिक पदार्थ, पीतक। The nutrient stored in the ovum.

Young's rule (यंग्सरूल) किसी बच्चे के लिए औषधि की मात्रा की गणना करने की एक विधि। इसके लिए बच्चे की आयु को उसकी आयु जमा 12 से भाग देते है। A method for calculating the dose of medicine for a child, divide the age of the child by his/her age plus 12.

Youth (यूथ) बचपन एवं परिपक्वता के बीच का काल। Period between childhood and maturity.

Z

Z (जैड) परमाणु-संख्या का प्रतीक। Symbol for atomic number.

Zea (ज़ीया) मक्का। Maize.

Zeimus (जीमस) अधिक मात्रा में मक्की खाने से होने वाला एक चर्म रोग। A skin disease caused by overuse of maize.

Zeis Glands (ज़ीस ग्लैण्ड्स) पलक की इसके स्वतन्त्र किनारे के पास स्थित त्वग्वसीय ग्रन्थियाँ। Sebaceous glands of the eyelid close to its free edge, each gland is associated with an eyelash.

Zenker's diverticulum (जींकर्स डाइवर्टिकुलम) ग्रासनलीय भित्ति के किसी दोष से होकर ग्रासनली की श्लेष्मिक कला का बहिःसरण होना। Herniation of the mucous membrane of the esophagus through a defect in the esophageal wall.

Zero (जीरो) शून्य, सिफर। The point from which thermometers are measured either in positive or negative direction.

Zinc (जिंक) यशद, जस्ता, नीले-श्वेत रंग की एक धातु। A metallic element, Zincum.

Zingiber (ज़िंजीबर) अदरक के पौधों का वंश। A genus of plants of ginger.

Zoanthropy (जोएन्थ्रोपी) जानवर होने की भ्रान्ति, स्वपश्वानुभूति। Delusion of being an animal.

Zollinger-Ellison syndrome (जोलिंगर एलिसन सिण्ड्रोम) अग्नाशय के इन्सुलिन अस्त्रावी अबुर्द द्वारा उत्पन्न एक रोग जिससे बहुत अधिक गैस्ट्रिन हार्मोन स्रावित होता है। यह आमाशय को अधिक मात्रा में हाइड्रोक्लोरिक एसिड तथा पैप्सिन स्रावित करने के लिए उद्दीप्त करता है जिससे फिर आमाशय एवं आँत का पैप्टिक अल्सर (उदरव्रण) बन जाता है। A condition caused by noninsulin secreting tumor of the pancreas, which secretes the gastrin hormone excessively. This stimulates the stomach to secrete a large amount of hydrochloric acid and pepsin, which in turn causes the formation of peptic ulcer of the stomach and intestine.

Zona (जोना) एक क्षेत्र या मण्डल पट्टा या बन्ध या मेखला,

वर्तुलाकार विसर्पिका। A zone, band, girdle, herpes zoster.

Zona Ciliaris (जोना सिलीयरीस) रोमक क्षेत्र। The ciliary processes collectively.

Zonal (ज़ोनल) क्षेत्रीय, मण्डलीय। Relating to a zone, zonal, zonary.

Zonary placenta (जोनरी प्लेसेन्टा) जरायु के चारों ओर चौड़े छल्ले के रूप में व्यवस्थित एक अपरा। A placenta arranged in the form of a broad ring around the chorion.

Zone (ज़ोन) चारों ओर से घेरने वाला स्थान अथवा सीमा, क्षेत्र मण्डल। An encircling area or boundary. (*i*) **Ciliary Zone** (सिलीयरी ज़ोन) नेत्र की परितारिका की अग्रज सतह का परिसरीय भाग। The peripheral part of anterior surface of the iris of the eye.

Zonesthesia (ज़ोनेस्थीसिया) ऐसा महसूस होना जैसे कोई रस्सा शरीर को भींच रहा हो। A sensation, as a cord in constricting the body.

Zonipetal (ज़ोनीपीटल) बाहर से किसी क्षेत्र या मण्डल में प्रवेश करने वाला। Passing towards a zone or region.

Zonula (ज़ोनुला) एक छोटा क्षेत्र या मण्डल, मण्डलिका। Zonule, a small zone.

Zonule (जोन्यूल) मण्डलिका अथवा पट्टी। A little zone, belt or girdle.

Zonulotomy (ज़ोन्यूलोटॉमी) रोमक मण्डलिका में चीरा लगाना। To make an incision into the ciliary zonule.

Zoodermic (जूडर्मिक) किसी जन्तु की त्वचा द्वारा सम्पादित जैसे त्वचा निरोपण में किया जाता है। Performed with the skin of an animal, as in skin grafting.

Zoogeny (जूजेनी) जन्तुओं का परिवर्धन एवं विकास। The development and evolution of animals.

Zoograft (जूग्राफ्ट) किसी जन्तु से उपलब्ध ऊतक का एक निरोप। A graft of tissue obtained from an animal.

Zooid (ज्वॉयड) पशु के समान। Animal-like.

Zoology (जूलॉजी) जन्तु-विज्ञान। The science of animals.

Zoomania (जूमैनिया) पशुओं या जानवरों को प्राप्त करने हेतु पागल बने रहना। Mania for obtaining the animals.

Zoonoses (जूनोसेज) जन्तुओं के रोग जो मनुष्य को संचारित हो सकते हैं। पशुजन्यरोग। Disease of animals transmissible to man.

Zoonotic (जूनोटिक) पशुजन्य रोगों से सम्बन्धित। Pertaining to zoonoses.

Zoophilia (जूफीलिया) पशुओं का शौक होना। Fondness of animals.

Zoophobia (जूफोबिया) जन्तुओं का विकृत भयः पशुभित्ति। Morbid fear of animals.

Zoospermia (जूस्पर्मिया) स्खलित वीर्य में जीवित शुक्राणुओं का पाया जाना। Presence of the living spermatozoa in the ejaculated semen.

Zootomy (जूटॉमी) जन्तुओं का विच्छेदन करना। Dissection of the animals.

Zootrophic (जूट्रॉफिक) जन्तु पोषण से सम्बन्धित। Concerning the animal nutrition.

Zygal (ज़ाइगल) दो रचनाओं को जोड़ने वाले ऊतक से सम्बन्धित। Pertaining to a tissue connecting two structures.

Zygapophysis (ज़ाइगापोफाइसिस) कषेरूका का सन्धायक प्रवर्ध।The articular process of a vertebra.

Zygoma (ज़ाइगोमा) शंखस्थि का गण्डास्थिक प्रवर्ध, गण्डास्थि। The zygomatic process of the temporal bone, malar bone.

Zygomaticoauricular (जाइगोमेटिको-ऑरिकुलर) गण्डास्थि एवं बाह्य कर्ण से सम्बन्धित। Pertaining to the zygomatic bone and auricle.

Zygomaticofrontal (जाइगोमेटिकोफ्रन्टल) जाइगोमा एवं ललाटीय हड्डी से सम्बन्धित। Pertaining to the zygoma and the frontal bone.

Zygomatico-orbital (जाइगोमेटिको-ऑर्बिटल) जाइगोमा एवं नेत्र-गुहा से सम्बन्धित।
Pertaining to the zygoma and the orbit.

Zygomatic Process (जाइगोमेटिक प्रोसेज) शंखस्थि के पट्टकी भाग का नीचे की ओर को जाने वाला एक पतला प्रक्षेपण, तथा गण्डास्थि का गण्ड चाप बनाने वाला एक भाग। A thin downward projection of squamous portion of the temporal bone and a portion of the zygomatic bone forming zygomatic arch.

Zygomycosis (ज़ाइगोमाइकोसिस) जाइगोमेटिक या गाल की हड्डी का कवक संक्रमण। Fungus infection of the zygomatic bone.

Zygosis (ज़ाइगोसिस) दो एककोशिकीय जन्तुओं का लैंगिक संयोग।
Sexual union of two unicellular animals.

Zygote (ज़ाइगोट) नर एवं मादा युग्मकों के संयोग से बनने वाली कोशिका, गर्भित डिम्ब. युग्मनज। The cell formed by the union of a male and female gamete, the fertilized ovum.

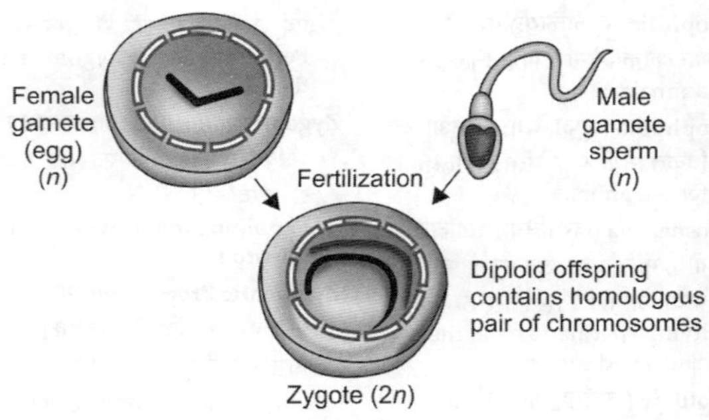

Zygote

Zymase (ज़ाइमेस) किण्वन या खमीरण करने वाला एन्जाइम। Fermenting enzyme.

Zyme (ज़ाइम) एन्जाइम अथवा किण्व (खमीर)। An enzyme or ferment.

Zymogen (ज़ाइमोजन) किण्वजन, खमीरजन, खमीर पैदा करने वाला। Producing the zyme.

Zymology (जाइमोलॉजी) किण्व-विज्ञान। The science of fermentation.

Zymolyte (जाइमोलाइट) वह पदार्थ जिस पर कोई किण्व या फर्मेन्ट क्रिया करता है। Substrate, substance upon which ferment acts.

Zymometer (ज़ाइमोमीटर) किण्वन की माप करने वाला एक उपकरण, किण्वनमापी यन्त्र। An apparatus for measuring fermentation.

Zymosis (जाइमोसिस) किण्वन या खमीरण, वह प्रक्रिया जिसके द्वारा कोई संक्रामक रोग उत्पन्न होता है। Fermentation, the process by which an infectious disease develops.

Zymotic (जाइमोटिक) किण्वन या खमीरण से संबंधित अथवा उसके द्वारा उत्पन्न। Pertaining to or produced by fermentation.